Dermatologic
Procedures
in Office Practice

Dermatologic Procedures
in Office Practice

SECOND EDITION

Richard P. Usatine, MD, FAAFP

Professor, Dermatology and Cutaneous Surgery
Professor, Family and Community Medicine
Fellowship Director, Underserved Dermatology Family Medicine Fellowship
Founding Director, Skin Clinic, University Health System
University of Texas Health San Antonio
San Antonio, Texas
United States

Daniel L. Stulberg, MD, FAAFP

Professor and Chair, Family & Community Medicine
Western Michigan University
Homer Stryker MD School of Medicine
Kalamazoo, Michigan
United States

ELSEVIER

Elsevier
1600 John F. Kennedy Blvd.
Ste 1800
Philadelphia, PA 19103-2899

Content Strategist: Lauren Boyle
Content Development Specialist: Ranjana Sharma
Publishing Services Manager: Shereen Jameel
Project Manager: Maria Shalini
Design Direction: Renee Duenow

Printed in India

Last digit is the print number: 9 8 7 6 5 4 3 2 1

Working together
to grow libraries in
developing countries

www.elsevier.com • www.bookaid.org

Contributors

Angela Abouassi
Skin Clinic
University Medical Associates, San Antonio
Texas
United States
Adjunct Faculty Assistant Professor
Department of Family & Community Medicine UT Health San Antonio
UT Health San Antonio, San Antonio
Texas
United States

Zeeshan Afzal, MD
MD
Dermatology
Doctors Dermatology, Edinburg
Texas
United States

Maria Bakirtzi, Dermatologist
Dermatologist
Dermatology
Private practice, Thessaloniki
Greece

Naiara S. Barbosa, MD
Assistant Professor
Department of Dermatology
Mayo Clinic, Jacksonville
Florida
United States

Elbert Belk, MD, FAAFP
Senior Physician
Dermatology
The Skin Clinics of Texas, Laredo
Texas
United States

Jimena Cervantes, MD
Associate Medical Director
Skin Clinic
University Medical Associates, San Antonio
Texas
United States
Adjunct Faculty Assistant Professor
Department of Family & Community Medicine UT Health San Antonio
UT Health San Antonio, San Antonio
Texas
United States

Wendy C. Coates, MD
Emeritus Professor of Emergency Medicine
Emergency Medicine
David Geffen School of Medicine at University of California, Los Angeles, Los Angeles
California
United States

Lucia Diaz, MD
Associate Professor
Pediatrics (Pediatric Dermatology) and Internal Medicine (Dermatology)
Dell Medical School at UT Austin, Austin
Texas
United States
Dermatology Residency Associate Program Director
Internal Medicine (Dermatology)
Austin
Texas
United States

Enzo Errichetti, Associate Professor
Prof.
Department of Medical Area
University of Udine, Udine
Italy

Robert Fawcett, MD
Retired, Former Associate Director
York Hospital Family Medicine Residency, York
Pennsylvania
United States

Regina Gallegos, MPT, CWS
CHILE Clinic - Center for Healing in the Lower Extremities
University of New Mexico
Albuquerque
New Mexico

Bernadatte Georga Gilbert, MD
Associate Dean for Admissions and Financial Aid
Family and Community Medicine
Penn State College of Medicine, Hershey
Pennsylvania
United States

Robert T. Gilson, MD
Associate Professor
Dermatology
UT Health San Antonio, San Antonio
Texas
United States

Jonathan Bradley Karnes, MD
Faculty Physician, Medical Director
Maine Dartmouth Dermatology
Maine Dartmouth Family Medicine Residency, Augusta
Maine
United States
Assistant Clinical Professor
Community and Family Medicine
Geisel School of Medicine at Dartmouth, Hanover
New Hampshire
United States

Nikki L. Katalanos, PhD, PA-C
Program Director (Retired)
Physician Assistant Program
University of New Mexico, Albuquerque
New Mexico
United States

Jennifer Krejci-Manwaring
Adjunct Professor
Dermatology
UT Health Science Center San Antonio, San Antonio
Texas
United States
Medical Director
Limmer Hair Transplant Center, San Antonio
Texas
United States
Staff Dermatologist
Audie Muphy Veterans Hospital, San Antonio
Texas
United States

Aimilios Lallas, MD, PhD
Associate Professor of Dermatology
First Department of Dermatology
Aristotle University, Thessaloniki
Greece
Associate Professor of Dermatology
First Department of Dermatology
Aristotle University of Thessaloniki, Thessaloniki
Greece

Eric J. Lew, DPM
Associate Professor
Orthopaedics
University of New Mexico Health Sciences Center,
    Albuquerque
New Mexico
United States

Ashfaq A. Marghoob, MD
Attending Physician
Dermatology
Memorial Sloan-Kettering Cancer Center, Hauppauge
New York
United States

Angela Martz, Physician Assistant, MS-PAS
Physician Assistant-Certified
Emergency Department
University of New Mexico, Albuquerque
New Mexico
United States

Ruby Gibson, MD
Tulane University School of Medicine, New Orleans,
    Louisiana
United States

Patrick Moran, DO
Central Washington Family Medicine
Yakima, Washington
United States

Christy Nwankwo, BA
Medical Student
School of Medicine
University of Missouri-Kansas City School of Medicine,
    Kansas City
United States

Ryan O'Quinn
Medical Director
South Texas Skin Cancer Center
San Antonio, Texas

Zaira Yazmin Ortega Orejel, MD
Physician
Dermatology
Elica Health Centers, Sacramento
California
United States

Ariadna Carolina Perez-Sanchez, MD
Assistant Professor
Internal Medicine
University of Texas Health Science Center at San Antonio,
    San Antonio
Texas
United States
Hospitalist
Hospital Medicine
University of Texas Health Science Center at San Antonio,
    San Antonio
Texas
United States

John L. Pfenninger, MD
President and Director, Founder
Family Medicine
The Medical Procedures Center, PC; The National Procedures
    Institute, Midland
Michigan
United States

Alba Posligua, MD
Dermatology Resident
Department of Dermatology
University of New Mexico, Albuquerque
New Mexico
United States

Hamid Qazi, MD, BSc Honors
Staff Physician
Family Medicine
Palomar Health Medical Group Graybill, San Diego
California
United States
Dermatology Fellow
Dermatology Care of Alabama, Tuscaloosa
Alabama
United States

Daniel Stulberg, MD FAAFP
Professor & Chair
Family and Community Medicine
Western Michigan University, Kalamazoo
Michigan
United States
Emeritus Professor
Family and Community Medicine
University of New Mexico, Albuquerque
United States

David L. Swanson, MD
Professor of Dermatology
Residency Program Director, Associate Director
    of Education
Mayo Clinic Arizona, Scottsdale
Arizona
United States

Richard P. Usatine, MD
Professor
Dermatology and Cutaneous Surgery
University of Texas Health San Antonio
Texas
United States
Professor
Family and Community Medicine
University of Texas Health San Antonio

Caroline Zhu, MD
University of Texas Southwestern
Dallas, Texas
United States

Foreword

As a family physician educator with a love of dermatology and skin procedures, it gives me great pleasure to write the forward for the 2nd edition of this wonderful book. As the editor and author of "The Essential Guide to Primary Care Procedures," Dr. Usatine's previous book on the subject, *Skin Surgery: A Practical Guide*, was a strong influence on me as I developed my expertise in skin work. Since then, I have had the pleasure to work with both authors of this new edition. Dr. Richard Usatine and I have been involved in planning and teaching the American Academy of Family Physicians (AAFP) Skin Problems and Diseases Course for over 24 years. In the last 18 years, Dr. Usatine has chaired this course, and I have worked directly with him in the course design and implementation. Dr. Usatine is a true leader in primary care dermatology education and especially for family physicians. Not only does he teach dermatology procedures in lectures and workshops, but he regularly publishes his work and photographs in the *Journal of Family Practice (JFP)*.

I also worked with Dr. Usatine on all three editions of the *Color Atlas of Family Medicine* and know the quality of his clinical photographs. With his permission, I regularly use his photos in my own teaching of dermatology topics and procedures. Dr. Usatine's photographic images have now been published in primary care and specialty books around the world. He has written the dermatology chapters for several of the best-selling family medicine textbooks. Dr. Usatine has been the family medicine editor for VisualDx and has provided over 20,000 photos to them for work in artificial intelligence and online publication. Dr. Usatine has also become a family medicine leader in dermoscopy education. He teaches alongside world experts in dermoscopy in the two largest dermoscopy courses in the US. Additionally, Dr. Usatine is a strong advocate for social justice and includes the full spectrum of skin colors in his writing and teaching. He is the column co-editor for "Dx Across the Skin Color Spectrum" in the journals *Cutis* and *JFP*. I know of no finer teacher of dermatology in Family Medicine.

Dr. Dan Stulberg has also taught with us for many years in the AAFP Skin Course. Dr. Stulberg has been teaching cryosurgery and electrosurgery for years in various AAFP conferences. His dermatology photographs and writings have been widely published in the *American Family Physician*. He maintains a strong interest in dermatology, procedural medicine and residency education. Dr. Stulberg was also a co-author with Dr. Usatine on the 4th edition of the book *Cryosurgery*. For many years Dr. Stulberg has been teaching dermatologic procedures to family medicine residents. Because of his skills in procedural dermatology, I asked him to contribute chapters to my own book.

Both lead authors continue to work as family physicians in addition to their work in dermatology. While Dr. Usatine spends 95% of his time in full-time dermatology he still gives back to his community through primary care work in student-run free clinics for individuals and families experiencing homelessness. He also has led medical missions to Ethiopia and Central America in which he supervised medical students interested in global health and caring for people living in extreme poverty. In addition to his role in teaching dermatology and procedures to residents, Dr. Stulberg has also expanded his role in family medicine leadership as a department chair in family medicine.

Together these two experts in dermatologic procedures have created a book with videos that will be a valuable guide for primary care providers worldwide. The photographs are excellent, and the videos are a great and modern way to learn or hone skills in these procedures. The skills you will learn from this book videos will help your patients and make your practice of medicine more enjoyable and rewarding.

Dr. EJ Mayeaux to 2nd edition

Preface

It is a great pleasure to release the second edition of our *Dermatologic Procedures in Office Practice* book with online videos and mobile application. The work on this book began in the 1990s when I had the great fortune of collaborating with leaders in dermatologic surgery to produce *Skin Surgery: A Practical Guide*. As a family physician, I was enthusiastic to learn these dermatologic procedures so that I could perform them well for my patients and teach them to other clinicians through photographs, writing, lectures, and workshops. Over the following 25 years, my additional experiences have led to a book and a mobile application that have better photographs, newer chapters and procedures, and high-definition video. *Dermatologic and Cosmetic Procedures in Office Practice* was published in 2012 by a team of four family physicians with additional expertise in dermatology. In this second edition, Dr. Stulberg and I decided to focus on core surgical procedures with the goal of diagnosing and treating skin cancers and benign skin conditions while maximizing the cosmetic outcome. We decided to not include lasers, fillers, and Botox as there are so many other available resources for these cosmetic procedures. We did add more content on dermoscopy, ultrasound, and procedures performed in challenging anatomical regions.

The book begins with a section entitled "Getting Started" and then follows with sections on basic procedures, advanced procedures, and a final section "Putting It All Together." The book with online videos and mobile application are especially directed toward family physicians and other primary care providers. Nurse practitioners and physician assistants practicing dermatology or primary care will also find the material useful. In addition, this set of resources has a lot to offer dermatology residents and dermatologists in their early stages of training.

The video segments have been developed over the past 14 years, mostly from surgeries performed in the University Health Skin Clinic in San Antonio. It is a unique clinic in which we train our dermatology fellows and family medicine residents to perform dermatologic procedures. It is the home of the first and only underserved family medicine dermatology fellowship in the country. I started this fellowship in 2009, and we now have three fellows a year training to provide dermatology care to communities that often lack access to dermatologists.

Whatever your current level of procedural skills, the videos, photographs, and text will take you to the next level. You and your patients will benefit greatly from the material presented. Start by reading the initial section on "Getting Started." Then learn to master all the "Basic Procedures" by providing these procedures for your patients as needed. If you are inclined to learn more advanced procedures, start with a few at a time and learn them well. Finally, use the "Putting It All Together" section to round out your procedural skills.

After 40 years as a family doctor including 17 years practicing full-time dermatology, I feel fortunate to be able to pass on my learning to the next generation of clinicians. Wishing you all a fulfilling career in medicine. We are all lucky to have opportunities to improve the lives of our patients through kind, compassionate, and competent healthcare delivery.

Richard P. Usatine, MD

Acknowledgments

I would like to acknowledge the support of my family. My children, Rebecca and Jeremy, are grown successful adults, but when I first began to write about dermatologic procedures, they were small children. In those years my photographs were 35mm slides often spread out on our dining room table. My family did not relish seeing these images but digital photography has revolutionized the capture of still photos and video so I now do all my publishing work on my computers in my home office. My wife of 40 years, Janna Lesser, has supported me throughout my career through her love and appreciation of the value of my work.

I want to thank Dr. Ash Marghoob for his mentorship in dermoscopy over the past 16 years. Dr. Marghoob is a world leader in dermoscopy research and education. He has co-authored many books and articles on dermoscopy. Dr. Marghoob began his career as a family physician and then became a board-certified dermatologist. He has taught dermoscopy to primary care providers for years. Together we teach dermoscopy yearly at the American Dermoscopy Meeting. Together we have written dermoscopy articles and created one popular free dermoscopy app.

I want to thank Dr David Swanson for his mentorship in dermatologic ultrasound. He encouraged me to get a portable ultrasound that plugs into my smartphone. Dr. Swanson wrote our ultrasound chapter, which is a great guide to how to use point-of-care ultrasound in dermatology.

I also want to thank Dr. Enzo Errichetti and Dr. Aimilios Lallas for their work on the dermoscopy chapter in general dermatology. Both dermatologists are international leaders in dermoscopy, and I was fortunate to work with them on a dermoscopy book focusing on non-neoplastic dermatoses across the skin color spectrum.

I want to acknowledge Dr. Daniel Stulberg as my partner in writing this book and two books before this. He has brought great knowledge and perspective to each of our collaborations and is a valued friend.

Finally, I would like to thank all my patients who have generously given of themselves to the creation of this book, mobile application, and videos. They have allowed me to photograph their procedures knowing that these photographs and videos will be used to train doctors and clinicians caring for people with skin diseases. It is only through their generosity that we have this resource today.

Richard P. Usatine, MD

I would like to thank all my patients for allowing me to share their stories and images of them to help others learn about skin care. I thank all my learners for the joy of teaching and watching them develop as physicians. I also want to express my sincere appreciation to Dr. Richard Usatine for his wonderful mentorship and guidance helping me advance my medical skills, teaching, conference presentations, editing, and publishing.

Daniel L. Stulberg, MD

We also want to thank the folks at Elsevier, especially Ranjana Sharma and Maria Shalini, for their hard work on the book.

Contents

SECTION ONE
Getting Started

1 *Preoperative Preparation* 2
RICHARD P. USATINE, MD, JENNIFER KREJCI-MANWARING, MD, AND RUBY GIBSON, MD

2 *Setting Up Your Office* 11
Facilities, Instruments, and Equipment
RICHARD P. USATINE, MD, AND MARION BELK, MD

3 *Anesthesia* 21
RICHARD P. USATINE, MD, AND ZEESHAN AFZAL, MD

4 *Hemostasis* 33
RICHARD P. USATINE, MD

5 *Selecting the Right Suture* 42
ALBA POSLIGUA, MD, NAIARA S. BARBOSA, MD, DANIEL L. STULBERG, MD, AND RICHARD P. USATINE, MD

6 *Suturing Techniques* 50
DANIEL L. STULBERG, MD, AND RICHARD P. USATINE, MD

SECTION TWO
Basic Procedures

7 *Laceration Repair* 70
RICHARD P. USATINE, MD, ANGELA MARTZ, PAC, WENDY C. COATES, MD, AND DANIEL STULBERG, MD

8 *Choosing the Biopsy Type* 83
RICHARD P. USATINE, MD, CAROLINE ZHU, MD, AND JOHN L. PFENNINGER, MD

9 *The Shave Biopsy* 101
RICHARD P. USATINE, MD, AND ZAIRA ORTEGA OREJEL, MD

10 *The Punch Biopsy* 114
RICHARD P. USATINE, MD, AND ANGELA ABOUASSI, MD

11 *The Elliptical Excision* 130
DANIEL L. STULBERG, MD, NIKKI KATTALANOS, PAC, AND RICHARD P. USATINE, MD

12 *Cysts and Lipomas* 152
JONATHAN KARNES, MD, AND RICHARD P. USATINE, MD

13 *Cryosurgery* 167
RICHARD P. USATINE, MD, AND DANIEL L. STULBERG, MD

14 *Electrosurgery* 185
RICHARD P. USATINE, MD, AND DANIEL L. STULBERG, MD

15 *Intralesional Injections* 206
RICHARD P. USATINE, MD, AND JIMENA CERVANTES, MD

16 *Incision and Drainage* 219
DANIEL L. STULBERG, MD, BERNADATTE G. GILBERT, MD, PATRICK MORAN, DO, AND RICHARD P. USATINE, MD

17 *Nail Procedures* 230
RICHARD P. USATINE, MD, ARIADNA PEREZ SANCHEZ, MD, AND ROBERT GILSON, MD

18 *Dermoscopy of Skin Cancer and Benign Neoplasia* 253
RICHARD P. USATINE, MD, AND ASHFAQ A. MARGHOOB, MD

19 *Dermoscopy in General Dermatology* 284
ENZO ERRICHETTI, MD, MARIA BAKIRTZI, AND AIMILIOS LALLAS

SECTION THREE
Advanced Procedures

20 *Biopsies and Excisions in Challenging Locations* 296
RICHARD P. USATINE, MD

21 *Flaps* 307
RYAN O'QUINN, MD, AND RICHARD P. USATINE, MD

22 *Ultrasound in Dermatology* 318
DAVID SWANSON, MD

SECTION FOUR
Putting It All Together

23 *Procedures to Treat Benign Conditions* 330
DANIEL STULBERG, MD, HAMID QAZI, MD, ROBERT FAWCETT, MD, AND RICHARD P. USATINE, MD

24 *Diagnosis and Treatment of Malignant and Premalignant Lesions* 354
RICHARD P. USATINE, MD, AND DANIEL L. STULBERG, MD

25 *Wound Care* 373
DANIEL STULBERG, MD, ERIC LEW, DPM, REGINA GALLEGOS, MPT, CWS, LUCIA DIAZ, MD, CHRISTY NWANKWO, BA, AND RICHARD P. USATINE, MD

26 *Complications* 387
Postprocedural Adverse Effects and Their Prevention
RICHARD P. USATINE, MD, AND DANIEL STULBERG, MD

27 *When to Refer/Mohs Surgery* 398
RYAN O'QUINN, MD, JOHN L. PFENNINGER, MD, AND RICHARD P. USATINE, MD

28 *Coding Common Skin Procedures* 406
JONATHAN B. KARNES, MD

APPENDIX A Consent Forms and Patient Information Handouts 415

APPENDIX B Procedures to Consider for Benign, Premalignant, and Malignant Conditions 421

Video Contents

Chapter 3: Anesthesia

3.1 Anesthesia for Shave Biopsy
3.2 Anesthesia for Punch Biopsy
3.3 Anesthesia for Elliptical Excision
3.4 Digital Block
3.5 Cyst Excision Behind Ear With Ring Block
3.6 Epidermal Cyst Excision From Back With Ring Block

Chapter 4: Hemostasis

4.1 Hemostasis With Aluminum Chloride After Shave Biopsy
4.2 Electrosurgical Hemostasis After Removing an Ellipse
4.3 Using Electrosurgery in an Undermined Area
4.4 Hemostasis With Forceps and Electrosurgery
4.5 Figure of Eight Suture for Hemostasis

Chapter 6: Suturing Techniques

6.1 Loading the Needle Holder
6.2 Instrument Tie
6.3 Simple Interrupted Suture
6.4 Simple Running Suture on Face
6.5 Simple Running Suture on Arm
6.6 Deep Vertical Mattress Suture With Skin Hook
6.7 Deep Vertical Mattress Suture With Skin Hook After Rotation Flap
6.8 Deep Vertical Mattress Suture With Forceps
6.9 Deep Horizontal Mattress Suture

Chapter 9: The Shave Biopsy

9.1 Shave of Benign Nevus on Face With DermaBlade
9.2 Shave of Benign Nevus on Neck With DermaBlade
9.3 Shave of Scalp Nevus With DermaBlade
9.4 Shave Excision of Keloid From Earlobe With DermaBlade
9.5 Shave Biopsy of Small BCC With DermaBlade
9.6 Shave Biopsy on Neck of Suspicious Lesion With DermaBlade
9.7 Shave of Nevus With #15 Blade
9.8 Shave a Benign Nevus With DermaBlade and Electrosurgery of Remaining Edge
9.9 Snip Excision of Two Skin Tags With Anesthesia
9.10 Snip Excision of One Skin Tag Without Anesthesia
9.11 Shave Biopsy of Lentigo Maligna Melanoma
9.12 Shave Biopsy on Scalp
9.13 Shave Biopsy Overview

Chapter 10: The Punch Biopsy

10.1 Punch Biopsy of Suspected Melanoma – Not Sutured
10.2 Punch Biopsy of Pityriasis Rosea With One Suture
10.3 Punch Biopsy of Palmar Psoriasis With Two Sutures Placed
10.4 Overview of the Punch Biopsy
10.5 Bullous Drug Eruption Biopsy Double Punch
10.6 Punch Biopsy Blue Nevus
10.7 Punch BCC Nose Surgifoam
10.8 Punch Closed With Figure of 8 Suture
10.9 Punch Biopsy of Malar Rash

Chapter 11: The Elliptical Excision

11.1 Ellipse Overview
11.2 Elliptical Excision of SCC on Thigh
11.3 Elliptical Excision of BCC on Arm
11.4 Elliptical Excision of SCC on Face
11.5 Elliptical Excision of Chondrodermatitis
11.6 Repair of Standing Cone (Dog Ear)

Chapter 12: Cysts and Lipomas

12.1 Epidermal Cyst Removed Intact on Abdomen
12.2 Pilar Cyst Excision
12.3 Cyst Removal Overview
12.4 Epidermal Cyst Excision From Back With Ring Block
12.5 Cyst Excision Behind Ear With Ring Block
12.6 Digital Mucous Cyst Excision
12.7 Lipoma Overview
12.8 Lipoma Excision – Full Procedure
12.9 Lipoma Expressed Manually
12.10 Lipoma Excision – Skin of Color

Chapter 13: Cryosurgery

13.1 Cryotherapy Overview
13.2 Liquid Nitrogen Removed From Dewar Using Withdrawal Tube
13.3 Cryo-Spray of Seborrheic Keratosis on Face – Long Bent Spray Tip
13.4 Pulsatile Spray of Seborrheic Keratosis on Neck – Aperture C Tip
13.5 Cryo-Spray of Flat Warts
13.6 Cryo-Spray of Actinic Keratosis With Bent Spray Tip
13.7 Keloid Treated With Cryo-Spray Then Intralesional Injection
13.8 Cryo-Tweezer-Skin-Tag
13.9 Cryo-Tweezer of Warts on Face
13.10 Cryo-Spray With Straight Short-Tip (Banana Model)
13.11 Cryo-Spray With Aperture C Tip (Banana Model)
13.12 Cryo-Spray With Bent Spray Tip (Banana Model)
13.13 Small Closed Probe With Liquid Nitrogen (Banana Model)
13.14 Large Closed Probe With Liquid Nitrogen (Banana Model)

Chapter 14: Electrosurgery

14.1 Electrosurgery Overview
14.2 Electrosurgery – Review of Hyfrecator
14.3 Electrosurgery of Cherry Angioma
14.4 Electrosurgery Loop Shave of Nevus With Feathering
14.5 Electrosurgery After Shave of Pyogenic Granuloma
14.6 ED&C of BCC
14.7 Electrodessication and Curettage of SCC in Situ on Dorsum of Hand

14.8 Electrosurgery With Sharp Tip Electrode (Banana Model)

14.9 Electrofulguration and Electrodessication With Blunt Tip Electrode (Banana Model)

14.10 Bipolar Electrode (Banana Model)

Chapter 15: Intralesional Injections

15.1 Injection Overview

15.2 Injecting Lichen Planopilaris With Steroid

15.3 Keloid Treated With Cryo-Spray Then Intralesional Injection

15.4 Injecting Hidradenitis With Steroid

15.5 Intralesional Steroid Psoriasis

15.6 Intralesional Steroid Psoriatic Nails

Chapter 16: Incision and Drainage

16.1 Paronychia I&D

16.2 Deroofing Hidradenitis

16.3 I and D of Cyst on Back

Chapter 17: Nail Procedures

17.1 Removal of Ingrown Toenail With Digital Block and Electrosurgery

17.2 Toenail Matrix Ablation With Phenol and Electrosurgery

17.3 Ingrown toenail surgery

17.4 Nail Matrix Shave Biopsy

Chapter 18: Dermoscopy of Skin Cancer and Benign Neoplasia

18.1 Dermoscopy Overview

18.2 Blink Sign Seborrheic Keratosis

18.3 Wobble Sign Intradermal Nevus

Chapter 19: Dermoscopy in General Dermatology

19.1 Scabies Mites Moving Under Dermoscopy

Chapter 20: Biopsies and Excisions in Challenging Locations

20.1 Punch Biopsies Scalp

20.2 Scalp Pilar Cyst

20.3 Elliptical Excision of Chondrodermatitis

20.4 Wedge Excision on the Ear After Mohs Surgery

20.5 Lip Mucocele Excision

20.6 Punch Biopsy on Foot

20.7 Shave Biopsy on Foot

Chapter 21: Flaps

21.1 Rotation Flap on Cheek After Mohs Surgery

Chapter 22: Ultrasound in Dermatology

22.1 Epidermal Cyst

22.2 Lipoma

22.3 Cellulitis

Chapter 23: Procedures to Treat Benign Conditions

23.1 Snip Excision of Skin Tags on Neck

23.2 Snip Excision of One Acrochordon Without Anesthesia

23.3 Electrosurgery of Cherry Angioma

23.4 Elliptical Excision of Chondrodermatitis

23.5 Shave Excision of Keloid From Earlobe With DermaBlade

23.6 Milia Extraction

23.7 Shave of Benign Nevus on Face With DermaBlade

23.8 Shave of Benign Nevus on Neck With DermaBlade

23.9 Shave of Scalp Nevus With DermaBlade

23.10 Shave of Nevus With #15 Blade

23.11 Electrosurgery Loop Shave of Nevus With Feathering

23.12 Sebaceous Hyperplasia Electrosurgery

23.13 Cryo-Spray of Seborrheic Keratosis on Face – Long Bent Spray Tip

23.14 Pulsatile Spray of Seborrheic Keratosis on Neck – Aperture C Tip

23.15 Electrosurgery of Dermatosis Papulosa Nigra

Chapter 24: Diagnosis and Treatment of Malignant and Premalignant Lesions

24.1 Cryo-Spray With Long Bent Spray Tip of Actinic Keratosis

24.2 Cryo-Spray of Actinic Keratosis With Aperture C Tip

24.3 Electrodessication and Curettage of SCC in Situ on Dorsum of Hand

24.4 Elliptical Excision of SCC on Thigh

24.5 Elliptical Excision of SCC on Face

24.6 Shave Biopsy of Small BCC With DermaBlade

24.7 Elliptical Excision of BCC on Arm

24.8 Shave Biopsy of Lentigo Maligna Melanoma on Forehead

Chapter 27: When to Refer/Mohs Surgery

27.1 Mohs Surgery and Repair of SCC on Neck

27.2 Mohs Surgery and Repair of BCC on Face

Getting Started

SECTION OUTLINE

1 *Preoperative Preparation*

2 *Setting Up Your Office: Facilities, Instruments, and Equipment*

3 *Anesthesia*

4 *Hemostasis*

5 *Selecting the Right Suture*

6 *Suturing Techniques*

1 Preoperative Preparation

RICHARD P. USATINE, MD, JENNIFER KREJCI-MANWARING, MD, and RUBY GIBSON, MD

SUMMARY

- Surgical planning consists of many steps, from office scheduling to preoperative patient preparation and sterile technique.
- A preoperative medical evaluation can prevent complications. It helps to get a blood pressure before starting surgery because severely elevated blood pressure can lead to increased bleeding and other complications.
- Informed consent and universal precautions are discussed.
- While we do not suggest stopping anticoagulation, it does help to be aware of whether a patient is anticoagulated before making the first cut with a scalpel.
- Antibiotic prophylaxis is reviewed by making use of minimal existing evidence and when it might be appropriate to consider their use based on risk assessment.
- Tips for preoperative preparation and sterile technique are provided.

The practice of skin surgery in the office requires careful planning and a team of well-instructed support personnel. Other keys to success are thorough patient education and informed consent, preoperative screening, good surgical technique, and sterile surgical instruments. The use of universal precautions to prevent the transmission of infectious diseases is paramount to protecting the clinician, the medical staff, and the patient.

Surgical Planning

Surgical planning should consist of the following:

- Office scheduling
- Preoperative medical evaluation
- Informed consent
- Universal precautions
- Preoperative medications
- Standby medications and equipment
- Preoperative patient preparation (skin, hair, drapes)
- Sterilization of instruments
- Sterile technique

Scheduling of Complex Surgeries

Simple surgical procedures, such as shave or punch biopsies, need no special scheduling. These procedures can be done rapidly as the need arises. However, clinicians contemplating performing more complex surgical procedures in the office will benefit from careful, deliberate consideration of how best to integrate the surgeries into the office schedule. Proper scheduling is critical to producing the efficient,

unhurried surgical atmosphere that is reassuring to both the patient and the staff.

Some offices schedule more complex surgeries at the end of the morning or the end of the afternoon to avoid being rushed by other patient responsibilities. This allows the clinician to approach surgery in an unhurried manner. Another strategy is to designate certain half-days for surgical procedures only.

Surgeons may also choose to perform more complex surgeries early in the week and avoid surgery on Friday so that patients can be seen the day after surgery for a postoperative check. This type of schedule helps prevent weekend calls or unneeded trips to the emergency center if a patient develops a hematoma or other complication that can be easily handled in the office.

Preoperative Medical Evaluation

MEDICAL HISTORY

A complete medical history and review of systems before minor surgery may not be necessary. Before a more complex skin procedure, however, the following information should be taken during the medical history:

- Current medications, especially anticoagulants, aspirin, and other nonsteroidal antiinflammatory
- Allergies, especially to antibiotics, tapes/adhesives, iodine, anesthetics (lidocaine)
- Cardiac disease (e.g., any condition requiring endocarditis prophylaxis such as a prosthetic heart valve), uncontrolled hypertension, epinephrine sensitivity, angina. The presence of a pacemaker or implantable defibrillator has implications for electrosurgery (see Chapter 14, *Electrosurgery*)

- Other illnesses and medical conditions (e.g., diabetes, seizure disorder, hematologic disorder or bleeding diathesis, joint replacement [positioning of grounding pad with electrosurgical device], high-risk groups for infectious diseases [e.g., injection drug users])
- Pregnancy, lactation
- Keloids or hypertrophic scars
- Infectious diseases (e.g., hepatitis B or C, HIV/AIDS, methicillin-resistant *Staphylococcus aureus*, tuberculosis)

For minor skin surgery under local anesthesia, blood pressure should be measured but does not need to be monitored unless the patient has a history of hypertension that is not controlled. Uncontrolled hypertension may lead to increased bleeding during surgery. If the blood pressure is significantly elevated, consider postponing the procedure or giving a dose of an appropriate antihypertensive agent prior to the start of the procedure. It is prudent to be more careful with fragile patients, such as the elderly, and to be particularly careful with the use of epinephrine-containing anesthetics in patients with a history of angina, cardiac disease, or sensitivity to epinephrine. It may help to warn these patients that they may develop an increased heart rate or a feeling of anxiety after injection of lidocaine with epinephrine.

Medical Contraindications

Skin surgery is not recommended on patients who have unstable angina because the epinephrine in the local anesthetic can precipitate angina. Although this is unlikely, it is worth having nitroglycerin in the office to deal with this potential situation. Patients who have uncontrolled diabetes mellitus may experience impaired wound healing. Closer follow-up after surgery may help avoid potential problems with these patients.

Informed Consent

Thorough discussion with patients regarding the benefits and risks of any planned surgical procedure and the alternatives to surgery is essential before surgery. It is always best to devote adequate time to this discussion so that all of the patient's questions can be answered in an unhurried manner. Although the optimal situation is to have the clinician who will perform the procedure provide the informed consent, a well-trained assistant can start the process, and the clinician can answer any questions beyond the skills of the assistant. Risks include pain, bleeding, infection, scarring, change in pigmentation, regrowth, slow healing, change in anatomic appearance, skin indentation, skin protrusion, local nerve damage/numbness, loss of muscle function, and need for further treatment. A complete list of risks is listed in Appendix A on the sample consent form titled "Disclosure and Consent: Medical and Surgical Procedures."

For many routine minor procedures, such as cryotherapy, a written consent may not be needed. However, clinicians may want to consider obtaining a written consent for any procedure, even as small as cryotherapy, if the procedure is to be performed on a cosmetically sensitive area such as the face or on those for whom scarring may be more of a concern. Written consent is always obtained for procedures that may have more significant adverse consequences, such as scarring or functional effects. Feel free to use or modify the form supplied in Appendix A for your own office. The informed consent must be signed by the patient's designated surrogate if the patient lacks decision-making capacity.[1]

For larger surgeries, show patients the planned excision before you begin the surgery. You can show the patient and any family in attendance your surgical markings before you start. Keep a handheld mirror nearby for excisions on the face so that your patient knows what you plan to do. This is a helpful method to make sure you truly have informed consent.

Universal Precautions

With the identification of AIDS in the 1980s, measures to prevent the transmission of contagious diseases to medical personnel have come to be known as universal precautions, and their use has been incorporated into every medical clinic, surgical center, or hospital. Diseases of chief concern are hepatitis B, hepatitis C, and HIV/AIDS. However, other contagious diseases, such as tuberculosis and syphilis, also present some potential risk to medical personnel.

The basics of universal precautions include the use of surgical gloves and the use of barrier clothing such as gowns, face masks, and eye protection; proper disposal of sharp, disposable surgical instruments, such as needles and scalpel blades, in special puncture-proof containers; disposal of all contaminated drapes and other soft items in specially marked biohazard containers; and collection and disposal of this material by professional hazardous-waste removal companies.

For skin surgery we have found it especially helpful to practice choreographed surgery, with particular attention paid to any sharp instruments. We handle only one sharp instrument at a time and are aware of its position at all times. All sharps should be counted as they are placed on and removed from the surgical tray. Avoid recapping needles that have been used with a patient. If a recap must be done, use the one-handed recap technique in which the needle sheath is positioned against an inanimate object. When suturing, use an instrument such as Adson forceps to load the needle onto the needle driver rather than your fingers. We take particular care to avoid rushing when performing surgery and also attempt to have extra help available – within earshot – at all times.

Medications

ANTICOAGULATION/ANTIPLATELET THERAPY

The clinician needs to find out which medications the patient is taking in order to determine if there will be an increased risk of bleeding in the intraoperative or postoperative period. This includes warfarin, aspirin, NSAIDs, clopidogrel, direct and indirect thrombin inhibitors, and factor Xa inhibitors. For larger surgeries, one might query patients about their use of any vitamin, herbal, or other over-the-counter supplements because some of these can alter the coagulation profile.

There are few official guidelines regarding the management of anticoagulation/antiplatelet therapies before cutaneous surgery; however, there is increasing evidence for continuing these medications.[2]

One large study of 2394 patients with 5950 lesions found four independent risk factors for postoperative bleeding:

1. Age 67 years or older (odds ratio [OR] 4.7)
2. Warfarin therapy (OR 2.9)
3. Surgery on or around the ear (OR 2.6)
4. Closure with a skin flap or graft (OR 2.7).[3]

Aspirin therapy was not an independent risk factor for bleeding. The researchers concluded that "most postoperative bleeds were inconvenient but not life threatening, unlike the potential risk of thromboembolism after stopping warfarin or aspirin." They recommended not to discontinue aspirin before skin surgery.[3] In 2326 patients operated on by a single surgeon, warfarin was used by 28 patients, 228 took aspirin, and the remainder took neither. There was no difference in the complication rate among the three groups. Researchers concluded that patients taking aspirin or warfarin do not need to discontinue these medications before minor dermatologic procedures.[4]

Warfarin is a vitamin K antagonist used frequently for preventing thrombotic and thromboembolic complications in patients with atrial fibrillation, prosthetic valve, and deep vein thrombosis prophylaxis and treatment. Although some studies have shown a lack of bleeding complications in patients taking warfarin, a metaanalysis with a total of 1373 dermatologic surgery patients found that those taking warfarin were nearly seven times as likely to have moderate to severe bleeding-related complications compared to controls.[5] Patients taking aspirin or NSAIDs were more than twice as likely to have a moderate-to-severe complication compared to controls. Furthermore, recent studies have demonstrated a statistically significant increase in bleeding in patients taking warfarin. Despite the increased risk of bleeding, the studies recommend continuing warfarin throughout surgery to prevent thrombotic complications.[6,7] In a prospective study of 51 patients undergoing a range of minor cutaneous surgical procedures, including excision biopsies, local flaps, and skin grafts, patients continued their normal warfarin regimen. The international normalized ratio (INR) was checked on the day of surgery, and it ranged from 1.1 to 4.0. No problems were encountered during surgery, but two patients presented with bleeding postoperatively a few days later. The study concluded that it is not necessary to modify warfarin regimens for minor cutaneous surgery.[8] In a prospective controlled observational study, 65 patients on warfarin underwent excision of 70 cutaneous tumors. There was no increase in bleeding tendency during surgery with those on warfarin when compared with controls. Five patients on warfarin (8%) reported moderate or severe postoperative bleeding. All patients on warfarin with bleeding complications had an INR of <2.6 at the time of surgery.[9] Bleeding risk could not be correlated with INR. The researchers suggested that it is crucial to observe meticulous hemostasis in all patients on warfarin regardless of INR.[9] If a patient's INR is supra-therapeutic (>3.5), the clinician should consider postponing the surgery and discuss management with the patient's cardiologist.[2]

A prospective study evaluated the safety of dermatologic surgery and found a 0.89% risk of hemorrhage. Of the 1911 patients, 38% were on one anticoagulant or antiplatelet medication, and 8.0% were on two or more. The study concludes that the rate of complications in dermatologic surgery is low even with patients on multiple oral anticoagulant and antiplatelet medications. The study also reported that complex repair, graft repair, flap repair, and partial repair were more likely to result in bleeding than intermediate repair.[7] This study also reported an increase in bleeding risk with clopidogrel. However, the authors still recommended continuing the medication during dermatologic surgery.[7] In a retrospective study of 220 patients taking clopidogrel-containing anticoagulation, patients were six times more likely to experience severe complications than aspirin monotherapy.[10] However, another prospective study found that patients taking clopidogrel did not experience a greater rate of complications compared to the other groups.[11]

A retrospective study was conducted for patients who underwent Mohs micrographic surgery or a basic excision while taking dabigatran or rivaroxaban. Twenty-seven patients taking dabigatran underwent 41 cutaneous surgeries; only one mild bleeding complication was observed and was resolved with a pressure dressing. Four patients on rivaroxaban underwent five cutaneous surgeries without complication. The study concluded that there were no severe hemorrhagic complications during cutaneous surgery and these medications could be continued during cutaneous surgery.[12]

The risk of bleeding must be balanced by the risk of not remaining on anticoagulants. There have been several reports of patients having thromboembolic events after stopping anticoagulation.[13-15] A survey of 504 members of the American College of Mohs Micrographic Surgery and Cutaneous Oncology were surveyed for thrombotic complications when anticoagulants were stopped. A total of 168 responding physicians reported 46 patients who had a thrombotic event. Thrombotic complications included stroke (24), transient ischemic attack (8), myocardial infarction (5), cerebral embolism (3), death (3), deep vein thrombosis (3), pulmonary embolism (2), and blindness (1). The authors reported a thrombotic risk of 1 in 6219 operations when warfarin was discontinued and 1 in 21,448 when aspirin was discontinued.[16]

In conclusion, the patient's medical conditions, cardiovascular protection, bleeding risk, and the procedure type and location must be taken into consideration when approaching the management of antithrombotic agents. Given the risk of potentially lethal thromboembolic events from discontinuing these medications and the minimal clinical significance of bleeding, the evidence suggests continuing anticoagulants in a vast majority of dermatologic procedures.[2,4,6-8,10,17-20] Exceptional care must be taken to prevent bleeding by using electrosurgery, epinephrine, tying off vessels, and applying handheld pressure for hemostasis. Pressure dressings can also help minimize the risk of hematoma. Lastly, patients should be made aware of the small but increased risk of postoperative bleeding and given verbal and written postoperative instructions.

ANTIBIOTIC PROPHYLAXIS

Clean, noncontaminated dermatologic surgeries have a low risk of surgical site infections at rate of 0.7% to 3% in patients without the use of prophylactic antibiotics.[21–25] The routine and indiscriminate use of prophylactic antibiotics for cutaneous procedures is not recommended because overuse results in multidrug-resistant pathogens, increased costs, and adverse events.[22] Preoperative antibiotics such as oral cephalexin, dicloxacillin, or clindamycin may be recommended for use with patients who have a higher risk of infection.[23] These situations might include a patient who has a contaminated or infected lesion; a lesion in an area of increased bacteria, such as the axilla, ear, or mouth; a lesion on a hand or foot, especially in patients with peripheral vascular disease; a situation in which the operation might take more than 1 hour or if the wound was open for more than 1 hour; a patient for whom complete sterile technique was not optimal; or any situation in which an infection would have serious consequences, such as in a patient with diabetes or neutropenia.

See Table 1.1 for classification of wound infection risk and the need for antibiotic prophylaxis. The 2008 Advisory Statement from the American Academy of Dermatology (AAD) on antibiotic prophylaxis in dermatologic surgery stated that antibiotics may be indicated for the prevention of surgical site infections for:

- Procedures on the lower extremities or groin
- Wedge excisions of the lip and ear (Figure 1.1)
- Skin flaps on the nose
- Skin grafts
- Patients with extensive inflammatory skin disease[23]

In addition, antibiotic prophylaxis may be indicated for infective endocarditis and prosthetic joint infection when the procedure involves oral mucosa or infected skin.[22,23] Table 1.2 provides recommendations for antibiotic prophylaxis in patients at increased risk of surgical site infection.

Diabetes is considered an independent risk factor for surgical site infection.[26] In a 5-year prospective observational study, infection incidence was significantly higher in patients

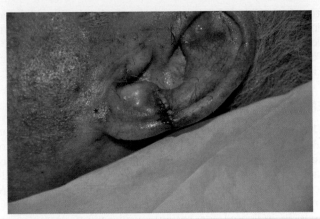

Figure 1.1 Completed repair of a wedge excision to remove a squamous cell carcinoma from the ear. Consider using prophylactic antibiotics with such a surgery because there is a higher risk of infection after a wedge excision of the ear. (Copyright Richard P. Usatine, MD.)

Table 1.2 Antibiotic Prophylaxis for Patients at Increased Risk of Surgical-Site Infection

Surgical Site	Medication	Dose*
Wedge on lip or ear, flap on nose, all grafts	Cephalexin or dicloxacillin	2 g
Groin or lower extremity	Cephalexin or TMP-SMX-DS or Levofloxacin	2 g 1 tablet 500 mg
ALLERGIC TO PCN		
Lip, ear, flap on nose, all grafts	Clindamycin, or	600 mg
Groin or lower extremity	Azithromycin, clarithromycin or TMP-SMX-DS or Levofloxacin	500 mg 1 tablet 500 mg
UNABLE TO TAKE ORAL MEDICATION		
Lip, ear, flap on nose, all grafts	Cefazolin, ceftriaxone	1 g IM/ IV
Groin or lower extremity	Ceftriaxone	1-2 g IV
UNABLE TO TAKE ORAL MEDICATION AND ALLERGIC TO PCN		
Lip, ear, flap on nose, all grafts	Clindamycin	600 mg IM/ IV
Groin or lower extremity	Clindamycin + gentamicin	600 mg, 2 mg/kg IV

*Give one hour before surgery.
IM, intramuscular; IV, intravenous; PCN, penicillin; TMP-SMX-DS, trimethoprim-sulfamethoxazole double strength.
Adapted from Wright TI, Baddour LM, Berbari EF, et al. Antibiotic prophylaxis in dermatologic surgery: advisory statement 2008. *J Am Acad Dermatol.* 2008;59:464-473.

Table 1.1 Classification of Wound Infection Risk

Class	Antibiotic Prophylaxis Needed?
Clean: noncontaminated skin, sterile technique = 5% infection	No
Clean contaminated: wounds in oral cavity, respiratory tract, axilla/perineum; breaks in aseptic technique = 10% infection rate	Consider
Contaminated: trauma, acute nonpurulent inflammation, major breaks in aseptic technique (intact, inflamed cysts; tumors with clinical inflammation) = 20% to 30% infection rate	Yes
Infected: gross contamination with foreign bodies, devitalized tissue (ruptured cysts; tumors with purulent, necrotic material) = 30% to 40% infection rate	Yes

From Haas AF, Grekin RC. Antibiotic prophylaxis in dermatologic surgery. *J Am Acad Dermatol.* 1995;32:155-176.

with diabetes (4.2%, 23/551) than in those without (2.0%, 135/6673) $(P < .001)$.[8] Noninfective complications were similar. Although this study demonstrates the increased risk, it does not prove that antibiotic prophylaxis will decrease this risk. The decision to use antibiotic prophylaxis is complex and must be based on all available data and the balance of the known patient risks with the potential antibiotic adverse effects.

The use of topical antibiotics for postsurgical wound infection is not indicated for prophylactic use. A metaanalysis from four trials did not show a statistically significant difference in the incidence of postsurgical wound infections between topical antibiotics and petrolatum/paraffin.[27] Petrolatum is recommended in place of topical antibiotics for routine postoperative care of clean surgical wounds.[28]

ENDOCARDITIS PROPHYLAXIS

The recommendations of the American Heart Association (AHA) for the prevention of bacterial endocarditis were last published in 2007.[29] Endocarditis prophylaxis is not indicated for incision or biopsy of noninfected, surgically scrubbed skin no matter what endocarditis risk factors are present. The 2007 guidelines state that antibiotic prophylaxis is indicated for patients undergoing dermatologic surgery on infected skin or surgery that involves breach of oral mucosa for patients with underlying cardiac conditions associated with the highest risk of an adverse outcome from infective endocarditis.

For individuals at highest risk for endocarditis who undergo a surgical procedure that involves infected skin or skin structures, it is reasonable for the therapeutic regimen administered for treatment of the infection to contain an agent active against staphylococci and beta-hemolytic streptococci, such as an antistaphylococcal penicillin or a cephalosporin (SOR C).[29] Vancomycin or clindamycin may be administered to patients unable to tolerate a beta-lactam antibiotic or who are known or suspected to have an infection caused by methicillin-resistant *Staphylococcus aureus*.[29] Suggested antibiotic prophylaxis regimens for dermatologic surgical procedures that breach the oral mucosa or involve infected skin in patients at high risk for infective endocarditis or hematogenous total joint infection are recommended in Table 1.3, Box 1.1.[23]

One published mnemonic to help remember when and how to use prophylactic antibiotics in skin surgery is I PREVENT. This represents Immunosuppressed patients; patients with a Prosthetic valve; some patients with a joint Replacement; a history of infective Endocarditis; a Valvulopathy in cardiac transplant recipients; Endocrine disorders

> **Box 1.1 High-Risk Cardiac Conditions for Which Antibiotic Prophylaxis Is Indicated With Infected Skin or Breach of Oral Mucosa**
> - Prosthetic cardiac valve
> - Previous infective endocarditis
> - Congenital heart disease (CHD)
> - Unrepaired cyanotic CHD, including palliative shunts and conduits
> - Completely repaired congenital heart defects with prosthetic material or device, whether placed by a surgical or catheter intervention, during the first 6 months after procedure
> - Repaired CHD with residual defects at site or adjacent to site of prosthetic patch or prosthetic device (which inhibits endothelialization)
> - Cardiac transplantation recipients who develop cardiac valvulopathy[29]

such as uncontrolled diabetes mellitus; Neonatal disorders including unrepaired cyanotic heart disorders (CHDs), repaired CHD with prosthetic material, or repaired CHD with residual defects; and the Tetrad of antibiotics: amoxicillin, cephalexin, clindamycin, and ciprofloxacin.[30]

INTERVENTIONS TO REDUCE ANXIETY AT TIME OF SURGERY

Smartphones are so ubiquitous today that they can be used to relax or distract patients before or during surgery. The patient could be asked if they would like to listen to music from their own phone or use their phone for reading or playing games if their hands will be free. Children often can be distracted by playing a game on smartphone during a procedure. Of course, the clinician can also offer their own phone to play relaxing music during the procedure including the administration of local anesthesia.

There are studies that demonstrate that music reduces pain and anxiety in patients undergoing surgery.[12,31,32]

Antianxiety medications such as alprazolam, diazepam, midazolam, or lorazepam can be useful in the very anxious

Table 1.3 Regimens to Prevent Infective Endocarditis in a Dermatologic Procedure[a]

	SINGLE DOSE GIVEN 30 TO 60 MIN BEFORE PROCEDURE		
Situation	Agent	Adults	Children
Oral	Amoxicillin	2 g	50 mg/kg
Unable to take oral medication	Ampicillin or	2 g IM or IV	50 mg/kg IM or IV
	Cefazolin or ceftriaxone	1 g IM or IV	50 mg/kg IM or IV
Allergic to penicillins or ampicillin (oral)	Cephalexin[b,c] or	2 g	50 mg/kg
	Clindamycin or	600 mg	20 mg/kg
	Azithromycin, clarithromycin	500 mg	15 mg/kg
Allergic to penicillins or ampicillin and unable to take oral medication	Cefazolin or ceftriaxone[c]	1 g IM or IV	50 mg/kg IM or IV
	Clindamycin	600 mg IM or IV	20 mg/kg IM or IV

IM, intramuscular; IV, intravenous.

[a]Antibiotic prophylaxis is indicated for patients undergoing dermatologic surgery on infected skin or that involves breach of oral mucosa for patients with underlying cardiac conditions associated with the highest risk of adverse outcome from infective endocarditis. See Box 1.1.

[b]Or other first- or second-generation oral cephalosporin in equivalent adult or pediatric dosage.

[c]Cephalosporins should not be used in an individual with a history of anaphylaxis, angioedema, or urticaria with penicillins or ampicillin.

Source: From Wilson W, Taubert KA, Gewitz M, et al. Prevention of infective endocarditis: guidelines from the American Heart Association: a guideline from the American Heart Association Rheumatic Fever, Endocarditis, and Kawasaki Disease Committee, Council on Cardiovascular Disease in the Young, and the Council on Clinical Cardiology, Council on Cardiovascular Surgery and Anesthesia, and the Quality of Care and Outcomes Research Interdisciplinary Working Group. *Circulation.* 2007;116:1736-1754.

patient who does not respond to nonpharmacologic methods of relaxation (such as slow abdominal breathing). These medications have been shown to decrease patient anxiety when undergoing dermatologic inpatient and outpatient procedures including Mohs micrographic surgery and hair transplantation.[33–35] If these medications are administered sublingually, the onset of action can be quicker than when they are administered orally. These medications should not be given to a patient who will be driving home. All patients given intraoperative or preoperative sedatives must be accompanied by an adult, must be counseled not to drive on the day of the surgery, must be observed postoperatively until the sedative effect has sufficiently diminished, and must be counseled that their mental capacities may be diminished for a prolonged period after surgery.

Standby Medications and Equipment

It is helpful to have injectable diphenhydramine and epinephrine available for subcutaneous injection in case of an anaphylactic reaction to anesthesia, latex, or other medication. It may also be helpful to have an Ambu-bag, an insertable airway, oxygen, a cardiac monitor, and a defibrillator in your office, but these items are not absolutely necessary.

Preoperative Patient Preparation

PREPARATION OF THE SKIN

The most common preoperative preparations to be used on the skin include alcohol, Betadine (povidone-iodine), and Hibiclens (chlorhexidine). The main advantages of using chlorhexidine are that it has a longer-lasting antibacterial effect than povidone-iodine and the risk of contact sensitivity may be less. One disadvantage of using chlorhexidine, however, is that it is more toxic to the eye if it accidentally drops into it. However, if the eye is flushed immediately, no damage may be done. Caution must be taken when using alcohol to be sure that all of the alcohol has evaporated before any electrosurgery is performed in the area.

The most important part of the preoperative preparation of the skin is the mechanical rubbing of the antiseptic onto the skin with the gauze. Although the gauze may not need to be sterile for the first prep, it might help to use sterile gauze in the last prep. It is actually impossible to sterilize the skin because bacteria can extend into hair follicles. The goal of the preoperative preparation of the skin is to reduce the bacteria on the skin surface by scrubbing the skin with a good antiseptic such as povidone-iodine or chlorhexidine. Povidone-iodine must be allowed to dry on the skin for its effect to be optimal. Chlorhexidine has the advantage of not staining the skin and being easy to wash off. Povidone-iodine has the advantage of being easy to see where it was applied but should be avoided in persons with iodine allergies. However, Darouiche et al. found a greater than 40% reduction in total surgical site infections among patients undergoing clean-contaminated surgery who had received a single chlorhexidine-alcohol scrub as compared with a povidone-iodine scrub.[36]

An 8-oz pump bottle of chlorhexidine can be kept in each examination/procedure room and can be used repeatedly by pumping the solution onto clean or sterile gauze. Povidone-iodine swab sticks are convenient but a bit more expensive than povidone-iodine in a bottle applied with gauze.

One extensive evidence review for the effectiveness of skin antiseptics in the prevention of surgical site infection concluded that chlorhexidine is a dominant strategy over povidone-iodine for preoperative skin antisepsis to prevent surgical site infection.[37]

A survey of MMS surgeons found that CHG is their most commonly used skin antiseptic except during periocular procedures, during which povidone-iodine is more often used.[38]

PREPARATION OF HAIR

The best method of hair removal over a surgical site is to use scissors to cut the hair. Using scissors to clip hair is now the preferred method for preoperative hair removal because a close shave with a razor causes minute abrasions of the skin that can increase the chance of infection.[39] A depilatory cream may also be used but this is messy and more time consuming. A chemical depilatory could be used by the patient the day before surgery if desired. The scalp is the area of the body in which the hairs can most interfere with surgery. Plastering down the hair with petrolatum or other ointment can decrease the number of hairs that interfere with surgery without causing a noticeable loss of hair during the postoperative period. Hair ties and bobby pins are invaluable items to have in the office (Figure 1.2).

Drapes

The use of sterile fenestrated aperture drapes (drapes with a hole) is recommended when suturing is performed so that the sutures do not drag over nonsterile skin (Figure 1.3). Sterile drapes are not necessary for small procedures, such as a shave biopsy, where suturing is not performed. Disposable or linen-quality sterile drapes are adequate for the procedures described in this book. You can create your own

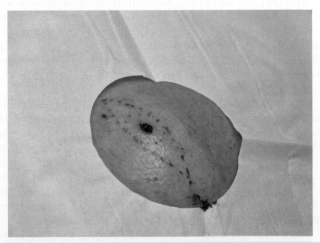

Figure 1.2 A fenestrated drape is used to produce a sterile field for the surgical removal of a basal cell carcinoma. (Copyright Richard P. Usatine, MD.)

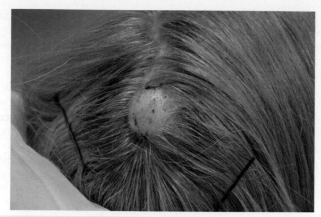

Figure 1.3 Hair on the scalp was cut short with clean scissors to make it easier to excise this ellipse over a pilar cyst. Note how the hairs surrounding the surgical site are held down with bobby pins. Petrolatum ointment can also be used to keep the surrounding hair out of the surgical field. (Copyright Richard P. Usatine, MD.)

aperture drapes by cutting a hole in a sterile disposable drape. This allows you to customize the size of the hole you need. This should be done with sterile suture scissors and not tissue scissors to avoid dulling your more expensive instruments. You can also use the paper that is used to wrap surgical trays before sterilization for this purpose to save money. Drapes can be cut in a variety of sizes with a variety of holes and then sterilized alone or as part of a packet. Some prepackaged disposable sterile drapes come with adhesive around the aperture to stabilize the drape and isolate the field.

Sterile Technique

Absolute sterile technique is not necessary for most minor skin surgical procedures. This is true not only for cryosurgery and electrosurgery but also for shave biopsies of the skin, curettage, incision and drainage, and other small surgical procedures in which the wounds are left open to heal without suturing. We no longer use sterile gloves for punch biopsies including those that are closed with sutures. Although all instruments must be sterile before use for these procedures, the clinician may use nonsterile gloves. Sterile drapes are not needed for these procedures. Of course, it is standard policy to use razor blades, scalpel blades, and needles that are disposed of at the end of the procedure.

Sterile technique is commonly used when performing surgery in which the wound will be closed, such as with suturing or staples. However, several studies have shown no difference in infection rates between the use of clean, nonsterile and sterile gloves in outpatient skin surgeries and Mohs surgery.[40-44] One study reported no difference in the prevalence of infection in cases with sterile gloves and nonsterile gloves but also reported that the use of sterile gloves was 3.5 times more expensive than nonsterile gloves.[42]

Physicians typically wear masks during procedures in the operating room. There have been some studies that masks and head coverings have not been shown to reduce the surgical site infection.[45] This includes a prospective

study of 508 laceration repairs in the emergency department where they found no difference in infection rate between cases where the physicians were wearing surgical caps and masks compared to the unmasked and uncapped group.[46] However, after the onset of the COVID-19 pandemic the use of face masks may remain a standard practice while seeing patients, regardless of whether surgery is being performed.

STERILIZATION OF INSTRUMENTS

Before sterilization, instruments must be cleaned of blood and debris. This can be done manually with a soft toothbrush, an ultrasonic cleaner, or a combination of these procedures.

A steam sterilizer (autoclave) is necessary to sterilize instruments and ensure that diseases such as viral hepatitis or HIV are not transmitted from patient to patient. Holding solutions should not be used to sterilize instruments. They are inadequate for proper sterilization and can only be used to temporarily hold or clean instruments. The instruments should be placed in sterilization bags with indicator strips to ensure the sterilization process is effective. These bags come in a variety of sizes to accommodate different instrument sets. Self-sealing bags cost a bit more than those that must be taped, but the convenience outweighs the cost.

Instruments can be packaged in sets for specific procedures such as punch biopsies, elliptical excisions, or nail surgery. Instruments can also be sterilized separately, but they need to be moved in a sterile manner onto the sterile surgical stand. It can be helpful to create surgical packs that contain a number of cotton-tipped applicators and gauze or just include these in the sets of instruments. This can save one the time of opening individually sterilized packets and can save money by allowing one to buy applicators and gauze in bulk.

Time-Out

With the encouragement of The Joint Commission (previously JCAHO, The Joint Commission on Accreditation of Healthcare Organizations), most hospitals are now mandating surgical time-outs prior to all surgery to reduce errors. This consists of identifying the patient by two forms of identification and confirming that the consent has been obtained, any required studies have been done, required equipment and required staff are present, and the surgical site has been identified prior to proceeding with the surgery. This is typically documented in writing or the electronic medical record (EMR) by the clinician or another member of the team present and prior to the start of the procedure. At any time or with any concern, any member of the team or staff may request a time-out to confirm that all is in order.

POSTOPERATIVE MANAGEMENT

Clinicians should provide patients with expectations during the immediate postoperative period including wound care and potential issues including swelling, bleeding, and pain. Postoperative pain after a dermatologic procedure is typically of low intensity and duration. Postoperative pain after most uncomplicated procedures can be adequately managed with nonnarcotic medications including acetaminophen and/or ibuprofen.[47] However, more extensive surgeries including flaps and grafts are associated with higher pain scores. In 2019, the expert panel consensus on opioid-prescribing guidelines for dermatologic procedures identified no dermatologic procedure that routinely requires more than 15 oxycodone 5-mg oral equivalents for postoperative pain.[47]

Conclusion

Outpatient skin surgery requires careful preparation to ensure the safety of the patient and medical personnel and optimal results. Strict adherence to universal precautions to prevent the transmission of contagious disease is now standard operating procedure. Brief medical evaluation by the clinician before performing procedures is recommended, and preoperative medications including antibiotic prophylaxis should be reviewed. Informed patient consent, standby medications and equipment, preparation of the operative site, sterilization of equipment, and sterile technique are all areas that require preoperative consideration. Proper preoperative planning is essential for all successful office procedures.

References

1. American Medical Association. *Informed Consent*. Accessed April 30, 2020. Available at: https://www.ama-assn.org/delivering-care/ethics/informed-consent.
2. Bunick CG, Aasi SZ. Hemorrhagic complications in dermatologic surgery. *Dermatol Ther*. 2011;24(6):537-550. doi:10.1111/j.1529-8019.2012.01454.x.
3. Dixon AJ, Dixon MP, Dixon JB. Bleeding complications in skin cancer surgery are associated with warfarin but not aspirin therapy. *Br J Surg*. 2007;94(11):1356-1360. doi:10.1002/bjs.5864.
4. Shalom A, Klein D, Friedman T, Westreich M. Lack of complications in minor skin lesion excisions in patients taking aspirin or warfarin products. *Am Surg*. 2008;74(4):354-357. Accessed April 30, 2020. Available at: https://pubmed.ncbi.nlm.nih.gov/18453305/.
5. Lewis KG, Dufresne RG. A meta-analysis of complications attributed to anticoagulation among patients following cutaneous surgery. *Dermatologic Surg*. 2008;34(2):160-165. doi:10.1111/j.1524-4725.2007.34033.x.
6. Kraft CT, Bellile E, Baker SR, Kim JC, Moyer JS. Anticoagulant complications in facial plastic and reconstructive surgery. *JAMA Facial Plast Surg*. 2015;17(2):103-107. doi:10.1001/jamafacial.2014.1147.
7. Bordeaux JS, Martires KJ, Goldberg D, Pattee SF, Fu P, Maloney ME. Prospective evaluation of dermatologic surgery complications including patients on multiple antiplatelet and anticoagulant medications. *J Am Acad Dermatol*. 2011;65(3):576-583. doi:10.1016/j.jaad.2011.02.012.
8. Sugden P, Siddiqui H. Continuing warfarin during cutaneous surgery. *Surgeon*. 2008;6(3):148-150. doi:10.1016/S1479-666X(08)80110-2.
9. Blasdale C, Lawrence CM. Perioperative international normalized ratio level is a poor predictor of postoperative bleeding complications in dermatological surgery patients taking warfarin. *Br J Dermatol*. 2008;158(3):522-526. doi:10.1111/j.1365-2133.2007.08419.x.
10. Cook-Norris RH, Michaels JD, Weaver AL, et al. Complications of cutaneous surgery in patients taking clopidogrel-containing anticoagulation. *J Am Acad Dermatol*. 2011;65(3):584-591. doi:10.1016/j.jaad.2011.02.013.
11. Kramer E, Hadad E, Westreich M, Shalom A. Lack of complications in skin surgery of patients receiving clopidogrel as compared with patients taking aspirin, warfarin, and controls. *Am Surg*.
12. Wan AY, Biro M, Scott JF. Pharmacologic and nonpharmacologic interventions for perioperative anxiety in patients undergoing Mohs micrographic surgery. *Dermatologic Surg*. 2020;46(3):299-304. doi:10.1097/DSS.0000000000002062.
13. Khalifeh MR, Redett RJ. The management of patients on anticoagulants prior to cutaneous surgery: case report of a thromboembolic complication, review of the literature, and evidence-based recommendations. *Plast Reconstr Surg*. 2006;118(5):110e-117e. doi:10.1097/01.prs.0000221114.01290.85.
14. Alam M, Goldberg LH. Serious adverse vascular events associated with perioperative interruption of antiplatelet and anticoagulant therapy. *Dermatologic Surg*. 2002;28(11):992-998. doi:10.1046/j.1524-4725.2002.02085.x.
15. Schanbacher CF, Bennett RG. Postoperative stroke after stropping warfarin for cutaneous surgery. *Dermatologic Surg*. 2000;26(8):785-789. doi:10.1046/j.1524-4725.2000.00079.x.
16. Kovich O, Otley CC. Thrombotic complications related to discontinuation of warfarin and aspirin therapy perioperatively for cutaneous operation. *J Am Acad Dermatol*. 2003;48(2):233-237. doi:10.1067/mjd.2003.47.
17. Callahan S, Goldsberry A, Kim G, Yoo S. The management of antithrombotic medication in skin surgery. *Dermatologic Surg*. 2012;38(9):1417-1426. doi:10.1111/j.1524-4725.2012.02490.x.
18. Hurst EA, Yu SS, Grekin RC, Neuhaus IM. Bleeding complications in dermatologic surgery. *Semin Cutan Med Surg*. 2007;26(4):189-195. doi:10.1016/j.sder.2008.03.002.
19. Kramer E, Hadad E, Westreich M, Shalom A. Lack of complications in skin surgery of patients receiving clopidogrel as compared with patients taking aspirin, warfarin, and controls. *Am Surg*. 2010;76(1):11-14. doi:10.1016/j.yder.2010.12.050.
20. Chang TW, Arpey CJ, Baum CL, et al. Complications with new oral anticoagulants dabigatran and rivaroxaban in cutaneous surgery. *Dermatologic Surg*. 2015;41(7):784-793. doi:10.1097/DSS.0000000000000392.
21. Rosengren H, Dixon A. Antibacterial prophylaxis in dermatologic surgery: an evidence-based review. *Am J Clin Dermatol*. 2010;11(1):35-44. doi:10.2165/11311090-000000000-00000.
22. Johnson-Jahangir H, Agrawal N. Perioperative antibiotic use in cutaneous surgery. *Dermatol Clin*. 2019;37(3):329-340. doi:10.1016/j.det.2019.03.003.
23. Wright TI, Baddour LM, Berbari EF, et al. Antibiotic prophylaxis in dermatologic surgery: advisory statement 2008. *J Am Acad Dermatol*. 2008;59(3):464-473. doi:10.1016/j.jaad.2008.04.031.
24. Rogers HD, Desciak EB, Marcus RP, Wang S, MacKay-Wiggan J, Eliezri YD. Prospective study of wound infections in Mohs micrographic surgery using clean surgical technique in the absence of prophylactic antibiotics. *J Am Acad Dermatol*. 2010;63(5):842-851. doi:10.1016/j.jaad.2010.07.029.
25. Maragh SLH, Brown MD. Prospective evaluation of surgical site infection rate among patients with Mohs micrographic surgery without the use of prophylactic antibiotics. *J Am Acad Dermatol*. 2008;59(2):275-278. doi:10.1016/j.jaad.2008.03.042.
26. Martin ET, Kaye KS, Knott C, et al. Diabetes and risk of surgical site infection: a systematic review and meta-analysis. *Infect Control Hosp Epidemiol*. 2016;37(1):88-99. doi:10.1017/ice.2015.249.
27. Saco M, Howe N, Nathoo R, Cherpelis B. Topical antibiotic prophylaxis for prevention of surgical wound infections from dermatologic procedures: a systematic review and meta-analysis. *J Dermatolog Treat*. 2015;26(2):151-158. doi:10.3109/09546634.2014.906547.
28. Levender MM, Davis SA, Kwatra SG, Williford PM, Feldman SR. Use of topical antibiotics as prophylaxis in clean dermatologic procedures. *J Am Acad Dermatol*. 2012;66(3):P445-P451.e3. doi:10.1016/j.jaad.2011.02.005.
29. Wilson W, Taubert KA, Gewitz M, et al. Prevention of infective endocarditis: guidelines from the American Heart Association: a guideline from the American Heart Association Rheumatic Fever, Endocarditis and Kawasaki Disease Committee, Council on Cardiovascular Disease in the Young, and the Council on Clinical Cardiology, Council on Cardiovascular Surgery and Anesthesia, and the Quality of Care and Outcomes Research Interdisciplinary Working Group. *J Am Dent Assoc*. 2008;139(suppl 1S):3S-24S. doi:10.1161/CIRCULATIONAHA.106.183095.

30. Moorhead C, Torres A. I prevent bacterial resistance. An update on the use of antibiotics in dermatologic surgery. *Dermatologic Surg.* 2009;35(10):1532-1538. doi:10.1111/j.1524-4725.2009.01269.x.

31. Kühlmann AYR, de Rooij A, Kroese LF, van Dijk M, Hunink MGM, Jeekel J. Meta-analysis evaluating music interventions for anxiety and pain in surgery. *Br J Surg.* 2018;105(7):773-783. doi:10.1002/bjs.10853.

32. Vachiramon V, Sobanko JF, Rattanaumpawan P, Miller CJ. Music reduces patient anxiety during Mohs surgery: an open-label randomized controlled trial. *Dermatologic Surg.* 2013;39(2):298-305. doi:10.1111/dsu.12047.

33. Ravitskiy L, Phillips PK, Roenigk RK, et al. The use of oral midazolam for perioperative anxiolysis of healthy patients undergoing Mohs surgery: conclusions from randomized controlled and prospective studies. *J Am Acad Dermatol.* 2011;64(2):310-322. doi:10.1016/j.jaad.2010.02.038.

34. Guo D, Kossintseva I. Periprocedural anxiolytic agents in dermatologic surgery: quantitative experience and systematic literature review of the effective differences. *J Am Acad Dermatol.* 2017;76(6):AB195. doi:10.1016/j.jaad.2017.04.760.

35. Lee MP, Zullo SW, Sobanko JF, Etzkorn JR. Patient-centered care in dermatologic surgery: practical strategies to improve the patient experience and visit satisfaction. *Dermatol Clin.* 2019;37(3):367-374. doi:10.1016/j.det.2019.03.006.

36. Darouiche RO, Wall MJ Jr, Itani KM, et al. Chlorhexidine-alcohol versus povidone-iodine for surgical-site antisepsis. *N Engl J Med.* 2010;362(1):18-26. doi:10.1056/NEJMoa0810988.

37. *Evidence Review for the Effectiveness of Skin Antiseptics in the Prevention of Surgical Site Infection: Surgical Site Infections: Prevention And Treatment: Evidence Review B.* National Institute for Health and Care Excellence (NICE); 2019. (NICE Guideline, No. 125.) https://www.ncbi.nlm.nih.gov/books/NBK569835/, 2019. [Accessed January 5, 2023].

38. Collins LK, Knackstedt TJ, Samie FH. Antiseptic use in Mohs and reconstructive surgery: an American College of Mohs Surgery member survey. *Dermatol Surg.* 2015;41:164-166.

39. Tanner J, Woodings D, Moncaster K, eds. Preoperative hair removal to reduce surgical site infection. In: *Cochrane Database of Systematic Reviews.* John Wiley & Sons, Ltd; 2006. doi:10.1002/14651858.cd004122.pub2.

40. Heal C, Sriharan S, Buttner PG, Kimber D. Comparing non-sterile with sterile gloves for minor surgery: a prospective randomised controlled non-inferiority trial. *Med J Aust.* 2015;202(1):27-32. doi:10.5694/mja14.00314.

41. Brewer JD, Gonzalez AB, Baum CL, et al. Comparison of sterile vs nonsterile gloves in cutaneous surgery and common outpatient dental procedures a systematic review and meta-analysis. *JAMA Dermatology.* 2016;152(9):1008-1014. doi:10.1001/jamadermatol.2016.1965.

42. Mehta D, Chambers N, Adams B, Gloster H. Comparison of the prevalence of surgical site infection with use of sterile versus nonsterile gloves for resection and reconstruction during Mohs surgery. *Dermatologic Surg.* 2014;40(3):234-239. doi:10.1111/dsu.12438.

43. Xia Y, Cho S, Greenway HT, Zelac DE, Kelley B. Infection rates of wound repairs during Mohs micrographic surgery using sterile versus nonsterile gloves: a prospective randomized pilot study. *Dermatologic Surg.* 2011;37(5):651-656. doi:10.1111/j.1524-4725.2011.01949.x.

44. Rhinehart BM, Murphy ME, Farley MF, Albertini JG. Sterile versus nonsterile gloves during Mohs micrographic surgery: infection rate is not affected. *Dermatologic Surg.* 2006;32(2):170-176. doi:10.1111/j.1524-4725.2006.32031.x.

45. Eisen DB. Surgeon's garb and infection control: what's the evidence? *J Am Acad Dermatol.* 2011;64(5):960.e1-e20. doi:10.1016/j.jaad.2010.04.037.

46. Ruthman JC, Hendricksen D, Miller RF, Quigg DL. Effect of cap and mask on infection rates in wounds sutured in the emergency department. *IMJ Ill Med J.* 1984;165(6):397-399. https://pubmed.ncbi.nlm.nih.gov/6146589/. Accessed May 13, 2020.

47. McLawhorn JM, Stephany MP, Bruhn WE, et al. An expert panel consensus on opioid-prescribing guidelines for dermatologic procedures. *J Am Acad Dermatol.* 2020;82(3):700-708. doi:10.1016/j.jaad.2019.09.080.

2 Setting Up Your Office

RICHARD P. USATINE, MD, and MARION BELK, MD

FACILITIES, INSTRUMENTS, AND EQUIPMENT

SUMMARY	
	■ The goal of this chapter is to help you set up your office for doing dermatologic procedures.
	■ Tips for adequate lighting and procedure chairs are provided.
	■ Other equipment reviewed includes floor lamps, stools, and Mayo stands.
	■ Hand instruments are reviewed in detail.
	■ Pointers are provided on injectable medications and chemicals that are most useful for dermatologic procedures.
	■ Cryosurgical and electrosurgical equipment are discussed.

When planning your office environment keep in mind the principle of setting yourself up for success. This means that you must stock your office with the equipment you will need to perform your procedures in a timely fashion with expertise and minimal complications. After receiving the proper training this will require researching the needed equipment as well as thoughtful placement of such in your office. It is advisable to purchase the best equipment you can afford in the beginning; equipment made in Germany, the United Kingdom, or the United States can be expected to function properly and remain sharp for the life of the instrument. An old saying is, "buy once, cry once."

It isn't necessary to purchase new equipment, however, as used medical supply stores abound in larger cities. An excellent way to find a reliable used medical equipment store is by simply asking other physicians in the area. Chances are they will be able to direct you to such a business. Another outstanding way to stock your office is to locate a physician who is retiring who will be happy to help you get started and will sell you his or her equipment for literally pennies on the dollar. A plethora of used medical equipment can be found by a simple Google search, and of course eBay will have everything you could wish for, but the reliability of such vendors could be questionable. The retiring physician option and the used equipment store carry the advantage of your being able to see and test the equipment prior to purchase, which justifies a slightly higher price. Remember also that starting out you do not want to over-purchase. It is fine to start small and grow your instrumentation as your practice grows.

A successful operating suite will have adequate lighting, a procedure chair that is adjustable in height and position, and high-quality surgical equipment. In this chapter, we will share what equipment we have found useful for success and how to save time and money while setting up your office.

Lighting

Simple surgical procedures can be performed in almost any office if the lighting is adequate. Standard office lighting is often too dim to allow proper visualization of the operative field. When setting up a new facility, consider doubling the number of light fixtures to improve illumination. For many clinicians, this will provide adequate lighting for performing simple surgical procedures.

Headlamps can also be used as an adjunct in the operative area. When used in conjunction with loupes, headlamps are valuable when performing finely detailed procedures. Often a good headlamp with magnification can be obtained at a hobby/crafts store for significantly less money than a medical supply company, and the quality is comparable. A phone light, otoscope, or dermatoscope can be helpful to illuminate a specific area during an exam.

SURGICAL LAMPS

Adequate lighting is paramount and is best achieved by using surgical lamps that are either ceiling mounted or on a rolling base. Great surgical lights can be purchased with LED bulbs for better energy efficiency and bright light with little heat. If you have a main procedure room, look into installing a ceiling-mounted lamp. A tall maneuverable floor lamp may be adequate and work well in your other exam rooms.

FLOOR LAMPS

You should have at least one good-quality movable floor lamp for your exam rooms. One per room is optimal but one good movable lamp is a good start. Look for a lamp that provides excellent illumination, ease of movement, and stability. The Burton Nova Exam® LED exam light (Figure 2.1) is one floor lamp that works well for us, but other floor lamps are available that provide similar features. The LED light

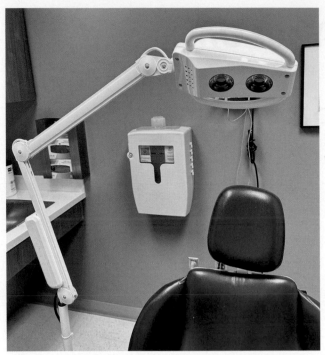

Figure 2.1 Nova LED lamp. Great lamp with two settings for procedures. (Copyright Richard P. Usatine, MD.)

source produces a cool light that enhances physician/patient comfort while delivering a uniform beam pattern and two possible illumination levels. The K-arm moves smoothly with no drifting for easy and reliable positioning.

WOOD'S LAMP

The Wood's lamp is an ultraviolet light that is useful for diagnosing or evaluating:

- Fungal infections including Microsporum canis and Malassezia furfur
- Vitiligo
- Erythrasma
- Melasma
- Lentigo maligna melanoma

There are many types, from those that are built in a unit with an accompanying magnifying lens to simpler, less expensive options. It is also helpful for identifying the coral red fluorescence of erythrasma. It can be used for accentuating the hypopigmentation of vitiligo. In melasma, it is used to see if the hyperpigmentation is within the epidermal or dermal layer. Melanin appears dark when in the epidermal layer but not in the dermal layer.[1] The Wood's lamp can be used to see the full extent of a lentigo maligna melanoma before biopsy or treatment.[1,2]

Surgical Table, Stools, and Mayo Stands

It is essential to have at least one good surgical table with a height adjustment. The best tables have preset positions that move the table to the optimal height for your work. Also, make sure that you find a table that allows the back and foot adjustments to move simultaneously as well as independently. If not, it can take a long time to get the patient in the proper position for procedures. It may also help to have a table that spins on a center axis for positioning the patient at the best angle in the room. Make sure that the table has stirrups. Even if you do not do gynecologic exams, stirrups can be helpful for skin procedures performed in the inguinal or genital area.

Individual preferences will determine if a clinician performs most procedures while sitting or standing. It is best to avoid bending over the surgical table for the health of your back and neck. It helps to adjust your table and stool for good body ergonomics. An easily adjustable pneumatic stool is advantageous. Ideally, the stool has foot-actuated controls that allow you to change the height while you are scrubbed in. Otherwise, a large hand control for the height adjustment is better than a small one.

Each room should have a Mayo stand to hold surgical instruments during surgery. Make sure these stands are stable and that the height can be adjusted.

Hand Instruments

Small surgical instruments can be categorized by their purpose in surgery, such as the following.

- *Cutting:* scalpels, razor blades, scissors, punches, curettes
- *Tissue holding:* forceps, skin hooks
- *Undermining:* scissors
- *Hemostasis:* hemostats or mosquitos
- *Suturing and wound closure:* needle holders, scissors, staplers

Instruments used to perform excisions include scalpel handles with blades, forceps, skin hooks, hemostats, scissors, and a needle holder. High-quality instruments that will last and perform well during surgical procedures should be purchased. A high-quality needle holder is important because a poorly manufactured one will not hold needles properly. The best surgical instruments are often made in Germany, England, and the United States. Some of the less expensive surgical instruments are manufactured in Pakistan, and the quality is comparable to the cost. Poorly made disposable hand instruments should be avoided.

CUTTING

Scalpels

A scalpel has two parts, the handle and blade. The four most useful blades (Figure 2.2) for skin surgery are given as follows.

- *No. 15 blade:* most commonly used blade for skin surgery
- *No. 15C blade:* shorter and thinner blade with a finer point than the traditional No. 15 blade. It is useful for fine plastics work on the face but is not needed in most offices
- *No. 11 blade:* sharply pointed with a cutting blade on both sides, making it useful for incision and drainage of an abscess or cyst
- *No. 10 blade:* larger than a No. 15 blade with the same shape. It is useful for doing a shave biopsy of a large lesion or for cutting a thick callus on the foot. Some surgeons prefer it for large skin excisions on the back because the skin is so thick in this location.

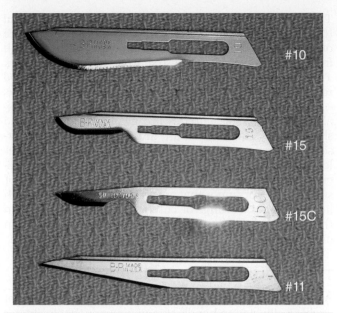

Figure 2.2 Scalpel blades used in skin surgery. (Copyright Richard P. Usatine, MD.)

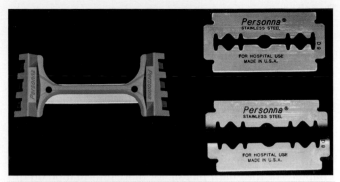

Figure 2.3 Razor blades for shave biopsies. The DermaBlade is the blue-handled blade to the left. The Personna double-edge blade is on the right. It needs to be broken in half, as seen on the bottom right, to be used as a single-edge blade for a shave biopsy. (Copyright Richard P. Usatine, MD.)

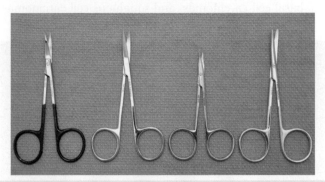

Figure 2.4 Assorted scissors for skin surgery: SuperCut iris scissor, gold-handled iris scissor, Gradle scissor, and a tissue undermining scissor. (Copyright Richard P. Usatine, MD.)

Blades are disposable and can be purchased separately or preattached to disposable plastic handles. The advantage of a totally disposable scalpel is that it eliminates the risk of being cut while attaching or removing a disposable blade from a nondisposable metal handle. The risk of being cut is low with good dexterity and experience. A needle holder or hemostat is helpful when placing a blade on the handle or taking it off. Blade-removal instruments can also be purchased. Although disposable scalpels are convenient, they are not as stable or as sharp as a metal scalpel handle with a disposable blade. For elliptical excisions and flaps, we prefer the sharp blades on a nondisposable metal handle. Consider buying metal scalpel handles that come with a ruler marking for measuring the size of your surgical incisions.

Personna Plus Microcoat blades are particularly sharp Teflon-coated blades. However, sharp disposable blades are also available from Bard-Parker, Cincinnati Surgical, and Swann-Morton. It may be worthwhile to try out more than one type to determine which one meets your personal needs and budget.

Razor Blades

We prefer razor blades rather than scalpels for most of our shave biopsies (Figure 2.3). The DermaBlade is a sharp Personna razor blade in an easy-to-use blue plastic handle. It is safe to handle for both the novice and the expert. A less expensive alternative is the Personna super double-edge blade that can be broken in half for use. Although these do not come in sterile packaging, they can be used for shave biopsies without putting them through the autoclave. At pennies a blade, these are the least expensive tool for shave biopsies but carry a higher risk of cutting yourself while breaking them in half and performing the shave biopsy. They can be broken in half within their paper container to avoid cutting your hand prior to use.

Scissors

Figure 2.4 shows different types of scissors used in skin surgery. The most versatile and affordable scissor for snip

excisions and cutting the base of a punch biopsy is the iris scissor, a small, sharp-tipped scissor that may be straight or curved. Use of the straight or curved iris is a matter of personal preference. The curved scissor is somewhat more expensive and may become dull more quickly than the flat scissor. Scissor length varies from 3 to 5 inches. The iris scissor can be used for suture removal and cutting sutures, but the ones used for this purpose should be kept separate from tissue-cutting scissors to avoid dulling your best surgical scissors. The iris scissor can also be used for blunt dissection and undermining. Scissors need periodic sharpening, but properly cleaned and treated instruments will generally last a long time and are worth the investment.

Gradle scissors have very small blades for fine cutting and undermining. These scissors can be invaluable with a punch biopsy of the nail matrix in which the tissue is friable and would be easy to crush if a less fine pair of scissors were used. Gradle scissors are more expensive than standard iris scissors.

Many companies make specific undermining scissors with sharp or blunt tips and sharp blades. Some of these are tenotomy scissors or Metzenbaum scissors. These could be used instead of the all-purpose iris scissor. New technologies are being used to make the blades of scissors sharper. For a premium price you can now buy scissors that are as sharp as a scalpel (e.g., SuperCut scissors). Endarterectomy scissors, which have a longer handle with blunt tips, also provide excellent control and precision for delicate work, but at a somewhat higher price.[3]

Punches

Punches come in sizes ranging from 2 to 10 mm. Clinicians may choose between disposable, one-use punches and reusable steel punches. Disposable punches are presterilized and need no maintenance (Figure 2.5). Reusable punches require cleaning and sterilization between procedures and must be sharpened periodically. We use disposable punches only because they are always sharp and convenient.

Although a wide range of punch instruments are produced by many manufacturers from 2 to 10 mm, the most useful punch biopsy instruments range from 3 to 6 mm. See Chapter 10, *The Punch Biopsy*, for more information on this surgical tool.

Curettes

Dermal curettes (Figure 2.6) are useful for treating pyogenic granulomas, molluscum contagiosum, seborrheic keratoses, basal cell carcinomas, and squamous cell carcinomas.

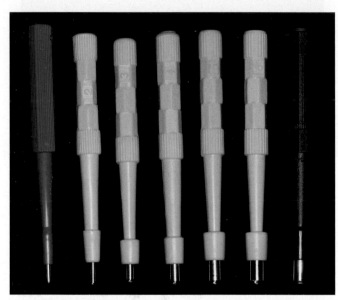

Figure 2.5 Assortment of punch types from 2 mm at the left to 6 mm at the right. (Copyright Richard P. Usatine, MD.)

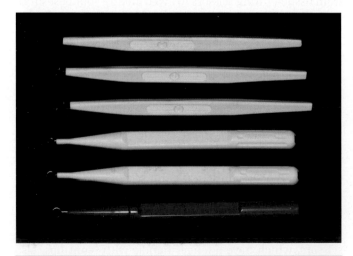

Figure 2.6 Skin curettes ranging from 3 mm to 7 mm. (Copyright Richard P. Usatine, MD.)

The head of the curette may be round (Fox curette) or oval (Piffard curette). One side of the curette head is dull. The other side has a sharp blade that is designed to cut through friable or soft tissue but is not so sharp as to cut normal skin. This allows the curette to distinguish between abnormal and normal tissue and to selectively remove the abnormal tissue.

Skin curettes range in size from 2 to 7 mm. Nondisposable and disposable curettes are available. The size and shape of the curette used are in part determined by personal preference. Larger curettes allow for removal of larger lesions with fewer strokes. Smaller curettes are more precise and can be used on smaller lesions and for curettage of small pockets of tumor that are more difficult to reach with larger curettes. A range of curettes should be available in the office. We keep 3-, 5-, and 7-mm disposable curettes in our offices and find that this covers our needs (Figure 2.6).

TISSUE HOLDING

A large variety of forceps and skin hooks are available that enable a clinician to handle skin in a means that facilitates cutting, undermining, and suturing. The goal of tissue holding is to provide the most stability during these procedures while minimizing skin trauma and scarring.

Forceps

Basic types of forceps include tissue forceps, dressing forceps, and splinter forceps. To aid in removing splinters, splinter forceps have sharp tips and no teeth. Dressing and tissue forceps are available with and without teeth. Opinions vary about the value of teeth on forceps. Some clinicians believe that they can handle skin more atraumatically when forceps have teeth, whereas others believe there is less tissue trauma without teeth. This is an issue that may be determined by personal preference.

The most used type of forceps in skin surgery is the Adson forceps, which has a broad handle and a long narrow tip (Figure 2.7). One common configuration is one tooth on one tip fitting into two teeth on the other tip. Many variations of this configuration exist. We suggest that you start with the basic 4¾-inch Adson forceps, with and without teeth, and experiment with others as needed. We prefer the teeth for suturing and the forceps without teeth when lifting a punch specimen up to cut the base. Adson forceps without teeth may tend to crush healthy tissue if one is applying a strong force to hold skin under tension.

The use of good-quality forceps with small teeth and accurate apposition is important. This allows you to pass the suture needle back and forth between the forceps and needle holder without touching the needle with your fingers, thereby decreasing your risks for a needlestick. Most disposable forceps do not hold suture needles well.

Skin Hooks

Skin hooks are capable of holding tissue in the least traumatic manner. They are better than forceps for reflecting skin while undermining without crushing skin edges. Skin hooks are especially useful for holding skin while undermining and while placing deep sutures. Skin hooks are available with single- or double-pronged hooks and with sharp or blunt prongs (Figure 2.8). Single, sharp-pronged hooks are the most versatile type of skin hook. The double-pronged

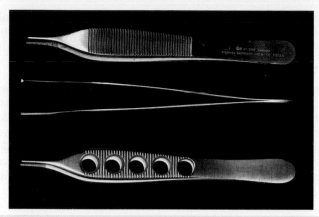
Figure 2.7 Adson forceps without teeth on top, microfine teeth in middle, and without teeth and with fenestrated handle on bottom. (Copyright Richard P. Usatine, MD.)

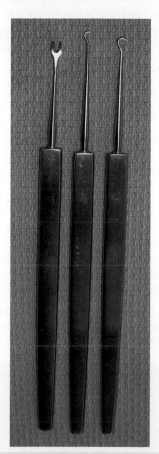
Figure 2.8 Different types of skin hooks that are used to hold up skin atraumatically while providing visualization for undermining tissue. (Copyright Richard P. Usatine, MD.)

skin hook can be useful in retracting the proximal nail fold and in office gynecologic surgery.

Skin hooks may be used for many of the same purposes as forceps and for additional procedures such as the following:

- Holding a wound edge while undermining the skin
- Retracting a skin edge to expose bleeding sites and to obtain hemostasis
- Pulling together the edges of an ellipse to see if there was sufficient undermining to allow for closure

- Moving a flap into place while placing the key suture
- Determining the degree of skin redundancy while treating dog ears (standing cones)
- Holding traction on the corners of an ellipse while placing sutures or staples

UNDERMINING

The skin may be undermined with any type of sharp tissue scissor. Blunt dissection will cause less trauma to the tissue and less bleeding by displacing vessels and nerves rather than cutting through them. Undermining with a scalpel is more likely to cut vessels and nerves but can be performed more rapidly. A sharp iris scissor is a good affordable choice for blunt dissection and cutting tissue while undermining. Other options include tenotomy scissors, Gradle scissors, Metzenbaum scissors, endarterectomy scissors, and specific undermining scissors (Figure 2.5).

Hemostasis

Hemostats are useful to clamp bleeding vessels selected for electrocoagulation or ligation. Hemostats may also be used to break up loculations after opening an abscess or for blunt dissection around cysts and lipomas. Hemostats may be curved or straight and are useful for clamping and tying bleeding vessels and tissue (Figure 2.9). These come in sizes between 3.5 and 5 inches. Larger hemostats are known as Kelly clamps, and smaller hemostats are called mosquitos. Personal preference determines the size and shape used. Curved hemostats are particularly useful for blunt dissection around subcutaneous masses and for reaching inside an abscess to break up loculations. Straight heavy-duty hemostats can be useful in partial and full toenail removal surgeries.

WOUND CLOSURE

Needle Holders

Needle holders for skin surgery should be relatively short because the suturing is not being done in a deep cavity.

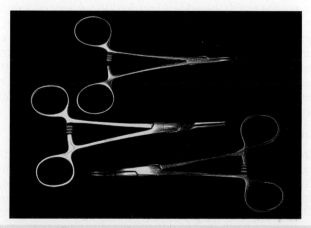
Figure 2.9 Different types of hemostats used for hemostasis, incision and drainage, and nail surgery. The Mosquito hemostat (*top*) is small, with a curved end; the straight Crile hemostat is at center. The bottom one is a curved hemostat larger than a mosquito. (Copyright Richard P. Usatine, MD.)

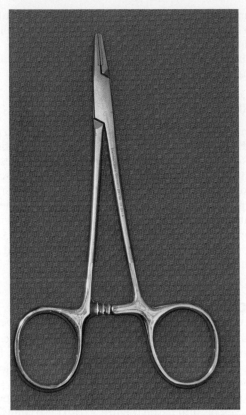

Figure 2.10 High-quality needle holder with gold-plated finger rings and tungsten carbide inserts for stable needle holding. (Copyright Richard P. Usatine, MD.)

A short handle allows for more precise needle handling. Smooth rather than serrated jaws are less likely to fray sutures while doing instrument ties. The Webster needle holder with smooth jaws is commonly used in skin surgery and is available in 4¾- and 5-inch sizes. Larger and heavier needle holders may be helpful when suturing tougher, thicker skin (e.g., on the back). Small, fine-needle holders are useful for fine work on the face and other delicate areas. It is important to have good-quality needle holders. Needle holders with gold-plated finger rings and tungsten carbide inserts are worth the price if you do skin surgery on a regular basis (Figure 2.10). The gold-plated handle is often a sign that the needle holder is of excellent quality, but this is not always true. The tungsten carbide insert does improve needle holding by limiting either twisting or rotation of the clamped needle. In addition, compression of sutures by these needle holders does not reduce suture breaking strength.[4]

Suture-Cutting Scissors

Virtually any type of scissor may be used to cut sutures during surgery or remove sutures after some wound healing has occurred. There may be an advantage to using a designated pair of scissors for suture cutting because tissue-cutting scissors will become dull if often used to cut sutures. Iris scissors work well to cut sutures during surgery or to remove sutures postoperatively. These fine, sharp-tipped scissors can easily go under the suture to cut it for removal. Special suture-removal scissors have a hook on the end of one blade that is designed to slip under the suture and cut it

without traumatizing the underlying skin. Examples of suture-cutting scissors include the Spencer, Shortbent, and Littauer stitch scissors.

Staplers

Staples are more expensive for wound closure than sutures and are generally not used in cosmetically sensitive areas. Staples are best applied to long incisions on the scalp, trunk, or extremities. In these areas, wounds can be closed more rapidly with staples than sutures. Staplers may be reusable or disposable. Reusable staplers are autoclavable and are used with sterile staple cartridges. This is not an essential item for the office.

SMALL INSTRUMENT SETS

To save time and expense, it helps to establish standard instrument sets for use in the office. Suggested sets for different surgical needs include the following:

Punch or Small Excision Set (Figure 2.11)

- Iris scissors
- Adson forceps (with and without teeth)
- Webster needle holder (smooth)
- Cotton-tipped applicators (CTAs) and gauze (may be added before autoclaving)

Ellipse or Large Excision Set (Figure 2.12)

- Blade handle
- Two hemostats
- Adson forceps (with and without teeth)
- Two skin hooks (single, sharp prong) (optional)
- Webster needle holder
- Iris scissors (or another scissor for undermining)
- Designated suture scissors (optional)
- Metal basin (optional, used for cleaning and irrigating with sterile saline)
- CTAs and gauze (may be added before autoclaving)

Adding clean CTAs and clean cotton gauze (purchased in bulk packs) to be autoclaved in surgical sets is an efficient way to prepare for surgery and save money. This saves setup

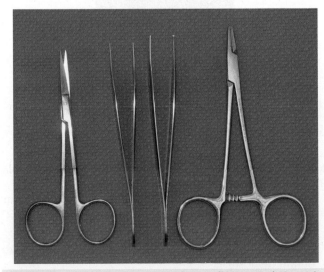

Figure 2.11 Instruments to be used with a punch biopsy tool. (Copyright Richard P. Usatine, MD.)

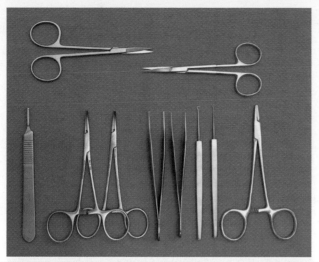

Figure 2.12 Elliptical excision set. (Copyright Richard P. Usatine, MD.)

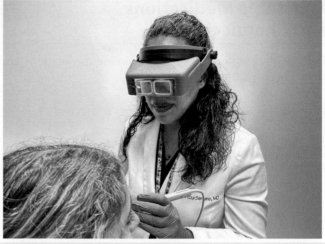

Figure 2.13 OptiVISOR loop providing 2× magnification and some eye protection. (Copyright Richard P. Usatine, MD.)

time and money over individually packaged sterile gauze and CTAs. It also avoids wasting of the paper that covers individually wrapped sterile gauze and CTAs, making for a greener office.

Information on nail surgery equipment is found in Chapter 17, *Nail Procedures*.

SURGICAL SKIN MARKERS

It is extremely helpful to draw lines where you intend to cut. This is true for all types of biopsies and excisions and not just for large ellipses and flaps. It is best to mark the skin before administering anesthesia because the anesthesia may distort the lesion or make it less visible.

A number of various types of surgical markers are available. A fine-point marker is most useful. The standard markers use gentian violet and do not tattoo the skin. Preoperative prepping with alcohol may rub off the gentian violet, but povidone-iodine and chlorhexidine will not. For biopsies, the alcohol prep should be applied gently to avoid rubbing off the markings.

Surgical markers can be purchased in sterile packages for single use in a sterile procedure, but this is rarely needed since the marking is usually done before injecting the local anesthetic and prepping the area for cutting. A sterile marker is more costly than a nonsterile marker. A surgical marker can be used over again as long as it has not touched body fluids.

Magnification Devices

It is helpful to have at least one device available to magnify lesions. A wide range of magnifying lenses are available, from inexpensive handheld magnifying lenses to expensive binocular loupes. Good-quality magnification with good lighting will allow the clinician to see small features, such as telangiectasias, that may not be visible to the naked eye. Keeping a small magnifying glass in your office or pocket is a great way to start. A small handheld lighted magnifying loupe (5× to 10×) is a compact and inexpensive option available in most hobby or electronic stores.

The advantage of loupes that are mounted to eyeglasses or a headband is that the clinician is able to use both hands in a procedure while getting the benefit of magnification. Magnification levels range from 1.5× to 6×. Two times magnification should be sufficient for most skin lesion diagnoses and procedures and provides a comfortable working distance from the lesion in focus (about 10 inches). The OptiVISOR is a good starting device, and various clip-on lights can be added to this product (Figure 2.13). Customized binocular loupes are expensive, high-quality optical instruments that are used by oral surgeons and in the operating room.

DERMATOSCOPE

If you plan to purchase only one instrument to improve dermatologic diagnosis, make it the dermatoscope and take at least one course to learn how to use it. This will save your patients countless biopsies and will help you as the clinician to detect melanoma and other skin cancers at an earlier stage.[5,6] Without a doubt you will be a better physician, and your patients will benefit if you perform dermoscopy in your office. See Chapters 18 and 19 for further information.

Personal Protective Equipment

Since the COVID-19 pandemic we are all very cognizant of the importance of personal protective equipment (PPE). To be protected from blood and fluids during surgery, clinicians must wear surgical gloves and eye protection. Surgical masks and eye protection are especially important for surgeries on known high-risk individuals or for surgeries in which the risk of exposure to blood or fluid is greatest. Although eyeglasses offer some protection, a face shield provides the best coverage. In our office, it seems that the number of postoperative skin infections has gone down since we all started wearing face masks during surgery. Faceshields are very important to protect the eyes and mouth from squirting cysts and body fluids. Nonsterile surgical gowns can be quite useful for keeping the clothing clean.

Injectable Medications and Chemicals

Medical offices should keep the following medications and chemicals on hand:

ANESTHETICS (SEE CHAPTER 3)

- Lidocaine with epinephrine (1%)
- Lidocaine without epinephrine (1% or 2%)
- Lidocaine/prilocaine cream and other topical anesthetics as needed

CHEMICALS (FIGURE 2.14)

- Aluminum chloride (70% in water for hemostasis) (see Chapter 4, *Hemostasis*)
- Trichloroacetic acid (TCA) (see Chapter 17, *Nail Procedures*) (We have moved from phenol to 90% TCA to destroy the matrix in ingrown nail surgeries.)
- Fungal stain (chlorazol black) helps with doing KOH preps looking for fungal infections.

INJECTABLES (FIGURE 2.15)

- 8.4% Bicarbonate (for buffering lidocaine) (see Chapter 3, *Anesthesia*)
- Sterile saline (for diluting injectable triamcinolone)
- Triamcinolone for injection (Kenalog), 10 and 40 mg/mL (see Chapter 15, *Intralesional Injections*)

Equipment

CRYOTHERAPY EQUIPMENT

Cryotherapy equipment for liquid nitrogen includes the following:

- Storage tank (Dewar) with a device to dispense the liquid nitrogen (Figure 2.16)

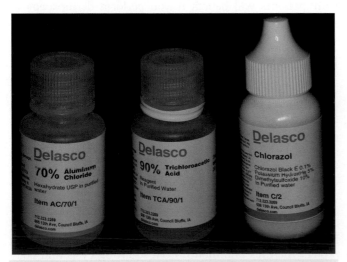

Figure 2.14 Useful chemicals to have in the office: aluminum chloride, trichloroacetic acid, and a fungal stain. (Copyright Richard P. Usatine, MD.)

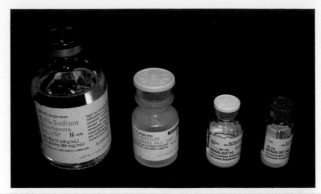

Figure 2.15 Injectables: bicarbonate, sterile saline, and triamcinolone. (Copyright Richard P. Usatine, MD.)

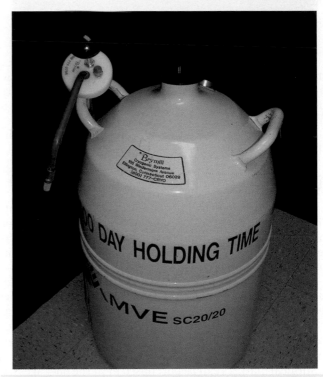

Figure 2.16 Storage tank (Dewar) with method to remove liquid nitrogen. (Copyright Richard P. Usatine, MD.)

- Cryogun (Figure 2.17)
- Cryo tweezers (Figure 2.18) are great for easy treatment of skin tags, especially those around the eyelids

Although this equipment can cost from $1000 to $1500, it will pay for itself many times over and allow you to treat actinic keratoses, warts, condyloma, seborrheic keratoses, and other benign lesions. While most offices will sign a monthly on-site service contract for liquid nitrogen delivery, it is possible to pick up the liquid nitrogen off-site for a significant saving. Just be sure to specify that you need medical-grade liquid nitrogen. See Chapter 14, *Cryosurgery*, for more tips on equipment.

ELECTROSURGERY EQUIPMENT

Having at least one electrosurgical instrument is essential before performing skin surgery (see Chapter 13, *Electrosurgery*).

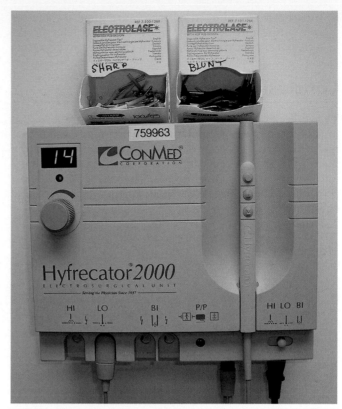

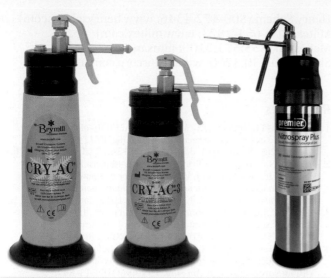

Figure 2.17 Cryoguns for cryosurgery. (Copyright Richard P. Usatine, MD.)

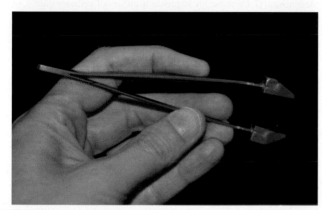

Figure 2.18 Cryo tweezer for skin tags and pedunculated warts. (Copyright Richard P. Usatine, MD.)

Figure 2.19 Electrosurgical instrument mounted on the wall. (Copyright Richard P. Usatine, MD.)

While the bleeding of shave biopsies can usually be stopped with chemicals, deeper excisions will often require electrocoagulation to obtain adequate hemostasis. This instrument will pay for itself with electrodesiccation and curettage (ED&C) of skin cancers and the destruction of lesions such as sebaceous hyperplasia and dermatosis papulosis nigra (benign lesions usually considered cosmetic and a cash-pay option for patients).

One only needs an electrosurgical unit that is capable of electrocoagulation and ED&C, not a cutting device. These can be obtained for about $1000 new (significantly less if used). If placed on wheels it can be easily moved from one exam room to another. The next step up is to have multiple units of this type mounted in each exam room (Figure 2.19). For many thousands of dollars an electrosurgical unit with cutting capability can be purchased. A smoke evacuator is especially important (and will be much appreciated by other staff members) if a cutting unit is used because cutting produces more smoke (plume). Most dermatologists do not purchase cutting units or smoke evacuators and do their cutting with scalpels and blades.

Electrosurgery Without Cutting (Essential)

- Conmed® Hyfrecator® 2000 (https://www.conmed.com/en/products/patient-care/office-based-electrosurgery/electrosurgical-unit/the-hyfrecator-2000-electrosurgical-system)
- Bovie Derm 942 (https://shop.symmetrysurgical.com/en/product/portfolios-electrosurgery-generators/A942)

AUTOCLAVE

Without an autoclave your office will grind to a halt unless you have chosen to use only disposable instruments. An adequate autoclave will cost around $2500 new but as above, there are multiple sources for used equipment that will allow you to purchase one for less. If you opt for a used autoclave, be sure to evaluate it prior to purchase: run it through at least one cycle. You will need trays for the autoclave as well as sterilization pouches for the instruments, which can be obtained through any medical supply company.

What to Have in Each Exam Room

- Alcohol wipes, nonsterile 4 × 4 gauze, tape, gloves, slides, adhesive bandages, cotton-tip applicators, petrolatum
- Small, easy-to-access portable plastic drawers to keep the above items in one place. Well-stocked built-in cabinets are an acceptable alternative.
- Mayo stand

■ Inexpensive hand mirrors, which are great to have for communication with patients before and after procedures. If the mirror disappears, it can be easily replaced.

Conclusion

To achieve excellence in skin surgeries and procedures it is important to have the appropriate instruments and equipment for these procedures. Good instruments and equipment that are well maintained will facilitate the diagnosis and treatment of skin disorders. The resource list below provides some sources for instruments, supplies, and equipment.

Resources

Acuderm (800-327-0015; www.acuderm.com)

Delasco Dermatologic Buying Guide, a comprehensive selection of dermatologic supplies and equipment (833-907-1791; www.delasco.com)

Ethicon (www.ethicon.com)

George Tiemann & Co. (www.georgetiemann.com)

Henry Schein (800-472-4346; www.henryschein.com)

Miltex (800-654-2873; www.miltex.com)

McKesson (855.571.2100; mms.mckesson.com/)

Sklar (610.430.3200; www.sklarcorp.com/)

References

1. Paraskevas LR, Halpern AC, Marghoob AA. Utility of the Wood's light: five cases from a pigmented lesion clinic. *Br J Dermatol*. 2005;152(5):1039-1044. doi:10.1111/j.1365-2133.2005.06346.x.
2. Navarro-Navarro I, Ortiz-Prieto A, Villegas-Romero I, Valenzuela-Ubiña S, Linares-Barrios M. Wood's lamp for delineating surgical margins in lentigo maligna and lentigo maligna melanoma. *Actas Dermosifiliogr*. 2022;113:642-645. doi:10.1016/j.ad.2021.06.011.
3. Kannler C, Jellinek N, Maloney ME. Surgical pearl: the use of endarterectomy scissors in dermatologic surgery. *J Am Acad Dermatol*. 2005;53(5):873-874. doi:10.1016/j.jaad.2005.06.047.
4. Abidin MR, Dunlapp JA, Towler MA, et al. Metallurgically bonded needle holder jaws. A technique to enhance needle holding security without sutural damage. *Am Surg*. 1990;56(10):643-647.
5. Dinnes J, Deeks JJ, Chuchu N, et al. Dermoscopy, with and without visual inspection, for diagnosing melanoma in adults. *Cochrane Database Syst Rev*. 2018;12(12):CD011902. doi:10.1002/14651858.CD011902.pub2.
6. Argenziano G. Dermoscopy improves accuracy of primary care physicians to triage lesions suggestive of skin cancer. *J Clin Oncol*. 2006;24:1877-1882.

3 Anesthesia

RICHARD P. USATINE, MD, and ZEESHAN AFZAL, MD

SUMMARY

- Most dermatologic procedures are performed with local anesthesia by injection or topical application.
- Topical anesthetics work well on mucous membranes but can also be used for intact skin.
- All the topical anesthetics are reviewed and compared.
- For most skin surgery procedures, the recommended anesthetic is 1% lidocaine with epinephrine.
- How to calculate the maximal dose of lidocaine is provided.
- Tips for how to decrease the pain of local anesthesia are provided.
- Epinephrine is safe to use with local anesthesia in all areas.
- How to perform nerve blocks such as digital and regional blocks is included.
- Field blocks (ring blocks) are described. The ring block is especially useful before draining an abscess or removing a deep epidermal cyst.

Local anesthesia is the reversible loss of sensation to a localized area achieved by the injection or topical application of anesthetic agents. Regional anesthesia involves larger areas and is achieved by nerve block and/or field blocks through the use of injectable anesthetic agents. Local anesthetics block the pain fibers of a nerve better than those fibers that carry sensations of pressure, touch, and temperature. Therefore if the patient feels pressure or pulling but no pain, the patient should be reassured that this is not unusual. There are many anesthetic agents that can be injected or applied topically.

Topical Anesthetics (Figure 3.1)

- EMLA (2.5% lidocaine and 2.5% prilocaine cream) (Rx)
- ELA Max (4% to 5% liposomal lidocaine) – penetration and quick-acting anesthesia, longer duration of action due to antidegradation properties
- LMX 4 and LMX 5 (liposome-encapsulated lidocaine 4% and 5% cream) (OTC)
- Topical lidocaine (2% and 4% gel or viscous solution, 5% ointment, 10% spray)
- Tridocaine gel (benzocaine 20%, lidocaine 6%, tetracaine 4%) (available from Canada)
- Ametop™ (4% tetracaine gel)
- LET (lidocaine 4%, epinephrine 1:2,000, and tetracaine 0.5%) – does not require occlusion, onset of action 15 to 30 minutes

Table 3.1 shows the onset of action for the most commonly used topical anesthetics in skin procedures. EMLA (eutectic mixture of local anesthetics) cream consists of 2.5% lidocaine and 2.5% prilocaine in an oil-in-water emulsion. This anesthetic cream works best if applied 30 minutes under occlusion or 60 minutes without occlusion before anesthesia is needed. It can be used to treat children and adults. EMLA cream is used for some laser procedures, superficial light electrodesiccation of benign growths, and curettage of molluscum contagiosum. In Figure 3.1B the EMLA has been applied to the condyloma prior to cryosurgery. The patient noted a major decrease in pain with a 2 minute application over previous cryosurgery without the EMLA.

EMLA is generic, affordable, and available in 30 g tubes. EMLA should not be used in infants younger than 3 months because the metabolites of prilocaine form methemoglobin. In one randomized control trial, EMLA and LMX 4 provided comparable levels of anesthesia after a single 30-minute application under occlusion prior to electrodesiccation of dermatosis papulosa nigra.[1] In a prospective double-blind study, EMLA, LMX4, and 4% tetracaine gel had comparable anesthetic efficacy and patient satisfaction scores for dermatologic laser and skin microneedling procedures.[1]

Topical lidocaine is available as a 2% and 4% gel or viscous solution, a 5% ointment, or a 10% spray. Regardless of the vehicle, topical lidocaine takes 15 to 30 minutes to produce anesthesia on mucosal surfaces. The degree of anesthesia is not comparable to injectable lidocaine, and unless it is combined with another agent such as phenylephrine, it has no vasoconstrictive action. Therefore for mucosal surgery in the mouth, it is best to inject 1% lidocaine with epinephrine after the topical lidocaine has numbed the surface. For this purpose, it is easy to put topical lidocaine gel on a cotton swab and have the patient hold it against the mucous membrane before the subsequent injection. This technique might be used to anesthetize a mucocele or fibroma on the lip.

Tridocaine (benzocaine 20%, lidocaine 6%, tetracaine 4%) is a local analgesic, anesthetic, and antipruritic. It is used to prevent pain associated with laser surgery, superficial skin surgery, needle insertion, and intravenous cannulation. It is indicated for intact skin only, and anesthesia is obtained in 10 to 15 minutes. It can be purchased online from Canadian sources or be created by a compounding pharmacy.

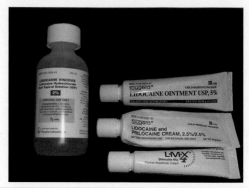

Figure 3.1 An assortment of topical anesthetics for skin surgery. (Copyright Richard P. Usatine, MD.)

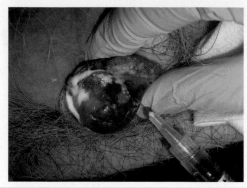

Figure 3.2 EMLA cream was applied for local anesthetic of extensive condyloma and a penis suspicious for Bowen's disease before he was given an injection of lidocaine and epinephrine for the biopsy and cryosurgery for the condyloma. (Copyright Richard P. Usatine, MD.)

Ametop (4% tetracaine gel) is a local anesthetic containing 40 mg tetracaine per gram. It can be used for needle cannulation, blood sampling, and superficial skin procedures. It is expected to provide anesthetic effect for 4 to 6 hours after 30 to 45 minutes of application. It is available in 1.5-g formulations and can be obtained online.

EMLA Technique for Intact Skin

1. Use alcohol wipes to remove oil from the area of skin to be anesthetized.
2. Apply EMLA in a thick layer to skin. Occlusive dressing (Tegaderm, Op-Site, or plastic wrap) may be placed on top of the EMLA. Either way, wait for about 30 to 60 minutes. Thicker skin may take over 1 hour to achieve anesthesia.
3. Remove EMLA with alcohol or with a tissue.
4. Perform the procedure or additional anesthesia without delay. Topical anesthesia will last only minutes after the EMLA is removed.

EMLA for Mucosa (Figure 3.2)

EMLA cream can work very rapidly for mucosa of the genitals or mouth. In Figure 3.2, a patient with extensive condyloma and a penis suspicious for Bowen's disease was treated with EMLA cream before being given an injection of lidocaine and epinephrine for the biopsy and cryosurgery for the condyloma.

- Apply EMLA cream generously.

- Wipe off in 2 to 10 minutes based on patient's perception of numbness.
- Perform procedure or inject lidocaine/epinephrine if needed.

Topical Refrigerants/Cryoanesthesia

- Ethyl chloride spray
- McKesson anesthetic spray – pentafluoropropane/tetrafluoroethane
- Liquid nitrogen

Topical refrigerants make the skin cold and provide some anesthesia for the removal of small superficial skin lesions such as skin tags and molluscum. These agents provide some cryoanesthesia before snip excisions of skin tags or curettage of molluscum. Cryoanesthesia does not provide adequate anesthesia for the removal of larger lesions. These agents are sprayed on the skin until a white frost develops. The numbing effect is partial at best and disappears in seconds. Refrigerant sprays may be used before injecting local anesthesia with a needle in a needle-phobic patient. While these sprays are probably less effective than EMLA, they work faster and therefore more convenient if the patient will tolerate the subsequent procedure.

Ethyl chloride is the only one of the refrigerants listed that is flammable, so it must not be used before electrosurgery. The label on ethyl chloride warns against inhaling too much of the product. The pentafluoropropane/tetrafluoroethane

Table 3.1 Topical Anesthetics			
Topical Anesthetic	**Ingredients**	**Vehicle**	**Onset of Action (minutes)**
EMLA	2.5% lidocaine and 2.5% prilocaine	Cream	60–120
LMX 4 LMX 5	Liposome-encapsulated lidocaine 4% and 5%	Liposome-encapsulated cream	30–60
Topical lidocaine	2% and 4% viscous solution, 5% ointment, 10% spray	Viscous solution, ointment, spray	30–60
Tridocaine gel (available from Canada) (AKA BLT)	Benzocaine 20%, lidocaine 6%, tetracaine 4%	Gel	30–60

Table 3.2 Local Anesthetics for Injection

Generic Name	Brand Name	Onset	Duration Plain	Duration With Epinephrine	Maximum Dose Plain (mg/kg) for Adults	Maximum Dose With Epinephrine (mg/kg) for Adults
Lidocaine	Xylocaine	<1 min	0.5–2 h	1–6 h	5	7
Ropivacaine	Naropin	1–15 min	2–6 h	–	3.5	–
Bupivacaine	Marcaine	2–10 min	2–4 h	4–8 h	2.5	3

product can be used with electrosurgery and claims to be nontoxic.

Liquid nitrogen can freeze the skin to cause a numbing effect; however, its use causes immediate pain and little real anesthesia. Rather than using liquid nitrogen for local anesthesia for skin tag excision, it is easier and less painful to use the liquid nitrogen with a Cryo Tweezer to treat the skin tags directly (see Chapter 14, *Cryosurgery*). Also, liquid nitrogen can be sprayed or directly applied to skin tags or molluscum rather than using it as anesthesia. This also avoids the need to deal with blood and hemostasis issues.

Contact cooling devices and assistive external devices are frequently used in laser treatments and are covered in Chapter 20, *Anesthesia for Cosmetic Procedures*.

LOCAL ANESTHESIA BY INJECTION

Lidocaine is the most widely used local anesthetic for injection in skin surgery. Bupivacaine (Marcaine) is used occasionally when long-lasting anesthesia is desired. Lidocaine has the advantage of having a more rapid onset (within 1 minute) and shorter duration of anesthesia. This shorter duration is sufficient and preferable for most skin surgery. When lidocaine is mixed with epinephrine, it lasts almost as long as bupivacaine and is less painful.[2] See Table 3.2 for a comparison of amide local anesthetics.

Epinephrine

Epinephrine is a vasoconstrictor while lidocaine alone is a vasodilator. Epinephrine with lidocaine decreases bleeding during surgery. Also, the vasoconstriction of epinephrine keeps the lidocaine in the area where it was injected, thereby decreasing immediate systemic absorption and toxicity while increasing the duration of anesthesia. This allows greater amounts of lidocaine to be used safely for local anesthesia by reducing systemic absorption and increasing the local action of the lidocaine.

1% Lidocaine With Epinephrine

For most skin surgery procedures, the recommended anesthetic is 1% lidocaine with epinephrine. Its advantages include almost immediate anesthesia, adequate duration of anesthesia, and decreased bleeding because of the epinephrine. There are only a negligible number of incidences of true allergies. Lidocaine without epinephrine has a duration of 0.5 to 2 hours, whereas lidocaine with epinephrine has a duration of 1 to 6.6 hours.[3] In one study of subcutaneous digital block with lidocaine, duration of anesthesia was 50 minutes without epinephrine and 280 minutes with epinephrine. In this study, it was also noted that onset of action was significantly shorter with epinephrine by 1.2 minutes ($P < .05$).[4] The most common commercial preparation contains 1% lidocaine (10 mg/mL) with 1:100,000 epinephrine. At this concentration, studies using laser-based and diffuse reflectance spectroscopy techniques demonstrate that time to maximum hypoperfusion ranges from 75 seconds to 2 minutes in human and porcine flaps. Blood perfusion plateaus at 20% to 25%, supporting the safe use of epinephrine in flaps with narrow pedicles.[5-6] This is also supportive of the use of epinephrine in appendages. In a study that measured the effect of subdermal injection of lidocaine combined with epinephrine on cutaneous blood flow, laser Doppler imaging demonstrated an immediate decrease in cutaneous blood flow which was maximal at 10 minutes in the forearm and 8 minutes in the face.[4] See "Debunking the Myth of Epinephrine Induced Necrosis" below.

Note that the initial skin blanching with injection is due to hydrostatic pressure along with the immediate effect of epinephrine. When hemostasis is critical to the procedure, it is best to wait 10 minutes for the epinephrine to produce maximal vasoconstriction. Waiting is less important for shave biopsies of lesions that are not very vascular in patients that are not anticoagulated. Injecting enough anesthetic so that the skin is firm can limit the amount of bleeding because small blood vessels become compressed by the anesthetic fluid (Figure 3.3).

Maximal Doses of Lidocaine

Maximal safe doses of 1% lidocaine with or without epinephrine are found in Table 3.3. Above these doses there is a risk of neurotoxicity and seizures. In most adults (over 50 kg) up to 35 mL of 1% lidocaine with epinephrine will be safe. Use of 1% lidocaine is preferable to 2% in most cases because a larger volume of anesthesia produces greater hemostasis and makes most cutaneous surgery easier to perform. Two percent lidocaine without epinephrine is useful in various nerve blocks when less volume is needed. Some clinicians prefer 2% lidocaine with epinephrine when they want to avoid tissue distortion from too much anesthetic volume. In this case, toxicity is not an issue as less than 5 mL of anesthesia is being used.

Decreasing the Pain of Local Anesthesia

Techniques to decrease the pain caused by injection of local anesthesia include the following:

- Use a small-gauge needle (27 or 30 gauge)
- Add sodium bicarbonate to the lidocaine for buffering
- Pinch or vibrate the skin as the needle enters (based on the gate theory of pain)
- Distract the patient in conversation or with music
- Inject very slowly because tissue distension hurts
- Inject deeper at first as more shallow injections that cause peau d'orange hurt more. The needle can be

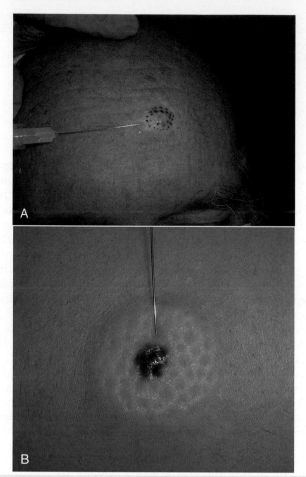

Figure 3.3 **(A)** Local anesthetic injected under a suspected BCC prior to shave biopsy. Note the blanching and swelling of the tissue in response to the volume injected and the epinephrine. **(B)** Local anesthetic injected under a suspicious pigmented lesion prior to a saucerization. Note the peau d'orange pattern due to the accentuation of the follicles when the anesthesia is given superficially. This hurts more than a slightly deeper injection seen in part A. (Copyright Richard P. Usatine, MD.)

It may be helpful to pinch or vibrate the skin as the needle enters and distract the patient in conversation. Although the needle should be inserted quickly, the injection will be less painful if the volume of anesthesia is injected slowly. The more superficial the injection, the more painful it is. For example, an injection bleb similar to that of a tuberculin skin test is more painful than a deeper subcutaneous injection. It is usually less painful if the injection is done slowly and deeply at first, followed by redirecting the needle for a more superficial, dermal, blanching type of injection. In this manner, a volume of 5 mL or more can be given slowly through one injection site. Skin blanching and visible tissue distention help determine the area that has been anesthetized. Also, tissue induration can be palpated to determine the distribution of the anesthesia. If need be, this area can be extended by reinjecting through another site that has already been anesthetized.

ADDING BICARBONATE

Acidic preservatives are added to lidocaine-epinephrine solutions to lower the pH to 3.5 to 5.5 because epinephrine is stable only in acidic environments.[8] This causes a burning pain by increasing local hydrogen ions responsible for activating nociceptors. Adding sodium bicarbonate (8.4% for injection) to the lidocaine-epinephrine anesthetic solution markedly decreases the pain caused by injection.[8-10] A new well-done study again demonstrated that adding $NaHCO_3$ to lidocaine-epinephrine effectively reduces burning pain during infiltration.[10] Most importantly they found that a 3:1 mixing ratio is significantly less painful than the 9:1 ratio used in earlier studies.[10] A cost analysis of the use of buffered lidocaine-epinephrine with bicarbonate in a 3:1 ratio over a 9:1 ratio showed a potential cost increase of $0.10 to $0.30 per injection.[11] They concluded that using the 3:1 ratio will minimize patient discomfort at a trivial increase in cost and equal time.[11] In our office we use Table 3.4 as our guide when mixing lidocaine-epinephrine with bicarbonate. While this takes more time and money, patients do appreciate that the injections are less painful.

ADDED BENEFIT TO WARMING THE ANESTHESIA

A warm (40°C) and neutral (pH 7.35) anesthetic preparation has been found to be less painful on injection than room-temperature nonneutral preparations.[12-16] One study suggests that warming and buffering have a synergistic effect.[13] Skin infiltration with warm buffered lidocaine was significantly less painful than infiltration with room-temperature unbuffered lidocaine, warm lidocaine, or buffered lidocaine.[13] In the other study, the mean pain scores for the four solutions were: 44.2 for plain lidocaine, 42.2 for

withdrawn partially and then angled more superficially to inject the upper dermis (like PPD).

■ Use only one injection site if possible, and if the area is large place subsequent injections into areas already anesthetized.

The main technique for decreasing the pain of injection is to inject the local anesthetic very slowly using a small-gauge needle (27 or 30 gauge). The larger the gauge number, the smaller the needle diameter and the less painful the injection. Use 30 gauge needles on the most sensitive areas including the face, the ears, the fingers, and the genitals. When injecting anesthesia for a laceration repair, injecting from within a laceration is less painful than injecting into intact skin.[7]

Table 3.3   Table of Maximal Doses of 1% Lidocaine (10 mg/mL)

Type of Lidocaine	Maximum Adult Dose (mg/kg)	Maximum Child Dose (mg/kg)	Maximum mL for 50 kg Adult	Maximum mL for 70 kg Adult	Maximum mL for 30 kg Child
1% Lidocaine without epinephrine	5	1.5–2	25	28	4.5–6
1% Lidocaine with epinephrine	7	3–4	35	49	9–12

Table 3.4	Lidocaine w/epinephrine + Bicarbonate (HCO₃⁻)
Formula	**3:1 ratio by Vent study***
Shave	3 mL syringe
	1.5 mL Lidocaine w/epinephrine
	0.5 mL Bicarbonate
	(alternative is 2.0 mL of Lid/epi in a 4:1 ratio)
Punch	5–6 mL syringe
	3 mL Lidocaine w/epinephrine
	1 mL Bicarbonate
or	
	4.5 mL Lidocaine w/epinephrine
	1.5 mL Bicarbonate
Excision	10–12 mL syringe
	6 mL Lidocaine w/epinephrine
	2 mL Bicarbonate
or	
	7.5 mL Lidocaine w/epinephrine
	2.5 mL Bicarbonate
or	
	9 mL Lidocaine w/epinephrine
	3 mL Bicarbonate

*Vent A, Surber C, Graf Johansen NT, et al. Buffered lidocaine 1%/epinephrine 1:100,000 with sodium bicarbonate (sodium hydrogen carbonate) in a 3:1 ratio is less painful than a 9:1 ratio: a double-blind, randomized, placebo-controlled, crossover trial. *J Am Acad Dermatol*. Jul 2020;83(1):159–165.

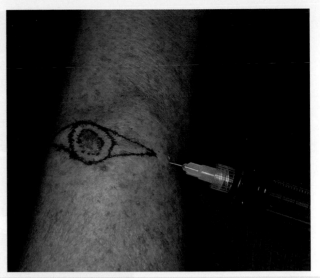

Figure 3.4 Injecting local anesthesia with lidocaine and epinephrine before an elliptical excision of a micronodular BCC on the forearm. Note the subtle blanching and swelling of the tissue in response to the volume injected and the epinephrine. Additional injections will be needed as the needle is not long enough to reach across the whole ellipse. (Copyright Richard P. Usatine, MD.)

warmed lidocaine, 36.7 for buffered lidocaine, and 29.2 for warmed buffered lidocaine (lower numbers equal less pain).[14] In one study, to reduce the pain of lidocaine infiltration, buffering was more effective than warming (warming was only to 38.9°C).[15] Due to the difficulty of warming these solutions in our office, we rely on buffering only to diminish the pain of anesthetic injections.

Injection Technique –

See Videos 3.1–3.3

The skin surface can be cleaned adequately with an alcohol wipe. Gloves should be clean but need not be sterile for the injections. When performing a biopsy or excision, it is helpful to mark the planned lines of incision with a surgical marker before doing the injection. This prevents losing sight of a nonpigmented lesion when the swelling and blanching occur from the anesthesia. The lines, circles, and ellipses (fusiform pattern) drawn provide a guide to the biopsy or excision. Start giving the local anesthesia by inserting the needle approximately 5 to 8 mm outside the area marked for biopsy or excision. If the needle is inserted exactly at the edge of the lesion or marked area, then the zone of anesthesia is more likely to be asymmetric when attempting to numb the area with a single injection. When starting the injection 5 to 8 mm outside the marked area, anesthesia for a shave or punch biopsy can be done with a single injection.

For shave and punch biopsies, the tip of the needle should reach the deep dermis so that an elevation and blanching of the tissue occurs (Figure 3.3). If the anesthetic is injected too deep into the subcutaneous tissue, no elevation will occur. It is usually not needed to pull back on the plunger before injecting as it is unlikely that the injection will go into a large vessel. When an injection is superficial in the dermis, you may see an accentuation of the follicles called peau d'orange (Figure 3.3B). This skin distention is more painful than the pain that occurs with a deeper dermis injection. However, if you intend to do a shave biopsy, you can start with a deeper dermis injection and finish with a more superficial injection to raise the lesion for biopsy. Starting deeper and adjusting the needle to a more superficial level is an effective technique (this can be done without removing the needle from the original injection site).

If the lesion to be removed is large (Figure 3.4), more injection sites are usually needed. Start each new injection in an area that has already received some anesthesia to diminish the pain with subsequent injections.

A smaller syringe requires less force for injections: 3 mL and 5 mL (or 6 mL) syringes are a good compromise between cost and comfort. These hold enough anesthetic for most small procedures and will be comfortable for the clinician. When using a larger 10 to 12 mL syringe, avoid the 30 gauge needle as the pressure needed to push the anesthesia through this small gauge needle on a larger syringe is uncomfortable for the clinician.

Dental Syringes

Using dental syringes to inject anesthesia can be very efficient and cost effective (Figure 3.5).

The benefits are:

1. Small diameter needle (30 gauge), less pain

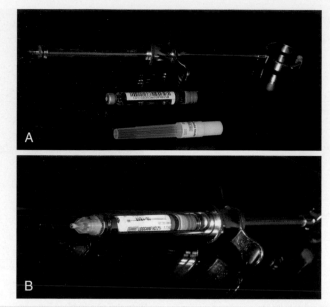

Figure 3.5 (A) Stainless steel dental aspirating syringe with the cartridge containing 1.7 mL 2% lidocaine with epinephrine and a 30 g ½ inch needle. **(B)** The 1.7 mL cartridge inserted into the dental syringe with the 30 g ½ inch needle in place. (Courtesy of André Jones DDS, AEGD, FADI.)

2. No anesthesia withdrawing (comes in prefilled vials of 2% lidocaine with epinephrine)
3. Available in 1.7 mL vials, so less wastage of leftover lidocaine, making it more cost effective
4. Due to metallic syringes, even with small size needles, administering anesthesia is steady and effortless even at high-resistance places like fingers, toes, and plantar feet
5. No risk of spillover or leakage from the syringe as needles are screwed over the syringe
6. No wastage of 18 gauge needle for withdrawing

Disadvantages:
Occur predominantly for larger excisions:

1. The needle length is a limiting factor as it is only available in ½ inch and 1 inch lengths. For larger and deeper lesions, a 1¼ to 1½ needle is preferred for sufficient and reliable anesthesia.
2. Vials of 1.7 mL are small and many would be needed.
3. 2% Lidocaine will reach toxic levels with ½ volume of 1% lidocaine.

A workaround is to also have multiuse vials of 1% lidocaine with epinephrine in the office with typical needles and syringes for larger procedures.

Adverse Reactions

Adverse reactions to lidocaine and epinephrine include the following.
Lidocaine:

- Allergy to lidocaine – extremely rare
- Central nervous system effects from too much lidocaine (tinnitus and excessive sedation may be early signs before progressing to major signs of toxicity including seizures, loss of consciousness)[17,18] – see Table 3.3 to avoid this
- Cardiovascular effects from too much lidocaine (myocardial depression, arrhythmias) – see Table 3.3 to avoid this

Epinephrine:

- Tachycardia
- Anxiety
- Tremulousness
- Decreased peripheral circulation

Debunking the Myth of Epinephrine-Induced Necrosis

For patients with normal circulation, it is safe to use epinephrine for local anesthesia in areas such as the tip of the nose, the fingers and toes, the ears, or the penis despite old dogma that epinephrine should not be used in these areas (Figure 3.6).[19-25] Many studies have even provided evidence to dispute the dogma that using epinephrine in a digital block produces digital necrosis.[20-25] Most cases of reported

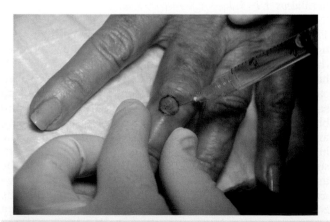

Figure 3.6 Lidocaine with epinephrine injected for local anesthesia prior to surgery on this squamous cell carcinoma. Multiple studies and our clinical practice indicate that use of epinephrine is safe on the fingers. (Copyright Richard P. Usatine, MD.)

digital necrosis were before 1950, and those cases were associated with procaine and cocaine injection with or without epinephrine.[20] Epinephrine-supplemented local anesthetics for ear and nose surgery were used without complications in more than 10,000 surgical procedures.[19] Using epinephrine with lidocaine results in a less bloody operating field and longer effectiveness of local anesthesia. The relative absence of blood in the operating field significantly reduces the duration of surgery and increases the healing rate, as less electrosurgery is needed.[19] The addition of epinephrine in digital blocks minimizes the need for the use of tourniquets and provides better and longer pain control during procedures on digits.[21] Evidence also suggests that epinephrine can safely be used in digital blocks even in patients with vascular disease.[22] A Cochrane Review of this issue found no reports of adverse events such as ischemia distal to the injection of epinephrine in digital nerve blocks.[23] In sum, the use of epinephrine with lidocaine in sites with end-arteries is beneficial for hemostasis and does not seem to pose a risk of ischemia. We have been using epinephrine in all of these areas for years with no complications.

There are a few patients who ask that no epinephrine be used because it makes them anxious. It is true that some patients may get tachycardia for a few minutes along with a feeling of anxiousness shortly after the injection. This can usually be handled by reassuring them that the feeling will pass in a few minutes. For most patients, this may have occurred in the past during a dental procedure (reason enough for anxiety in many people).

Rare adverse effects associated with too large a systemic dose of injectable anesthetics (injection into a vein or too large a dose of the anesthetic) include arrhythmias, cardiac arrest, and CNS effects such as dizziness, hallucinations, dysarthria, dysgeusia, tremors, twitching, seizures, and altered consciousness.[17]

LIDOCAINE ALLERGIES

Lidocaine allergies are extremely rare. Almost all patients who report an allergy actually have had a vasovagal reaction with lidocaine injections or sensitivity to the epinephrine effects. Other patients are actually allergic to the paraben preservative in the multidose vials of lidocaine or they had an allergic reaction to a local anesthetic ester such as Novocain (procaine, novocaine). Because the paraben is not added to the single-use vials, it may be helpful to try these vials when the patient reports a mild allergy and lidocaine is needed once again.

The ester forms of local anesthetics, such as novocaine, produce more allergic reactions. Fortunately, there is no cross-reactivity between novocaine and lidocaine. Therefore lidocaine use is safe in a patient with a true novocaine allergy. All dentists are now using lidocaine, not novocaine. Patients may think they are receiving novocaine in the dentist's office, but they are most likely receiving lidocaine or articaine, which has increased perfusion in bone.

The approach for a patient who reports a specific allergy to lidocaine is to take a careful history to determine if a vasovagal or epinephrine reaction may be the actual cause of the patient's adverse experience. As long as the reported allergy was not life-threatening, it is reasonable to try a test injection of a small amount of lidocaine (from a single-use vial), because true systemic lidocaine reactions are so rare.

Alternatives to lidocaine are injectable diphenhydramine (Benadryl) or injectable normal saline. Diphenhydramine provides adequate short-term anesthesia, but it may cause the patient to become drowsy. When normal saline is injected to induce a firm wheal, it provides a few minutes of anesthesia as well.

Nerve Blocks –

See Video 3.4

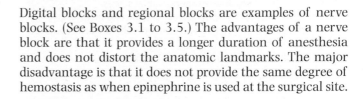

Digital blocks and regional blocks are examples of nerve blocks. (See Boxes 3.1 to 3.5.) The advantages of a nerve block are that it provides a longer duration of anesthesia and does not distort the anatomic landmarks. The major disadvantage is that it does not provide the same degree of hemostasis as when epinephrine is used at the surgical site.

Box 3.1 Nerve Blocks

Advantages

- Anesthetizes the nerve before it reaches the operative site
- Affects a large area with small amount of anesthetic
- No distortion of operative site

Disadvantages

- No vasoconstriction
- Longer onset
- Shorter duration
- Risk of nerve laceration

Technique – General Principles

- Lidocaine and/or longer-acting anesthetic
- 5-mL syringe
- 27- or 30-gauge ½-inch needle
- Inject slowly into subcutaneous plane in vicinity of nerve
- Avoid directly hitting the nerve (back off if sharp pain when inserting needle)
- Don't inject directly into the foramen
- Pull back on the plunger before infiltrating
- Wait 10–15 minutes for the full effect

Vidimos A, Ammirati C, Pobleti-Lopez C. *Dermatologic Surgery.* Elsevier; 2009.

Box 3.2 Supraorbital/Supratrochlear Nerve Block (V1)

Provides sensation to forehead

Indications

- Laser resurfacing
- Large surgical defects

Location

- Supraorbital nerve – midpupillary line along superior bony orbit
- Supratrochlear nerve – superior/medial corner of bony orbit

Inject about 1 mL lidocaine (± epinephrine) in subcutaneous fat overlying supraorbital foramen.

Inject about 1 mL at root of nose/medial border of orbit.

Vidimos A, Ammirati C, Pobleti-Lopez C. *Dermatologic Surgery.* Elsevier; 2009.

Box 3.3   Infraorbital Block (V2)

Provides sensation to lower eyelid, medial cheek, nose, and upper lip

Indications

- Fillers
- Laser resurfacing
- Large surgical defects

Location

- Foramen is 1 cm inferior to the infraorbital ridge along the midpupillary line.

Approach through the oral cavity.

The nerve is 0.5–1 cm above superior labial sulcus.

Anesthetize oral mucosa with topical benzocaine first.

Enter at apex of first bicuspid and direct needle toward estimated location of foramen.

Inject 1–2 mL with a ½-inch needle (27 or 30 gauge).

Vidimos A, Ammirati C, Pobleti-Lopez C. *Dermatologic Surgery*. Elsevier; 2009.

Box 3.4   Mental Nerve Block (V3)

Sensation to lower lip, chin, and mucous membranes

Indications

- Fillers
- Laser resurfacing
- Large surgical defects

Location

- Midway between upper and lower edge of mandible below second bicuspid (midpupillary line)

Approach through the oral cavity.

Anesthetize oral mucosa with topical benzocaine first.

27- or 30-gauge ½-inch needle

Enter inferior labial sulcus between first and second bicuspids.

Inject 1–2 mL around mental foramen.

Vidimos A, Ammirati C, Pobleti-Lopez C. *Dermatologic Surgery*. Elsevier; 2009.

Box 3.5   Digital Block

Paired dorsal and medial digital nerves

Indications

- Nail plate avulsion
- Nail unit biopsy
- Distal digit surgery
- Periungual warts

Lidocaine 1% or 2% with epinephrine

5-mL syringe

27- or 30-gauge needle

Topical anesthesia or ice prior to injecting

No more than 5 mL total volume

The digital block can be more effective than a local injection on the digit especially for surgery around the nail. Anesthetizing the digital nerves with lidocaine will almost always provide good anesthesia. Injection on each side of the digit with lidocaine will anesthetize both dorsal and ventral nerves on either side of the digit (Figure 3.7).

A 3-to-5 mL syringe may be used with 1% or 2% lidocaine and epinephrine, delivering 1.0 to 1.5 mL on each side of the digit and 1.0 mL on the top (Figure 3.8).

A wing block is an alternative or an adjunct to a digital block for surgery on any part of the nail unit (Figure 3.9). The main advantage over a digital block is that it provides better hemostasis at the site of surgery. Wing blocks work faster than a digital block but the injection usually hurts more at first. We prefer performing a wing block after a successful digital block to help with hemostasis and to ensure excellent anesthesia (see Chapter 17, *Nail Procedures*).

Regional blocks (i.e., infraorbital, supraorbital, or mental nerve blocks) are helpful when a larger area of the face is to be anesthetized and anatomic distortion is to be avoided. For that reason, facial regional blocks are very helpful for cosmetic procedures involving fillers and ablative lasers. These blocks can be done with a small amount of 1% or 2% lidocaine (0.5 to 1.0 mL) without or with epinephrine. See Figure 3.10 for a guide on where to inject for these blocks. It is important to be aware that these blocks do not assist in hemostasis, so some lidocaine with epinephrine may still be useful in the local area as an adjunct to the regional block. Regional blocks can be done through the skin as in Figure 3.10 or using an intraoral approach as in Figure 3.11. Oral surgeons regularly use the intraoral approach (Figure 3.12). See Chapter 20, *Anesthesia for Cosmetic Procedures*, for more additional information on these blocks.

Field or Ring Block –

See Video 3.5 and 3.6

A field block creates a "wall" of anesthesia around an area to be anesthetized. Rather than injecting the anesthetic directly into the area to be numbed, the anesthetic is injected around it to affect the nerves that normally transmit sensations of pain and touch (Figure 3.13). A field block is useful when it is necessary to avoid distorting the tissue to be cut, in cases of infection, and in locations where local anesthesia may not work adequately. Epinephrine is used with lidocaine to decrease bleeding.

The ring block is especially useful before draining an abscess or removing a deep epidermal cyst. The acid environment of the abscess can hydrolyze the anesthetic. The field block allows the anesthetic to work on normal surrounding tissue and avoids the problem of distending the abscess or cyst further by keeping the anesthetic out of the abscess cavity. A 27 gauge 1½-inch needle is useful for administering a field block. In Figure 3.13, the ring block injections are marked on the skin. Each subsequent injection goes into an area that was previously anesthetized. This method also minimizes the chance that you will be sprayed by the contents of a distended abscess or cyst.

Pregnancy and Lactation

Local anesthetics can cross the placental membrane by passive diffusion. Shave and punch biopsies involve such a small amount of local anesthetic that there is little risk to

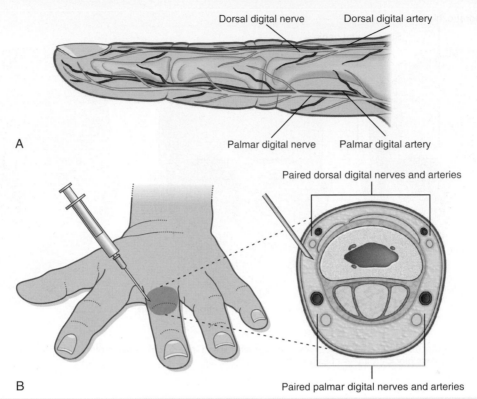

Figure 3.7 Digital innervation and nerve block. **(A)** Dorsal and palmar digital arteries and nerves run together. **(B)** Dorsal approach and administering digital nerve block allows anesthesia of dorsal and palmar bundles with one puncture. (Courtesy of Robinson, et al. Surgery of the Skin, Elsevier.)

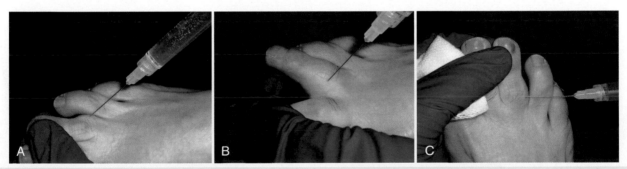

Figure 3.8 Three steps of a digital block prior to nail matrix biopsy for longitudinal melanonychia. **(A)** Injection into the affected side. **(B)** Injection into the other side of the digit. **(C)** Anesthetizing the nerves that run on the dorsum of the toe. Lidocaine with epinephrine is safely used. (Copyright Richard P. Usatine, MD.)

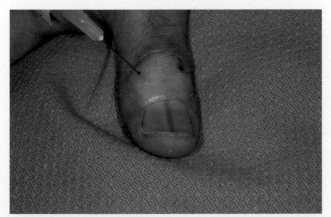

Figure 3.9 Prior to a nail matrix biopsy, a wing block ensures that the procedure is painless and minimizes bleeding during the procedure. Lidocaine with epinephrine is safely used. (Copyright Richard P. Usatine, MD.)

the fetus. Using the old rating systems, lidocaine is pregnancy category B, and epinephrine is pregnancy category C. Epinephrine should be used conservatively, as large doses can cause decreased placental perfusion. Elective and large procedures are best delayed until after delivery.[17]

Lidocaine and epinephrine are excreted in breast milk and should be used with caution in women who are nursing. If a procedure with local anesthesia is needed, the woman may pump her breast milk several hours after the procedure and discard the expressed milk.[17]

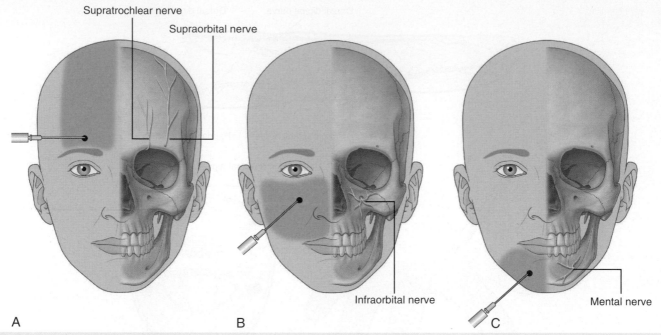

Supratrochlear nerve

Supraorbital nerve

Infraorbital nerve

Mental nerve

A

B

C

Figure 3.10 Location and sensory distribution for nerve blocks. **(A)** Supraorbital and supratrochlear nerve block. **(B)** Infraorbital nerve block (follow the midpupillary line). **(C)** Mental nerve block. (Courtesy of Surgery of the Skin, Elsevier.)

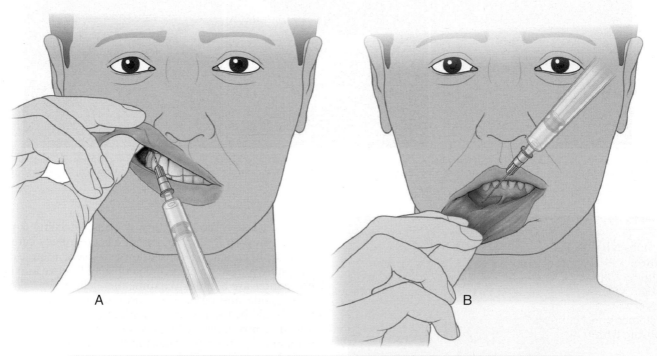

A

B

Figure 3.11 Intraoral route for blocking infraorbital and mental nerves. (Courtesy of Surgery of the Skin, Elsevier.)

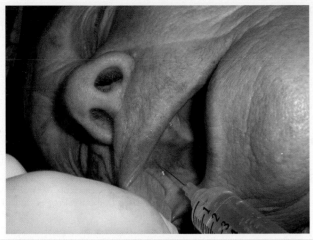

Figure 3.12 An intraoral infraorbital block performed using 2% lidocaine. Note that this patient is edentulous but this approach works well regardless of the state of the dentition. The amount of anesthetic needed is only 1 mL. (Copyright Richard P. Usatine, MD.)

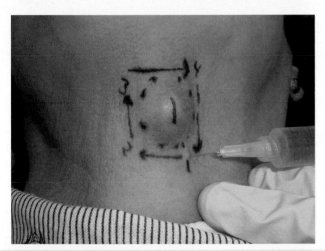

Figure 3.13 Ring block around an epidermal inclusion cyst. Arrows are marked to see where each of the four injections will be administered to create a circumferential block. This method helps to anesthetize the whole area and avoids injecting lidocaine directly into the cyst – which is not needed and increases the chance that the cyst will squirt fluid at the surgeon doing the procedure. (Copyright Richard P. Usatine, MD.)

Conclusion

A thorough understanding of the techniques for administering local anesthesia is essential for the performance of painless skin surgery. A safely and properly anesthetized patient will allow the most controlled and highest-quality surgery. Keeping the patient comfortable will create a happy customer and help to establish and maintain a good relationship with the healthcare provider.

Summary of Basic Materials Needed

Anesthetics (Most Useful)

- Topical anesthetics: EMLA cream, topical lidocaine gel
- Injectable anesthetic: 1% lidocaine with epinephrine

Needles

- 18 to 21 gauge for drawing up anesthetic from vial
- 27 and 30 gauge needles are optimal for most local injections, digital blocks, and field blocks (27 × 1.25 inch and 30 × 1 inch are excellent). (We use the 30 gauge needles on the face, genitalia, and any small procedure and reserve the 27 gauge needles for the trunk and extremities when larger volumes need to be injected.)

Syringes

- 3 mL syringe is optimal for most shave biopsies.
- 5 mL or 6 mL syringe is adequate for most punch biopsies.
- 10 mL or 12 mL syringe may be helpful with elliptical excisions.

See Chapter 1 for a list of distributors of surgical and anesthetic supplies.

References

1. Chiang YZ, Al-Niaimi F, Madan V. Comparative efficacy and patient preference of topical anaesthetics in dermatological laser treatments and skin microneedling. *J Cutan Aesthet Surg.* 2015;8(3):143-146.
2. Howe NR, Williams JM. Pain of injection and duration of anesthesia for intradermal infiltration of lidocaine, bupivacaine, and etidocaine. *J Dermatol Surg Oncol.* 1994;20:459-464.
3. Kouba DJ, LoPiccolo MC, Alam M, et al. Guidelines for the use of local anesthesia in office-based dermatologic surgery. *J Am Acad Dermatol.* 2016;74(6):1201-1219.
4. Sonohata M, Nagamine S, Maeda K, et al. Subcutaneous single injection digital block with epinephrine. *Anesthesiol Res Pract.* 2012;2012:487650.
5. Sheikh R, Memarzadeh K, Torbrand C, Blohme J, Malmsjo M. Hypoperfusion in response to epinephrine in local anaesthetics: investigation of dependence on epinephrine concentration, spread of hypoperfusion and time to maximal cutaneous vasoconstriction. *J Plast Reconstr Aesthet Surg.* 2017;70(3):322-329.
6. Sheikh R, Dahlstrand U, Memarzadeh K, Blohme J, Reistad N, Malmsjo M. Optimal epinephrine concentration and time delay to minimize perfusion in eyelid surgery: measured by laser-based methods and a novel form of extended-wavelength diffuse reflectance spectroscopy. *Ophthalmic Plast Reconstr Surg.* 2018;34(2):123-129.
7. Bartfield JM, Sokaris SJ, Raccio-Robak N. Local anesthesia for lacerations: pain of infiltration inside vs outside the wound. *Acad Emerg Med.* 1998;5:100-104.
8. Isedeh P, Forrest ML, Liu D, Aires D. Ensuring that injectable bicarbonate-buffered lidocaine-epinephrine complies with 2015 United States Pharmacopeia (USP) compounding provisions. *J Am Acad Dermatol.* 2016;75(2):454-455.
9. Cepeda MS, Tzortzopoulou A, Tackrey M. Adjusting the pH of lidocaine for reducing pain on injection. *Cochrane Database Syst Rev.* 2010;12:CD006581.
10. Vent A, Surber C, Graf Johansen NT, et al. Buffered lidocaine 1%/epinephrine 1:100,000 with sodium bicarbonate (sodium hydrogen carbonate) in a 3:1 ratio is less painful than a 9:1 ratio: a double-blind, randomized, placebo-controlled, crossover trial. *J Am Acad Dermatol.* 2020;83(1):159-165. doi:10.1016/j.jaad.2019.09.088.
11. Wu AG, Conway J, Roy B, et al. Cost analysis of the use of buffered lidocaine 1%, epinephrine 1:100,000 with sodium bicarbonate in a 3:1 ratio over a 9:1 ratio. *J Am Acad Dermatol.* 2021;85(1):e21-e22. doi:10.1016/j.jaad.2020.12.091.
12. Yang CH, Hsu HC, Shen SC, et al. Warm and neutral tumescent anesthetic solutions are essential factors for a less painful injection. *Dermatol Surg.* 2006;32:1119-1122.
13. Mader TJ, Playe SJ, Garb JL. Reducing the pain of local anesthetic infiltration: warming and buffering have a synergistic effect. *Ann Emerg Med.* 1994;23:550-554.
14. Colaric KB, Overton DT, Moore K. Pain reduction in lidocaine administration through buffering and warming. *Am J Emerg Med.* 1998;16:353-356.

15. Bartfield JM, Crisafulli KM, Raccio-Robak N, Salluzzo RF. The effects of warming and buffering on pain of infiltration of lidocaine. *Acad Emerg Med.* 1995;2:254-258.

16. Hogan ME, vanderVaart S, Perampaladas K, Machado M, Einarson TR, Taddio A. Systematic review and meta-analysis of the effect of warming local anesthetics on injection pain. *Ann Emerg Med.* 2011;58(1):86-98.

17. Lin Y, Liu SS. Local anesthetics. In: Barash PG, Cullen BF, Stoelting RK, eds. *Clinical Anesthesia.* New York: 7th ed. Wolters Kluwer Health/Lippincott Williams & Wilkins; 2013:575.

18. Vasques F, Behr AU, Weinberg G, Ori C, Di Gregorio G. A review of local anesthetic systemic toxicity cases since publication of the American Society of Regional Anesthesia recommendations. *Reg Anesth Pain Med.* 2015;40:698-705.

19. Häfner HM, Röcken M, Breuninger H. Epinephrine-supplemented local anesthetics for ear and nose surgery: clinical use without complications in more than 10,000 surgical procedures. *J Dtsch Dermatol Ges.* 2005;3(3):195-199.

20. Nielsen LJ, Lumholt P, Hölmich LR. Local anaesthesia with vasoconstrictor is safe to use in areas with end-arteries in fingers, toes, noses and ears. *Ugeskr Laeger.* 2014;176(44):V04140238.

21. Krunic AL, Wang LC, Soltani K, Weitzul S, Taylor RS. Digital anesthesia with epinephrine: an old myth revisited. *J Am Acad Dermatol.* 2004;51(5):755-759.

22. Ilicki J. Safety of epinephrine in digital nerve blocks: a literature review. *J Emerg Med.* 2015;49(5):799-809.

23. Prabhakar H, Rath S, Kalaivani M, Bhanderi N. Adrenaline with lidocaine for digital nerve blocks. *Cochrane Database Syst Rev.* 2015;(3):CD010645.

24. Thomson CJ, Lalonde DH, Denkler KA, Feicht AJ. A critical look at the evidence for and against elective epinephrine use in the finger. *Plast Reconstr Surg.* 2007;119:260-266.

25. Lalonde D, Bell M, Benoit P, Sparkes G, Denkler K, Chang P. A multicenter prospective study of 3,110 consecutive cases of elective epinephrine use in the fingers and hand: the Dalhousie Project clinical phase. *J Hand Surg Am.* 2005;30:1061-1067.

4 *Hemostasis*

RICHARD P. USATINE, MD

SUMMARY

- The goal of hemostasis in surgery is to control bleeding while avoiding unnecessary tissue destruction.
- Using epinephrine with lidocaine prevents some bleeding and may prevent issues with hemostasis.
- The types of hemostasis that are covered in detail include chemical/topical, electrocoagulation, pressure dressings, sutures and ties, tourniquets and clamps, and physical agents.
- The preferred chemical hemostatic agent for a shave biopsy or shave excision is aluminum chloride.
- Electrocoagulation is an ideal method to control bleeding during more extensive surgeries.
- Sutures are the most commonly used method for hemostasis in punch biopsies and excisional surgeries.
- Absorbable gelatin foam sponges are useful for punch biopsies.
- Tourniquets for digital surgery and chalazion clamps for lip surgery can be very helpful to control bleeding.

Achieving hemostasis is an essential component of all surgery. The goal of hemostasis in surgery is to control bleeding while avoiding unnecessary tissue destruction. It is important to understand the advantages and disadvantages of all methods of hemostasis to be able to choose the appropriate methods for each surgical situation. The first step is to attempt to prevent bleeding with the injection of epinephrine. After that, hemostasis can be achieved by chemical agents or electrocoagulation. Hemostasis may also be achieved by physical methods that involve pressure, sutures, gelatin sponges, and instruments.

Epinephrine – Step One

The first step in hemostasis for any dermatologic procedure that involves cutting the skin is to inject the area with lidocaine and epinephrine.

Time to wait:

- When injecting lidocaine and epinephrine the initial blanching occurs as a combination of hydrostatic pressure from the injection along with the initial effect of the epinephrine. However, recent studies have shown that the epinephrine reaches its full hemostatic potential for skin surgery at 7 minutes.[1-3]
- If the lesion is known to be particularly vascular such as a pyogenic granuloma, angioma, or vascular-appearing malignancy then it is best to wait for 7 to 10 minutes for the epinephrine to work. Also, if the area for biopsy or excision is very vascular such as the scalp or lip then it also helps to wait for the full effect of the epinephrine.

Safe to use in all sites:

- Lidocaine with epinephrine is safe to use for skin surgery in every location, including the areas in which medical students are taught to never use epinephrine. That is, evidence shows that epinephrine can be safely used on

the nose, toes, fingers, and hose (penis).[4-6] The epinephrine myth originated in the 1940s, when very acidic (pH 1) procaine-epinephrine was injected into the fingers, causing finger necrosis.[4] Strong evidence now exists for the safe use of epinephrine in fingers.[4-8] It can be safely used for digital blocks but may be avoided for digital blocks in patients with significant vasculopathy affecting the circulation of the digits. Epinephrine can also be used safely on the ear to help with hemostasis.[7-8]

Types of Hemostasis

- Chemical/topical
- Electrocoagulation
- Direct pressure or pressure dressing
- Sutures and ties
- Tourniquets and clamps (don't indent)
- Physical agents (gelatin sponge)

Chemical Hemostatic Agents

- Aluminum chloride – preferred agent (Figure 4.1)
- Monsel's solution (ferric subsulfate)
- Silver nitrate sticks are not recommended.

General Principles of Chemical Hemostasis

Chemical hemostatic agents work by causing protein precipitation, which stops the bleeding. These agents work best in a dry field, allowing the chemical to go directly to the bleeding tissue without being diluted by pooled blood. Chemical agents are useful after a shave biopsy or a small

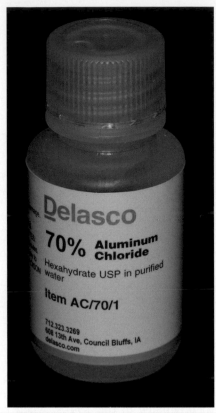

Figure 4.1 Aluminum chloride 70% in purified water is the most useful topical hemostatic agent. (Copyright Richard P. Usatine, MD.)

punch biopsy. Chemical agents should not be used in deep wounds that will be closed with sutures.

ALUMINUM CHLORIDE

Aluminum chloride comes in strengths from 20% to 70%, available in water- or alcohol-based solutions (Figure 4.1). Alcohol alone (anhydrous alcohol) will support a solution of up to 20%, so the stronger concentrations are either in water or a mixture of water and alcohol. I prefer to use aluminum chloride in an aqueous solution because it can be used safely with electrosurgery and comes in higher concentrations. With an alcohol-based solution, it is possible to ignite the alcohol when electrosurgery is performed in the same field. However, drying the field after applying the alcohol-based solution makes it safe to use with electrosurgery.

Aqueous aluminum chloride can be ordered as a 35% or 70% solution from Delasco (see end of chapter for ordering information). Both are inexpensive and excellent for hemostasis. No studies are available to determine whether one percentage is better than another. I use 70% with good results. These solutions have a 3-year shelf life. Drysol, a brand name of 20% aluminum chloride in anhydrous ethyl alcohol that is sold by prescription to treat hyperhidrosis, also produces hemostasis but is more expensive to purchase and messier to use.

The major advantage of aluminum chloride is that it is a clear solution that does not stain or tattoo the tissue. It does not cause tissue necrosis and does not damage the normal skin surrounding the wound. Aluminum chloride should not be used in deep wounds that will be sutured because it can delay healing and increase scarring.

When using aluminum chloride after a shave or punch biopsy (*see video 4.1*):

1. First prepare 2 to 3 cotton-tipped applicators (CTAs) with aluminum chloride by dipping them in the container and allowing them to sit on a nonsterile gauze pad (this will ensure that they are not too moist).
2. For a shave biopsy use the stick-end of the prepared CTA to stabilize the shave specimen instead of a forceps. Then after the specimen is removed, turn the CTA over to apply the aluminum chloride to the biopsy site.
3. The aluminum chloride should then be applied to the dry field by rolling or twisting the moist applicator against the open wound (Figure 4.2A).
4. It helps to hold the CTA perpendicular (Figure 4.2B) to the skin to apply firm pressure on the bleeding areas while twisting the aluminum chloride–soaked applicator clockwise and counterclockwise.

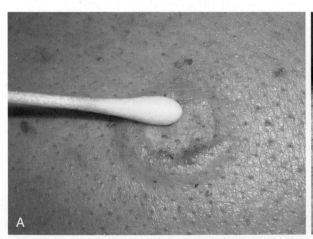
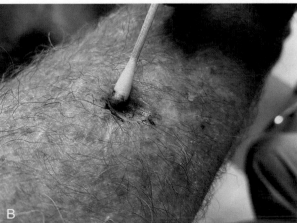

Figure 4.2 Clear aluminum chloride on a cotton-tipped applicator (CTA) being used to stop bleeding after shave biopsies. **(A)** Dabbing it on with some pressure. **(B)** Applying vertical pressure with a CTA can stop most bleeding. (Copyright Richard P. Usatine, MD.)

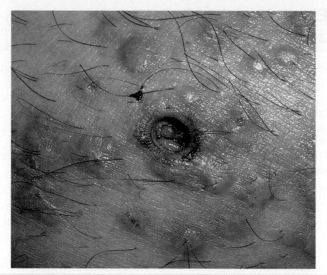

Figure 4.3 A 4-mm punch biopsy being left open to heal by secondary intention. Hemostasis was achieved using aluminum chloride. (Copyright Richard P. Usatine, MD.)

5. After a 2 to 4 mm punch biopsy, a dry cotton-tipped applicator can be held with downward pressure against the open hole to dry the field. Most CTAs will stay upright once inserted into a 3 to 4 mm punch biopsy hole.

6. For a punch biopsy in which a suture will not be used for hemostasis, the aluminum chloride should be applied with downward pressure and held against the wound until hemostasis is achieved (Figure 4.3).

MONSEL'S SOLUTION

Monsel's solution consists of 20% ferric subsulfate. It is used to produce hemostasis after biopsies of the skin and cervix. It is applied to the skin in the same manner as aluminum chloride. There is a small risk of tattooing the skin through iron deposition. One major nuisance in using Monsel's solution is that the iron precipitates around the top of the container, making it difficult to open. Aluminum chloride containers are always easy to open.

Monsel's solution can leave a histologic artifact in the skin. Therefore, when a repeat biopsy is performed in an area where Monsel's solution was previously used, it helps to warn the pathologist.[9]

SILVER NITRATE

Silver nitrate comes in easy-to-use sticks. However, its hemostatic action is slower and the response to it is more variable. Pain response to application for skin tag removal was greater with silver nitrate than with aluminum chloride or ferric subsulfate.[10] Compared with aluminum chloride and ferric subsulfate, silver nitrate has the highest risk of causing persistent pigmentary change after application.[10] Silver nitrate may permanently tattoo the skin black with silver. Silver nitrate has been used to treat umbilical granulomas in infants, but there are better and safer options for this and for skin hemostasis.[11]

Electrocoagulation

Electrocoagulation is an ideal method to control bleeding during surgery. *See videos 4.2–4.4.* Electrocoagulation is essential in most elliptical excisions and flaps. Some cyst and lipoma excisions will not need electrocoagulation, but it is best to be prepared with the electrosurgery instrument in the room. During surgery, electrocoagulation helps to produce a relatively bloodless field (Figure 4.4). This helps to see the landmarks for placing both deep and superficial sutures. Electrocoagulation can prevent postoperative bleeding and hematoma formation.

Electrocoagulation is an alternate method of hemostasis after a superficial or deep shave biopsy. It can also be used as a backup in the rare instance in which chemical agents fail to provide hemostasis after a shave biopsy or excision. First dry the surgical field with a cotton-tipped applicator or gauze before using electrocoagulation, especially after a chemical agent in an alcohol solution has been used. Use the minimum amount of current needed for hemostasis because more tissue destruction will increase the risk of scarring.

Electrosurgery is an ideal method for hemostasis when tissue destruction is desired. This is true when shaving off a pyogenic granuloma or hemangioma. The electrodestruction diminishes the likelihood of regrowth of vascular tissue while achieving hemostasis. Another example of this is during electrodesiccation and curettage of a basal cell carcinoma (BCC). The electrodesiccation simultaneously destroys malignant tissue and produces hemostasis. (See Chapter 14 for further information on this procedure.)

In surgical wounds that need closure, it is important not to use so much electrocoagulation that it produces large areas of char and tissue necrosis. This can increase the risk of wound infection. When a vessel is not responding to electrocoagulation, use a suture. A figure-of-eight suture is hemostatic when applied correctly around bleeding vessels and tissue (Figure 4.5). For example, if you are already

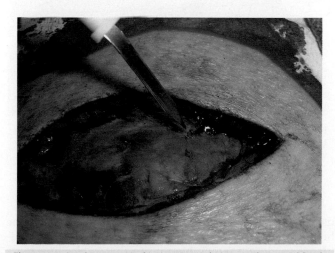

Figure 4.4 An electrosurgical instrument is being used to stop bleeders after undermining the wound edges. Note that the surgical assistant is using two skin hooks to hold open the undermined skin while the clinician is using the Hyfrecator to stop the bleeding. (Copyright Richard P. Usatine, MD.)

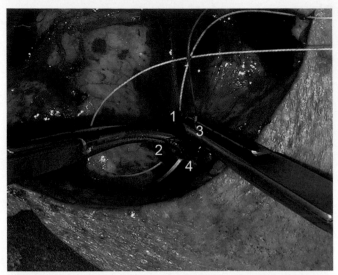

Figure 4.5 The figure-of-eight suture can be used to stop bleeding with a deep absorbable suture. A figure-of-eight suture pulls tissue together to tamponade bleeding vessels. Start the figure-of-eight by clamping the bleeding vessel or tissue with one or two hemostats. The bleeding should stop before proceeding with the suture. Insert the needle with absorbable suture at #1, going over the hemostat and exiting the tissue at #2. Reload the needle and insert the needle at #3 and exit at #4 with the second stitch parallel to the first. Then tie the suture between points #1 and #4, creating the crossover figure-of-eight suture. The hemostat may be released once the first or second tie is in place. (Copyright Richard P. Usatine, MD.)

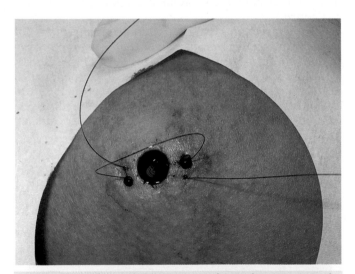

Figure 4.6 The figure-of-eight suture can be used to stop a punch biopsy from bleeding with nonabsorbable suture on the surface. (Copyright Richard P. Usatine, MD.)

using Vicryl for your deep sutures, just use this for the hemostatic stitch. Another use for the figure-of-eight suture is to close a punch biopsy site that is bleeding more than usual (Figure 4.6). This is accomplished with nonabsorbable suture. Any punch biopsy could be closed this way, and doing this can be an opportunity to practice the figure-of-eight suture.

Electrosurgical Equipment and Its Use

Electrosurgical equipment uses an alternating current transferred to the patient through cold electrodes. The tissue is heated through tissue resistance to the current. The current used can range from 0.5 MHz to 4 MHz (radiofrequency). There are many types of electrosurgical units, which are covered in detail in Chapter 13.

Regardless of the type of unit used, there are four major ways to produce electrocoagulation:

1. Electrode directly contacts the bleeding site or vessel.
2. Electrode is touched to a hemostat or forceps that is grasping the bleeding tissue or vessel and then activated.
3. Special bipolar forceps grasp the tissue and are activated with a foot peddle (Figure 4.7).
4. Cut with coagulation; a number of electrosurgical units can cut tissue and produce hemostasis simultaneously (see Chapter 14, *Electrosurgery*).

Working in a Bloody Field

Bipolar forceps have the advantage of potentially working in a bloody field that is not entirely dry. It is still best to dry the field as much as possible. The current can still pass through the bleeding tissue despite the presence of some blood (they will not work in a pool of blood). When a standard electrode is not working because the field has too much blood, it may help to grasp the bleeding tissue with a hemostat or forceps until the bleeding slows and then direct the current through the instrument to stop the bleeding (often a high current setting is needed for this). The bipolar forceps is safer than a monopolar electrode in a patient with a pacemaker or implantable defibrillator (see Chapter 14, *Electrosurgery*).

In Figure 4.8, a pyogenic granuloma was just shaved off the lip of a postpartum woman. A dry cotton-tipped applicator was rolled ahead of the electrode with pressure to dry

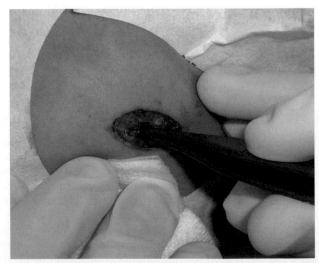

Figure 4.7 Bipolar forceps are useful for focused hemostasis and safer when the patient has a pacemaker. (Copyright Richard P. Usatine, MD.)

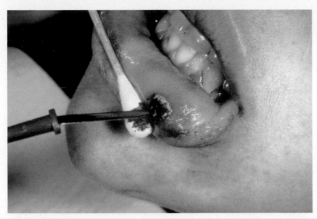

Figure 4.8 After excising a pyogenic granuloma from the lip, a Hyfrecator is being used to destroy any remaining abnormal tissue and to achieve hemostasis. Note that the cotton-tipped applicator is being rolled just ahead of the electrosurgical electrode. (Copyright Richard P. Usatine, MD.)

the field for electrocoagulation with a Hyfrecator electrode. Because this was a very vascular lesion, the electrocoagulation was applied as the cotton-tipped applicator was lifted from the bleeding site.

Sterile vs Nonsterile Procedures

Because a shave excision does not need to be a sterile procedure, the handpiece and the electrode should be clean but do not have to be sterile. However, when doing an excision in which sutures will be placed, it is optimal if the electrode is sterile, and the handpiece is either sterile or covered in a sterile sheath. Most cutting units have a handpiece that can be sterilized in an autoclave. Sterile handpiece sheaths for use in sterile surgical procedures are available for the Hyfrecator and similar units. A sterile surgical glove may also be used as a sterile sheath by placing the handpiece through one of the longer fingers on the glove.

When to use electrocoagulation:

- In a wound that will be closed with sutures
- To obtain a relatively bloodless field during surgery
- To prevent postoperative bleeding and hematomas
- When the chemical hemostatic agent fails after a shave biopsy or shave excision
- When tissue destruction is desired (e.g., with removal of a BCC or a pyogenic granuloma)

Hemostasis Around the Eye

All the hemostatic chemicals can be damaging to the eye. Exercise great caution when using chemical agents after a shave or snip (scissors) biopsy on the eyelids or near the eye. The chemical from a dripping CTA can run into the eye when the biopsy is close to the globe. The Cryo Tweezer described in Chapter 13 is a preferred method for treating skin

tags or warts around the eye to avoid chemical exposures. If aluminum chloride is to be used in this location, dry off the chemical agent on the cotton-tipped applicator with a gauze pad before carefully touching the cotton-tipped applicator to the eyelid or periocular skin. If any chemical does get into the eye, the eye should be flushed immediately. Using electrosurgery for hemostasis can also keep chemicals away from the eye.

When using electrocoagulation near the eye, the physician should be aware that the spark will arc to the area closest to the electrode. Make sure that the treatment area is closer to the electrode than the globe. A spark to the globe is potentially damaging to the eye.

Mechanical Hemostasis: Pressure and Sutures

The direct application of pressure works to slow and stop bleeding in many surgical procedures. A blood vessel or pumping arteriole that does not stop bleeding with electrocoagulation can be tied off with suture. Suturing a wound closed is another form of pressure application that brings the two open sides in direct opposition to each other. Packing an open wound with gauze (such as a drained abscess) also is a form of direct application of internal pressure.

FIGURE-OF-EIGHT SUTURE – *See Video 4.5*

Buried

In skin surgery, blood vessels or nonstop bleeding areas may require tying off with suture. It is usually quicker to use the electrosurgery unit for small bleeders, but larger blood vessels and pumping arterioles usually need to be ligated with sutures. These vessels can be clamped with 1 or 2 hemostats and tied off with absorbable sutures (such as Vicryl). The figure-of-eight suture is useful in this setting (Figure 4.5).

A figure-of-eight pulls tissue together to tamponade bleeding vessels and tissue.

- Start the figure-of-eight by clamping the bleeding vessel or tissue with a hemostat. The bleeding should stop before proceeding with the absorbable suture.
- Insert the suture needle close to and below the hemostat and grasp some tissue.
- Reload the needle and make a second pass close to and above the hemostat parallel to the first pass below.
- Tie the suture with an instrument tie, creating the crossover figure-of-eight suture.
- Release the hemostat carefully once the first or second instrument tie is in place and complete four instrument ties.

Superficial

The figure-of-eight suture is useful to close a punch biopsy that is bleeding more than usual (Figure 4.6). In fact, any punch biopsy may be closed this way to get practice with the figure-of-eight suture for when it is needed in the more tense situation of deeper nonstop bleeding.

Oozing on the Edges

Horizontal mattress sutures can be used to stop oozing on the edges of the wound and achieve wound eversion (Figure 4.9). Also, a running locked suture (Figure 4.10) provides more hemostasis than a running suture that is not locked. In most skin surgery the locking is not needed and increases the risk of necrosis of the wound edges. When bleeding is continuing despite other methods, the benefits may outweigh the risk of locking the sutures.

Pressure Dressing and Postoperative Care

After suturing an elliptical excision, it is wise to apply a pressure dressing to decrease the risk of hematoma formation. This can be left in place for 24 to 48 hours and is described further in Chapter 25, *Wound Care*. We recommend that patients apply direct pressure for 5 to 10 minutes by the clock if there is postoperative bleeding after leaving the office. Increasingly longer periods of time can be attempted as needed. Of course, if the bleeding continues patients will need to access direct care.

PHYSICAL AGENTS

Several physical agents produce hemostasis. These include the absorbable gelatin foam sponges such as Surgifoam (Figure 4.11A) and Gelfoam.[12,13] A piece of a gelatin sponge can be placed into the hole of a punch biopsy that is not sutured (Figure 4.11B). This can be very helpful when performing a punch biopsy on the scalp or on the edge of an ulcer (Figure 4.12).[14] These sponges can be used to stop the bleeding on the edge of an ulcer that was biopsied when the compromised tissue is not adequate to hold a suture (Figure 4.13C).

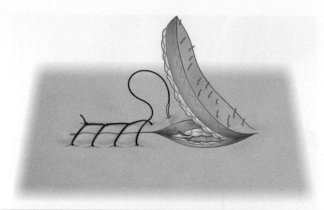

Figure 4.10 A running locked suture provides more hemostasis than a running suture that is not locked. (From Robinson J, Hanke W, Sengelmann R, Siegel D. *Surgery of the Skin. Procedural Dermatology.* 2nd ed. Mosby; 2010.)

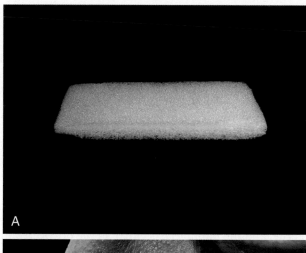

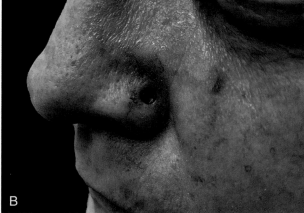

Figure 4.11 (A) Surgifoam (absorbable gelatin foam) comes in large white strips to be cut down as needed for hemostasis. **(B)** Surgifoam placed in this 3 mm punch biopsy on the nasal ala achieved hemostasis easily instead of a suture to avoid distortion of the anatomy. (Copyright Richard P. Usatine, MD.)

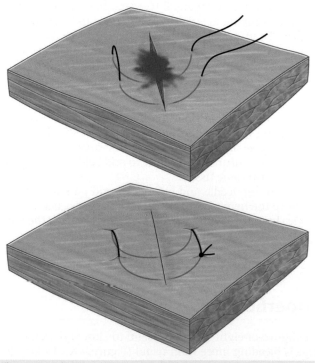

Figure 4.9 A horizontal mattress suture can be used to minimize oozing at the cut edges. (From Robinson J, Hanke W, Sengelmann R, Siegel D. *Surgery of the Skin: Procedural Dermatology.* 2nd ed. Mosby; 2010.)

- Absorbable Gelatin Foam Sponge (Ethicon Surgifoam™) is made from porcine gelatin. It provides a matrix for platelet aggregation and adhesion. It is also antibacterial. Surgifoam comes in various sizes and can be cut to place in and around biopsy sites for hemostasis in lieu of sutures.

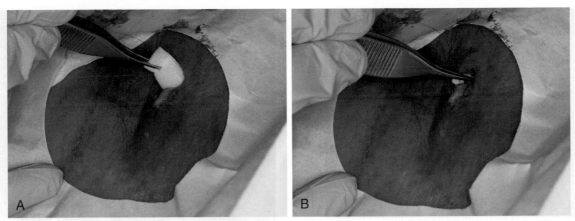

Figure 4.12 Surgifoam placed in this double punch biopsy on the edge of an ulcer achieved hemostasis instead of a suture as the tissue was not healthy enough to hold a suture. (Copyright Richard P. Usatine, MD.)

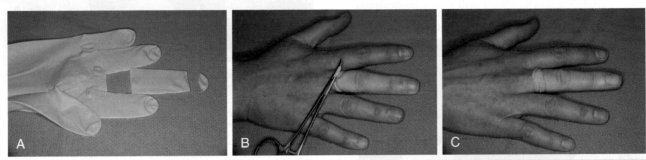

Figure 4.13 A tourniquet can be made with a surgical glove to create a bloodless field for finger or toe surgery. **(A)** A finger from a sterile surgical glove is severed at both its base and its tip. **(B)** The cylinder created is placed over the tip of the finger and rolled back proximally, forming the tourniquet. Note the finger blanching. **(C)** The tourniquet can be controlled easily with a curved hemostat. This provides additional compression and ensures the tourniquet is not forgotten at the end of the procedure. (Copyright Richard P. Usatine, MD.)

- Gelatin (Gelfoam™) is a hygroscopic absorbing material. It is available in foams/sponges, powders, and sheets/films. The sponge/foam may be tailored in strips to be applied in moist areas together with sutures. It may harbor infections.[15]
- Cellulose (Surgicel™, Oxycel™) is processed from plant fiber that is oxidized in the presence of nitrogen dioxide to form cellulosic acid. This absorbable material is trimmed in strips (mesh, gauze, sponge) and placed in the wound bed; it becomes gelatinous in 24 to 48 hours and degrades in 1 to 6 weeks. Occasionally, this material can lead to foreign body reaction.[15]
- Microfibrillar collagen (Avitene™, Instat™) is a bovine collagen derivative created by processing raw product into collagen fibrils. It comes in several forms including powder/flour, sheets, and sponges. It claims to be a more effective hemostatic material than gelatin or cellulose.[15]

Steps to follow for absorbable gelatin foam sponge in a punch biopsy:

- Cut a piece of absorbable gelatin foam sponge equal to 2 to 3 times the punch biopsy width before starting the procedure (Figure 4.12).
- Immediately after the punch specimen is removed insert the sponge.
- If there is brisk or arterial bleeding, a wider diameter of gelatin foam may be needed. Apply pressure until the foam expands and the bleeding stops.[14]

- If needed, an assistant may press a circular scissor handle firmly into the skin surrounding the site to slow the bleeding while the foam is inserted (see details below under instrument tamponade).[16]

Using Tourniquets, Clamps, and Instruments to Prevent Bleeding

- Tourniquets for digital surgery can be made with a surgical glove to decrease bleeding during finger and toe surgery (Figure 4.13).
- A chalazion clamp was designed to keep a bloodless field on the eyelid when removing a chalazion. Larger chalazion clamps are very useful for lip surgery to provide hemostasis and control the surgical field (Figure 4.14).
- Safe time duration for tourniquets and clamp use lacks evidence, so recommendations vary from 20 minutes to over 2 hours. In a large study of tourniquet use in hand surgery, even those 60 patients whose tourniquet time exceeded 2 hours showed no postoperative complications.[17] Durations of 20 to 30 minutes should be safe in most cases.
- Instrument tamponade is a method described by Whalen et al. for hemostasis during a punch biopsy of the scalp.[16] An assistant uses the circular handle of an instrument

5 Selecting the Right Suture

ALBA POSLIGUA, MD, NAIARA S. BARBOSA, MD, DANIEL L. STULBERG, MD, and
RICHARD P. USATINE, MD

SUMMARY

- Suture is a surgical material formed by a needle and a strand used for wound closure.
- For office practice, we will focus on sutures used for dermatologic wounds and procedures, including biopsies and excisions.
- Many types of sutures are available, each with its own properties, performance, and uses. Choosing among this wide variety of available materials depends on many factors including type and size of wound, site, surgeon's experience, suture's ease of use, and expected healing.
- Understanding the characteristics of each suture is crucial when deciding which material to use for any given wound.

Introduction

Suture is a surgical material formed by a needle and a strand used for wound closure. For office practice, we will focus on sutures used for dermatologic wounds and procedures, including biopsies and excisions. Many types of sutures are available, each with its own properties, performance, and uses. Choosing among this wide variety of available materials depends on many factors including type and size of wound, site, surgeon's experience, suture's ease of use, cost and expected healing.[1] Understanding the characteristics of each suture is crucial when deciding which material to use for any given wound.[2]

In this chapter, we will discuss the following.

- Wound healing and sutures
- Suture needle
  - Types of points/tips
  - Body of the needle
  - Swage or shank
- Suture material (strand)
  - Characteristics and mechanical properties
  - Types
- Other wound closure materials
  - Staples
  - Tissue adhesives
  - Skin tape or surgical strips
- Selecting the right suture
  - Properties
  - Advantages and disadvantages of commonly available sutures
  - Practical recommendations for outpatient practice
  - Alternative materials for wound closure

Wound Healing and Sutures

All sutures are foreign bodies and may increase the risk of wound infection if not used properly or left in place too long. The goal is to use the minimum suture required to keep the wound together until it heals. Deep (buried) or subcuticular sutures are beneficial in keeping wounds closed without leaving marks on the skin. External sutures are left in place just long enough to keep the wound closed because each extra day increases the risk of "railroad track" skin marking. Smaller sutures generally leave fewer skin marks and can lead to a better cosmetic result.

Wound healing is described by tensile strength, the force per unit area required to pull a wound apart. Studies show that a wound does not begin to gain significant tensile strength until about 3 weeks after closure, at which point it has only 10% of its final tensile strength. Tensile strength increases more quickly after 3 weeks and reaches its maximum strength at around 60 days. It never returns to more than 80% of normal skin.[3] Thus wounds subject to any tension should usually be closed in two layers: a deeper dermal layer with suture material that will maintain significant strength for 6 to 8 weeks and a second superficial skin suture that can be removed in 7 days or less without fear of wound disruption. A suture or staple left in the skin for more than 10 days will often allow epithelial cells to grow from the surface down into the dermis along the suture or staple tract, resulting in permanent scar tissue on each side of the incision scar itself and detracting from the final appearance of the healed wound. In addition, a suture that is tied too tight will cause necrosis and subsequent scarring of the enclosed tissue within the loop, resulting in cross-hatch marks, or "railroad tracks." The goal of the superficial suture layer is to carefully approximate the epidermis, not to add significant strength to the closure. The deeper dermal sutures should take nearly all tension off the epidermal closure.

SUTURE ANATOMY

Sutures are composed of the packaging, the needle, and the strand.[1] The packaging is important to keep the suture sterile and to avoid physical damage. It is composed of an inner and outer package, and it provides information regarding the type and size of suture strand and needle (Figure 5.1).

SUTURE NEEDLE

Suture needles are composed of three parts: the point or tip, the body, and the swage or shank (Figure 5.2). The ideal needle should be sharp and firm to allow entry into the tissue yet bend before breaking and be as atraumatic as possible. Most needles are made of stainless steel, with different available alloys including nickel, titanium, and molybdenum. Some are coated with a micro layer of silicon that helps to decrease the force needed to pass through the tissue and retain sharpness longer. The point goes from the tip to the maximum cross-section of the body and is the first portion of the suture that penetrates the tissue.[4]

Types of Points/Tips

Needle tips can be round (blunt) or triangular (cutting). The round tip lacks a cutting edge, and its taper ratio determines its sharpness (8:1–12:1). These are best for tissue that might easily tear, such as subcutaneous fat, and not as useful for dermis and epidermis. Therefore round-tip needles are infrequently used in dermatologic procedures. The

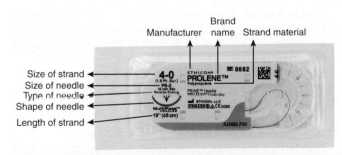

Figure 5.1 Suture package information.

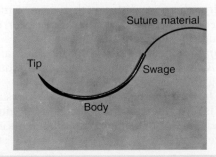

Figure 5.2 Suture parts, note the reverse cutting tip.

triangular tip, more commonly used, is further classified as conventional cutting and reverse cutting (Figure 5.3).[4]

- Conventional cutting tip has three sharp edges, and the major cutting edge is on the inner portion of the needle. It cuts tissue as it passes, and it has an increased risk of tissue tearing and strand damage. It is useful for suturing skin, but it should be avoided in friable tissue such as mucosa and tendon.[4]
- Reverse cutting tip possesses three sharp edges, and the major cutting edge is on the outer portion of the needle. It cuts the tissue as it passes but it has a decreased risk of tissue tearing. It is useful for suturing skin, and it is the most popular needle in dermatology.

Needles from Ethicon used in skin surgery are named with the following nomenclature:

- **P or PS** (plastic): fine reverse-cutting plastics needle
- **PC** (precision cosmetic): fine conventional cutting plastics needle
- **FS** (for skin): basic reverse-cutting skin needle – not as sharp as the plastics needles

Body of the Needle

The body of the needle is the distance along the arc between the tip to the end of the shank. This is the portion that is grasped by the needle holder for the placement of a stitch. This area should be as close as possible to the diameter of the suture strand to avoid trauma. It may be rectangular or flattened to improve the grasping and decrease the risk of needle bending. Its curvature can be 1/4, 3/8, 1/2, or 5/8 of a circle. The most common needle curvatures used in dermatologic surgery are 3/8 followed by 1/2.[4,5]

In our practice, PS-2 and P-3 needles are the most commonly used for biopsies and excisions. PS-2 needles are bigger and therefore better for thicker sutures (often used on trunk and extremities), such as 3-0 and 4-0, while P-3 needles are smaller and better for finer sutures (often used on the face and neck), such as 5-0 and 6-0.

NEEDLE LENGTH

Needle length is chosen based on the skin thickness and the desired length of the placed sutures. When closing thin skin on the face or genital area, a 13-mm needle length is a good choice for both the absorbable and nonabsorbable sutures. When suturing the back, it helps to have a longer needle such as one that is 19 mm in length. For other areas of intermediate skin thickness, a 16-mm needle length should be adequate.

Keep in mind that a larger needle allows for larger and fewer stitches when running a suture whether it is external or subcuticular. A 16-mm needle is a good length for closing a punch biopsy regardless of the location. With experience, your choices may vary and be different based on personal preference (Figure 5.4).

Swage or Shank

The needle swage or shank is connected to the strand through a laser-drilled swage that minimizes skin trauma. In the past, the suture was threaded through the eye of the needle, which due to its thickness, could lead to significant skin trauma.[4]

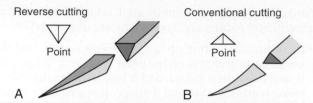

Figure 5.3 (A) Reverse-cutting needles. **(B)** Conventional cutting needles. (Redrawn from and courtesy of Ethicon product catalog Sutures/Adhesives/Drains/Hernia Repair.)

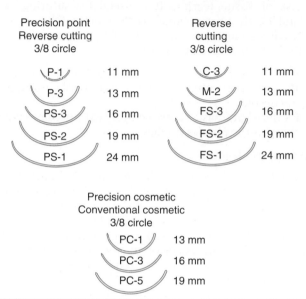

Figure 5.4 Needles for skin surgery. (Adapted from Ethicon product catalog Sutures/Adhesives/Drains/Hernia Repair.)

SUTURE MATERIAL (STRAND)

The ideal suture strand should be strong, easy to handle, visible, and able to stretch and coil with the swelling of the tissue and have good knot security with little tissue reaction, risk of trauma, or infection. Suture materials can be classified by their configuration (monofilament vs multifilament or braided), origin (natural vs synthetic), or by their degradation ability (absorbable vs nonabsorbable).[2]

Suture Material Characteristics and Properties

Size: suture strand size is determined using the United States Pharmacopeia (USP) system. The more zeros after the USP number, the smaller the suture is. A 6-0 suture is smaller than a 3-0.[1] Another important factor that determines the diameter of a suture is its chemical composition; for example, a 5-0 nylon is smaller than a 5-0 surgical gut.

A procedure on the trunk or extremities will likely require a larger suture size (3-0 or 4-0 suture) compared to a procedure on the face or neck (5-0 or 6-0 suture).[5]

Origin: suture strand origin is based on whether a suture is derived from natural sources (e.g., silk, surgical gut) versus synthetic (e.g., polypropylene, nylon). Natural suture materials produce a higher inflammatory reaction and are degraded by proteolysis. Absorbable synthetic materials are degraded by hydrolysis.[1]

Coating: suture strands can be coated with antibiotics (triclosan). This theoretically reduces the colonization of the material. Nevertheless, studies have been inconclusive regarding reduction of surgical site infection. Sutures with antibiotic coating often will have "Plus" as part of their name, such as Vicryl Plus™, Monocryl Plus™, and PDS™ II Plus.[6]

Configuration: sutures can be monofilament or multifilament (also known as braided). If composed of one single strand, it is called monofilament; if composed of braided strands, this is a multifilament.[7] A monofilament suture in general has the benefits of having lower coefficient of friction, tissue reactivity, capillarity, and risk of infection, but they must be handled carefully due to the risk of breakage, less knot security, and ease of handling.[1,6]

Tensile strength: the ability to approximate the tissue wound edges without breaking the suture strand. Larger sutures (e.g., 3-0) have increased tensile strength compared to smaller ones (e.g., 6-0); synthetic materials are generally stronger than natural ones. Multifilaments have greater tensile strength than monofilaments.[5]

Visibility: the ability to readily see the suture when placing it. Polypropylene (Prolene™) is blue and polyglactin 910 (Vicryl™) is white; but polyglecaprone-25 (Monocryl™) and polydioxanone (PDS™) are usually see through. These undyed strands have the benefit of avoiding an unsightly show through the skin when placed intradermally.[1,8]

Capillarity: the capacity to absorb the bodily fluids where it will be immersed. Multifilaments have increased capillarity which may promote more organism accumulation and therefore more infections compared to monofilaments.[9]

Coefficient of friction: the ease of passing a suture through the tissue. It is directly related to the knot stability. A monofilament has less coefficient of friction compared to a multifilament.[2]

Elasticity: the capacity of a material to return to its original length after being stretched. This is relevant when the tissue develops edema after a procedure; an elastic suture would not cut the skin or create necrosis, and it will approximate once this phenomenon subsides.[2]

Plasticity: the ability of a suture to be permanently altered to a new shape or length. This is important because if there is tissue edema, the suture will stretch, but in contrast to an elastic material, this strand will be loose after this event.[2]

Pliability: the ease with which a given suture bends. Multifilaments have more pliability, are easier to handle, and have higher knot security.[6]

Memory: the capability of a suture to maintain its original shape. A suture with an increased memory has less ease of handling and knot security.[2]

Ease of handling: the ability to handle the suture comfortably. It is directly related to pliability and knot security, and inversely related to memory. Multifilaments are usually easier to work with.[1]

Knot security: the likelihood that a knot will hold without slipping.[2] The knot remains tied due to the suture configuration and coefficient of friction. A multifilament suture with intrinsic high coefficient of friction has a more secure knot compared to a monofilament. It is inversely related to memory. The minimum number of throws that a multifilament knot should have is two; if this is a monofilament, more throws should be made.[10]

Tissue reactivity: all sutures are foreign body materials that will elicit different levels of tissue reactions. Multifilament, natural material, such as silk (nonabsorbable) or catgut (absorbable), will have more tissue reactivity than the monofilament synthetic sutures.[2]

Spitting potential: the likelihood that the suture will be extruded from the tissue (for buried absorbable materials). Polyglactin-910 (Vicryl™) has an increased spitting potential (Figure 5.5).[1]

Suture Material Types by Their Degradation Ability

Absorbable Sutures. Absorbable sutures are usually used as intradermal/subcutaneous sutures for decreasing the tension, dead space, and increasing the wound edge approximation. They are often referred to as "deep or subcutaneous sutures." A material is considered absorbable if it loses most of its tensile strength within 60 days after placing the suture.[11] The degradation of a suture may be affected by different factors including in what part of the body it is placed (e.g., faster in mucosa/moist areas), if a patient is febrile, protein deficient, stressed, has diabetes, or other systemic diseases.[2]

The most commonly used sutures for dermatologic procedures are polyglactin-910 (Vicryl™), polyglecaprone-25 (Monocryl™), and polydioxanone (PDS™).[12]

Monocryl™ and PDS™ are synthetic monofilaments, and as discussed before, their advantages include decreased coefficient of friction, tissue reactivity, capillarity, and risk of infection. Monocryl™ has increased ease of handling, pliability, knot security, and less memory compared to PDS™.

Vicryl™ is a synthetic multifilament and the most used absorbable suture. Its benefits include ease of handling, knot security, pliability, and is not as reactive as the natural origin sutures. Its disadvantages include less elasticity and increased risk of spitting suture.[1]

Surgical gut is a natural origin multifilament suture, and it has increased tissue reactivity. It may be helpful as superficial skin sutures in low tension areas, for placement of skin grafts, or in a small defect or punch biopsy site when patients are unable to return for suture removal.[13] Absorbable sutures are further characterized in Table 5.1.

NONABSORBABLE SUTURES

Nonabsorbable sutures are frequently used for surface sutures, and their purpose is to approximate the superficial portion of a wound and are referred to as "top or skin sutures." These are resistant to degradation and require manual removal. Usually, they are removed within 5 to 7 days when on the face or neck, and 10 to 14 days when on the trunk or extremities. The most commonly used nonabsorbable sutures for dermatologic procedures are nylon (Ethilon™), polypropylene (Prolene™), and silk.[2] Ethilon™ is the most used synthetic nonabsorbable suture. It has similar ease of handling and knot security versus the more expensive Prolene™; nevertheless, the latter has the least tissue reactivity, it is helpful for running subcuticular placement, and its plasticity allows it to stretch to accommodate postsurgical edema without cutting/traumatizing the surrounding tissue. Silk is an organic nonabsorbable suture that is easy to handle and has great knot security, but it generates high tissue reactivity. It is the most commonly used suture in mucosal repairs due to its cost-effectiveness, softness, and comfort on these areas.[9] Nonabsorbable sutures are further characterized in Table 5.2.

ALTERNATIVE WOUND CLOSURE MATERIALS

Staples

The nonabsorbable (Proximate™) staples are made of stainless steel, which is one of the least reactive materials, but its price can be higher. These are helpful in high-tension and thicker skin areas, such as the scalp.[14] The absorbable (Insorb™) staples are for subcuticular placement and are composed of a polylactide/polyglycolide absorbable copolymer. These are useful in areas with increased risk of infection and can be time-saving in place of sutures.[15] Most often, we reserve the use of staples for larger incisions (>7.5 cm) on the scalp, trunk, or extremities.

Tissue Adhesives

Adhesives are practical in low-tension areas where the deep dermis has been already well approximated. These materials keep the epidermis intact, are easy and fast to apply, avoid risk of suture track marks, and do not require

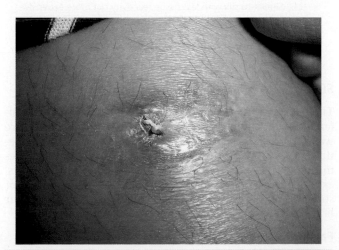

Figure 5.5 Spitting suture of Vicryl after a two-layer repair on the leg. (Copyright Richard P. Usatine, MD.)

Table 5.1   Characteristics of Absorbable Sutures

Suture	Absorption	Ease of Handling	Knot Security	Tissue Reactivity	Comments
MONOFILAMENTS					
Polyglecaprone-25 (Monocryl™)	90–120 days	↑	↑	↓↓	Least reactive, more elastic. Used in cosmetically sensitive and lower tension wounds.
Polydioxanone (PDS™)	180–240 days	↓	↓	↓	Longest-lasting absorbable material. Used in wounds with moderate to high tension.
Polyglyconate, glycolic acid (Maxon™)	180 days	↑	↑	↓	Better ease of handling and knot security than PDS™. Used in higher tension wounds.
Glycomer 631 (Byosin™)	90–110 days	↑	↓	↓	Useful in higher tension areas.
MULTIFILAMENTS					
Fast-absorbing gut	21–42 days	↑	↓	↓	Used as dissolving top sutures.
Plain gut	70 days	↑	↓	↑↑↑	Most reactive suture.
Chromic gut	90 days	↓	↓	↑↑	Lasts longer and less reactive than plain gut.
Fast-absorbing polyglactin 910 (Vicryl Rapide™)	42 days	↑↑	↑↑	↓	Useful for skin grafts.
Polyglactin 910 (Vicryl™)	56–70 days	↑↑	↑↑	↓	Increased risk of suture spitting. Used in high tension wounds.
Polyglycolic acid (Dexon™)	90 days	↑↑	↑↑	↓	

Table 5.2   Characteristics of Nonabsorbable Sutures

Suture	Ease of Handling	Knot Security	Tissue Reactivity	Comments
MONOFILAMENTS				
Nylon (Ethilon™)	↑	↓↓	↓↓	Most commonly used top suture.
Polypropylene (Prolene™)	↑	↓↓	↓↓↓	Least reactive of all nonabsorbable sutures. High plasticity. Used in cosmetically sensitive areas and sites with high risk of infection. Blue color makes it more visible on scalp.
Polybuster (Novafil™)	↑	↓↓	↓↓	Most elastic of nonabsorbable sutures.
MULTIFILAMENTS				
Silk	↑↑↑	↑↑	↑↑↑	Most easy-to-handle suture. Second most reactive suture, after surgical gut. Used in mucosa due to its soft nature.
Polyester (Ethibond™, Mersilene™)	↑↑	↑↑	↓↓	Similar to silk with less tissue reactivity but more expensive. Highest tensile strength of nonabsorbable sutures.

removal.[16] These should not be used in open, deep, mucosal, or infected wounds.[17] Most commonly, we reserve the use of adhesives for cosmetically sensitive incisions that are low-tension and fully approximated with subcutaneous sutures.

Available adhesive products include 2-octylcyanoacrylate (Dermabond™, Band-Aid Liquid Bandage™), butyl cyanoacrylate (LiquiBand™), N-butyl-2-cyanoacrylate (GluSeal™), and gum mastic (Mastisol™), which is frequently used in conjunction with surgical strips.

Skin Tape or Surgical Strips

Surgical strips have the benefit of keeping the epidermis intact, similar to the tissue adhesives. The most used brand is Steri-Strips™.[18]

SELECTING THE RIGHT SUTURE

The sutures or wound closure material will depend on different factors including its location, what kind of procedure was performed, the tension that it may have, and sometimes even the patient's ability to return for suture removal.[14] The suggestions below are based on the authors' experience (see also Tables 5.3 and 5.4). The examples of sutures included are the ones available for this particular brand, but many comparable alternatives are available.

Face

- Deep – Polyglactin (Vicryl) or polyglecaprone-25 (Monocryl) 4-0 and 5-0 with 13- and 16-mm needles
- Surface – Nylon (Ethilon) or polypropylene (Prolene), 5-0 (6-0 optional) with 13- and 16-mm needles

Table 5.3 Suggested Suture Selections by Location for Excision

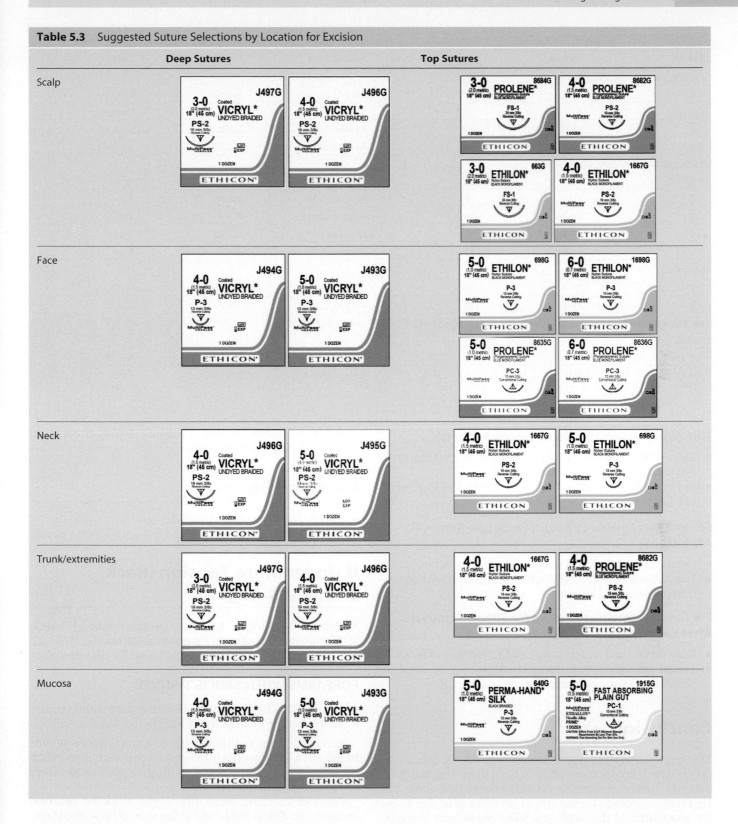

Scalp, Extremities or Trunk

- Deep – Polyglactin (Vicryl) or polyglecaprone-25 (Monocryl) 4-0 with 16-mm needle
- Surface – Nylon or polypropylene 4-0 and 5-0 with 16-mm needle

If Under More Tension (Back, Shoulders, Legs)

- Deep – Polyglactin (Vicryl), 4-0 with 16-mm needle (3-0 with 19-mm needle optional for greatest tension)
- Surface – Nylon and/or Prolene 4-0 with 16- to 19-mm needle

Table 5.4   Details of Some Recommended Sutures

Suture	Needle	Needle Size (mm)	Needle Type	Order #	Color
COATED VICRYL (POLYGLACTIN)					
5-0	P-3	13	Reverse cutting	J493G	Undyed
4-0	P-3	13	Reverse cutting	J494G	Undyed
5-0	PS-3	16	Reverse cutting	J500G	Undyed
3-0	PS-2	19	Reverse cutting	J427H	Undyed
PROLENE (POLYPROPYLENE)					
6-0	P-3	13	Reverse cutting	8695G	Blue
5-0	P-3	13	Reverse cutting	8698G	Blue
6-0	PS-3	16	Reverse cutting	8680G	Blue
5-0	PS-3	16	Reverse cutting	8681G	Blue
4-0	PS-2	19	Reverse cutting	8682G	Blue
Nylon					
5-0	PS-3	16	Reverse cutting	1668G	Black
4-0	PS-2	19	Reverse cutting	1667G	Black
BIOPSY SUTURE FOR PUNCH BIOPSIES WITH 9-INCH LENGTH SUTURE (DELASCO BRAND)					
Nylon					
5-0	FS-3	16	Reverse cutting	BDL-50B	Black
4-0	FS-3	16	Reverse cutting	BDL-40B	Black

Thin Skin (Forearms in Some Elderly Patients)

- Deep – Polyglactin (Vicryl) or polyglecaprone-25 (Monocryl) 4-0 with 13-mm reverse cutting needle
- Surface – Nylon and/or Prolene 4-0 with 16- to 19-mm needle

For Patients Unable to Return for Suture Removal After Biopsy

- Gut can be used for top sutures for small punches.
- WoundSeal™ is a cost-effective and well-tolerated option for nonfacial biopsies.

For Patients Unable to Return for Suture Removal After Excision

- Gut can be used for top suture in low-tension closures.
- Tissue adhesive (+/− surgical strips) can be used in place of top sutures in appropriate wounds.

Conclusion

The large variety of sutures available makes it difficult to decide which products are going to be right for you and your patients. Table 5.5 contains detailed information about the commonly stocked skin sutures in an office practice. To do the procedures in this book, you will need at least one type of absorbable and one type of nonabsorbable suture.

The minimum starting set of sutures should probably include:

Face

- Deep – Polyglactin (Vicryl), 4-0 and 5-0 with 13- and 16-mm needles

- Surface – Polypropylene (Prolene), 5-0 (6-0 optional) with 13- and 16-mm needles

Neck and Below

- Polyglactin (Vicryl), 4-0 with 16-mm
- Nylon or polypropylene 4-0 and 5-0 with 16-mm needle

If Under More Tension (Back, Shoulders, Legs)

- Polyglactin (Vicryl), 4-0 with 16-mm needle (3-0 with 19-mm needle optional for greatest tension)
- Nylon and/or Prolene 4-0 with 16- to 19-mm needle

FOREARMS WHEN SKIN IS THINNED

- Polyglactin (Vicryl), 4-0 with 13-mm reverse cutting needle
- Nylon and/or Prolene 4-0 with 16- to 19-mm needle

Reverse cutting is probably the best starting needle type because it will be less likely to inadvertently cut tissue. Then consider trying conventional cutting needles to see what works best in your hands.

Consider carrying some silk if you work on mucosal membranes. Silk is softer inside the mouth. Fast-absorbing sutures such as fast-absorbing gut, or Vicryl Rapide, can be used for patients who may not be able to return easily for suture removal and can also be used inside the mouth.

Add a monofilament absorbable suture such as Monocryl if you will be doing subcuticular closures in which the suture will remain in place to dissolve over time. Do not buy too many boxes of sutures at first until you settle on the sutures that will be best in your practice.

Table 5.5 Recommendation of Suture by Location

Location	Suture	Comments	Suture Removal*
Scalp	Skin: interrupted or running 3-0 or 4-0 Prolene or Nylon Galea: 3-0 Vicryl	Skin – avoid dermal sutures as these may injure hair follicles. Blue color of Prolene will allow easier suture placement and removal, especially in the midst of dark hair. (optional) Suturing galea will alleviate tension	7–10 days
Face	Deep: interrupted 4-0 or 5-0 Vicryl Surface: interrupted or running 5-0 or 6-0 Prolene or Nylon	Closure of the dermis with absorbable suture allows early skin suture removal and avoids cross-hatch marks	5–7 days
Ear	Skin: interrupted 5-0 or 6-0 Prolene or Nylon	There is no need to suture ear cartilage for routine through and through ear lacerations – closing the skin on both the anterior and posterior surface of the ear is sufficient to re-establish stability	5–7 days
Lip	Orbicularis muscle: 4-0 Vicryl Dermis: 4-0 or 5-0 Vicryl Skin: interrupted or running 5-0 or 6-0 Prolene or Nylon Oral mucosa: interrupted 5-0 Vicryl or silk	Mark the vermilion border prior to infiltration of local anesthetic – the first dermal stitch should be at this point	5–7 days for the skin sutures
Intraoral	3-0, 4-0, or 5-0 chromic gut (silk is an alternative that will require suture removal)	Size of chromic used is dependent on the tension of the closure	None
Neck	Deep: 4-0 Vicryl Surface: interrupted or running 5-0 Prolene or Nylon, or 4-0 Monocryl or Prolene subcuticular	For small wounds or lacerations in elderly individuals with thin anterior neck skin, a single layer closure is acceptable. In this case, remove sutures in 7 days, and tape wound for additional 1–2 weeks	7 days
Trunk, arms, legs	Deep: interrupted 3-0 or 4-0 Vicryl Surface: 4-0 Nylon or Prolene interrupted or running	For elderly patients with thin forearm skin, try deep sutures with a 13-mm reverse cutting needle. If this tears, a single-layer closure with mattress sutures may help when there is tension.	7–14 days
Digits	Skin: interrupted 4-0 Nylon or Prolene	Usually a single-layer closure is preferred due to the thick epidermal layer	10–14 days

*Increased time may be necessary for patients on chronic corticosteroids or in high-tension wounds.

Resources

Delasco, for ordering sutures, especially for the special punch biopsy suture – www.delasco.com

Ethicon, for an excellent online catalog of all Ethicon sutures, which can be searched by suture type or needle type – https://www.ethicon.com/na/epc/search/platform/wound%20closure?lang=en-default

References

1. Byrne M, Aly A. The surgical suture. *Aesthet Surg J*. 2019;39(suppl 2):S67-S72. doi:10.1093/asj/sjz036.
2. Hochberg J, Meyer KM, Marion MD. Suture choice and other methods of skin closure. *Surg Clin North Am*. 2009;89(3):627-641. doi:10.1016/j.suc.2009.03.001.
3. Levenson SM, Geever EF, Crowley LV, Oates JF, Berard CW, Rosen H. The healing of rat skin wounds. *Ann Surg*. 1965;161(2):293-308. doi:10.1097/00000658-196502000-00019.
4. Byrne M, Aly A. The surgical needle. *Aesthet Surg J*. 2019;39 (suppl 2):S73-S77. doi:10.1093/asj/sjz035.
5. Yag-Howard C. Sutures, needles, and tissue adhesives: a review for dermatologic surgery. *Dermatol Surg*. 2014;40(suppl 9):S3-S15. doi:10.1097/01.DSS.0000452738.23278.2d.
6. Butt E, Ashraf I, Veitch D, Wernham A. Dermatological surgery: an update on suture materials and techniques. Part 2. *Clin Exp Dermatol*. 2021;46(8):1411-1419. doi:10.1111/ced.14812.
7. Regan T, Lawrence N. Comparison of poliglecaprone-25 and polyglactin-910 in cutaneous surgery. *Dermatol Surg*. 2013;39(9):1340-1344. doi:10.1111/dsu.12265.
8. Albertini JG. Surgical pearl: gentian violet – dyed sutures improve intraoperative visualization. *J Am Acad Dermatol*. 2001;45(3):453-455. doi:10.1067/mjd.2001.113472.
9. Tajirian AL, Goldberg DJ. A review of sutures and other skin closure materials. *J Cosmet Laser Ther*. 2010;12(6):296-302. doi:10.3109/14764172.2010.538413.
10. Trimbos JB. Security of various knots commonly used in surgical practice. *Obstet Gynecol*. 1984;64(2):274-280.
11. Moy RL, Waldman B, Hein DW. A review of sutures and suturing techniques. *J Dermatol Surg Oncol*. 1992;18(9):785-795. doi:10.1111/j.1524-4725.1992.tb03036.x.
12. Lu LK, Ko JM, Lee J, et al. A randomized, prospective trial evaluating surgeon preference in selection of absorbable suture material. *J Drugs Dermatol*. 2012;11(2):196-201.
13. Ashraf I, Butt E, Veitch D, Wernham A. Dermatological surgery: an update on suture materials and techniques. Part 1. *Clin Exp Dermatol*. 2021;46(8):1400-1410. doi:10.1111/ced.14770.
14. Regula CG, Yag-Howard C. Suture products and techniques: what to use, where, and why. *Dermatol Surg*. 2015;41(10):S187-S200. doi:10.1097/DSS.0000000000000492.
15. Iavazzo C, Gkegkes ID, Vouloumanou EK, Mamais I, Peppas G, Falagas ME. Sutures versus staples for the management of surgical wounds: a meta-analysis of randomized controlled trials. *Am Surg*. 2011;77(9):1206-1221. doi:10.1177/000313481107700935.
16. Beam JW. Tissue adhesives for simple traumatic lacerations. *J Athl Train*. 2008;43(2):222-224. doi:10.4085/1062-6050-43.2.222.
17. Palm MD, Altman JS. Topical hemostatic agents: a review. *Dermatol Surg*. 2008;34(4):431-445. doi:10.1111/j.1524-4725.2007.34090.x.
18. Davis M, Nakhdjevani A, Lidder S. Suture/Steri-Strip combination for the management of lacerations in thin-skinned individuals. *J Emerg Med*. 2011;40(3):322-323. doi:10.1016/j.jemermed.2010.05.077.

6 · Suturing Techniques

DANIEL L. STULBERG, MD, and RICHARD P. USATINE, MD

SUMMARY

- Appropriate suturing techniques underly the ability to remove skin lesions and successfully repair the defects.
- Use of correct instruments facilitates suturing.
- Step-by-step instructions for simple, running, mattress, buried, figure eight, corner, and specialized techniques and closures are described.
- Undermining and attention to fragile skin and the patient's risk factors and activities help with closure and prevention of dehiscence.
- Suture removal timing and management of complications are delineated.
- Practice on simulated or animal skin models and starting with basic skills advances one's technique with experience.

Suturing techniques are a key part of the global picture of removing lesions and skillfully repairing the defect to obtain good healing and cosmetic results. Prior to starting the incision, the clinician will assess the lesion for excision and consider the margin required and its relation to adjacent structures and the relaxed skin tension lines. After this inspection, the provider will plan the excision and the anticipated repair and then select the appropriate suture to place on the surgical tray before cutting. Small punch excisions can be repaired by one or more simple interrupted sutures or an inverted figure-of-eight suture. Larger wounds may be optimally closed with a combination of buried deep sutures, mattress sutures, and simple interrupted or simple running sutures.

A good closure result depends on multiple steps. In general, the first aspect in a large excision is to make sure that there is enough stretch in the skin to close the skin edges with minimal tension. After adequate undermining, close the deep tissues with absorbable sutures to help approximate the skin edges, reduce the dead space, help with hemostasis, and reduce the risk of hematoma formation. If the skin edges are fragile or there is some tension, mattress sutures can help close the wound successfully. The final closure is most commonly performed with interrupted sutures, running simple, running horizontal mattress sutures, or running subcuticular sutures.

Basic Skills

 See Videos 6.1–6.9.

The clinician must acquire certain basic suturing skills as discussed next.

LOADING THE NEEDLE HOLDER (DRIVER)

- Even though a needle holder has holes in the handle for the thumb and a finger, it is usually easier to place sutures at the correct angle and with the correct wrist rotation by placing the needle holder in the palm of your hand instead of putting your thumb and finger in the holes (Figure 6.1).
- Grasp the needle two-thirds of the way from the point to the swaged-on thread. In most cases the needle will be loaded perpendicular to the needle holder, but for some techniques it helps to use another angle.
- Needles used for skin surgery are curved in the arc of a circle (usually 3/8 of the circle). Work with the curve of the needle and follow the arc to prevent bending the needle.

USING FORCEPS IN THE NONDOMINANT HAND

Learn to suture with a good pair of Adson forceps in the nondominant hand (Figure 6.2). The forceps can be used to:

- Hold the skin edge gently when inserting the suture needle.
- Provide some stability of the skin on the opposite side while pushing the needle through and out of the skin.
- Grasp the needle once it is pushed through the skin (this is a better method than holding the needle with the fingers). Note, that disposable Adson forceps usually do not have the ability to grasp a needle for this maneuver. This is one reason for using higher-quality instruments whenever possible.
- Hold the needle when reloading the needle holder.

PERFORMING AN INSTRUMENT TIE

See Video 6.2.

To perform a secure instrument tie (Figure 6.3A–F):

- Wrap the first throw of the knot twice around the tip of the needle holder as a surgeon's or friction knot (especially if the suture is monofilament) to hold the skin edge together better.

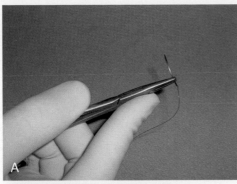

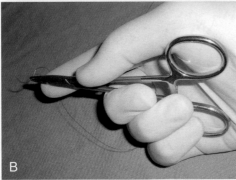

Figure 6.1 (A) Needle holder with the needle correctly loaded. **(B)** Although some surgeons prefer to put their fingers in the loops, holding the needle holder in the palm of the hand offers maximum dexterity. (Copyright Richard P. Usatine, MD.)

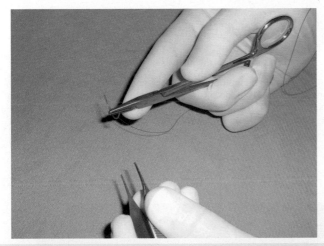

Figure 6.2 Using Adson forceps in the nondominant hand while suturing. (Copyright Richard P. Usatine, MD.)

- For external skin sutures, pull the suture with enough tension for the skin edges to just meet and not cause any puckering.
- Place the second throw and pull until it meets the first throw squarely, but do not tighten yet. Too much tension can cause a railroad or cross-hatch pattern of scarring perpendicular to the suture line.
- Place the third throw and now tighten to cinch the knot.
- For deep sutures or hemostatic sutures, pull each of the knot throws tight and secure. In general, place four throws for knots with nylon and Prolene since they have "memory" and will spring back sometimes untying the knot. Five throws

are a good idea at the beginning and end of a running suture because if it opens the whole length of the suture can be lost.
- 2 to 3 throws are adequate for braided sutures including Vicryl, but 3 to 4 throws are suggested for deep sutures under tension.

Specific Suturing Techniques

See Video 6.3.

SIMPLE INTERRUPTED SUTURE

The simple interrupted suture (Figure 6.4A) is the most basic suturing technique to master and is used to close anything from small incisions under little tension to a large excision under tension in conjunction with deep sutures.

- Pronate the wrist to place the point of the needle perpendicular (or even 10 degrees more than perpendicular away from the wound margin) to the skin.
- Rotate the needle through the skin. One mental picture for beginners is to punch the needle straight down then rotate the needle through the tissue following the arc of the needle.
- The needle should enter and exit the skin at the same depth from the skin surface on both sides to maintain good apposition.
- The needle should enter and exit the epidermis equidistant from the wound margin on each side.

The reason for creating a flask shape path is to promote eversion of the wound edge. Eversion will heal in a flat scar when the fibrosis of healing pulls the skin edges downward. Without wound eversion the scar may be depressed (Figure 6.5). While this belief in wound eversion is longstanding, one RCT seems to have put this practice into question. In this split-wound intervention, wound eversion was not significantly associated with improved overall scar assessments by blinded observers or patient assessment.[1]

As this is still controversial,[2,3] we still teach methods of obtaining eversion including the following (Figure 6.6A and B):

- Over-accentuating the arc of the needle's path to point slightly away from the skin edge and then rotating it through the skin
- Indenting the skin lateral to the wound with the forceps to deflect the skin edge upward while suturing
- Gently elevating the edge of the wound with a forceps or skin hook while placing the sutures

If the skin edges are uneven, this can be corrected by keeping the depth from the surface equal on both sides (Figure 6.7).

Simple interrupted sutures are useful for small wounds as well as for excellent control and lining up larger wounds with the rule of halves. The rule of halves is to place the first suture at the midpoint of the wound halfway from each end of the defect. Then place subsequent sutures halfway between the first suture and the end of the wound and

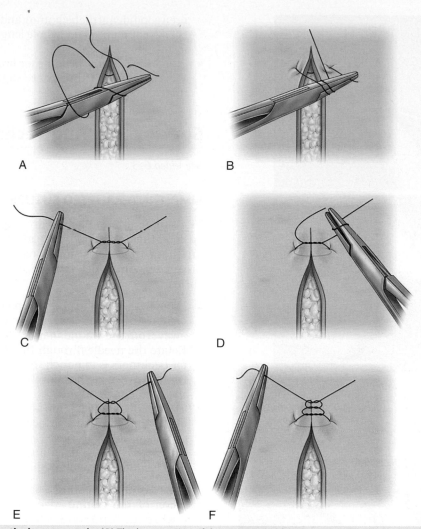

E   F

Figure 6.3 How to perform the instrument tie. (A) The long portion of the suture is held in the non-dominant hand and wrapped twice around the end of the needle driver. **(B)** The needle driver grasps the short end of the suture. The two ends of the suture are pulled taught in opposite directions **(C)**, causing the tied suture to lie flat against the closing incision. **(D)** The long end is wrapped once around the jaws of the needle holder. **(E)** The suture is again pulled taught in opposite directions. **(F)** A third throw is placed in the same fashion. (Adapted from Taylor RS. Needles, sutures, and suturing. *Atlas Office Proced.* 1999;2:53–74.)

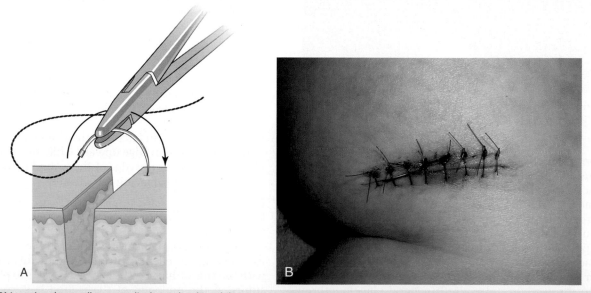

Figure 6.4 (A) Inserting the needle perpendicular to the skin while initiating a simple interrupted suture. (From Vidimos A, Ammirati C, Poblete-Lopez C. *Dermatologic Surgery.* Saunders; 2008.) **(B)** Final repair showing simple interrupted sutures all lined up with all the knots on the same side of the incision. (Copyright Richard P. Usatine, MD.)

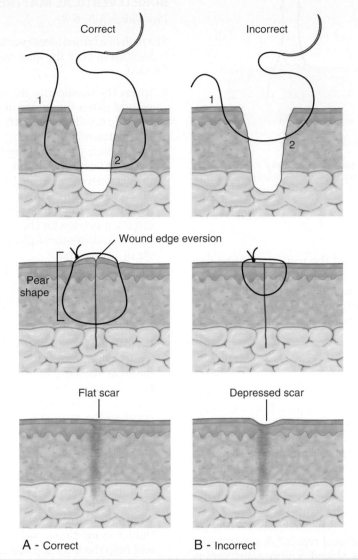

Figure 6.5 Proper placement of epidermal sutures involves looping a larger portion of the dermis and/or subcutis than the epidermis. This creates a pear-shaped suture which everts wound edges **(A)**. Failure of wound edge eversion often leads to a more depressed, noticeable scar **(B)**. Numbers indicate entry points of the needle. (Adapted from Taylor RS. Needles, sutures, and suturing. *Atlas Office Proced.* 1999;2:53–74.) (From Robinson J, Hanke W, Sengelmann R, Siegel D. *Surgery of the Skin: Procedural Dermatology.* 2nd ed. Mosby; 2010.)

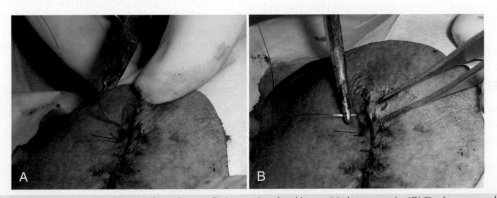

Figure 6.6 Methods for obtaining eversion. **(A)** Note how the needle is entering the skin at a 90-degree angle. **(B)** The forceps are being used to push against the skin and ensure that the needle leaves the skin at a 90-degree angle. (Copyright Richard P. Usatine, MD.)

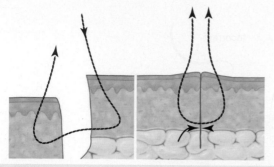

Figure 6.7 Using a simple interrupted suture to make even any skin edges that are uneven. Place the suture deep on the low side and shallow on the high side. (From Vidimos A, Ammirati C, Poblete-Lopez C. *Dermatologic Surgery*. Saunders; 2008.)

proceed in a similar fashion until the wound is closed (see Figure 11.23 in Chapter 11, *The Elliptical Excision*). This technique is useful to avoid standing cones (dog ears) at the ends from uneven suturing and can also be used to even out an asymmetrical defect where one side is longer than the other.

SPACING BETWEEN SUTURES

Sutures should be placed close enough together to preventing gapping of the skin margins. In general, this requires closer sutures in thinner versus thicker skin. The downside of more sutures is the additional time required and the risk of additional scars from needle punctures and cross hatching if the sutures are placed or become too tight due to swelling or remaining in place for longer periods. A study of face and neck repairs compared repairing one half of the suture line with running cuticular sutures placed 2 mm apart versus 5 mm apart for the other half. They found no difference in cosmesis or successful repair.[4] A general surgery study compared sutures placed 5 mm apart versus 10 mm apart in a similar fashion showed no difference in cosmesis or successful repairs for repairs on the trunk and extremities.[5] Regarding distance placing sutures away from the wound margin, a third similarly performed split study found no difference in outcomes with sutures placed 2 mm from the wound margin and 5 mm from the wound margin in head and neck repairs.[6] The provider should use this evidence along with their experience and the results as they close the wound to judge the exact suture placement within these parameters.

DEEP OR BURIED SUTURE

Deep or buried sutures are placed using absorbable suture materials. Most deep sutures are placed vertically, but deep horizontal mattress sutures may also be used, especially if there is tension.

Deep sutures perform five important functions:

- Relieve tension
- Close dead space
- Provide hemostasis
- Oppose dermis
- Produce eversion.

BURIED VERTICAL MATTRESS SUTURE
(See Videos 6.6–6.8)

The path of a buried (deep) vertical mattress suture (Figure 6.8) is designed to bury the knot and keep it from poking through the skin.

- Insert the needle into the deep dermis at the base of the wound (often the undermined area).
- Pass the needle through the tissue away from the midline of the wound and come up in the superficial dermis (approximately the dermal-epidermal junction).
- Hold the needle with your Adson forceps and let go of the needle with your needle holder.
- To avoid touching the needle with your fingers, pass the needle from the forceps back to the needle holder in the direction needed for the second half of the stitch.
- Pull the suture through, leaving a short end in the middle of the wound.
- Insert the needle at the same level in the superficial dermis directly opposite from the exit point of the first pass of the needle. Rotate the needle through the tissue coming out at the base of the wound in the undermined area at the same depth as the first suture.
- If closing a large defect with significant undermining of wound edges, use the needle to pass under a small amount of tissue at the base of the defect to attach the dermis to the underlying tissue to prevent hematoma formation.
- Tie this off with square-knot throws and cut the ends short so the knot stays deep within the wound. When tying the knot make sure both ends of the suture are on the same side of the line of the suture or the knot will not bury.
- Start with a surgeon's knot of two wraps.
- First, pull the suture perpendicular to the wound.
- Next rotate the suture 90 degrees and parallel to the wound, pulling firmly until the wound edges close tighter. Sometimes rocking the suture back and forth will help the knot slip tighter. Avoid breaking the suture as that requires starting all over again.
- Cinch the knot down tightly before starting the second throw.
- If the wound is under tension and the knot is slipping, a surgical assistant may help by holding the tissue together between the first and second knot.
- Another technique to help tie with tension on the suture is to lift the suture ends up vertically after the first throw and have an assistant pinch the suture ends together to prevent slippage until the second throw is secured.[7]

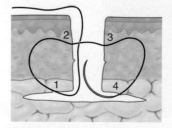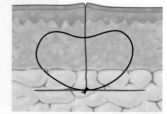

Figure 6.8 Buried vertical mattress suture. Numbers indicate entry points of the needle. (Adapted from Robinson J, Hanke W, Sengelmann R, Siegel D. *Surgery of the Skin: Procedural Dermatology*. 2nd ed. Mosby; 2010.)

BURIED VERTICAL MATTRESS SUTURE (WITH ACCENTUATED HEART SHAPE)

The buried vertical mattress suture (Figure 6.9) is created using a technique that produces a heart-shaped pattern in the deep tissue to improve wound eversion. The needle is placed as described above for a buried deep suture but will go up to the dermal-epidermal junction (DEJ) and then come out 2 mm below the DEJ. If you merely make a circle with the deep stitch, the tension vectors may pull the edges down and invert the wound.

DEEP HORIZONTAL MATTRESS SUTURE

See Video 6.9.

The deep or buried horizontal mattress suture (Figure 6.10) can be useful when it is desirable to take tension off the wound but the skin is not very thick, such as that on the face.

- Place the absorbable suture horizontally parallel to the skin surface.

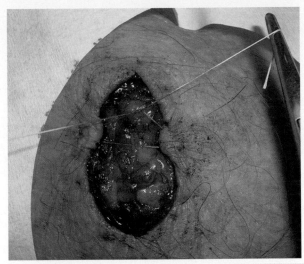

Figure 6.10 Buried (deep) horizontal mattress suture. (Copyright Richard P. Usatine, MD.)

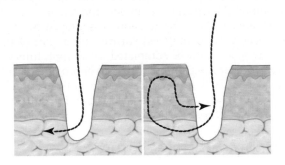

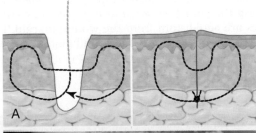

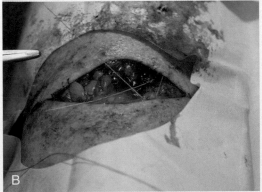

Figure 6.9 (A) This buried vertical mattress suture is a variation of the simple buried suture with the intent of increasing wound eversion. This schematic is done in an incision without undermining but can be done with an undermined excision, too. The path of the suture creates a more extreme heart shape than the previous figure. (From Vidimos A, Ammirati C, Poblete-Lopez C. *Dermatologic Surgery*. Saunders; 2008.) **(B)** Buried (deep) vertical mattress suture (Copyright Richard P. Usatine, MD.)

- Mirror the pattern through the dermis at the same level on the opposite side of the incision.
- Tie in the same manner as the deep vertical mattress suture.

This suture does not close dead space as well as the deep vertical mattress suture, but it can be easier to place when the skin is thin and not much undermining is needed.

REMOVING A DEEP SUTURE

If any deep suture does not come out as planned, it is better to remove it and start over than to allow the suture to cause anatomic distortion or inadequate closure. Practice will help, but even the best skin surgeons will need to remove a suture that does not perform its duty well.

RUNNING SIMPLE SUTURE

See Videos 6.4–6.5.

A running simple suture (Figure 6.11) is an efficient way to close long repairs that are not under tension or no longer under tension after the deep sutures are placed.

- Start by placing a simple interrupted suture at one end of the wound, and tie it with at least four or five throws.
- Instead of cutting both ends of the suture, cut only the short free end, and preserve the length of the suture with the needle attached.
- Continue the repair by placing the next stitch farther along the wound.
- Pass the needle through the skin on both sides of the wound, and repeat the process along the length of the defect.
- Insert the needle vertically/perpendicular to the skin to promote wound eversion.
- Suture until the length of the wound is closed. Be careful to not create too much tension along the wound as this will lead to increased risk of scarring.

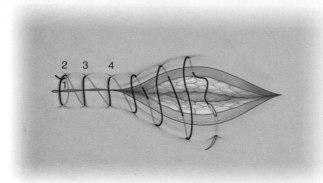

Figure 6.11 Running simple suture (running cuticular suture). Multiple simple sutures are placed in succession, allowing for rapid closure of wounds. Numbers indicate entry points of the needle. (Adapted from Taylor RS. Needles, sutures, and suturing. *Atlas Office Proced.* 1999;2:53–74.) (From Robinson J, Hanke W, Sengelmann R, Siegel D. *Surgery of the Skin: Procedural Dermatology.* 2nd ed. Mosby; 2010.)

- Passing the suture at a 45-degree angle under the skin along the length of the incision will lay the suture across the wound at a right angle to the incision. Moving the suture under the skin at 90 degrees will lay the suture across the wound at a 45-degree angle (Figure 6.12A and B). Either technique works well.
- Instead of pulling the last loop tight, leave a loop long enough to use it as an end to tie to the end with the needle (Figure 6.13).
- Tie the suture to this loop, and then cut the loop and the needle end of the suture. Three cut ends will be present.

VERTICAL MATTRESS SUTURE

Vertical mattress sutures (Figure 6.14A–C) distribute some of the stress and cutting force of the suture over a broader

area. The vertical mattress suture shifts much of the tension away from the skin edge and promotes eversion.

- Place the suture similarly to a simple interrupted suture but farther from the skin margin.
- Emerges equidistant on the other side of the wound often referred to as *far-far*
- Reverse the course of the needle, and place it closer to the skin edge on the same side where the needle just emerged.
- Advance the needle to come out equidistant from the wound on the opposite side of the wound and back toward the first insertion of the needle. These are placed close to the skin edge, *near-near*.
- Tie the two ends with the knot lying away from the skin edge.

This allows the skin edges to evert while placing the greatest amount of tension between the far and near entrance points of the suture instead of directly on the skin margin. To learn/remember the sequence of steps in this technique, it may be helpful to remember the saying *far-far, near-near*. Additional vertical mattress sutures may be placed along the wound to complete the repair.

Alternatively, once the tension is managed by strategically placed vertical mattress sutures, the repair of the intervening spaces may be completed with simple interrupted sutures or a running simple suture to approximate the skin edges. Use care to not inadvertently cut the previously placed sutures with the needle of the running suture when sewing close to those sutures.

HORIZONTAL MATTRESS SUTURES

Horizontal mattress sutures (Figure 6.15) are another option for placing tension away from the skin edges. Instead of placing the suture *far-far, near-near*, the four entrance/exit sites are equidistant from the wound margin, but the two lines of suture crossing the wound margin are parallel

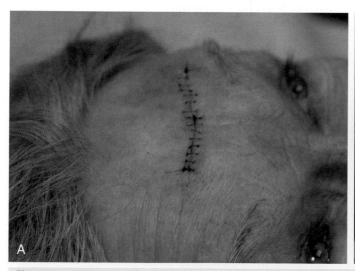

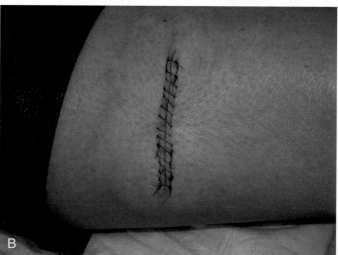

Figure 6.12 (A) Running simple suture advancing deep with suture line perpendicular over the wound. (Copyright Daniel L. Stulberg, MD.) **(B)** Running simple suture advancing over the skin with a 45-degree angle appearance. (Copyright Richard P. Usatine, MD.)

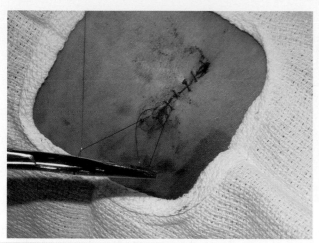

Figure 6.13 Leaving a loop near the end to tie off to. (Copyright Daniel L. Stulberg, MD.)

in a horizontal plane, in contrast to the two lines of suture in the vertical mattress, which are in a vertical plane.

- Start the horizontal mattress suture on one side of the wound as in a simple interrupted suture.
- Exit on the opposite side of the wound equidistant from the wound.
- Reverse the needle, insert it equidistant from the wound edge several millimeters lateral to the exit site, and then emerge equidistant on the opposite side of the wound.
- Finally, tie the suture on the side of initial needle entry.

This places the tension mostly along the section of the suture where the open loop is and the segment with the knot that is parallel to the wound margin. As above, the repair can be completed with additional horizontal mattress sutures, simple interrupted sutures, or a running simple suture to approximate the skin edges.

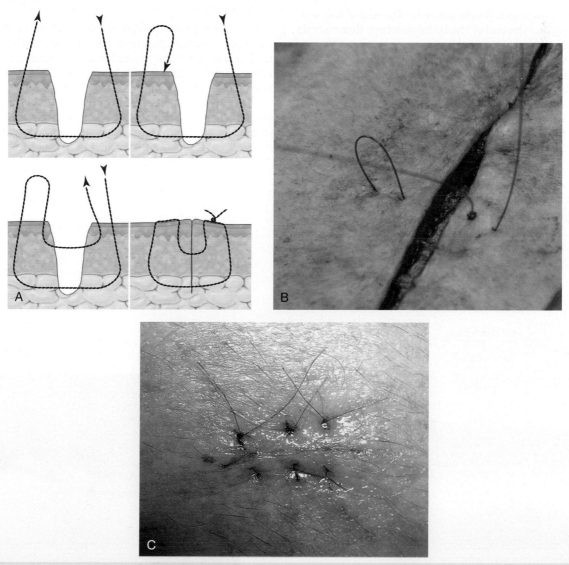

Figure 6.14 (A) The vertical mattress suture. **(B)** The vertical mattress suture prior to tying the knot. **(C)** Vertical mattress sutures on the face. (**A**: From Vidimos A, Ammirati C, Poblete-Lopez C. *Dermatologic Surgery*. Saunders; 2008; (**B, C**: Copyright Richard P. Usatine, MD.)

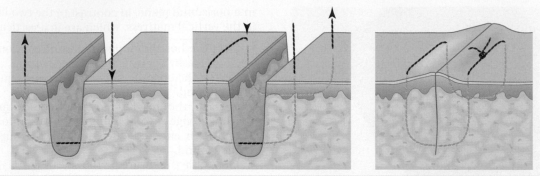

Figure 6.15 The horizontal mattress suture. (From Vidimos A, Ammirati C, Poblete-Lopez C. *Dermatologic Surgery*. Saunders; 2008.)

RUNNING HORIZONTAL MATTRESS SUTURE

This variation combines the distribution of tension away from the wound edge, which is possible with a traditional horizontal mattress suture with some of the speed of a running simple suture (Figure 6.16).

- Start the suture as a simple suture at the end of the incision or beyond the end of the incision where there is little or no tension.
- Tie the suture and cut only the short nonneedle end.
- Insert the needle several millimeters away from the exit of the first suture on the same side of the incision with the line parallel to the incision.
- Place the suture through the skin and subcutaneous tissues across the incision to emerge equidistant on the other side of the incision.

- Repeat the process several millimeters further along with the needle going in opposite directions for each new stitch. This will create a series of alternating dashes on either side of the incision.
- At the end of the incision, tie the needle end of the suture to the last loop of suture as in the simple running suture above.

The horizontal running suture will carry the tension parallel to and removed from the wound edge instead of the tension being on the wound edges themselves. The suture material will traverse the wound incision perpendicular and deep to the incision.

If the repair is long, removal can be facilitated by occasionally placing a simple suture across and over the incision instead of under it.[8] This segment can be easier to cut in contrast to the segments parallel to the incision, which due

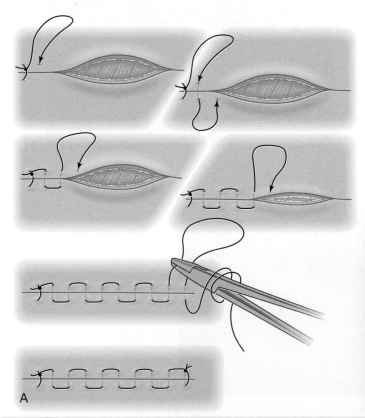

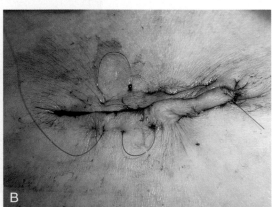

Figure 6.16 (A) The running horizontal mattress suture. **(B)** The running horizontal mattress suture causes eversion of the skin. (**A** From Vidimos A, Ammirati C, Poblete-Lopez C. *Dermatologic Surgery*. Saunders; 2008; **B** Copyright Richard P. Usatine, MD.)

to the tension on them may be difficult to elevate. This tension is also what helps to approximate the wound, evert the skin edges, and avoid undue tension at the skin edges. Because there are only two knots to tie (one at each end), it is relatively quick to place.

Tips for Working With Fragile Skin

Due to age or chronic systemic steroid use, some patients have very thin fragile skin. Using tightly pulled thin suture in fragile skin can cut through the skin just like a cheese wire cuts through cheese. It is important to distribute the tension away from the skin edges and to disburse it along the wound to get a good closure and avoid lacerating the wound margins.

In addition to using deep stitches in the dermis and mattress sutures as above, in extremely thin skin the clinician can place wound closure tapes parallel to the wound margins and then suture through the wound closure tapes (Figure 6.17). This supports the skin and further distributes the tension. The sutures can be removed at the appropriate time for the body location and the patient's risk factors (age, nutritional deficit, systemic steroids, etc.) If the wound closure tapes are still well adhered, they can be left in place to fall off on their own or removed gently or with the aid of adhesive remover. Use care to avoid damaging the skin or opening the wound by aggressive removal of the strips.

CORNER (TIP) STITCH

The corner, or tip, stitch (Figure 6.18) is useful in more complex wounds, advancements, and Z-plasties where a point needs to be sutured into a corner. This suture is very similar to the horizontal mattress suture, and it distributes tension away from the point of the flap or similar tissue.

- Start the needle on the side of the wound opposite the point but lateral to where the point of tissue is to reside.
- Pass the needle through the tissue emerging in the dermis.
- Enter into the corresponding portion of the point of tissue in the same level of the dermis and travel through it, remaining in the dermis and coming out on the other side of the point.
- Return to the original side of the wound via the dermis, and tie the initial and emerging suture ends on the wound edge opposite from the point of loose tissue.

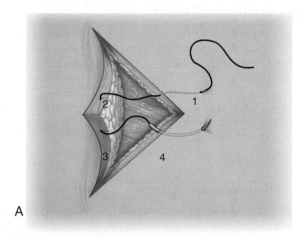

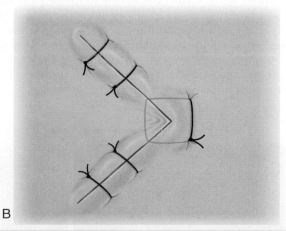

Figure 6.18 The three-point corner (tip) suture (half-buried horizontal mattress tip stitch). **(A)** This suture is started as an interrupted suture (1) on the V portion of the wound crossing over to the tip of the flap (2). A horizontal bite is made through the dermis of the tip (3). The needle is then directed back across the wound and tied (4). **(B)** Final appearance of this suture after placement. Numbers indicate entry points of the needle. (Adapted with permission from Robinson JK. Technique of suture placement. In Robinson J, Hanke W, Sengelmann R, Siegel D. *Surgery of the Skin: Procedural Dermatology.* 2nd ed. Mosby; 2010.)

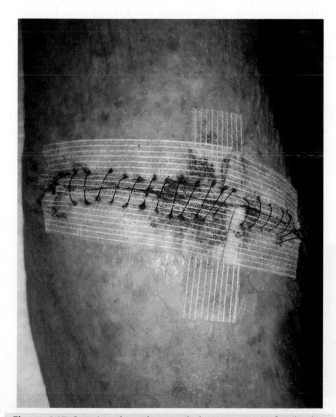

Figure 6.17 Suturing through wound closure tapes in fragile skin. (Copyright Daniel L. Stulberg, MD.)

The suture never emerges through the epidermis of the point of tissue, and the tension is distributed somewhat away from the fragile point of tissue and its blood supply.

INVERTED FIGURE-OF-EIGHT SUTURE AND FIGURE-OF-EIGHT SUTURE

The advantage of a figure-of-eight suture (Figure 6.19A–C) is that it gives the strength and placement effect of two interrupted sutures but only has one knot to tie. The traditional figure-of-eight suture is good for hemostasis of a bleeding blood vessel but crosses at the top of the placement centering all of the tension to one point crossing the skin. The inverted figure-of-eight is well suited for skin sutures crossing underneath the tissue and distributing the tension with two segments of suture over the skin. The inverted figure-of-eight is an excellent choice for medium-sized punch biopsies 4 to 6 mm in diameter in thin skin or up to 8 mm in thick skin, as in the back, that can be closed with a single inverted figure-of-eight suture. It can also be used to close the small defects from the minimal cyst excision technique in Chapter 12.

Inverted figure-of-eight:

- Start the suture 1/3 from the end of the defect and diagonally across the wound, emerging on the other skin edge 1/3 from the opposite end of the defect.
- Return the needle to the original side opposite the exit point of the initial suture placement.
- Advance the suture diagonally crossing the first suture under the skin to the opposite side, emerging directly across from the first entry point and tie.
- This will place the cross deep and two parallel lines of suture over the skin.

Traditional figure-of-eight:

- Start the needle on one side of the bleeding vessel or wound and emerge equidistant on the other side of the bleeding vessel or wound.
- Without tying, return the needle to the original side of the wound, and insert it further along the area of bleeding or the wound equidistant from the wound margin as the first site, and emerge equidistant on the other side.
- Tying the suture from the entry point to the final point will pull the wound together, and the suture will cross over itself in an X or figure-of-eight pattern.

- If performing for hemostasis in deep tissues, observe to see if the bleeding resolves before cutting the suture ends.
- If bleeding persists, pull gently upward with the suture ends to elevate the tissue, throw another simple stitch deeper around the area of bleeding, and tie to the original suture end.
- Repeat the process until hemostasis is achieved, and then cut the suture ends.

RUNNING SUBCUTICULAR SUTURE

A running subcuticular stitch (Figure 6.20A and B) is used to avoid making punctures through the epidermis and may leave less scarring. It can be performed with absorbable suture remaining in the tissues or utilizing nonabsorbable suture with knots at both ends above the skin for removing the suture at a later time. One advantage of a completely buried absorbable suture is that there is no need for suture removal.

- Before placing this suture, ensure hemostasis and approximate the wound with deep sutures as described above to reduce any tension on the skin edges. With absorbable suture, anchor one end with a suture around a small amount of dermis deep in the dermis near the end of the wound.
- Secure a knot at that point around, and cut the short end retaining the needle on the long end.
- Place the needle through the subcutaneous tissue to bury the knot, and emerge at the apex of the wound.
- With the needle in a plane parallel to the skin surface, enter one side of the dermis inside the wound margin, traveling horizontally along the wound, and emerge a short distance away in the dermis still within the wound margin.
- Repeat the process on the other side of the wound with the entry point directly opposite the emerging point. The suture should be placed at the same level in the dermis to maintain the skin repair level.
- Some clinicians will rotate the skin edge vertically with forceps to facilitate suturing in a vertical motion rather than horizontally.
- Proceed to the other end of the wound until it is nearly closed, leaving the last suture loop long to tie to (Figure 6.20C).

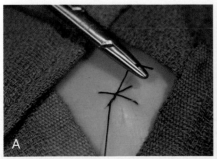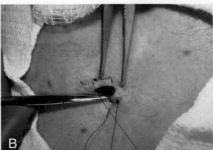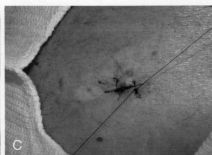

Figure 6.19 (A) A standard figure-of-eight suture with the crossing of suture above the wound in an artificial skin model. **(B)** Suturing an inverted figure-of-eight in the suture crossed below the skin. **(C)** This produces two parallel sutures above the skin with the convenience of only one knot to tie. (Copyright Daniel L. Stulberg, MD.)

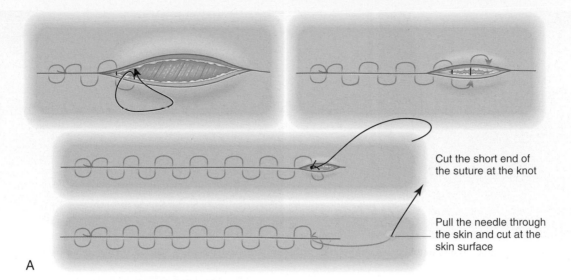

Cut the short end of
the suture at the knot

Pull the needle through
the skin and cut at the
skin surface

A

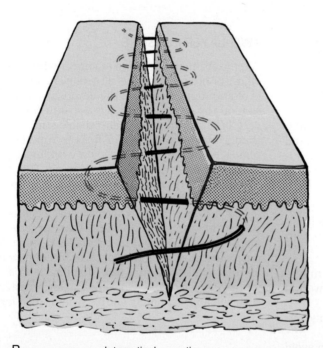

B   Intracuticular continuous

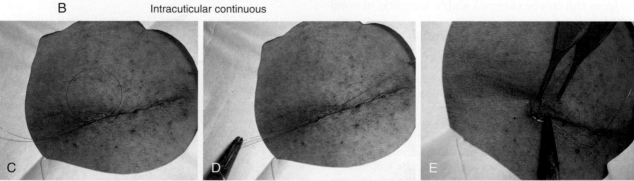

Figure 6.20 **(A)** Running subcuticular suture performed with absorbable suture. In this case the knots on both ends are buried. The suture is initiated with a simple dermal interrupted suture. Cut only the short end after tying the knot. After completing the running subcuticular suture, the suture end is tied off with another dermal interrupted suture. Cut only the short end. The needle end is then passed through the end of the incision and exited distal to the incision. The needle is pulled with tension. This pulls the knot deeper into the wound. The suture is then cut at the skin surface. (From Vidimos A, Ammirati C, Poblete-Lopez C. *Dermatologic Surgery*. Saunders; 2008.) **(B)** Running subcuticular suture is placed at the level of the upper dermis. (Baker SR. *Local Flaps in Facial Reconstruction*. 2nd ed. Mosby; 2007.) **(C)** Subcuticular suture leaving the last loop long for tying. (Figures C-G Copyright Richard P. Usatine, MD.) **(D)** Subcuticular suture tying the knot within the wound. **(E)** Subcuticular suture burying the final knot.

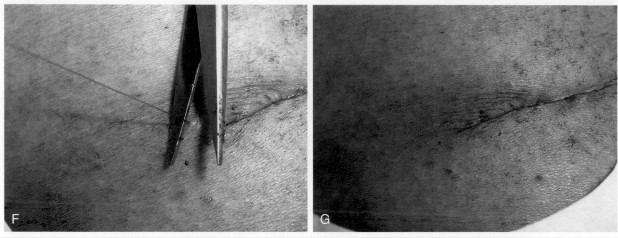

Figure 6.20 cont'd **(F)** Subcuticular suture cutting the suture outside of the wound burying the suture. **(G)** Subcuticular suture invisible from the surface.

- Tie the suture back to the last loop as described in the simple running suture and within the wound (Figure 6.20D).
- Cut the loop, but keep the needle attached to the other end.
- Being careful not to cut the newly placed suture, place the needle deep through the wound and emerge through the skin approximately 1 cm outside the wound (Figure 6.20E). This will bury the knot deeply. The suture is cut at the skin surface, allowing the end to drop under the skin and leaving the suture invisible from the surface (Figure 6.20F, G).

To make a running subcuticular suture completely removable, achieve hemostasis, and relieve skin tension with deep sutures:

- Start the skin repair by placing a nonabsorbable monofilament suture beyond the end of the surgical wound and emerging at the apex of the wound.
- No knot is made at this time, so be careful not to inadvertently pull the loose end into the wound.
- The loose end can be clamped with a hemostat to avoid losing it.
- Proceed as above, suturing along the length of the wound.
- If the wound is long, it can be helpful to create an extracutaneous loop that can be cut so that the entire length of the suture does not need to be pulled only from one end.
- To make an extracutaneous loop, place a suture through the dermis and epidermis across from the last suture emerging from the dermis.
- Across from this stitch place the suture through the epidermis, and emerge in the dermis to resume the subcuticular suture until you reach the end of the wound.
- Place the last suture through the apex of the wound, and emerge beyond the apex.
- Loop the suture around the needle holder several times, and then grasp the suture at the skin surface to create a knot at the skin to hold it in place.
- Repeat for several throws to hold it in place.
- Repeat the knotting process at the original entry beyond the apex of the wound.

TWO-LAYER CLOSURE

After excising a skin lesion or cancer with margins using an ellipse or other technique, a two-layer closure (Figure 6.21) is often required to close the empty space and reduce tension on the skin edges. This is a strong closure for skin surgery because the buried absorbable suture will take more than 1 month to dissolve. After the superficial sutures are removed, the deep sutures go on working to prevent dehiscence and unattractive scar widening. This method also is the best at preventing hematomas because it effectively closes the dead space.

Learn to use the two-layer closure because it should be the workhorse for performing skin surgery beyond small biopsies. Additionally, the two-layer closure, if used to reduce skin tension, empty space, or bleeding, can be billed as an intermediate closure (see Chapter 28, *Coding and Billing for Dermatologic Procedures*). Billing for an intermediate closure will approximately double what is paid for the surgical

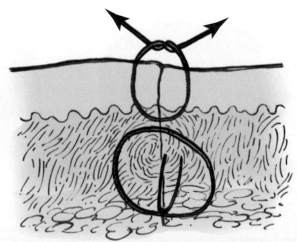

Figure 6.21 The two-layer closure consists of a deep absorbable suture with a more superficial nonabsorbable suture. (From Baker SR. *Local Flaps in Facial Reconstruction*. 2nd ed. Mosby; 2007.)

excision alone. Some insurance companies will require prior approval for an intermediate closure, so keep this in mind when scheduling an excision that will require a two-layer closure. Most importantly, this closure provides the best result for many skin excisions.

Intermediate closure:

- The easiest way to put in the deep sutures is to start on the end of the ellipse furthest from you and work toward yourself.
- This will allow you to start with sutures where there is least tension and remove tension from the central wound as sutures move to the middle of the ellipse.
- Once the deep sutures have gone beyond the middle region, most of the tension will be removed. When this works well, a running stitch can be used for the external nonabsorbable sutures to save time.
- For small ellipses, it can be difficult to place additional deep sutures after tying the first one. Consider placing the deep sutures and leaving enough suture length to tie later after all of the deep sutures are placed. Additionally, tying from alternating ends until getting to the middle can reduce the amount of tension and difficulty trying to tie the middle stitch, which has to close the furthest width of the ellipse.

Suture Removal

Nonabsorbable cutaneous sutures can be safely removed early on when good deep sutures have been placed. The typical time periods used are 5 to 6 days on the face and 7 to 10 days for the trunk and 10 to 14 days for the extremities. There is a balance between the risk of dehiscence if the sutures are removed too soon and scarring at the site of the sutures if they are left in too long. At suture removal, wound closure tapes may be placed across the wound for protection and to provide a small amount of support to the wound closure. We find this is rarely needed when the suturing was done well. Let the patient know that the wound closure tapes usually fall off spontaneously.

PURSE STRING SUTURE

Resecting skin cancers, especially melanomas, with their associated margins requires large excisions of skin. An ellipse is usually 3 times longer than its width, leading to a minimum 6 cm length if a 1-cm margin is indicated. Using a purse string suture can be an excellent alternative to avoid large ellipses (Figure 6.22A–D). This is a good choice for the back and dorsum of the hand.

Technique for Purse String Suture (Figure 6.23A–d)

- Counsel the patient regarding the option of a larger amount of tissue removed and a linear closure versus an initially wrinkled up smaller closure that will settle down over time.
- After pathology confirms the diagnosis, ink the margin of the lesion.
- Draw a line at the indicated margin around the lesion based on the diagnosis.
- Incise sharply along the drawn margin, undermine and remove the lesion with margins.
- Widely undermine circumferentially beyond the margins to allow the skin to stretch.

- Using a strong absorbable suture, start the suture in the mid dermis, getting a solid portion/depth of dermis peripheral to the defect, and emerge several millimeters along the defect.
- Repeat this step every several millimeters along the length of the defect until emerging at the initial suture entry.
- Using a friction/surgeon's knot, firmly but gently pull the suture ends, puckering the skin together like the top of a leather pouch coin purse.
- Tighten the suture until the defect approaches a small elliptical shape, and complete the knot.
- Using simple interrupted sutures or vertical mattress sutures if needed for tension, close the elliptical defect into a mostly linear closure with anticipated puckering.
- Remove the superficial sutures at the return visit, leaving the intradermal purse string suture intact to resorb over time.
- A second option is to use nonabsorbable suture, placing the purse string outside the wound (Figure 6.23D).

COMPRESSIVE SUTURES

With the minimal cyst excision technique and lipoma removal via small incisions, there is often a defect below the skin and no easy access to place deep sutures to close the empty space due to the small incision (Figure 6.24A and B).

- Using a large needle, suture wide from the incision and pass deep to the empty space to compress the underlying tissues to the overlying skin.
- Based on the size of the excision, place additional compressive sutures.

This usually obviates the need for cutaneous sutures, so utilize the techniques above to make sure there is good skin approximation with wound edge eversion. If needed, place interrupted skin sutures. This technique can also be used if there is active bleeding that cannot be visualized to place a deep figure-of-eight stitch.

Alternative Closure Techniques

WOUND CLOSURE TAPES

Wound closure tapes may be used as an adjunct for skin closure in addition to deep sutures and skin sutures. Some clinicians will use wound closure tapes alone for linear excisions of small lipomas or cysts when there is no tension on the wound edges. For elliptical excisions, it is important to close the dermis and relieve wound tension if wound closure tapes are to be the only epidermal closure used.

It helps to apply a liquid adhesive (tincture of benzoin or Mastisol) to facilitate adherence of the wound closure tapes. Wound closure tapes, which come in ⅛-, ¼-, and ½-inch widths, can be cut in half transversely so they are not as long for small wounds typical in the office setting (Figure 6.25).

In addition to providing support to healing skin, overlapped wound closure tapes also provide an occlusive dressing and a moist healing environment. This is convenient because the patient does not need to change any dressings at all. The disadvantage is that if there is any bleeding or drainage, the tapes will get discolored and may dislodge. If the edges start to curl up or are nonadherent, they can be trimmed with nail clippers or scissors to reduce the likelihood of their getting inadvertently pulled off.

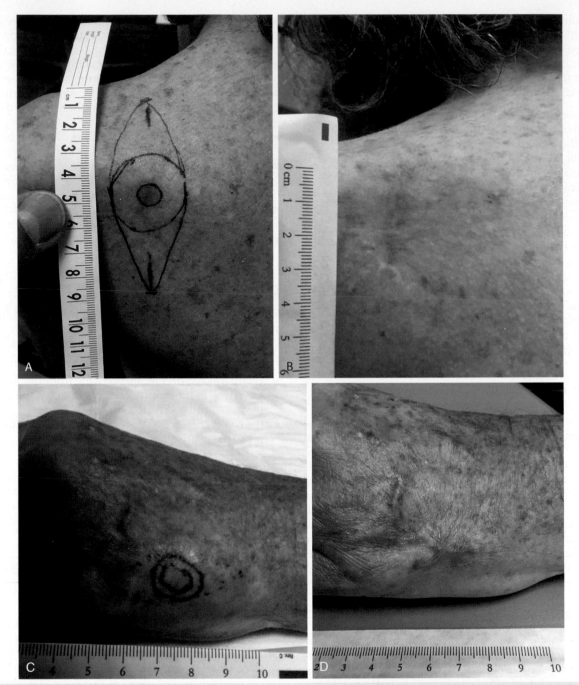

Figure 6.22 **(A)** This re-excision of melanoma with 1-centimeter margins would require an ellipse 3 by 9 centimeters. (Copyright Daniel L. Stulberg, MD.) **(B)** At 4 months, 3-centimeter scar from purse string suture instead of minimum 9-centimeter scar. (Copyright Daniel L. Stulberg, MD.) **(C)** The dotted lines show the usual excision margins needed for an elliptical removal of a skin cancer. The inner solid line shows the extent of the cancer, and the larger circle shows the 5 mm required surgical margins. (Copyright Daniel L. Stulberg, MD.) **(D)** Healed postoperative result. (Copyright Daniel L. Stulberg, MD.)

GLUES

Cyanoacrylate glues (2-octylcyanoacrylate, Dermabond) have been used for years for closure of wounds due to lacerations when there is no tension on the skin edges. A review of their use in the operating room found no increased rate of infection or dehiscence, but the studies excluded wounds under high tension.[9] If a surgical wound of an excision is approximated with no significant tension due to well-placed deep sutures, then skin glue is an option for the final skin closure[10] (see Chapter 7, *Laceration Repair*).

Learning the Techniques: Suggestions on How to Practice

Pig's or cow's feet (fresh or previously frozen, not smoked) and artificial skin pads provide a good medium for practice (Figure 6.26A and B). Nectarines or bananas can be sutured to practice a deft touch because their skin is fragile and care is needed to follow the curve of the needle and avoid tension or it will tear (similar to the fragile skin of the elderly).

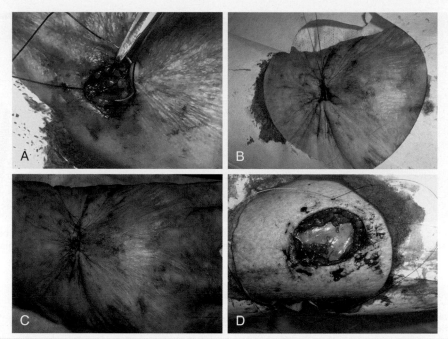

Figure 6.23 (A) The skin cancer with margins was removed, and a purse string/gathering suture is being placed with multiple small bites around the perimeter of the defect ending adjacent to the start of the stitch. (Copyright Richard P. Usatine, MD.) **(B)** The purse string is tightened until the defect is almost closed and may appear linear or elliptical. (Copyright Richard P. Usatine, MD.) **(C)** Interrupted sutures completed the closure. (Copyright Richard P. Usatine, MD.) **(D)** Using nonabsorbable suture, placing the purse string outside the wound. (Copyright Richard P. Usatine, MD.)

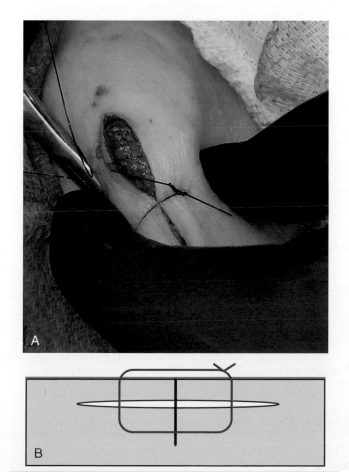

Figure 6.24 (A) Compressive sutures. **(B)** Compressive suture diagram. (Copyright Daniel L. Stulberg, MD.)

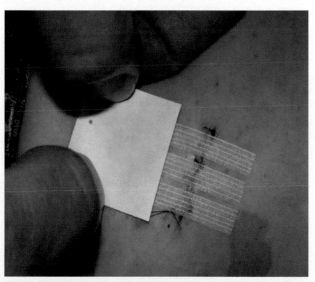

Figure 6.25 Wound closure tapes. (Copyright Daniel L. Stulberg, MD.)

Conclusion

Skin can be sutured in various ways to achieve good healing and cosmesis. Clinicians should be familiar with several techniques so they can use them – or often a combination of them – as the situation requires to achieve good approximation of the deep tissues, reduction or distribution of tension, and apposition of the dermis with slight eversion of the skin to reduce the risk of dehiscence and unnecessary scarring. Table 6.1 summarizes the advantages and disadvantages of the suturing techniques discussed in this chapter.

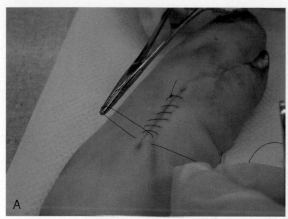 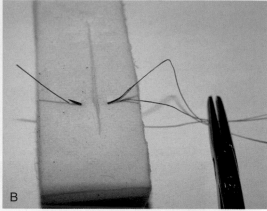

Figure 6.26 (A) Using a pig's foot to practice a simple running suture. This figure is demonstrating how the final knot will be tied to a loop of suture material. (Copyright Richard P. Usatine, MD.) **(B)** Practicing a vertical mattress stitch on an artificial skin pad. (Copyright Daniel L. Stulberg, MD.)

Table 6.1 Advantages and Disadvantages of Suturing Techniques

Suture Technique	Advantage for Clinician	Disadvantage for Clinician	Advantage for Patient	Disadvantage for Patient	Well Suited for
Simple interrupted	Accurate control of depth, placement, and tension.	Time consuming, each one needs to be tied.	Can line up wounds better when there is a mismatch in height or length of the two sides.	Potential for "railroad track" scarring.	Small wounds and to line up larger wounds.
Simple deep or buried vertical mattress	Relieves tension, closes dead space, provides hemostasis, opposes dermis, produces eversion.	Takes more skill and experience to do well.	Decreased chance of dehiscence and hematoma.	Suture material retained in tissues can cause spitting sutures or suture granulomas.	Closing wounds that have some tension and/or dead space.
Deep horizontal mattress	Opposes dermis in areas where skin is thin. Less undermining is needed.	Takes more skill and experience to do well, does not close dead space as well as buried vertical mattress.	Decreased chance of dehiscence.	Spitting sutures or suture granulomas.	Closing wounds under tension that are not very deep.
Vertical mattress	Excellent wound eversion, decreased wound tension. Adds support to wounds under stress.	Requires more time to place than simple interrupted suture – not as good as deep sutures for relieving tension.	Wound eversion can prevent depressed scarring.	Potential for "railroad track" scarring but not as obvious as with simple interrupted sutures.	Closing wounds under tension when not using deep sutures or in addition to deep sutures when extra eversion is desired.
Horizontal mattress	Distributes tension away from skin edge.	More time consuming than running sutures. Suture removal is more difficult.	Wound eversion can prevent depressed scarring.	Risk of ischemia at wound edge if too tight.	Closing short wounds or part of a long wound under tension with good eversion.
Running horizontal mattress	Faster than individual horizontal mattress sutures and achieves good wound eversion.	Requires more time to place than simple running suture.	Wound eversion can prevent depressed scarring.	Suture can sink into the skin, which can be uncomfortable to remove.	Closing long wounds under tension with good eversion.
Inverted figure-of-eight	Faster than two simple interrupted sutures.	N/A	Faster completion of procedure.	N/A	Closing punch biopsies and small excisions.
Deep figure-of-eight	Ideal suture to stop bleeding during skin surgery.	Is more time consuming than electrocoagulation.	Effective way to get hemostasis.	Can produce scarring if used for skin closure after punch biopsy.	Hemostasis, alternative for closing punch biopsies.
Running subcuticular – absorbable	Can produce a very good cosmetic result.	Takes more time and skill to place. Not for wounds under tension.	No "railroad track" scars. No suture removal.	Suture material retained in tissues as possible nidus of inflammation or infection.	Cosmetically sensitive areas or if suture removal is an issue.
Running subcuticular – nonabsorbable	Can produce a very good cosmetic result.	Takes more time and skill to place. Not for wounds under tension.	No "railroad track" scars.	Requires suture removal.	Cosmetically sensitive areas.
Staples	Quick to place.	Less control than sutures, higher cost.	Quick to place.	Multiple entry points, hard material in skin, can leave more scarring.	Large scalp wounds where cosmesis is not an issue.

References

1. Kappel S, Kleinerman R, King TH, et al. Does wound eversion improve cosmetic outcome? Results of a randomized, split-scar, comparative trial. *J Am Acad Dermatol.* 2015;72(4):668-673. doi:10.1016/j.jaad.2014.11.032.

2. Dzubow L. Wound edge eversion: tradition or science? *J Am Acad Dermatol.* 2015;73(2):e63. doi:10.1016/j.jaad.2015.04.042.

3. Wang AS, Kappel S, Eisen DB. Reply to: "Wound edge eversion: tradition or science?" *J Am Acad Dermatol.* 2015;73(2):e65. doi:10.1016/j.jaad.2015.04.043.

4. Sklar LR, Pourang A, Armstrong AW, Dhaliwal SK, Sivamani RK, Eisen DB. Comparison of running cutaneous suture spacing during linear wound closures and the effect on wound cosmesis of the face and neck: a randomized clinical trial. *JAMA Dermatol.* 2019;155(3):321-326. doi:10.1001/jamadermatol.2018.5057.

5. Stoecker A, Blattner CM, Howerter S, Fancher W, Young J, Lear W. Effect of simple interrupted suture spacing on aesthetic and functional outcomes of skin closures. *J Cutan Med Surg.* 2019;23(6):580-585. doi:10.1177/1203475419861077.

6. Weinkle A, Harrington A, Kang A, Armstrong AW, Eisen DB. Aesthetic outcome of simple cuticular suture distance from the wound edge on the closure of linear wounds on the head and neck: a randomized evaluator blinded split-wound comparative effect trial. *J Am Acad Dermatol.* 2022;86(4):863-867. doi:10.1016/j.jaad.2021.10.036.

7. Farshchian M, Sklar LR. The pinch stitch: a pearl for suturing wounds under tension. *J Drugs Dermatol.* 2020;19(12):1262. doi:10.36849/JDD.2020.5461.

8. Chacon AH, Shiman MI, Strozier N, Zaiac MN. Horizontal running mattress suture modified with intermittent simple loops. *J Cutan Aesthet Surg.* 2013;6(1):54-56. doi:10.4103/0974-2077.110102.

9. Coulthard P, Esposito M, Worthington HV, et al. Tissue adhesives for closure of surgical incisions. *Cochrane Database Syst Rev.* 2002;3: CD004287.

10. Toriumi DM, Bagal AA. Cyanoacrylate tissue adhesives for skin closure in the outpatient setting. *Otolaryngol Clin North Am.* 2002; 35(1):103-118, vi-vii.

Laceration Repair

RICHARD P. USATINE, MD, ANGELA MARTZ, PAC, WENDY C. COATES, MD, and DANIEL STULBERG, MD

SUMMARY

- Repair lacerations to restore function, achieve hemostasis, and facilitate healing and cosmesis.
- Lacerations should be repaired as soon as feasible to reduce the likelihood of infection.
- Injected or topical anesthesia facilitates cleaning and closure of lacerations.
- Regional and field blocks provide excellent anesthesia and are less likely to cause distortion.
- Nonabsorbable sutures provide strength to the repair and take tension off the skin while healing.
- Mattress sutures can reduce tension on the skin edges and are useful in fragile skin and areas of movement.
- Wound tapes and glues may be used in lacerations with tension on the wound and are less painful.
- Staples are a quick, effective option that is used in less visible repairs.
- Antibiotics are usually not indicated unless grossly contaminated or at very high risk.
- Special structures, namely lips, eyelids, ears, and nose, require special attention for optimal repair.

When lacerations require intervention, they may be repaired with sutures, surgical adhesive strips, tissue adhesives, or staples. The goals of laceration repair are as follows:

- Achieve hemostasis
- Prevent infection
- Preserve function
- Restore appearance
- Minimize patient discomfort

In repairing skin, it is helpful to understand the three phases of wound healing.

- Phase 1: Initial Lag Phase (Days 0 to 5)
  - No gain in wound strength
- Phase 2: Fibroplasia Phase (Days 5 to 14)
  - Increase in wound strength occurs
  - At 2 weeks, the wound has achieved only 7% of its final strength.
- Phase 3: Final Maturation Phase (Day 14 Until Healing Is Complete)
  - Further connective tissue remodeling
  - Up to 80% of normal skin strength

Nonabsorbable skin sutures, skin adhesives, or staples are used to give the wound strength during the first two phases. After the nonabsorbable skin sutures or staples are removed, surgical adhesive strips or previously placed deep absorbable sutures play an important role in the final phases of wound healing.

Patients should be asked about their tetanus immune status, and prophylaxis should be considered. Analgesic medication may need to be provided in the acute setting and for a few days thereafter depending on the extent of the trauma and patient preferences. For most patients, acetaminophen or ibuprofen should be sufficient, but in selected patients, prescription narcotics may be indicated.

Indications for Repair

- Lacerations that are open and less than 12 hours old
- Wounds greater than 24 hours old require special consideration but may be closed for function or cosmesis, especially on the face[1]
- Some bite wounds in cosmetically important areas (close follow-up recommended)
- Traumatic amputations of the fingertips and nail bed laceration repairs

Contraindications for Repair

- Wounds more than 12 hours old (more than 24 hours old on the face)
- Animal and human bite wounds (exceptions: facial wounds, dog bite wounds)
- Puncture wounds

Supplies and Equipment

- Surgical prep: povidone-iodine (Betadine), chlorhexidine (Hibiclens), or copious soap and water
- Ruler marked in centimeters used for overall size, documentation of findings, and billing purposes
- Irrigation device for contaminated wounds: 30-mL syringe with 18-gauge angiocatheter or commercially manufactured splash shield device (Figure 7.1) and sterile saline
  - 1% or 2% lidocaine with or without epinephrine (see Chapter 3, *Anesthesia*)
  - Topical LET (lidocaine, epinephrine, tetracaine has 73% effective anesthesia vs 40% with EMLA [eutectic mixture local anesthetic][2]) may also be considered.

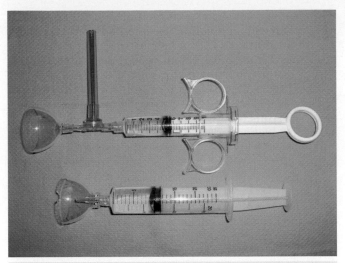

Figure 7.1 Many useful devices are available for irrigating dirty wounds, including the Zerowet Klenzalac system, which has a special syringe attached to a splash shield, and the more simple Zerowet Supershield for use on a standard syringe. (Copyright Richard P. Usatine, MD.)

- Syringes and 27- or 30-gauge needle (small-gauge needles are preferred to administer anesthesia)
- Sterile drapes; fenestrated drape (applied so that the hole is over the laceration)
- 4 inch × 4 inch gauze sponges; cotton-tipped applicators are useful for hemostasis.
- Sterile instruments: 4.5-inch needle holder, curved or straight iris scissors, one mosquito hemostat, suture scissors, Adson forceps with teeth
- No. 15 blade (for trimming devascularized or macerated tissues) with scalpel handle (single disposable unit also available)
- Sutures (see Chapter 5, *Suture Material*), surgical adhesive strips, staples, or tissue adhesive
- Skin-marking pen (if wound revision is needed)
- Electrosurgical unit may be considered for electrocoagulation
- Protective mask with plastic shield for eyes or other types of personal protective equipment

Preprocedure Patient Preparation

The patient should be informed of the nature of his or her lacerations. If the laceration is in a cosmetically important area, consider offering the option of a specialist, such as a plastic surgeon or ophthalmologist, for the repair. Advise the patient about the risks of pain, bleeding, dehiscence, infection, and scarring. Inform the patient that most repairs cause some permanent scarring, although attempts will be made to optimize the appearance. Wounds can always be revised or cosmetically altered if needed.[3] Warn patients of the risks of hyperpigmentation or hypopigmentation, hypertrophic scars, keloids, nerve damage, alopecia, and distortion of the original anatomy. Those with a history of keloids or scar hypertrophy are at high risk of keloid or

hypertrophic scar at the repair. After a discussion of risks and benefits, have the patient sign a consent form or document verbal consent before beginning the procedure (see Chapter 1, *Preoperative Preparation*).

INITIAL ASSESSMENT

The initial evaluation before anesthesia should include a history of how the wound was sustained, factors that might impair healing, tetanus immunization history, and an assessment of peripheral neurovascular and functional movement status. See Table 7.1 for essentials of wound assessment. The clinician should consider the possibility of domestic violence in patients with traumatic wounds, especially if lacerations appear on the face or if multiple injuries of varying ages are noted.

ARE ANTIBIOTICS NEEDED?

In general, antibiotics are not needed for either wound infection prophylaxis or subacute bacterial endocarditis (SBE) prophylaxis when dealing with cutaneous procedures (see Chapter 1).[4] Consideration should be given to coverage for *Staphylococcus aureus* and methicillin-resistant *S. aureus* (MRSA) infection in special situations.

The following are major goals for prescribing antibiotics (when indicated) before or after skin surgery:

- Prevention of a new wound infection in high-risk situations
- Prevention of the spread of an existing local infection
- Treatment of an existing infection
- Prevention of bacterial endocarditis

Grossly contaminated wounds may require antibiotic prophylaxis, but in general thorough wound cleansing and preparation is all that is necessary for the majority of lacerations.[5] The clinician must consider host factors, the anatomic location of the surgery, the sources that might contaminate the wound, and method of wound injury. The multiple factors to be considered when making a decision about antibiotic prophylaxis for skin procedures are:

COEXISTING CONDITIONS

- Diabetes mellitus
- Peripheral vascular disease
- Frail elderly patients

Table 7.1 Essentials of Wound Assessment

Parameters	Factors to Consider
Mechanism of injury	Sharp vs. blunt trauma, bite
Dirty vs. clean	Outdoors vs. kitchen sink
Time since injury	Suture up to 12 hours; 24 hours on face
Foreign body	Explore and obtain radiograph for metal or glass
Functional examination	Neurovascular, muscular, tendons
Need for prophylactic antibiotics	If needed, give ASAP and cover *Staphylococcus aureus*; irrigate well

- Immunocompromised
- Previous radiation to the site
- Malnutrition (e.g., alcoholism, chemotherapy)
- History of previous infection or slow healing
- Chronic steroid use
- Morbid obesity

LOCATIONS

- Axilla, mouth, and anogenital areas have higher levels of bacterial colonization
- End arterial locations (fingers, toes) with diseases of vascular compromise[6]
- Over joint spaces where there is a possibility of entering the joint (e.g., metacarpal-phalangeal joints)

CONTAMINATION

- Dirty wounds, especially in barnyards, meatpacking plants, etc.
- Less than optimal sterile technique (should be rare)
- Deep puncture wounds
- Bites (especially human and cat bites)
- Presence of a nonremovable retained foreign body[7]

METHOD OF WOUND INJURY

- Crush injury (10-fold increase in infection with devitalized skin)
- Penetrating injury

The recommendations of the American Heart Association (AHA) for the prevention of bacterial endocarditis (as of 2021, last published in 2007) are discussed in Chapter 1.[4] Endocarditis prophylaxis is not needed for incision or biopsy of surgically scrubbed noninfected skin no matter what endocarditis risk factors are present. The 2007 guidelines state that antibiotic prophylaxis is recommended for procedures on infected skin and skin structures for patients with underlying cardiac conditions associated with the highest risk of adverse outcome from infective endocarditis (see Table 1.3).[4]

Cummings et al. performed a metaanalysis of randomized studies on the use of antibiotics to prevent infection of simple wounds.[8] They concluded that there is no evidence in published trials that prophylactic antibiotics offer protection against infection of nonbite wounds in patients treated in emergency departments. However, prophylactic antibiotics did reduce the incidence of infection in patients with dog-bite wounds in another metaanalysis.[9] The authors concluded that it may be reasonable to limit prophylactic antibiotics to patients with dog-bite wounds that are at highest risk for infection.[9]

Cat and dog bite injuries carry the risk of infection with *Pasteurella multocida*, and human-bite injuries carry the risk of infection with *Eikenella corrodens* and *S. aureus*. Based on the microbiology of these wounds, amoxicillin/clavulanate provides good prophylactic coverage for the bacteria affecting most bite injuries. Alternatives include second-generation cephalosporins or clindamycin with a fluoroquinolone.

Related to the question of antibiotic use in lacerations is the question of using antibiotics in abscesses. The first line treatment for skin abscesses is incision and drainage (I&D) rather than with antibiotics. The question of whether adding an antibiotic to I&D is helpful was undertaken in a randomized trial at five US emergency departments. They gave trimethoprim-sulfamethoxazole 2 DS twice daily, for 7 days, to a random selection of outpatients who had an uncomplicated abscess that was being treated with drainage. The trimethoprim-sulfamethoxazole treatment resulted in a higher cure rate among patients with a drained cutaneous abscess than placebo. This suggests that in settings with high MRSA prevalence, the addition of trimethoprim-sulfamethoxazole should be considered to the standard I&D.[10]

The best method for prevention of wound infections is to clean and irrigate traumatic wounds well, rather than relying on prophylactic antibiotics. The clinician needs to weigh the benefits and the risks of antibiotic use based on the individual patient and the circumstances of the wound repair or skin surgery.

LOCAL AND REGIONAL ANESTHESIA

In traumatic wounds, neurovascular integrity should be assessed prior to administration of anesthesia. The wound should then be fully anesthetized to allow for painless examination of the tissue damage, thorough irrigation, and adequate closure. Many wounds can be adequately anesthetized with 1% or 2% lidocaine. Consider using lidocaine with epinephrine to provide increased hemostasis if there are no contraindications to epinephrine use in the patient or the wound itself (see Chapter 3, *Anesthesia*). Lidocaine with epinephrine has the advantage of staying more local, thereby allowing more volume to be used with less risk of lidocaine toxicity. The use of epinephrine will also typically double the duration of anesthesia extending it from 1 hour with plain lidocaine to 2 hours with epinephrine. This can be helpful if extensive cleaning, debriding, or a time-consuming repair is needed. Topical anesthetics are effective for wounds that do not involve mucosal surfaces. A combination of lidocaine, epinephrine, and tetracaine (LET) applied with a saturated cotton ball or as a gel formulation directly into the wound provides adequate anesthesia for many wounds.[1] LET is also useful for abscesses.[11,12]

Regional anesthesia may be desirable in cases where the volume of locally infiltrated anesthesia might exceed the safe maximum dosage (see Chapter 3, Table 3.3) or in cosmetically important areas where a local infiltration might distort the anatomy and impair a meticulous closure. If a regional anesthetic technique is employed, lidocaine without epinephrine is the optimal choice, because epinephrine's role as a vasoconstrictor is not needed at a site remote to the traumatic wound.

Follow these instructions to minimize the pain of injecting local anesthetic:

- Use a small-gauge needle (27 or 30 gauge).
- Injecting slowly has been recommended but a recent study found no difference in pain between 15, 30, and 45 seconds[13]
- Inject directly into the subcutaneous tissues through the open wound (not through intact skin)
- Warm anesthetic to body temperature (optional)

- Buffer the anesthetic with sodium bicarbonate (1 part bicarbonate for 3 parts lidocaine is more effective than the previously touted 1:9 ratio[14]) (*optional*)

WOUND PREPARATION

After the initial assessment and administration of local or regional anesthetic, and antibiotics if indicated, wounds should be cleansed and inspected thoroughly for foreign bodies, deep tissue layer damage, and injury to nerve, vessel, or tendon. Underlying bone or joint injury should be considered in wounds sustained as a result of traumatic force. A radiograph should be obtained to look for retained glass or metal in wounds sustained from broken glass or metal and to assess for joint integrity or fractures in traumatic injuries. Complex wounds or those in cosmetically important areas should be closed by a practitioner with the appropriate expertise. This is also helpful if the wound may require revision in the future.

DETERMINE IF THE WOUND NEEDS INTERVENTION TO CLOSE

One study assessed the difference in clinical outcome between lacerations of the hand closed with sutures and those treated conservatively.[15] Consecutive patients with uncomplicated lacerations of the hand (full thickness <2 cm; without tendon, joint, fracture, or nerve complications) who would normally require sutures were randomized to suturing or conservative treatment. The mean time to resume normal activities was the same in both groups (3.4 days). Patients treated conservatively had less pain, and treatment time was 14 (10 to 18) minutes shorter. The groups did not differ significantly in the assessment of cosmetic appearance on the visual analogue scale. Conservative treatment was faster and less painful.[14]

CLEANSING

After the wound is anesthetized, cleansing of the wound should be performed by irrigation with normal saline at 8 to 12 psi of pressure. This can be accomplished by attaching an 18-gauge angiocatheter or a commercially available splash shield to a 20- or 30-mL syringe. At least 200 mL of irrigation is recommended. Irrijet and Zerowet were superior to an angiocatheter in preventing splatter during wound model irrigation.[9] Zerowet was particularly effective in preventing splatter onto the irrigator's face (Figure 7.1).[9]

A multicenter comparison of tap water versus sterile saline for wound irrigation showed equivalent rates of wound infection in immunocompetent patients.[16] The tap water group irrigated their own wounds under the water tap for a minimum of 2 minutes after they had the wound anesthetized. Higher-risk wounds were excluded from the study, indicating that tap water is a reasonable cleansing alternative for low-risk lacerations. In one randomized clinical trial, warmed saline was more comfortable and soothing than room-temperature saline as a wound irrigant among patients with linear lacerations.[17]

Chemical compounds such as hexachlorophene (Phisohex), chlorhexidine gluconate (Hibiclens), or povidone-iodine (Betadine) should not be used inside wounds but may be applied to external, intact skin if desired. Greasy contaminants can be removed with any petroleum-based product, such as petrolatum or bacitracin ointment. To prevent a road rash tattoo, wrap petroleum gauze around the fingers and wipe off the asphalt and other foreign material embedded in the skin after anesthesia. Topical and regional anesthetic techniques are particularly effective in this situation.

DEBRIDEMENT

After the cleansing process, wounds should be examined for devitalized tissue that needs removal or debridement. This debridement may convert a jagged, contaminated wound into a clean surgical one and can be accomplished with a scalpel or sharp tissue scissors. As much tissue as possible should be preserved in case future scar revision is necessary. After debridement, wound edges should be held together to see if they are under any tension. Wounds under significant tension are best repaired by a two-layer closure. In dirty wounds, however, this may increase the incidence of infection.

UNDERMINING

Undermining can significantly reduce skin tension when there is a gap to be closed. Undermining may increase the risk of infection and thus should be avoided in dirty wounds. Care should be taken to minimize the use of this technique in areas with poor blood supply because the process of undermining reduces it further. Extreme care is also needed when undermining around vital structures. Approximately one-third to one-half of the undermined tissue is freed up to be brought into the defect. When needed and if possible, undermine bilaterally as far back as the wound is wide (or until primary closure can be achieved).

Closure Technique

Ideally, four principles should be incorporated into the process of closing any wound:

1. *Control all bleeding before closure.* This can be accomplished by applying direct pressure for at least 5 minutes, injecting lidocaine *with* epinephrine, with electrocoagulation, or by tying off bleeders with absorbable figure-8 sutures or applying an external ice pack.
2. *Eliminate "dead space."* Eliminate areas where tissue fluid and blood can accumulate. Deep sutures are particularly useful in this regard.
3. *Accurately approximate tissue layers to each other.* Scars are most visible when shadows are created by depressed or elevated tissue. Also be sure that anatomic areas match on each side in critical areas such as the vermilion border of the lip or the eyebrows.
4. *Approximate the wound with minimal skin tension.* If the amount of tension will be significant, undermining and/or deep, inverted, buried sutures are used to decrease the tension on the skin margin.

CHOICE OF SUTURES

Most lacerations will be closed with nylon, polypropylene (Prolene), or similar nonabsorbable suture. If a two-layer closure is needed, an absorbable suture such as polyglactin 910 (Vicryl) or a synthetic absorbable monofilament suture (Monocryl) is a good choice for the deep layer. Vicryl, silk, or Monocryl are useful for closure in the mouth or other areas where the nylon ends will be bothersome.[18]

Alternately, rapidly absorbing Vicryl Rapide may be used in oral lacerations without the need for suture removal. In one study, otherwise healthy children with facial lacerations were randomized to repair using fast-absorbing catgut or nylon suture.[19] There were no significant differences in the rates of infection, wound dehiscence, keloid formation, and parental satisfaction between the absorbable catgut and the nylon suture.[18] Fast-absorbing catgut suture is not as easy to work with as nylon but does have the advantage of not requiring suture removal in children who may be very fearful of the suture removal process. Dermabond (cyanoacrylate tissue adhesive) was compared to suture in facial lacerations, especially chin lacerations, and found to have a similar outcome.[20]

Suggested suture size and time of removal based on anatomic areas is found in Table 7.2.

SUTURED REPAIRS

Lacerations are approximated with sutures using a variety of techniques (see Chapter 6, *Suturing Techniques*), as discussed in the following subsections.

SIMPLE INTERRUPTED SUTURE

On completion of a simple interrupted suture (Figure 7.2), the skin margins should be flat to slightly everted. The needle should enter the skin surface at a 90-degree angle. The stitch should be as wide as it is deep. The suture on both sides of the wound should be equal distance from the wound margin and of equal depth. The final shape should appear like that of a pear (see Chapter 6, Figure 6.5). Previously, 2-mm spacing between sutures was used in fine plastic closure of the face and farther apart in other types of closures. Recent studies comparing 2-mm vs 5-mm spacing for opposite ends of sutured repairs showed no difference in

outcomes at 3 months[21] and patient and provider preference for the 5-mm spacing.[22] Suturing 5 mm vs 2 mm from the wound margin showed no difference in outcomes.[23] Additional sutures take longer to place, and based on these studies, placing sutures less than 5 mm apart does not improve outcomes. The provider should consider less closely spaced sutures and rely more on the clinical results of good apposition of the wound margins without gapping to determine spacing.

Avoid tying the knots too tightly. The knots should be lined up on the same side of the wound, usually the one with the best blood supply or least interference with comfort (e.g., away from eyelid).

SIMPLE RUNNING STITCH

The advantages of the simple running stitch (Figure 7.3) in sterile wounds under little or no tension are that it is quick, it distributes tension evenly, and it provides excellent cosmetic results. If there is significant gaping of the wound, interrupted suture methods should be used. Because the risk of contamination is increased with traumatic lacerations, the simple running stitch is less desirable in these wounds. In case of infection, the entire wound closure would need to be removed. The relative disadvantage of removing the entire stitch at one time also poses a problem in wounds under some increased tension. With interrupted techniques, some sutures may be removed early for better cosmesis, whereas a few remaining ones can be left for prevention of dehiscence and removed at a later date. The simple running stitch is ideal in the scalp and is often used in elliptical excision repairs.

DEEP SUTURE WITH INVERTED KNOT OR BURIED STITCH

Deeper wounds or wounds under tension are best closed by providing structural support and not relying solely on nonabsorbable superficial sutures. Well-placed deep absorbable sutures (Figure 7.4 and Chapter 6, Figure 6.9A and B) can do much to aid in closing a wound, remove tension from the superficial skin sutures, and decrease scarring by providing increased wound support long after the epidermal sutures have been removed. Deep sutures also close dead space, which decreases the risk of hematomas and dehiscence.

Table 7.2   Suture Size and Time of Removal

Anatomic Area	Days Until Removal	External Suture Size	Buried Absorbable Suture Size
Face	3–6	5-0 or 6-0	4-0 or 5-0
Scalp	10–14	4-0, staples	3-0 or 4-0
Upper body	7–10	4-0	4-0
Hand	7–10	4-0 or 5-0	4-0
Lower body	10–14	4-0	3-0 or 4-0
Over joint (splint recommended)	14–21	4-0	3-0 or 4-0

Source: Adapted from Coates WC. Lacerations to the face. In Tintinalli JE, Kellen GD, Stapczynski JS. *Emergency Medicine, A Comprehensive Study Guide.* 6th ed. New York: McGraw-Hill; 2004.

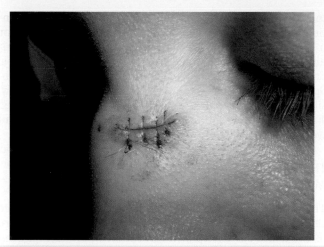

Figure 7.2 Simple interrupted suture of a small nose laceration. (Copyright Richard P. Usatine, MD.) **From 1st edition**

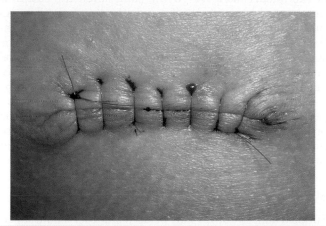

Figure 7.3 Running stitch. Always keep the depth of the suture placement the same on each side. (Copyright Richard P. Usatine, MD.) **From 1st edition**

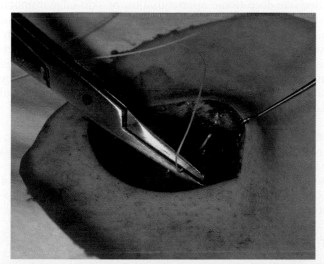

Figure 7.4 Deep stitch with absorbable suture material. The suture needle should enter deep in the skin below the dermis where the undermining was accomplished and exit in the upper dermis. (Copyright Richard P. Usatine, MD.) **From 1st edition**

The inverted knot technique places the knot as far below the skin margins as possible to avoid suture spitting (migration of deep sutures to the skin surface). It also keeps the ends of the cut suture from protruding through the wound margin. To start the stitch, begin at the bottom of the wound (in the undermined area if undermining was used) and come up usually just below the epidermal-dermal junction. Go straight across the incision, entering at the same level on the opposite side, then go down to the base at the same depth the initial suture was started and tie. Care should be taken to achieve symmetry of depth and width on both sides of the laceration. For a more detailed discussion of the deep vertical mattress suture, see Chapter 6, *Suturing Techniques*, for details and examples. The epidermis is then fully closed with a closure of choice (nonabsorbable suture, wound closure strips, or tissue adhesive).

VERTICAL MATTRESS SUTURE

The vertical mattress suture (Figure 7.5 and Chapter 6, Figure 6.14A–C) promotes eversion of the wound edges of the skin. It is also useful when the natural tendency of loose skin is to create inversion of the wound margins, which should be avoided. A good example is the loose skin under the triceps muscle and thin skin in older people. The stitch is also appropriate when the skin is very thin and interrupted sutures have a tendency to pull through.

HORIZONTAL MATTRESS SUTURE

The horizontal mattress suture (Figure 7.6) is helpful in wounds under a moderate amount of tension or movement and also promotes wound edge eversion. It is especially useful on the palms or soles and in patients who are poor candidates for deep sutures because of susceptibility to wound infections. It is also helpful over joints due to the amount of movement with activity. It is not recommended in wounds that are located in cosmetically important areas.

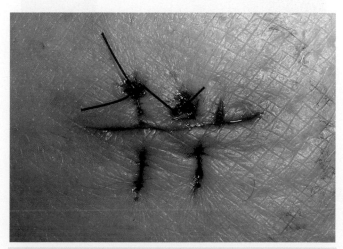

Figure 7.5 Vertical mattress suture. (Copyright Richard P. Usatine, MD.) **From 1st edition**

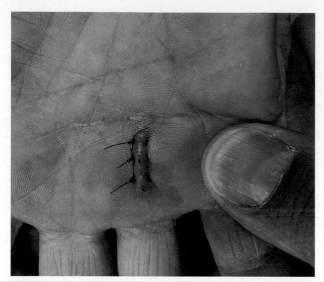

Figure 7.6 Horizontal mattress stitch. (Copyright Daniel L. Stulberg, MD.)

SUBCUTICULAR RUNNING SUTURE

The subcuticular running suture (Figure 7.7 and Chapter 6, Figure 6.20A–G) is used to close linear wounds that are under minimal tension. It yields an excellent cosmetic result. It is advantageous in patients who tend to form hypertrophic scars or keloids, because it minimizes the number of times the skin's surface must be perforated with the suture needle. Meticulous alignment of each stitch is critical to prevent gaps in the linear wound. The ends of the suture

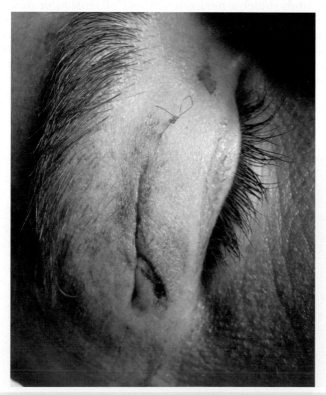

Figure 7.7 Subcuticular running suture. (Courtesy of Joe Deng, MD.)
From 1st edition

may be taped under slight tension to preserve approximation. If desired, the two ends can be tied over the wound, or a knot can be placed at each end to prevent slippage. Usually a polypropylene-coated nylon works best. Steri-Strips, or tissue glue, can be used to supplement this type of stitch. Special care must be taken to avoid pressure on the wound, since this stitch separates easily. Subcuticular interrupted sutures are also a fine choice for smaller wounds and wounds with little tension.

THREE-POINT OR HALF-BURIED MATTRESS SUTURE

The three-point or half-buried mattress suture (see Chapter 6, Figure 6.18A, B) is designed to permit closure of the acute corner tip of a laceration without impairing blood flow to the tip. It is an intradermal stitch in which the needle is inserted initially into the intact skin on the nonflap portion of the wound and passed through the skin at the middermis level. At the same level, the suture is then passed transversely through the tip of the flap, returned on the opposite side of the wound, and brought through the skin, paralleling the point of entrance. The suture is tied and draws the tip snugly into place in good approximation. Care should be taken not to have the knot tied over the point of the flap. This same approach can be used in closing a stellate laceration, drawing the tips together in a purse-string fashion. The resulting knot should be placed over the segment of the stellate laceration with the best blood supply. Repair of a "T" laceration also uses this technique.

SURGICAL ADHESIVE STRIPS (STERI-STRIPS)

Surgical adhesive strips may be used alone for small, superficial wounds (especially in young children).[24,25] When these strips suffice to close a wound, they are more easily placed without physical or psychological trauma to the child. However, surgical adhesive strips alone are not appropriate for deep lacerations because they do not provide adequate deep-tissue approximation or skin-edge eversion when used alone. Surgical adhesive strips with or without gum mastic did not provide any additional strength to wounds closed by subcuticular continuous suture.[26] Surgical adhesive strips are especially helpful after suture removal to prevent dehiscence and may be left on until they fall off. Patients may shower with them on after the initial 24 hours.

Surgical adhesive strips adhere better to the skin when a sticky substance is applied to the skin first. Tincture of benzoin and gum mastic (Mastisol) are both helpful. Studies have shown that gum mastic offers superior adhesive qualities compared with benzoin and has a lower incidence of postoperative contact dermatitis and subsequent skin discoloration.[27]

TISSUE ADHESIVES

Tissue adhesives may be used to close certain wounds that are not under any tension and are not at risk for infection. Tissue adhesive can also be used when deep sutures have relieved the tension on the skin in cosmetically important areas. These can be purchased as octylcyanoacrylate (Dermabond) and butylcyanoacrylate (SkinStitch). A Cochrane systematic review provides evidence that tissue adhesives are an option for sutures, staples, and adhesive strips for the management of simple traumatic lacerations that are not under tension nor prone to wound infection.[28] Overall, no significant differences were found in cosmetic scores at the reported assessment periods between tissue adhesives and these other methods. At 1 to 3 months, a subgroup analysis significantly favored butylcyanoacrylate over all other skin closure methods. Tissue adhesives significantly lowered the time to complete the procedure, the levels of pain, and the incidence of erythema. However, the data revealed a significant increase in the rate of dehiscence with the use of tissue adhesives when compared with the other methods of skin closure.[29]

Tissue adhesives and surgical adhesive strips are both excellent "no needle" alternatives for the closure of suitable pediatric lacerations.[20] These two techniques are similar in efficacy, parental acceptability, and cosmetic outcome. Appropriate wound preparation techniques, such as irrigation under local or topical anesthesia, are still necessary. Nail bed repair performed using tissue adhesives is significantly faster than suture repair.[30] Tissue adhesives provide similar cosmetic and functional results in the management of acute nail bed lacerations.

Tissue adhesives should be avoided on any wound that has any tension. They should not be used on any area that can be flexed (i.e., a knuckle or wrist). If it is necessary to use on a jointed area, immobilize the joint with a splint. Cover eyes with gauze when working on the forehead or near the eye. Consider using petrolatum to create a barrier between the cut and the eyes to minimize the chance of the product running into the eye. If the product enters the eye, it may be removed by applying an ophthalmic ointment, which will eventually dissolve the adhesive. This can be followed by gentle irrigation, often performed several hours later by the patient at home using water in their hands over a sink. Appropriate treatment for any resulting corneal abrasion should be followed.

Follow these guidelines, which are adapted from SkinStitch information, when using tissue adhesives (Figure 7.8A–C) and an example of Dermabond usage (Figure 7.8D and E):

- Tap glue down into the bottom bulb of the applicator.
- Holding the applicator tip upright, snip the tip as close to the end as possible.
- Never put the glue in the wound.
- Apply a thin layer of adhesive along the edge of the area to be treated, or use the multiple dot technique.
- Pull the adhesive across to the other side of the wound, using the applicator as a hockey stick. In effect, you are building a bridge over the minor cut or wound.
- Hold the wound edges together for 30 to 60 seconds.
- Apply a second and third thin coat. Remember, two or three thin layers are actually stronger than one thick coat. Dermabond recommends three layers.
- Some patients may experience mild burning; this is normal, but warn patients so that they do not move and ruin the adhesion.
- A Steri-Strip can be used for extra strength or to keep a child from picking at the wound.

STAPLES

Staples are most often used to repair scalp lacerations. They are also useful on extremity wounds or in mass casualty events where wound closure is used to control bleeding. In one randomized trial of children (ages 1 to 16 years) with simple scalp lacerations, patients were randomly assigned to either a stapling or suturing procedure.[31] Procedure time was significantly lower in the stapling group ($P = 0.001$). There were no significant differences in the final follow-up cosmetic score between the two groups.[27] Although staples are faster to apply to the scalp, the cost of the materials is greater. Scalp stapling should not be attempted in men who are already bald or in wounds that extend to the forehead.

DELAYED PRIMARY CLOSURE (TERTIARY INTENTION)

Primary closure is defined by the use of sutures, strips, or adhesives to close the wound at the time of initial surgery or evaluation. Healing by secondary intention occurs when no attempt is made to close the wound and the wound heals naturally by granulation. This method is used after a simple shave biopsy, in grossly contaminated or infected wounds, or in wounds that present far too late to consider closure.

Delayed primary closure is healing by tertiary intention. This technique is used for wounds that are greater than 12 hours old (24 hours for facial lacerations) but would cosmetically benefit from closure in a few days. After anesthetizing, evaluating, and irrigating the wound, insert a small piece of petroleum gauze between the wound edges and place the patient on an antibiotic, such as cephalexin, for 5 days. On the third day, the patient should return for definitive repair. If the wound appears clean and free of infection and has not started the granulation process, the repair can proceed. The wound is reanesthetized, reirrigated, and closed primarily with nonabsorbable sutures (i.e., no deep sutures because they increase the chance of infection). Debridement of nonviable tissue is of utmost importance in delayed closure. The patient continues the course of prescribed antibiotics, and suture removal occurs at the interval beginning at the time of suturing (Table 7.2).

Complications

The complications of laceration repair are the same as when a biopsy or surgical excision is performed (bleeding, infection, dehiscence, etc.). The main differences relate to coexisting trauma such as crush injuries that can devitalize tissue around the laceration or lead to underlying injuries to tendons, vessels, bones, or joints. For discussion of complications and their treatment and prevention see Chapter 26, *Complications*.

Postprocedure Patient Education

Most wounds are best protected with a dressing during the first 24 to 48 hours after closure. Continued oozing might be expected, or pressure might be needed. For hemostasis, a pressure dressing should be applied. This could be a folded

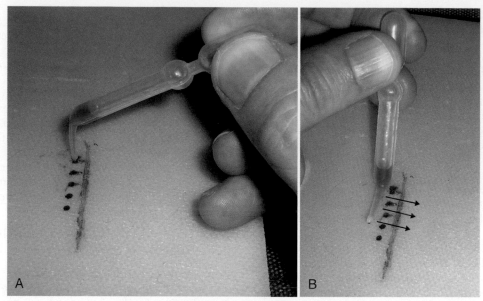

How to apply skinstitch skin adhesive

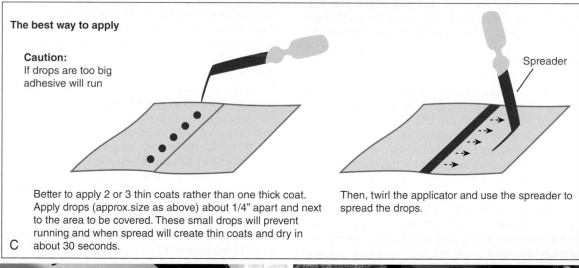

The best way to apply

Caution:
If drops are too big
adhesive will run

Better to apply 2 or 3 thin coats rather than one thick coat.
Apply drops (approx.size as above) about 1/4" apart and next
to the area to be covered. These small drops will prevent
running and when spread will create thin coats and dry in
about 30 seconds.

Spreader

Then, twirl the applicator and use the spreader to
spread the drops.

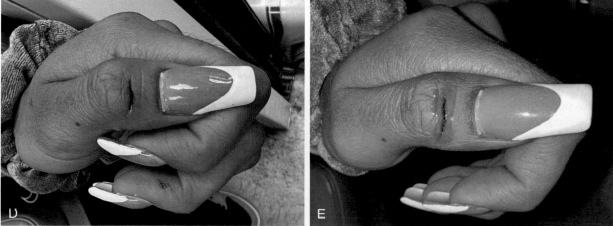

Figure 7.8 Use of tissue adhesive to close a laceration not under tension. **(A)** Better to apply two or three thin coats rather than one thick coat. Apply drops (approx. size as above) about ¼" apart and next to the area to be covered. These small drops will prevent running and when spread will create thin coats and dry in about 30 minutes. **(B)** Then, twirl the applicator and use the spreader to spread the drops. (Photographs courtesy of Richard P. Usatine, MD. Device courtesy of SkinStitch Corp, Massena, NY.) **(C)** Laceration of thumb. **(D)** Laceration of thumb repaired with Dermabond. **(C** and **D** Copyright of Vickie McCoskey PAC.)

gauze over a thin strip of sterile ointment over the suture line with tape over it, or a nonstick type of gauze dressing covered with gauze and tape. Trade names for nonstick dressings include Xeroform, Adaptic, and Telfa. It is not usually necessary to keep a wound completely dry after 24 hours, because the epidermis has formed a seal by this time. Therefore, patients may shower after 24 hours and redress the wound after gently drying it. Immersion of the laceration should be avoided because the sutures provide an avenue to introduce into the wound the bacteria present in a body of water (e.g., bath, hot tub, swimming pool, lake, ocean, kitchen sink).

Moist healing (application of petrolatum after gentle daily washing) aids in quicker healing. Although antibiotic ointments were traditionally used for dressings postsurgically, Smack et al. determined that clean wounds heal just as well when white petrolatum is applied.[32] Neomycin and bacitracin are frequent contact allergens and have not been proven to prevent infections after a laceration is repaired. Application of any of these products should be limited to the smallest possible area over the suture line. Extension over the wound edges may lead to maceration of the skin and reduce its ability to hold the sutures securely in place, thus causing them to pull through and lead to wound dehiscence. Suggestions for the timing for skin suture removal are listed in Table 7.2.

Wounds on the face or scalp may be dressed with a thin layer of antibiotic ointment or petrolatum in lieu of a mechanical dressing. It is best to cover them at night to avoid drying. Instruct patients to return if signs of wound infection appear, including spreading erythema, pus, lymphangitis, or fever. A routine wound check is not necessary for patients who understand the importance of monitoring the wound for signs of infection. All wounds should be covered with sunscreen for at least 6 months following the repair if they are located on areas exposed to the sun.

Considerations for Specific Anatomic Repairs

LIP

When evaluating a patient with a superficial lip laceration, it is important to note whether the laceration extends through the vermilion border. In this instance, the vermilion border should be approximated first with a 6-0 nylon (or polypropylene) suture. There is no room for error in this area, because even a 1-mm discrepancy is a cosmetic problem.

For lip lacerations that extend through multiple layers, a more complex repair must be performed (Figure 7.9A–C). A through-and-through laceration is repaired in three steps. After ensuring the integrity of the teeth, the wound is gently irrigated. As above, when feasible the vermilion border is approximated, then the muscular layer is repaired with absorbable suture (4-0 Vicryl or Vicryl Rapide). Next, the mucosal layer is closed with a soft suture for comfort (4-0 chromic, Vicryl or Vicryl Rapide). Finally, the wound is reirrigated from the outside, and the skin is closed with simple interrupted sutures. It is reasonable to consider an infraorbital regional nerve block for an upper lip laceration or a mandibular regional nerve block for a lower lip laceration (see Chapter 3, *Anesthesia*).

EYELID

Lacerations around the eye require careful examination of ocular structures. The integrity of the globe should be carefully assessed, and a thorough eye exam is warranted. If a visual abnormality, lacrimal system defect, or globe rupture is suspected, immediate referral is indicated. Repair by an ophthalmologist or oculoplastic specialist is warranted in wounds that involve the lacrimal system, lid lacerations that extend through the tarsal plate, or wounds that cross the palpebral margins.

For an uncomplicated lid laceration, a small (6-0) suture is used. Care must be taken to place the suture through the skin only and to avoid penetration through the tarsal plate or globe (Figure 7.7). Regional anesthesia with a supraorbital nerve block for the upper lid or an infraorbital nerve block for the lower lid may be useful (see Chapter 3, *Anesthesia*).

NOSE

Nasal lacerations can be repaired using standard techniques after careful evaluation for underlying injury. In many cases an underlying nasal bone fracture or cartilage disruption is present. If the nasal bone is fractured and a laceration is present, it should be treated as an open

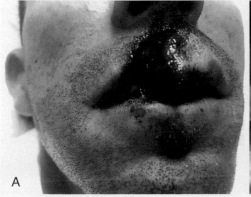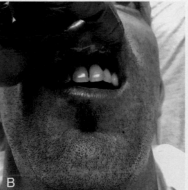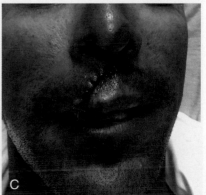

Figure 7.9 Lip laceration repair. **(A)** Evaluation of full-thickness lip laceration with attention to lining up the vermillion border. **(B)** Repair of muscle, then mucosa. **(C)** Repair of skin as final step of full-thickness lip laceration repair. (Copyright Angela Martz, PAC.)

fracture and appropriate antibiotics prescribed. Nasal cartilage rarely requires suturing, because it is held in place by surrounding anatomic structures and regains stability when the overlying skin is sutured. Lacerations to the alar margins must be aligned carefully. When a blunt force trauma causes a nasal laceration, a careful examination for a septal hematoma should be undertaken. Epistaxis should be controlled prior to the repair and may involve packing or referral to an ENT specialist.

EAR

Ear lacerations through the cartilage are managed similarly to the nose as above with slight adjustments. Due to the thin skin over the cartilage, some providers do not place deep or subcutaneous sutures as the suture material remains palpable and possibly visible after healing. The cartilage is repaired with nylon or polypropylene by suturing through the skin, cartilage, and the skin on the opposite side of the cartilage, then returning the suture to the original side. This allows the entire nonabsorbable suture to be removed after 5 to 7 days. Other providers will use deep Monocryl or other absorbable sutures to reapproximate the perichondrium. Additional 5-0 or 6-0 sutures are then used to reapproximate the skin defect (Figure 7.10A–C). After the repair, use commercial bolsters or rolled gauze over petrolatum or a nonadherent dressing to apply pressure to the ear to prevent accumulation of blood adjacent to the cartilage, which can lead to inflammation of the cartilage and a "cauliflower ear" appearance.

NAIL BED

Nail bed lacerations can be grossly apparent or be suspected when there has been blunt trauma to the nail area and a subungual hematoma occupies greater than 50% of the surface under the nail. If the nail is loose, it should be removed and the underlying nail bed laceration repaired. It is important to preserve the natural smoothness of the nail bed when an underlying laceration has occurred and avoid scarring as in Figure 7.11. The practitioner can also consider removing the nail of the patient who has a >50% subungual

hematoma. The wound is repaired with a rapidly absorbing suture, such as Vicryl Rapide, or with tissue adhesive.

Alternatively, a patient with a nail bed laceration can have a partial nail removal on the distal side of the laceration. Using an 18-gauge needle, two or three holes are bored into the proximal end of the nail bed laceration. The sutures are directed through these holes on the proximal nail and into the soft tissue on the distal side of the nail bed.

Thorough anesthesia is required and is best achieved using a digital or metacarpal block. If the nail is removed, it can be used as the resulting dressing postprocedure. It can be reinserted into the eponychium to ensure that new nail growth can occur. In the event that the nail itself cannot be replaced, future nail growth can be promoted by inserting a small piece of nonadherent gauze or a foil stent into the eponychium. To protect the sensitive nail bed area, a bulky finger dressing can be applied over a single layer of nonadherent gauze. Alternatively, a commercially available synthetic nail product can be placed over the area to afford protection against painful trauma.[33]

CPT/Billing Codes and ICD-9-CM Diagnostic Codes

Coding and billing becomes very complex for laceration repair and excisions. Important factors to list for billing personnel are as follows:

- Location
- Length of closure
- Intermediate repair includes either undermining or placement of deep-buried sutures. Intermediate repair increases the amount that can be billed significantly. Do not forget to bill for this portion if your repair is truly an intermediate one.
- Suture removal is included in the initial charge if the original sutures were placed by members of the same clinical practice.
- Suture removal can be billed if performed by an unassociated clinician or group from the clinician or group that performed the repair.

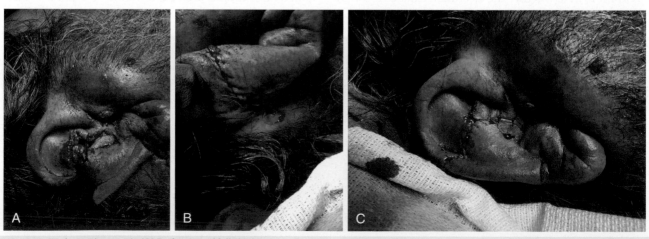

Figure 7.10 Ear laceration repair. **(A)** Evaluation of full-thickness ear laceration. **(B)** Repair of posterior aspect of ear. **(C)** Repair of anterior aspect of ear. (Copyright Angela Martz, PAC.)

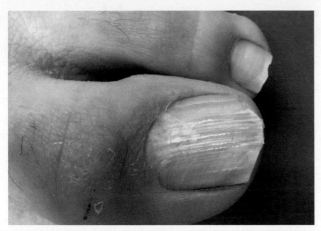
Figure 7.11 Cuticle scarred to nail post trauma. (Copyright Daniel L. Stulberg, MD.)

Box 7.1 Suturing Pearls for Lacerations

- Use 27- to 30-gauge needle for anesthesia, into the open laceration.
- Use 1% lidocaine with epi (epinephrine is helpful to achieve hemostasis).
- Undermine only when needed.
- Eliminate dead space with deep sutures.
- Use deep inverted buried absorbable sutures to reduce skin tension.
- Evert skin edges slightly ("Build pyramids, not ditches").
- Place interrupted sutures half to equally as far apart as they are across. The more tension, the more the sutures needed. Follow the Erlenmeyer flask (or pear) shape. The finer the suture, the more the sutures needed, but the less the scarring.
- Edema occurs after closure. Only approximate tissues; do not strangulate the skin.
- Begin gentle washing of wound after 12 to 24 hours; if Steri-Strips and/or tissue glues are not used, apply an ointment to keep the wound moist to speed healing.
- Apply Steri-Strips after suture removal in wounds under tension.

Conclusion

In the treatment of lacerations, careful inspection, adequate irrigation, skilled closure, and appropriate wound care can produce the best functional and cosmetic results. See Box 7.1 for a list of suturing pearls for lacerations. The principles and steps covered in this chapter show how lacerations can be repaired with maximal skill and minimal discomfort to the patient.

Resources

Splash Shield covers the full face with clear plastic on a comfortable headband (800-536-6686; www.splashshield.org).

Zerowet Supershield and Zerowet Klenzalac irrigation system (www.zerowet.com; 800-438-0938).

The remainder of the equipment can be obtained from any medical supplier, including those listed in Chapter 2.

References

1. Rahim K, Saleha S, Zhu X, Huo L, Basit A, Franco OL. Bacterial contribution in chronicity of wounds. *Microb Ecol.* 2017;73(3):710-721. doi:10.1007/s00248-016-0867-9.
2. Singer AJ, Stark MJ. LET versus EMLA for pretreating lacerations: a randomized trial. *Acad Emerg Med.* 2001;8(3):223-230. doi:10.1111/j.1553-2712.2001.tb01297.x.
3. Newberry CI, Thomas JR, Cerrati EW. Facial scar improvement procedures. *Facial Plast Surg.* 2018;34(5):448-457. doi:10.1055/s-0038-1669400.
4. Wilson W, Taubert KA, Gewitz M, et al. Prevention of infective endocarditis: guidelines from the American Heart Association: a guideline from the American Heart Association Rheumatic Fever, Endocarditis, and Kawasaki Disease Committee, Council on Cardiovascular Disease in the Young, and the Council on Clinical Cardiology, Council on Cardiovascular Surgery and Anesthesia, and the Quality of Care and Outcomes Research Interdisciplinary Working Group. *Circulation.* 2007;116:1736-1754.
5. Barnes S, D'Amore K, Propersi M, Reyes M. Acute traumatic wounds: evaluation, cleansing, and repair in the ED. *Emerg Med Pract.* 2021;23(suppl 12):1-43.
6. Kawaiah A, Thakur M, Garg S, Kawasmi SH, Hassan A. Fingertip injuries and amputations: a review of the literature. *Cureus.* 2020;12(5):e8291. doi:10.7759/cureus.8291.
7. Rupert J, Honeycutt JD, Odom MR. Foreign bodies in the skin: evaluation and management. *Am Fam Physician.* 2020;101(12):740-747.
8. Cummings P, Del Beccaro MA. Antibiotics to prevent infection of simple wounds: a meta-analysis of randomized studies. *Am J Emerg Med.* 1995;13:396-400.
9. Cummings P. Antibiotics to prevent infection in patients with dog bite wounds: a meta-analysis of randomized trials. *Ann Emerg Med.* 1994;23:535-540.
10. Talan DA, Mower WR, Krishnadasan A, et al. Trimethoprim-sulfamethoxazole versus placebo for uncomplicated skin abscess. *N Engl J Med.* 2016;374(9):823-832. doi:10.1056/NEJMoa1507476.
11. Adler AJ, Dubinsky I, Eisen J. Does the use of topical lidocaine, epinephrine, and tetracaine solution provide sufficient anesthesia for laceration repair? *Acad Emerg Med.* 1998;5:108-112.
12. Resch K, Schilling C, Borchert BD, et al. Topical anesthesia for pediatric lacerations: a randomized trial of lidocaine-epinephrine-tetracaine solution versus gel. *Ann Emerg Med.* 1998;32:693-697.
13. Tangen LF, Lundbom JS, Skarsvåg TI, et al. The influence of injection speed on pain during injection of local anaesthetic. *J Plast Surg Hand Surg.* 2016;50(1):7-9. doi:10.3109/2000656X.2015.1058269.
14. Vent A, Surber C, Graf Johansen NT, et al. Buffered lidocaine 1%/epinephrine 1:100,000 with sodium bicarbonate (sodium hydrogen carbonate) in a 3:1 ratio is less painful than a 9:1 ratio: a double-blind, randomized, placebo-controlled, crossover trial. *J Am Acad Dermatol.* 2020;83(1):159-165. doi:10.1016/j.jaad.2019.09.088.
15. Quinn J, Cummings S, Callaham M, Sellers K. Suturing versus conservative management of lacerations of the hand: randomised controlled trial. *Br Med J.* 2002;325:299.
16. Moscati RM, Mayrose J, Reardon RF, et al. A multicenter comparison of tap water versus sterile saline for wound irrigation. *Acad Emerg Med.* 2007;14:404-409.
17. Ernst AA, Gershoff L, Miller P, et al. Warmed versus room temperature saline for laceration irrigation: a randomized clinical trial. *South Med J.* 2003;96:436-439.
18. Kim H, Hwang K, Yun SM. Catgut and its use in plastic surgery. *J Craniofac Surg.* 2020;31(3):876-878. doi:10.1097/SCS.0000000000006149.
19. Luck RP, Flood R, Eyal D, et al. Cosmetic outcomes of absorbable versus nonabsorbable sutures in pediatric facial lacerations. *Pediatr Emerg Care.* 2008;24:137-142.
20. Mikhail GR, Selak L, Salo S. Reinforcement of surgical adhesive strips. *J Dermatol Surg Oncol.* 1986;12:904-905, 908.
21. Sklar LR, Pourang A, Armstrong AW, Dhaliwal SK, Sivamani RK, Eisen DB. Comparison of running cutaneous suture spacing during linear wound closures and the effect on wound cosmesis of the face and neck: a randomized clinical trial. *JAMA Dermatol.* 2019;155(3):321-326. doi:10.1001/jamadermatol.2018.5057.
22. Stoecker A, Blattner CM, Howerter S, Fancher W, Young J, Lear W. Effect of simple interrupted suture spacing on aesthetic and functional outcomes of skin closures. *J Cutan Med Surg.* 2019;23(6):580-585. doi:10.1177/1203475419861077.

23. Weinkle A, Harrington A, Kang A, Armstrong AW, Eisen DB. Aesthetic outcome of simple cuticular suture distance from the wound edge on the closure of linear wounds on the head and neck: A randomized evaluator blinded split-wound comparative effect trial. *J Am Acad Dermatol.* 2022;86(4):863-867. Erratum in: J Am Acad Dermatol. 2023 Jul;89(1):195. doi: 10.1016/j.jaad.2021.10.036.

24. Mattick A, Clegg G, Beattie T, Ahmad T. A randomised, controlled trial comparing a tissue adhesive (2-octylcyanoacrylate) with adhesive strips (Steristrips) for paediatric laceration repair. *Emerg Med J.* 2002;19:405-407.

25. Zempsky WT, Parrotti D, Grem C, Nichols J. Randomized controlled comparison of cosmetic outcomes of simple facial lacerations closed with Steri-Strip skin closures or Dermabond tissue adhesive. *Pediatr Emerg Care.* 2004;20:519-524.

26. Yavuzer R, Kelly C, Durrani N, et al. Reinforcement of subcuticular continuous suture closure with surgical adhesive strips and gum mastic: is there any additional strength provided? *Am J Surg.* 2005;189:315-318.

27. Lesesne CB. The postoperative use of wound adhesives. Gum mastic versus benzoin, USP. *J Dermatol Surg Oncol.* 1992;18:990.

28. Farion K, Osmond BV, Hartling L, et al. Tissue adhesives for traumatic lacerations in children and adults. *Cochrane Database Syst Rev.* 2002;2002(3):CD003326. doi:10.1002/14651858. CD003326.

29. Beam JW. Tissue adhesives for simple traumatic lacerations. *J Athl Train.* 2008;43:222-224.

30. Strauss EJ, Weil WM, Jordan C, Paksima N. A prospective, randomized, controlled trial of 2-octylcyanoacrylate versus suture repair for nail bed injuries. *J Hand Surg Am.* 2008;33:250-253.

31. Khan AN, Dayan PS, Miller S, et al. Cosmetic outcome of scalp wound closure with staples in the pediatric emergency department: a prospective, randomized trial. *Pediatr Emerg Care.* 2002;18: 171-173.

32. Smack DP, Harrington AC, Dunn C, et al. Infection and allergy incidence in ambulatory surgery patients using white petrolatum vs bacitracin ointment. A randomized controlled trial. *JAMA.* 1996; 276:972-977.

33. Hawken JB, Giladi AM. Primary management of nail bed and fingertip injuries in the emergency department. *Hand Clin.* 2021;37(1): 1-10. doi:10.1016/j.hcl.2020.09.001.

8

Choosing the Biopsy Type

RICHARD P. USATINE, MD, CAROLINE ZHU, MD, and JOHN L. PFENNINGER, MD

SUMMARY Skin biopsies can be categorized into five types: shave, punch, excisional, incisional, and curettement.

- Most skin biopsies are performed with a shave or punch technique; these are covered in detail in this chapter and in the chapters that follow.
- A deep shave (saucerization) biopsy is an accepted and desirable method to obtain a complete full depth biopsy of many melanomas.
- The risk of a false-negative partial biopsy is present when punch or shallow shave biopsies are used for assessment of large lesions suspicious for melanoma.
- Tips on how to choose the best lesion and biopsy site are provided for widespread rashes where biopsy site choice can influence the quality of the result.
- Specific biopsy recommendations are made for commonly encountered conditions such as suspected skin cancers and common skin growths and eruptions.
- Considerations for specific anatomic areas are included.
- Information on the best practices for submitting a pathologic specimen are provided.

Skin biopsies can be categorized into five types (Figure 8.1):

1. Shave
2. Punch
3. Excisional (elliptical)
4. Incisional (wedge)
5. Curettement

Most skin biopsies are performed with a shave or punch biopsy technique. Choosing which type of biopsy to perform influences the diagnostic yield, the cosmetic result, cost, and the time required for the clinician to perform the procedure. It is also important to understand the parameters for selecting that portion of a lesion which will provide the most information for the pathologist.[1-3]

General Principles

SHAVE BIOPSY (SEE CHAPTER 9, *THE SHAVE BIOPSY*)

Choice of biopsy technique has much to do with the clinician's initial assessment of the lesion. It is particularly important to consider the depth of involvement within the skin. The shave method is particularly suited to lesions confined to the epidermis and upper dermis, such as thin melanomas, basal cell carcinomas (BCCs), and squamous cell carcinomas (SCCs).

SUPERFICIAL VERSUS DEEP SHAVE BIOPSY (SAUCERIZATION, SCOOP)

The original "shave biopsy" term referred to a superficial shave that was used to remove lesions that stuck up or were no deeper than the epidermis/upper dermis. This was easily performed with a scalpel. With the advent of the flexible razor blade as a common tool for shave biopsies, these biopsies may easily be "deep" and described as "saucerization" or "scoop" biopsies.

The fear of transecting a melanoma stemmed from the earlier practice of a shave biopsy being so superficial that important depth information would be lost using a shave technique with a scalpel. Now a saucerization biopsy is an accepted and desirable method to obtain a complete full depth biopsy of many melanomas. (Figures 8.2 and 8.3).[4,5] We can put aside the myth that a suspected melanoma should not be biopsied using a "shave" technique; we just need to realize that the shave must be a saucerization with adequate depth.[4,6]

Figure 8.2
Figure 8.3
Important *advantages* of shave biopsy include the following:

- Minimal equipment is needed.
- Minimal risk of bleeding (even for patients on anticoagulants)
- Speed (because no sutures are required)
- Rapid healing (because a full-thickness wound is not created)

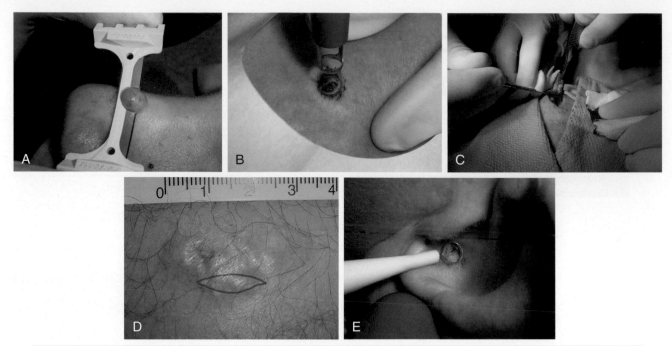

Figure 8.1 Five biopsy methods: **(A)** shave, **(B)** punch, **(C)** excision, **(D)** incisional, **(E)** curettement. (Copyright Richard P. Usatine, MD.)

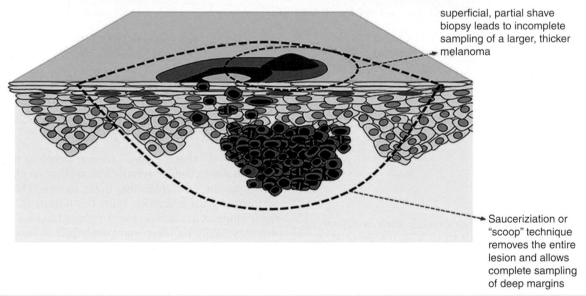

superficial, partial shave
biopsy leads to incomplete
sampling of a larger, thicker
melanoma

Sauceriziation or
"scoop" technique
removes the entire
lesion and allows
complete sampling
of deep margins

Figure 8.2 Diagnostic excisional biopsy with deep shave/saucerization technique. (Courtesy of Swetter SM, et al. Guidelines of care for the management of primary cutaneous melanoma. *J Am Acad Dermatol.* 2019;80(1):208–250.)

- Raised lesions up to 1 cm can be easily biopsied with deep shave biopsy. With the entire lesion removed, there's much less risk of missing an abnormality as can happen with a small punch biopsy that may not remove the entire lesion.[7]

  Particularly useful in certain anatomic areas, such as the back and the shin, that are difficult to suture due to skin tension

- Cosmetic results of a shave biopsy are generally excellent; in many cases, but not all, results will be superior to those achieved with full-thickness excision biopsy with suture closure.

- For lesions suspicious for melanoma, a deep shave biopsy provides ideal breadth and depth for pathology. Breadth is crucial to a biopsy to demonstrate the epidermis for pathologists to search for potential pagetoid spread of melanocytes, a finding suggestive of melanoma. Depth is significant as it is relied upon for clinicians to determine prognosis and management. For instance, a sentinel lymph node biopsy (SLNB) should be considered for melanoma extending 0.8 mm to 1 mm deep and is recommended for those thicker than 1 mm.[5,8]

- Deep shave biopsies can be performed quickly, with the whole process taking less than 5 minutes. We advocate performing them the same day that melanoma is

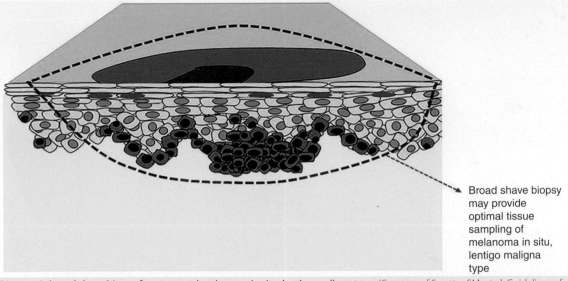

Broad shave biopsy may provide optimal tissue sampling of melanoma in situ, lentigo maligna type

Figure 8.3 Diagnostic broad shave biopsy for suspected melanoma in situ, lentigo maligna type. (Courtesy of Swetter SM, et al. Guidelines of care for the management of primary cutaneous melanoma. *J Am Acad Dermatol.* 2019;80(1):208–250.)

suspected as the evidence has shown that deep shave biopsies of melanoma are reliable and accurate in 97% of cases.[9]

- If there is visible residual pigment at the base of a shave biopsy, a second pass should be performed with a shave or punch technique. Ideally, the full depth should be obtained with the initial saucerization.

Disadvantages include:

- A possible indentation scar if a deep shave is performed. However, there have been several reports showing the results of shave biopsies of melanocytic lesions are cosmetically acceptable to patients.[10,11]
- Recurrence of the lesion if not followed by an additional excisional or destructive procedure
- Not shaving deep enough and thus not providing the pathologist with enough material for evaluation. Therefore to ensure a depth greater than 1 mm, the clinician should aim to get a tissue specimen that is at least as thick as a dime (1.3 mm).[6]

PUNCH BIOPSY (SEE CHAPTER 10, *THE PUNCH BIOPSY*)

Punch biopsy is the method of choice for the tissue diagnosis of most inflammatory or infiltrative diseases and for other lesions in which the predominant pathology lies in the dermis, such as a dermatofibroma. Punch biopsy produces a full-thickness specimen of the skin that, when done properly, extends to the subcutaneous fat.

It is important to note a common misconception regarding the use of punch biopsy in cases of suspected melanoma – while some mistakenly believe that punch biopsy is always the preferred procedure for these lesions, a deep shave biopsy, or saucerization, is often the best diagnostic method. One exception is when the punch biopsy can obtain a 0- to 1-mm margin around the entirety of a suspected melanoma. This would be possible with a 6- to 8-mm punch and a small melanoma. The saucerization

technique is preferred in most other instances. A punch might be preferred in a large thick melanoma in which a saucerization will get neither sufficient breadth nor depth (Figure 8.4). The only caveat is that if the punch is negative in a suspicious lesion, a second larger biopsy should be performed.

Advantages:

- Quick, easy, simple
- Minimal equipment needed
- Full depth specimen

Disadvantages:

- Bleeding may be more of a problem than with a shave biopsy but usually is controlled with sutures or topical hemostatic agents.
- Care must be taken not to penetrate too deeply over nerves, arteries, and thin skin.
- Sampling error can result in a missed diagnosis, such as in a melanoma when only a portion of a pigmented lesion is cancer.[7]

PARTIAL BIOPSIES

- The risk of partial biopsy is present when punch biopsies are used for assessment of large lesions suspicious for melanoma, and a negative biopsy result is obtained.
- It is reassuring that a partial biopsy does *not* contribute to local recurrence or metastatic potential of a malignant neoplasm.[12]

INCISIONAL AND EXCISIONAL BIOPSY (SEE CHAPTER 11, *ELLIPTICAL EXCISION*)

Incisional biopsy refers to excising a portion of a lesion using full-thickness excision techniques. It is used for obtaining a large sample of a large lesion (but not the entire lesion). *Excisional* biopsy refers to full-thickness excision of the entire lesion usually with an elliptical pattern. Both

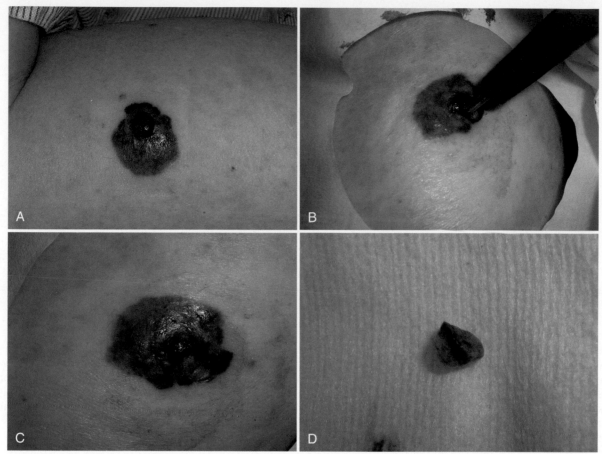

Figure 8.4 (A) A 37-year-old woman presents with a large pigmented lesion on the lower leg suspicious for melanoma. **(B)** The lesion was too large for a full excisional biopsy by any technique so decision was made that a punch biopsy through the thickest portion might provide the most information. A 4-mm punch biopsy in action. A larger punch biopsy could be justified. However, sufficient tissue was obtained with the 4-mm punch. **(C)** Melanoma showing how the punch biopsy cut down to the subcutaneous fat. **(D)** Punch specimen seen on edge showing the darkly pigmented melanoma. If the pathologist did not see melanoma in this specimen, then additional sampling should be performed with more tissue sent for analysis. (Copyright Richard P. Usatine, MD.)

require suturing. An incisional biopsy (Figure 8.1D) is a great way to biopsy suspicious lesions on the sole because these are easier to close than a round punch.

Excisional elliptical biopsies were considered the method of choice for lesions highly suggestive of malignant melanoma by many in the past and some even now (Figure 8.5 and 8.6). Many dermatologists and dermatopathologists now prefer the deep shave biopsies as the procedure of choice for suspicious lesions. There is no consensus on this choice, and as long as the correct diagnosis is obtained both options are valid.

When performing an elliptical excisional biopsy of a pigmented lesion, the recommendation is to align the ellipse along the axis of lymphatic drainage and to not exceed a 3-mm margin (Figure 8.5).[4,5] This helps perform a better SLNB if needed as a future step.

The advantages include providing a full depth sample of the whole lesion.

- The disadvantages of elliptically excising all "suspicious" lesions are:
  - (1) It is often overtreatment if the lesion turns out to be benign such as a seborrheic keratosis. More tissue is removed than what is needed, which adds to the cost and increases scarring and other complications (e.g., excising a totally benign nevus or minimally atypical one).
  - (2) Another surgery is still required if the lesion is a melanoma because the initial ellipse is performed with margins smaller than recommended for definitive treatment.

The elliptical biopsy method is also used to diagnose and remove dermal lesions (e.g., dermatofibroma) and subcutaneous cysts and tumors (epidermal cysts and lipomas). (See Chapter 12, *Cysts and Lipomas*).

INCISIONAL BIOPSY

This is essentially an elliptical biopsy that does not remove the whole suspicious lesion because the size is too large at the time of biopsy. Incisional biopsies may be used to biopsy a large lesion suspicious for melanoma on the face or sole of the foot (Figure 8.1D). A narrow ellipse on the sole of the foot may be easier to close with sutures than some punch biopsies and can potentially provide more tissue for analysis.

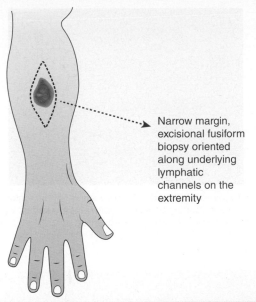

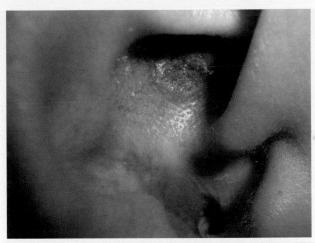

Narrow margin, excisional fusiform biopsy oriented along underlying lymphatic channels on the extremity

Figure 8.7 A suspicious lesion in the ear was biopsied with a curette and turned out to be a squamous cell carcinoma. (Copyright Richard P. Usatine, MD.)

Figure 8.5 Longitudinal/axial orientation of diagnostic elliptical/fusiform excisional biopsy on the extremity. (Adapted from Swetter SM, et al. Guidelines of care for the management of primary cutaneous melanoma. *J Am Acad Dermatol.* 2019;80(1):208–250.)

CURETTEMENT BIOPSY

Using a sharp curette is another method of biopsy. It is the method of last resort because it can destroy the architecture of the lesion being sent for pathology. A disposable 3-mm curette is a good choice for this procedure. Curettage is best suited for difficult areas such as in the canthal folds where the skin is thin and mobile or in areas difficult to access such as an ear canal or nostril. Care must be taken not to go too deep and injure vital tissue. A small lesion can be curetted off and sent to pathology (Figure 8.7).

Choice of Site to Biopsy

When the decision has been made to biopsy a lesion, along with choosing the *method* of biopsy, the clinician must also choose the *site* that will be biopsied.

If a "rash" or inflammatory process is present, select a "fresh" lesion that has recently appeared rather than one that has been present longer. Many times older lesions have been excoriated or secondarily infected, obscuring the primary pathology. Choose a lesion on the upper body rather than the lower body whenever possible (Figure 8.8) as the histology may be easier to interpret, and the healing should be more rapid. Biopsies of the lower legs are more likely to have delayed healing or get infected. Also avoid the axilla and groin if possible because these areas are more prone to infections.

If a vesicular-bullous reaction is present, the biopsy should be taken at the margin of the lesion to include normal tissue. Excise a whole small bulla or vesicle if possible, and send in formalin for standard hematoxylin and eosin (H&E) staining (Figure 8.9). It is helpful for the pathologist to examine the area where the epithelium is lifted from the tissue below to determine the level of the split (dermal-epidermal junction vs a more superficial epidermal split).

If lesions are scattered throughout, choose a site where aesthetic considerations are less of a concern (e.g., avoid the face if possible) and where scarring is less likely. The sternum, shoulders, upper back, and areas of skin tension are

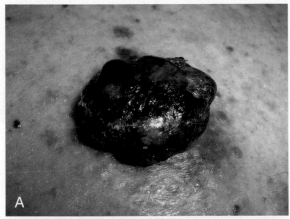

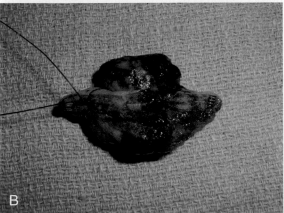

Figure 8.6 (A) Pigmented lesion highly suspicious for nodular melanoma. **(B)** Full-thickness elliptical biopsy confirmed the diagnosis for nodular melanoma, and the depth was 22 mm. Punch biopsy or partial saucerization would not have been able to provide this depth information but would have shown a depth of at least 4 mm if done correctly. This would lead to the correct management including an excision with 2 cm margins and a sentinel lymph node biopsy. (Copyright Richard P. Usatine, MD.)

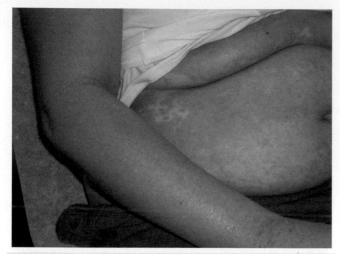

Figure 8.8 Erythroderma in a 19-year-old woman from head to toe. A 4-mm punch biopsy was performed on her arm rather than the leg. (Copyright Richard P. Usatine, MD.)

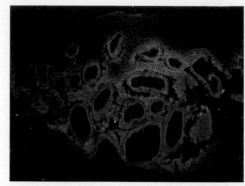

Figure 8.10 Direct immunofluorescence against immunoglobulin (Ig) G antibodies surrounding cells of the epidermis in a patient with pemphigus vulgaris. Note the chicken-wire appearance. (Reproduced with permission from Martin Fernandez, MD and Richard P. Usatine, MD.)

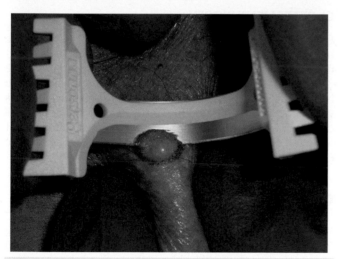

Figure 8.9 A shave biopsy of an intact blister in a patient with suspected *bullous pemphigoid.* (Copyright Richard P. Usatine, MD.)

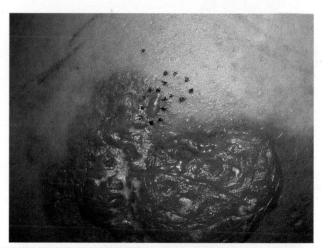

Figure 8.11 Bullous eruption suspicious for autoimmune bullous disease. Two punch biopsies will be performed. The circle around the small bulla will be sent for H&E, and the adjacent circle will be a perilesional punch biopsy for direct immunofluorescence (DIF). (Copyright Richard P. Usatine, MD.)

more likely to scar. Also, choose a lesion on the upper body rather than the lower body whenever possible.

- Direct immunofluorescence (DIF) studies are especially helpful for autoimmune bullous diseases because antibodies and complement will light up in the skin (Figure 8.10). When DIF testing is to be done, this biopsy is usually taken from perilesional skin. That means that this biopsy will not include the bulla or the erosion at all.
- The DIF specimen is generally obtained with a punch biopsy next to the visible pathology. One can draw two circles, first with one on the edge of the bulla and the other next to the edge (Figure 8.11). It is easy to anesthetize both areas with one injection. Make sure to not mix up the specimens when these are put in the containers. Note that the perilesional skin specimen should be sent in special Michel's media or sterile saline (sterile gauze in a sterile urine cup with some sterile saline on top), and let the lab know to transfer it to Michel's media when it arrives.

Another option is to do one shave biopsy that is cut into two parts:

- Take a shave biopsy that includes the bulla and the perilesional skin.
- Then cut it to send the bulla section for H&E and the perilesional skin for DIF (Figure 8.12).
- It is crucial to not mix up the specimens. For this reason, the double punch biopsy method may be easier and ensures that there is sufficient depth in each specimen.

In pemphigus vulgaris the antibody deposition is seen in the intercellular spaces of the epidermis. The pattern of the DIF fluorescence is described as chicken wire (Figure 8.10).

The DIF does not have to be done on the initial biopsy but may be performed to clarify and add data to a standard biopsy for H&E staining. There are only a few autoimmune diseases in which lesional skin is preferred (see Tables 8.1 and 8.2). A 4-mm punch is adequate. It must be sent to the lab in special Michel's media (or on saline-soaked gauze).

Useful tips on the DIF biopsy by suspected diagnosis:.

- **Autoimmune bullous diseases:** take normal-appearing perilesional skin less than 1 cm from a bulla. As false-negative

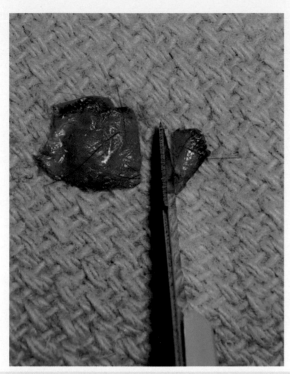

Figure 8.12 A broad shave biopsy on the edge of a bulla is cut to send the bulla section for H&E and the perilesional skin for DIF. (Copyright Richard P. Usatine, MD.)

results may arise from samples from the lower extremities, avoid these sites if possible.

- **Connective tissue diseases:** the biopsy should be taken from an established lesion (often in sun-exposed areas), ideally that is more than 6 months old but still active. An additional specimen is often taken in a sun-protected site.
- **Vasculitis:** for best results, take a punch biopsy or a deep-shave biopsy of a lesion that is less than 24 hours old.

If a basal cell carcinoma is suspected, it is often easy to shave off the whole lesion. If the lesion is large, almost any area can be biopsied, but it is better to select a raised-up border rather than an ulcerated portion. Biopsying the ulcer alone may inaccurately provide a pathology specimen showing only inflammation and reparative debris if not sampled deeply enough. A 4- to 6-mm punch biopsy is an option if the lesion is a flat sclerosing type of BCC.

If a squamous cell carcinoma is suspected and the lesion is too large to shave off in its entirety, biopsy a raised edge or any thick central location. The goal is to obtain a deep sample so the pathologist can determine extent of invasion. Some thin peripheral areas may only involve actinic change, missing the most advanced pathology. A broad deep shave is usually adequate for a biopsy. A second biopsy/excision may be needed if the pathologist reports that there is squamous dysplasia and an SCC cannot be ruled out.

Table 8.1 Location for Direct Immunofluorescence Biopsies

Disease	Where to Biopsy	Findings
Pemphigus vulgaris	Perilesional skin	Intercellular deposition of IgG
Pemphigus foliaceus	Perilesional	Intercellular deposition of IgG
IgA pemphigus	Perilesional	Intercellular deposition of IgA
Paraneoplastic pemphigus	Perilesional	Intercellular deposition of IgG Antibodies also directed to simple or transitional epithelium (rat bladder)
Bullous pemphigoid	Perilesional	Linear basement membrane staining with IgG and/or C3. Salt split samples will localize to the epidermal side.
Cicatricial pemphigoid (MMP)	Perilesional skin, mucosa, or conjunctiva	Linear basement membrane staining with IgG and/or C3. Salt split samples show variable localization.
Herpes gestationis	Perilesional	Linear basement membrane staining with C3. IgG is generally less pronounced.
Epidermolysis bullosa acquisita	Perilesional	Heavy IgG and/or C3 along the basement membrane zone. Salt split samples will localize to the dermal side.
Dermatitis herpetiformis	Lesional or normal skin from disease-prone area	Granular IgA within dermal papillae
Lichen planus	Inflamed, but nonulcerated mucosa or skin	Clumps of cytoid bodies and fibrinogen in the basement membrane zone
Lupus band test	Normal skin	Granular IgG or IgM along the basement membrane zone
Discoid lupus erythematosus	Lesional skin	Granular deposition of IgG, IgM, and/or IgA along the basement membrane zone in conjunction with cytoid bodies
Systemic lupus erythematosus	Lesional skin	Same as for discoid lupus.
Bullous lupus erythematosus	Perilesional skin	Heavy IgG and/or C3 along the basement membrane zone
Vasculitis	Early lesion (punch biopsy or deep shave)	Perivascular IgA: Henoch Schoenlein purpura Perivascular IgM/IgG/C3: other forms of vasculitis
Linear IgA dermatitis	Perilesional skin	Linear IgA deposition at the basement membrane zone
Porphyria/pseudoporphyria cutanea tarda	Perilesional skin	Linear IgG, IgM, and C3 around vessels and dermal-epidermal junction

Source: Courtesy of Robert Law, MD.

Table 8.2   Suspected Disease Entities With Recommended Biopsy Type, Size, and Requested Laboratory Tests

Disease	Recommended Biopsy Technique	Comments
Autoimmune bullous diseases	H&E – Saucerized removal of intact bulla if possible, or broad saucerization of periphery of bulla DIF – Perilesional skin ≤ 1 cm from bulla	Avoid lower extremity when possible because of delayed healing and greater risk of false-negative results.
Egidermolysis bullosa	Saucerized removal of intact bulla if possible, or broad saucerization of periphery of bulla	Blisters >12 hours old should be avoided; a fresh blister can be induced in clinically uninvolved skin near a site where the patient usually blisters. Topical anesthetics should be avoided because they may induce artificial blistering.
Vasculitis	H&E – Punch or deep shave of well-established purpuric lesion (>72 hours old) DIF – Punch or deep shave of acute lesion (<24 hours old)	IgA vasculitis is more likely to retain positive DIF findings in established lesions.
Panniculitis	Deep incisional biopsy	Punch biopsy specimens tend to fracture, leaving inflamed or necrotic fat behind. An electric rotary power punch can overcome this limitation. A 6-mm punch is the smallest size that should be divided for culture and H&E. The edge of a necrotic focus provides a high yield for culture and special stains. The skin surface should be prepped with alcohol and allowed to evaporate. Deliver the culture specimen to the desk that handles fungal and AFB specimens.
Lupus and dermatomyositis	H&E – Punch biopsy of an established lesion (>6 months old) that is still active DIF – Punch biopsy of lesional skin; choose an established lesion (>6 months old) that is still active	
SJS/TEN vs SSSS	Shave or punch biopsy including the full thickness of the epidermis	Desquamating sheets of skin may constitute an adequate specimen.
Scarring alopecia	H&E – ≥4-mm punch biopsy of an established lesion (>6 months old) that is still active DIF – ≥4-mm punch biopsy of lesion skin; choose an established lesion (>6 months old) that is still active	For all forms of alopecia, avoid the active advancing border. Established lesions are preferred. One specimen can be bisected transversely 1 mm above the dermal/SQ junction, or it can be submitted intact for the laboratory to section transversely or with the HoVert or Tyler techniques. One specimen can be bisected vertically – half submitted in Michel's medium for DIF and half added to the formalin bottle containing the transversely bisected or intact specimen.
Nonscarring alopecia	For pattern alopecia or telogen effluvium – ≥4-mm punch biopsy of an established area of alopecia For alopecia areata or syphilis – ≥4-mm punch biopsy of an active lesion of recent onset is preferred	If pattern alopecia or telogen effluvium is suspected, the specimen can be bisected transversely 1 mm above the dermal/SQ junction, or it can be submitted intact for the laboratory to section transversely or with the HoVert or Tyler techniques. For other forms of nonscarring alopecia, the specimen should be submitted intact.
BCC/SCC	Shave or punch biopsy of adequate depth to show the invasive pattern and to detect perineural invasion if present	In convex sites or thin facial skin, more superficial shave biopsy specimens may be appropriate. The skin should be pulled taught to provide greater control over depth. Avoid creating contour defects in sebaceous skin.
Suspected melanoma	Complete excisional removal whenever possible	This may take the form of a saucerization
DFSP	Deep incisional biopsy	
CTCL	Broad shave biopsy specimens below the depth of the DEJ are superior to punch biopsies	
Primary cutaneous B-cell lymphoma	Deep incisional biopsy whenever possible	A punch biopsy specimen or saucerization does not allow assessment of architecture.

AFB, Acid-fast bacilli; *BCC,* basal cell carcinoma; *CTCL,* cutaneous T-cell lymphoma; *DEJ,* dermoepidermal junctions; *DFSP,* dermatofibrosarcoma protuberans; *DIF,* direct immunofluorescence; *H&E,* hematoxylin and eosin; *IgA,* immunoglobulin A; *SCC,* squamous cell carcinoma; *S/S,* Stevens-Johnson syndrome; *SQ,* subcutaneous; *SSSS,* staphylococcal scalded skin syndrome; *TEN,* toxic epidermal necrolysis.

Courtesy of Elston DM, Stratman EJ, Miller SJ. Skin biopsy: biopsy issues in specific diseases. *J Am Acad Dermatol.* Jan 2016;74(1):1–16; quiz 17–18. doi:10.1016/j.jaad.2015.06.033. Erratum in: *J Am Acad Dermatol.* Oct 2016;75(4):854ss. PMID: 26702794.

If a melanoma is suspected, it is best to provide a specimen with adequate depth. In cases of suspected lentigo maligna melanoma on the face, a broad shave provides a better sample than a few punch biopsies and is less deforming than a large full-thickness elliptical excisional biopsy. It is not practical to perform an elliptical excision on every potentially malignant pigmented lesion. It may be better in most instances to sample the whole lesion with a broad deep shave (saucerization) than doing one or more punch biopsies (Figure 8.13). This broad shave is the recommended

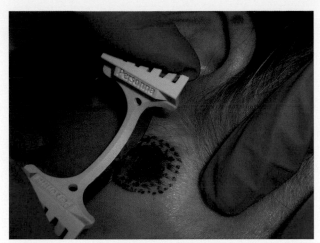

Figure 8.13 Saucerization of the whole growing pigmented lesion on the face of a 28-year-old woman. The biopsy revealed a 1.3-mm depth melanoma that was not transected at the base. (Copyright Richard P. Usatine, MD.)

biopsy technique for lentigo maligna melanoma on the face by the NCCN.[4] Dermoscopy is a tool that can help you choose the most suspicious area to biopsy in a large lesion if it is impractical to biopsy the whole lesion (see Chapter 18, *Dermoscopy*). Partial biopsies do not negatively influence melanoma patient survival, as these biopsies do not cause the melanoma to spread.[6,13]

If the lesion is predominantly an ulcer, take the biopsy at the edge of the ulcer, rather than in the ulcer bed. This may apply when trying to distinguish pyoderma gangrenosum from a stasis ulcer.

DOCUMENTATION OF BIOPSY SITE

With all biopsies (especially if multiple lesions are obtained), record a detailed description of the biopsy site, which can include an avatar and/or photo in the chart. Biopsy sites may heal quickly and can be difficult to find later when definitive treatment is necessary. Photos can aid in identifying correct locations. If it is not easy or desired to place photographs in the medical record, make sure the camera or phone camera is set to record the correct date of the photo. Then the prebiopsy photo can be found by searching by date. Make sure to keep these photos in a HIPAA compliant manner. These photos can be very important in planning definitive treatment for malignancies (including Mohs surgery – see Chapter 27). Some clinicians borrow the patient's phone camera and take a photo on this so the patient will have their own record of the lesion location if they need to see a Mohs surgeon or surgical oncologist.

Is It Cancer?

PIGMENTED LESIONS: MELANOMA AND ITS DIFFERENTIAL DIAGNOSES

Early detection and prompt removal of *melanoma* can be lifesaving. The clinical signs of melanoma were described using this mnemonic:

"ABCDE," where A = asymmetry, B = borders (irregular), C = color (variegated), D = diameter (greater than 6 mm),

and E = evolving and elevation.[14] Some have suggested adding an "F" for a change in **F**eeling since some melanomas present with onset of pruritus in a nevus.

However, not all melanomas show these signs, and our goal should be to pick up melanomas before the lesions reach 6 mm in diameter and even when it is symmetric or it does not have varied colors (some nodular melanomas). The dermatoscope is essential to increase the sensitivity and specificity for detecting melanoma (see Chapter 18, *Dermoscopy of Skin Cancer*).[15,16] Whether or not a dermatoscope is used, it is incumbent on the clinician to biopsy or do an immediate referral for any suspicious pigmented lesion. It cannot be over emphasized that patient history is of utmost importance in the evaluation of any lesion and should never be taken lightly. If a patient is concerned that a lesion has changed, it deserves a clinical and dermoscopic exam to decide upon a biopsy or referral. When dermoscopy is not available, it is probably best to err on the side of biopsying any potential malignancy.

The National Comprehensive Cancer Network (NCCN) has well-established guidelines for biopsy of pigmented lesions suspected of melanoma.[4] These include the following:

- Excisional biopsy (elliptical, punch, or saucerization) with 1- to 3-mm margins is preferred.
- Margins between 1 to 3 mm are recommended during biopsy, as wider margins may interfere with lymphatic mapping.
- Consider the orientation of wide local excision when planning an excisional biopsy. It is advised that for extremities, the biopsy be performed parallel to underlying lymphatics.
- When evaluating large lesions or those in certain areas of the body (for instance, the plantar surfaces, fingers, face, or ears), one can opt to biopsy what clinically appears to be the thickest or most atypical area of the lesion. Another way to approach large lesions is to take several "scouting" biopsies.
- Caution must be taken if one opts to take a superficial shave biopsy, as this may make it challenging to gauge the true Breslow depth, but clinicians can opt for this biopsy method for lesions of low suspicion for melanoma. Note though that for malignant lesions such as melanoma in situ or lentigo maligna, a broad shave biopsy is still preferred for optimal assessment on histopathology.
- In instances where an initial partial biopsy fails to provide sufficient tissue for diagnosis or microstaging – but *not* when SLN staging criteria are met – a repeat narrow-margin excisional biopsy should be performed.

If a melanoma is truly suspected, a deep shave biopsy may indeed be the ideal method of sampling. A punch biopsy can have significant sampling errors and false-negative results unless the whole lesion is removed or multiple biopsies are obtained from larger lesions. The object is to detect melanoma early and save lives. If a larger lesion is atypical in appearance, the entire lesion will need to be removed, but the initial biopsy will at least help determine required margins for excision or if a referral is indicated. A punch biopsy may be used as long as a negative (nonmalignant) biopsy of a suspicious lesion larger than the initial punch is followed up with an excision in which all the remaining tissue is excised and examined.

Lentigo Maligna (One Type of Melanoma In Situ)

Flat, macular lesions suspected of being lentigo maligna (LM) (Figure 8.14) present another problem because many of these lesions are very large (often over 2 cm in diameter) and frequently are present on the face. The radial growth phase may last for years, and the vertical (invasive) phase may never develop. A broad shave biopsy of suspected LM or LMM should provide a better tissue sample than one or more punch biopsies and will not cause the cosmetic deformities of a large full-thickness biopsy (Figure 8.14). A broad shave biopsy is recommended by the NCCN guidelines.[4]

Benign Nevi

Many patients will request mole removal purely for cosmetic reasons. Alternatively, the lesions may be in areas of repeated trauma (e.g., from shaving, combing, irritation from clothes or jewelry, etc.). Shave excision is the treatment of choice if the patient is requesting removal. The lesion should still be sent for histological examination. Removal of some nevi on the face may yield a better cosmetic result when accomplished by punch or meticulous excision when large. Size, location, age of the patient, history, and type of skin all are factored into the decision. Nevi with a deeper intradermal component (e.g., intradermal nevi, blue nevi) may recur or deeply pigment after shave removal especially in younger patients. A shave excision can still be performed but the patient should be forewarned as a part of informed consent that regrowth or pigment changes may still require full depth excision later. In general, deep nevi such as blue nevi should be removed down to SC fat and always sent for pathology. For nevi with hair (usually intradermal nevi or congenital nevi), a shave excision is too superficial to remove the hair follicles. In this instance, it is best to perform a deeper excision with a punch or ellipse.

Dermoscopy Findings of Nevi With Age

Age has been found to be a factor in individual patient's nevus dermoscopy pattern. Young prepubertal children often have nevi that demonstrate a globular or homogeneous pattern. This globular pattern is also commonly found in

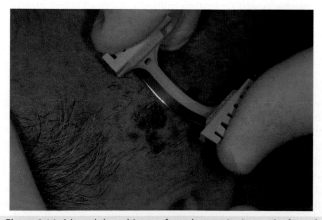

Figure 8.14 A broad shave biopsy of a melanoma in situ on the face of a 49-year-old man. A punch biopsy may have missed the melanoma, and elliptical excision may have been too aggressive if this turned out to be a seborrheic keratosis or solar lentigo. (Copyright Richard P. Usatine, MD.)

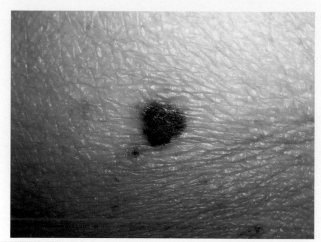

Figure 8.15 A seborrheic keratosis that is suspicious for melanoma. A shave biopsy proved this to be an SK only. Dermoscopy would also be helpful and might have prevented the need for a biopsy. (Copyright Richard P. Usatine, MD.)

adults older than 60 years of age. Adolescents tend to have nevi revealing a peripheral rim of globules. In contrast, adults most frequently exhibit a reticular pattern in their moles.[17] Nevi that differ from the expected patterns or stand out as "ugly ducklings" should be considered for biopsy. See Chapter 18, *Dermoscopy*.

Seborrheic Keratoses

Classic seborrheic keratoses will not need a biopsy. However, because some of these lesions mimic malignant tumors such as melanomas when they are darkly pigmented, biopsy should be performed if any doubt exists (Figure 8.15). Dermoscopy can help make this distinction and avoid a biopsy in many cases (see Chapter 18, *Dermoscopy*). When performing a biopsy on seborrheic keratoses, care should be taken to avoid unnecessarily deep or destructive techniques. Seborrheic keratoses are epidermal lesions. Shave biopsy or saucerization is the biopsy technique of choice. Treatment with cryotherapy without biopsy is very acceptable for lesions in which the clinical diagnosis is certain. However, lesions that fail to resolve after 6 weeks should be evaluated and a biopsy considered.

NONPIGMENTED LESIONS SUSPICIOUS FOR CANCER

Actinic Keratoses

Actinic keratoses can be very superficial or be hypertrophic. They are considered a precancerous lesion and as such, should be treated or biopsied. Thinner obvious lesions can be treated with topical agents, cryotherapy, or electrodesiccation without biopsy initially. If lesions persist after treatment, or if there is concern about a cancer at the base, then a shave biopsy is indicated. With high-risk lesions such as a *cutaneous horn*, a deeper saucerization is best to provide the pathologist with enough tissue to discern invasion (Figure 8.16).

Keratoacanthomas (KA)

The history and clinical appearance of these lesions are quite distinct. They grow rapidly in a matter of months and may appear like a BCC with central keratin plug (Figure 8.17).

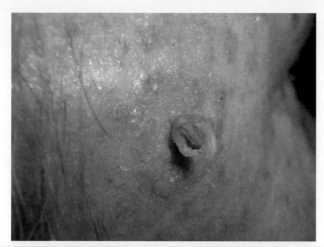

Figure 8.16 A cutaneous horn arising in a squamous cell carcinoma on the face. A saucerization provided the diagnosis. (Copyright Richard P. Usatine, MD.)

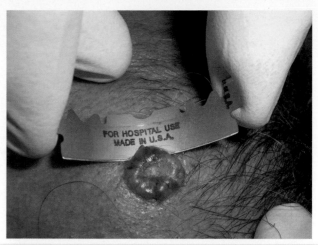

Figure 8.18 A razor blade being used for a shave biopsy of a nodular BCC. (Copyright Richard P. Usatine, MD.)

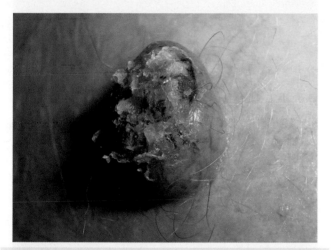

Figure 8.17 A keratoacanthoma with a pearly raised border and a keratin-like volcanic core. (Copyright Richard P. Usatine, MD.)

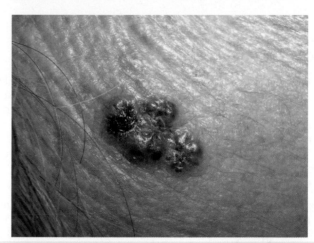

Figure 8.19 Pigmented BCC on the temple of an elderly woman. A deep shave biopsy was performed in case this turned out to be a melanoma. While doing the shave biopsy the tissue below the lesion was viewed to make sure that the shave was below the pigment. With the similar morphology throughout a punch biopsy should have provided adequate initial information whether or not this turned out to be a BCC or melanoma. (Copyright Richard P. Usatine, MD.)

It is a well-differentiated variant of SCC. If suspected, smaller lesions (8–10 mm) can be removed with a deep saucerization followed by ED&C. For larger lesions, full-thickness excision is the best method of biopsy/removal.

Basal Cell Carcinoma (BCC)

The majority of BCCs are relatively small (<1 cm) raised tumors on the face, head, neck, or exposed parts of the trunk and extremities. Nearly any method can be used to biopsy these lesions. The shave biopsy can be used for most of these tumors and has the advantage of not producing a deeper or full-thickness wound should the lesion prove not to be a cancer (Figure 8.18).

Sclerosing (morpheaform) BCCs are flat and more difficult to diagnose clinically and histopathologically. A punch specimen is one option, although a well done deep shave often is adequate to make the diagnosis.

Pigmented BCCs can appear very much like melanomas (Figure 8.19). Dermoscopy can help one differentiate these two diagnoses. A saucerization can then provide adequate tissue to make the histologic diagnosis.

Squamous Cell Carcinoma (SCC)

Squamous cell carcinoma (SCC) may be difficult to diagnose by histopathology as it is part of a spectrum from actinic keratosis to SCC in situ to invasive SCC. A deep shave biopsy should be taken to get a specimen with adequate depth to enable the pathologist to render an accurate opinion. When the shave is not deep enough, the pathologist may add to the reading of an AK or SCC in situ that invasive SCC cannot be ruled out. As with BCC, the clinician should carefully record the site of biopsy. For large lesions, particularly those in or around the oral cavity and ears, it is important to check for lymphadenopathy. Prompt treatment after diagnosis of SCC is essential because some of these lesions have the potential for metastasis (see Chapter 34).

Amelanotic Melanomas

Amelanotic melanomas can be more challenging to diagnose clinically. This is one strong reason that dermoscopy is an important skill to learn. (Figure 8.20).

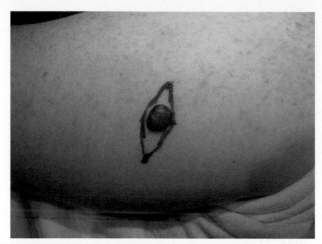

Figure 8.20 An amelanotic melanoma about to be excised. The diagnosis was not obvious, but the elliptical excision provided great tissue for diagnosis. (Courtesy of EJ Mayeaux.)

DIAGNOSING A "RASH" OR OTHER DERMATOLOGIC CONDITION

For most challenging rashes, a 4-mm punch biopsy will be helpful to make the diagnosis. Dermoscopy can help narrow down the differential diagnosis or make a definitive diagnosis. (See Chapter 19, *Dermoscopy* of other lesions in general dermatology.)

Table 8.2 is full of great recommendations on how to do a biopsy based on specific diagnoses.

Citation:

Elston DM, Stratman EJ, Miller SJ. Skin biopsy: biopsy issues in specific diseases. *J Am Acad Dermatol.* Jan 2016;74(1): 1–16; quiz 17–18. doi:10.1016/j.jaad.2015.06.033. Erratum in: *J Am Acad Dermatol.* Oct 2016;75(4):854. PMID: 26702794.

Inflammatory Disorders

Various inflammatory disorders present as unknown rashes, and a punch biopsy should provide adequate tissue for diagnosis (e.g., lichen planus, psoriasis, and cutaneous lupus erythematosus). The typical malar rash of *systemic lupus erythematosus (SLE)* in a patient with a strongly positive ANA does not require a biopsy for diagnosis. However, some cases of cutaneous lupus may need a biopsy for diagnosis (Figure 8.21). *Lichen planus* presents with different morphologies from atrophic to hypertrophic, from solid to bullous. A punch biopsy may be needed for definitive diagnosis if the clinical picture is not classic (Figure 8.22). A 4-mm punch biopsy or a deep shave should provide adequate tissue (see Chapter 10, *Punch Biopsy*).

Almost all inflammatory dermatoses have a dermal component. Punch biopsy is necessary to preserve the dermal architecture so the dermatopathologist can evaluate the cellular infiltrate, both as to its nature and its pattern. In most cases in which a punch biopsy is indicated, the biopsy need only go through the dermis, and the specimen is cut off at the top of the subcutaneous fat.

However, to diagnose *erythema nodosum* (Figure 8.23), the punch specimen should include as much of the subcutaneous fat as possible. This is because erythema nodosum

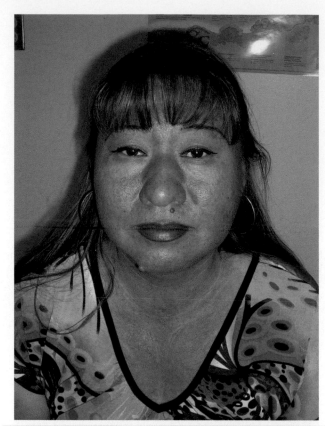

Figure 8.21 An erythematous eruption in photo-exposed areas turned out to be subacute cutaneous *lupus erythematosus* proven by a 4-mm punch biopsy on the anterior chest. (Copyright Richard P. Usatine, MD.)

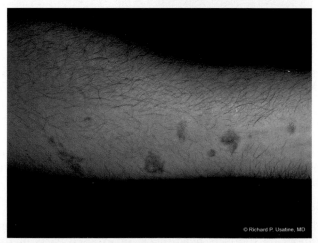

Figure 8.22 An atrophic variant of lichen planus in a 36-year-old man proven by a 4-mm punch biopsy. The biopsy was essential for diagnosis of this rare variant of lichen planus. (Copyright Richard P. Usatine, MD.)

is a panniculitis (inflammation of the fat), with the overlying dermis secondarily involved. A double punch may be performed in which a single 5- to 6-mm punch is performed and then a smaller 4-mm punch is used to get a second specimen in the deeper fat. While there are no studies to support the double punch method, some authors recommend a deep incisional or excisional biopsy with a generous portion of subcutaneous fat.[18] In many cases the clinical

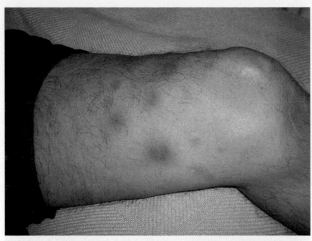

Figure 8.23 Erythema nodosum is a panniculitis. Therefore a punch biopsy should be deep and obtain subcutaneous fat. This patient had *erythema nodosum leprosum*. (Copyright Richard P. Usatine, MD.)

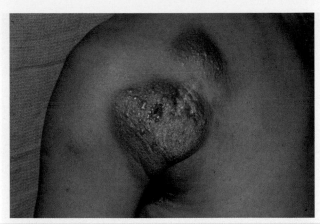

Figure 8.25 Cutaneous T-cell lymphoma in the more advanced tumor stage. A 4-mm punch biopsy was sufficient to make the diagnosis. (Copyright Richard P. Usatine, MD.)

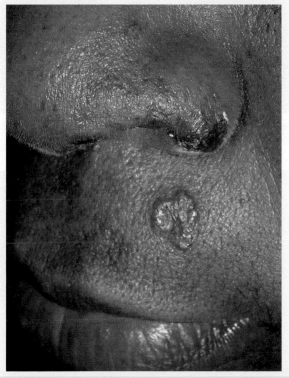

Figure 8.24 Sarcoidosis is an infiltrative disease found often on the face and nasal rim. While the morphology and distribution in a Black woman is highly suggestive of sarcoidosis, it is best to confirm the diagnosis with a biopsy. In this case it is best to biopsy the lesion below the nose rather than risk anatomic distortion of the nasal rim. A punch biopsy is generally preferred. (Copyright Richard P. Usatine, MD.)

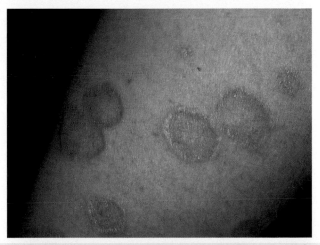

Figure 8.26 Disseminated granuloma annulare on the arm. A 4-mm punch biopsy of a granulomatous ring is recommended if the diagnosis is in question. (Copyright Richard P. Usatine, MD.)

picture supports the diagnosis without a biopsy. But if a biopsy is needed, the double punch is much less invasive and is a reasonable approach before doing a larger biopsy.

Infiltrative Disorders

Infiltrative disorders, such as *granulomas*, also require punch rather than shave biopsy to deliver a suitable specimen for dermatopathologic examination. Examples of infiltrative disorders include *sarcoidosis, cutaneous T-cell lymphoma*, and *granuloma annulare* (Figures 8.24 to 8.26).

Morphea and lichen sclerosus are diagnosed with punch biopsies as well (Figures 8.27 and 8.28).

Erythroderma

Erythroderma is a dangerous dermatologic condition in which most of the skin becomes severely inflamed (red showing better in lighter skin) and begins to peel off in flakes (Figure 8.29). The impaired skin barrier makes the person vulnerable to dehydration and infection. It is the dermatologic manifestation of a number of underlying disease processes, including various forms of dermatitis, drug reactions, and lymphoproliferative disorders. The key to proper diagnosis and treatment is contingent on a good biopsy.

A short differential diagnosis of erythroderma includes:

- Psoriasis
- Atopic and contact dermatitis
- Drug reaction
- Dermatomyositis
- Cutaneous T-cell lymphoma (CTCL)
- Idiopathic

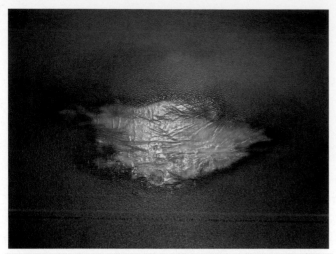

Figure 8.27 Morphea (localized scleroderma) on the abdomen of this Black woman. A 4-mm punch biopsy was used to make the diagnosis. (Copyright Richard P. Usatine, MD.)

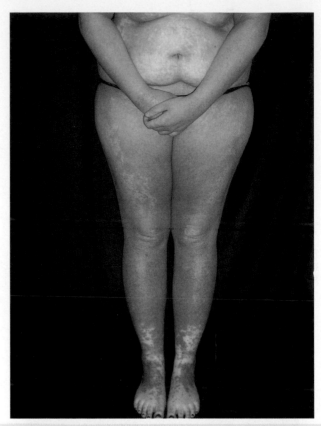

Figure 8.29 Erythroderma in a 19-year-old woman. A stat biopsy was done to obtain a diagnosis. (Copyright Richard P. Usatine, MD.)

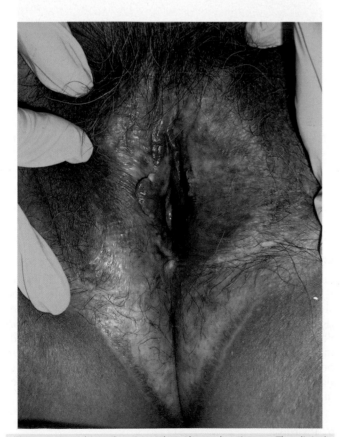

Figure 8.28 Lichen sclerosis on the vulva and perineum. The clinical impression was confirmed with a 3-mm punch biopsy that was left open to heal by second intention. Sutures in this area can be very uncomfortable, and the tissue heals well without suturing. The whitest area was chosen to rule out vulvar intraepithelial neoplasia. (Copyright Richard P. Usatine, MD.)

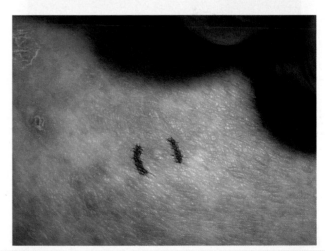

Figure 8.30 A close-up of a small pustule in a 67-year-old woman with erythroderma. A 4-mm punch biopsy of this site made the diagnosis of pustular psoriasis. (Copyright Richard P. Usatine, MD.)

Since erythroderma covers most of the body, there are many areas to choose from for the biopsy. Like most diagnostic challenges, the 4 mm punch biopsy is the standard method for obtaining tissue. Choose an area on the upper body such as the arm or trunk with significant skin involvement. If there are pustules as in pustular psoriasis, biopsy a pustule too (Figure 8.30). Ask the dermatopathologist to rush the processing and reading of this biopsy. Many patients will need hospitalization, but a quick biopsy in the office before transferring the patient to the hospital could

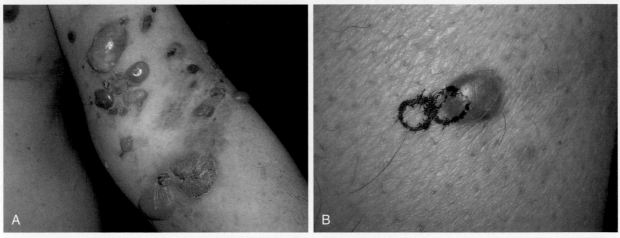

Figure 8.31 (A) New onset bullous eruption in a man recently started on linagliptin. **(B)** Two punch biopsies were planned. The punch on the edge of the intact bulla was sent for H&E, and the adjacent perilesional punch biopsy was sent for direct immunofluorescence (DIF). The results confirmed a diagnosis of *bullous pemphigoid*. (Copyright Richard P. Usatine, MD.)

help to get a quicker answer to guide treatment. Sometimes it might help to get two biopsies from different locations.

Bullous Lesions

There are many skin diseases that present with bullous lesions from *bullous impetigo* to *bullous pemphigoid* (Figure 8.31). While bullous impetigo can be diagnosed and treated based on history and physical exam, the immunobullous diseases such as bullous pemphigoid and pemphigus should be biopsied while initiating treatment. These diseases are often treated with prolonged courses of oral steroids and immunosuppressive medications, so it is essential to have the correct diagnosis from the start. It is standard to perform two biopsies, one sent in formalin for H&E staining and another biopsy sent for direct immunofluorescence (DIF). See earlier discussion under "Choice of Sites to Biopsy." See Table 8.1 for more detailed information on where and how to biopsy tissue for DIF.

Suspected Infectious Rash

In most cases of common infectious diseases the diagnosis can be made clinically, with a KOH preparation, a PCR test, or with a culture. Sometimes a 4-mm punch biopsy may be needed for bacterial and fungal stains. Fungal infections are often diagnosed with periodic acid Schiff (PAS) stains. If there may be an infectious origin and standard biopsies in formalin are not providing the answer, send fresh tissue in a sterile urine cup on top of a sterile gauze soaked with sterile saline, and ask for tissue cultures including bacterial, AFB, and fungal stains and cultures.

Considerations for Specific Anatomic Areas

ANTERIOR SHIN

The thin skin on the shin make both excision and punch biopsy more complicated. Shave biopsy is preferred when it is a reasonable alternative. Choose a different site if possible, and if not possible try to biopsy away from the bone.

HANDS AND FEET

Care must be taken when performing punch biopsies on the hands and feet because of proximity to vessels, tendons, bone, and nerves. The sensory nerves along the lateral sides of the fingers lie within potential damage by a biopsy punch. On the dorsum of the hand, tendons are vulnerable. When a punch biopsy is needed on the palm of the hand, it is best to choose an area that has sufficient soft tissue between the skin and the bones and tendons. The thenar eminence is a good choice if the rash involves this area.

CHEST AND BUTTOCKS

The chest and buttocks may be considered cosmetic areas and may require particular care to avoid scarring. Keloidal or hypertrophic scarring is common in both of these areas. Large, deep shave biopsies should be avoided if possible.

SCALP – ALOPECIA

A scalp biopsy may be needed to diagnose various forms of scarring alopecia (e.g., lichen planopilaris, folliculitis decalvans) (Figure 8.32) and some atypical nonscarring alopecia cases (e.g., androgenic alopecia, telogen effluvium, and alopecia areata). Of course, diagnosis begins with history and physical exam.

- Dermoscopy of the hair (trichoscopy) can lead to the diagnosis of many cases of alopecia without a biopsy. Some examples of the structures visible with the dermatoscope that lead to a diagnosis include:
  - Exclamation point hairs in alopecia areata
  - Miniaturized hairs in androgenic alopecia
  - Perifollicular scale in lichen planopilaris
- When the diagnosis is still not clear, a biopsy that includes involved hair follicles can help make the diagnosis. Biopsy can demonstrate inflammatory infiltrates of the follicular unit that help to classify the scarring alopecias:
  - Lymphocytic: discoid lupus erythematosus, lichen planopilaris and central centrifugal scarring alopecia

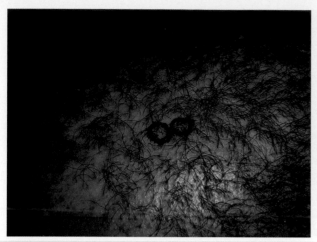

Figure 8.32 The patient presented with hair loss of unknown etiology. Two 4-mm punch biopsies were performed. The two biopsy sites were marked with a surgical marker around remaining hair follicles. It is important to give the pathologist remaining hair follicles and not completely bald scalp. (Copyright Richard P. Usatine, MD.)

- Neutrophilic: folliculitis decalvans and dissecting folliculitis
- Mixed: acne keloidalis nuchae

How to Do a Scalp Biopsy

- Usually two 4-mm punch biopsies are preferred so the pathologist can cut one specimen longitudinally and the other vertically. This gives additional information that may be needed for diagnosis.
- When doing two punch biopsies, close the first one before starting the second one because two simultaneously bleeding sites can be harder to deal with than one at a time.
- Use a 4-mm punch because it will allow for a cotton-tipped applicator to be inserted into the punch space to prevent bleeding before putting in a hemostatic stitch.
- An alternative approach involves using one 6- to 8-mm punch, and then once it has been removed bisecting the specimen with a scalpel running in the direction of the hair follicles.
- See Chapter 4 (Hemostasis) and Chapter 20 (Working in Challenging Locations) for more tips on scalp biopsies.
- Place both punches or one bisected punch in a single formalin container so that it can be cut horizontally and vertically for analysis.

EARS, EYELIDS, NOSE, AND LIPS

Shave biopsies are often preferred on the ears, eyelids, nose, and lips. If a punch biopsy is indicated, use of a 3-mm punch will avoid most problems with dog ears (see Chapter 10). On the ears it is best to avoid cutting into the cartilage unless it is necessary for the diagnosis. On the eyelids, care must be taken to avoid the conjunctival margin and the lacrimal ducts to avoid scarring that will lead to eye dysfunction. On the upper nose, a shave biopsy may be preferred but on the nasal ala a 3-mm punch biopsy may heal better. A punch

biopsy >4 mm can distort the anatomy of the nose. On the lips, care must be taken to align the vermilion border if any sutures are used.

How to Submit a Specimen to the Lab

To obtain the most accurate diagnosis from the pathologist, it is important to provide all the relevant information on the submission form that accompanies the specimen. Drs. Boyd and Neldner have developed the "five D's" mnemonic to remember the essential information to include on the requisition form:

- Description
- Demographics
- Duration
- Diameter
- Diagnosis[19]

DESCRIPTION

The clinician should write a description of the appearance of the lesion. Examples of common descriptive terms include erythema, scale, pearly, raised, pigmented, ulcerating, crusted, nodular, papular, macular, vesicular, and bullous.

DEMOGRAPHICS

The age and sex of the patient should be noted as well as travel history, ethnicity, family history, etc. Even an occupational history (gardener), or other personal history (extensive tanning bed use) can be immensely helpful.

DURATION

How long a lesion has been present will help define the possible diagnoses.

DIAMETER

Recording the size of the lesion is especially important if the clinician has not excised the entire lesion. Pigmented lesions larger than 6 mm are more likely to be melanoma. Unless recorded, the pathologist will not know the size of an incompletely excised lesion. For eruptions, one can record the distribution of the eruption.

DIAGNOSIS

A clinician should commit to the most likely diagnosis and record it on the lab requisition. In most cases alternative diagnoses should be included. Submitting the suspected diagnosis and differential diagnosis is helpful to the pathologist. It also helps the clinician improve diagnostic acumen. Always go back to the differential diagnosis when looking at the final result. This can actually be fun.

Two additional "D's" to consider include:

Diseases

Knowing of other significant diseases the patient has, such as SLE, RA, HIV, or immune suppression, can certainly aid the pathologist in discerning the nature of some lesions.

Drugs

Medications can alter the appearance of a lesion (e.g., topical steroids) or be the cause of an inflammatory change (e.g., allergy to neomycin). It is important then to note both what the patient is using/taking (if pertinent) and what may have been used to treat the lesion.

Following the "seven D's" approach to submitting a specimen will improve communication with the pathologist and maximize the accuracy of the final histologic diagnosis.

Margin Assessment

Margin examination may be requested on shave biopsies of suspected BCC. However, only the Mohs technique allows examination of 100% of the margin. For all other types of biopsies and excisions, margins are sampled only using a serial cross-sectioning (bread-loafing) technique. The greater the sampling, the higher the degree of confidence in the margin assessment. To increase the degree of sampling, larger specimens may be sectioned during grossing and then step sectioned to view multiple cuts on the slide. Pathologists report that the "examined margins are negative" or that the lesion extends to the deep or a lateral margin.

When a margin is positive, it is truly positive. However, a negative margin does not ensure that the lesion has been completely removed. For example, if you do a shave excision of a BCC, the report may say that the examined margins are negative. This means that on the two dimensions which can be examined on a slide, the margins are negative, not necessarily that the lesion has been fully removed.[20-23]

Some question whether pathologists should even report margins on shave biopsies. Others question whether it is acceptable to observe patients with positive margins on definitive BCC excision rather than always recommending re-excision.[22] More data should help define these areas in the future.

Box 8.1

Margin Assessment

Margin examination may be requested; however, only the Mohs technique allows examination of 100% of the margin. For all other types of biopsies and excisions, margins are sampled only. The greater the sampling, the higher the degree of confidence in the margin assessment. To increase the degree of sampling, larger specimens may be sectioned during grossing and then step sectioned to view multiple cuts on the slide. We report that the "examined margins are negative" or that the lesion extends to the deep or a lateral margin. It should be noted, however, that while a positive margin is positive, a negative margin does not ensure that the lesion has been completely removed. For example, if you do a shave excision of a BCC, we will say on the report that the examined margins are negative. This means that on the two dimensions which can be examined on a slide, the margins are negative, not necessarily that the lesion has been fully removed.

The above clarification is provided courtesy of Terry L. Barrett, M.D., Dermatopathologist.

Conclusion

The choice of biopsy technique can substantially affect the diagnostic information obtained, the time required to perform the procedure, the cosmetic result, and the cost. Shave, punch, incisional, excisional, and curettage biopsies each have advantages and disadvantages. (See Chapters 9, 10, and 11 for further information on these procedures.) Choosing among these biopsy techniques requires consideration of the size and morphology of the lesion in question, its anatomic location, the experience and skill of the clinician, and the initial assessment of the diagnosis. It is of utmost importance that clinicians feel comfortable performing skin biopsies. Although it may not affect patient survival with a short delay between diagnostic biopsy and definitive treatment for melanoma, delaying or not performing the initial biopsy itself may have grave consequences.[24,25]

References

1. Bergfield WF, Pfenninger JL, Weinstock MA. Skin biopsy: selecting an optimal technique. *Patient Care*. 2001;30:11-21.
2. Tran KT, Wright NA, Cockrell CJ. Biopsy of the pigmented lesion—When and how. *J Am Acad Dermatol*. 2008;59:852-871.
3. Achar S. Principles of skin biopsies for the primary care physician. *Am Fam Physician*. 1996;54(8):2411-2418.
4. Coit DG, Andtbacka R, Bichakjian CK, et al. Melanoma. *J Natl Compr Cancer Netw JNCCN*. 2009;7(3):250-275. doi:10.6004/jnccn.2009.0020.
5. Swetter SM, Tsao H, Bichakjian CK, et al. Guidelines of care for the management of primary cutaneous melanoma. *J Am Acad Dermatol*. 2019;80(1):208-250. doi:10.1016/j.jaad.2018.08.055.
6. Seiverling EV, Ahrns HT, Bacik LC, Usatine R. Biopsies for skin cancer detection: dispelling the myths. *J Fam Pract*. 2018;67(5):270-274.
7. Ng JC, Swain S, Dowling JP, Wolfe R, Simpson P, Kelly JW. The impact of partial biopsy on histopathologic diagnosis of cutaneous melanoma: experience of an Australian tertiary referral service. *Arch Dermatol*. 2010;146(3):234-239.
8. Swetter SM, Thompson JA, Albertini MR, et al. NCCN Guidelines® insights: melanoma: cutaneous, version 2.2021. *J Natl Compr Cancer Netw JNCCN*. 2021;19(4):364-376. doi:10.6004/jnccn.2021.0018.
9. Zager JS, Hochwald SN, Marzban SS. Shave biopsy is a safe and accurate method for the initial evaluation of melanoma. *J Am Coll Surg*. 2011;212(4):454-460.
10. Gambichler T, Senger E, Rapp S, Alamouti D, Altmeyer P, Hoffmann K. Deep shave excision of macular melanocytic nevi with the razor blade biopsy technique. *Dermatol Surg*. 2000;26(7):662-666.
11. Ferrandiz L, Moreno-Ramirez D, Camacho FM. Shave excision of common acquired melanocytic nevi: cosmetic outcome, recurrences, and complications. *Dermatol Surg*. 2005;31(9 Pt 1):1112-1115.
12. Kessinger A. Adverse effect of melanoma incision. *Curr Probl Cancer*. 1985;13(9):4-43.
13. Molenkamp BG, Sluijter BJR, Oosterhof B, Meijer S. Non-radical diagnostic biopsies do no negatively influence melanoma patient survival. *Ann Surg Oncol*. 2007;14(4):1424-1430.
14. McGovern TW, Litaker MS. Clinical predictors of malignant pigmented lesions: a comparison of the Glasgow seven-point checklist and the American Cancer Society's ABCDs of pigmented lesions. *J Dermatol Surg Oncol*. 1992;18:22-26.
15. Williams NM, Rojas KD, Reynolds JM, Kwon D, Shum-Tien J, Jaimes N. Assessment of diagnostic accuracy of dermoscopic structures and patterns used in melanoma detection: a systematic review and meta-analysis. *JAMA Dermatol*. 2021;157(9):1078-1088. doi:10.1001/jamadermatol.2021.2845.
16. Dinnes J, Deeks JJ, Chuchu N, et al. Dermoscopy, with and without visual inspection, for diagnosing melanoma in adults. *Cochrane Database Syst Rev*. 2018;12(12):CD011902. doi:10.1002/14651858.CD011902.pub2.

17. Zalaudek I, Docimo G, Argenziano G. Using dermoscopic criteria and patient-related factors for the management of pigmented melanocytic nevi. *Arch Dermatol.* 2009;145(7):816-826. doi:10.1001/archdermatol.2009.115.

18. Pérez-Garza DM, Chavez-Alvarez S, Ocampo-Candiani J, Gomez-Flores M. Erythema nodosum: a practical approach and diagnostic algorithm. *Am J Clin Dermatol.* 2021;22(3):367-378. doi:10.1007/s40257-021-00592-w.

19. Boyd A, Neldner K. How to submit a specimen for cutaneous pathology analysis. *Arch Fam Med.* 1997;6(1):64-66.

20. Brady MC, Hossler EW. Reliability of biopsy margin status for basal cell carcinoma: a retrospective study. *Cutis.* 2020;106(6):315-317. doi:10.12788/cutis.0123.

21. Purnell JC, Duncan JR, Stratton MS, Huang C, Phillips CB. Negative predictive value of biopsy margins in keratinocyte carcinoma: a literature review. *Dermatol Surg Off Publ Am Soc Dermatol Surg Al.* 2020;46(4):525-529. doi:10.1097/DSS.0000000000002171.

22. Ranganath B, Teixeira RM, Patel T, Garza R, Murphy RXJ. Clinical and financial implications of positive margins after nonmelanoma skin cancer resection: a longitudinal evaluation. *Ann Plast Surg.* 2021;87(1):80-84. doi:10.1097/SAP.0000000000002566.

23. Willardson HB, Lombardo J, Raines M, et al. Predictive value of basal cell carcinoma biopsies with negative margins: a retrospective cohort study. *J Am Acad Dermatol.* 2018;79(1):42-46. doi:10.1016/j.jaad.2017.12.071.

24. McKenna DB, Lee RJ, Prescott RJ, Doherty VR. The time from diagnostic excision biopsy to wide local excision for primary cutaneous malignant melanoma may not affect patient survival. *Br J Dermatol.* 2002;147(2):48-54.

25. Oppenheim EB. Failure to biopsy skin lesions prompts litigation. *Med Malpract Prev.* Published online April 1990.

9 *The Shave Biopsy*

RICHARD P. USATINE, MD, and ZAIRA ORTEGA OREJEL MD

SUMMARY

- The shave biopsy is one of the most useful approaches for obtaining tissue for diagnostic purposes and for the removal of benign surface neoplasms.
- A saucerization is a deep shave and is one recommended method for the diagnosis of melanoma.
- Indications and contraindications for shave biopsy are provided.
- Advantages and disadvantages are discussed.
- Most shave biopsies are performed with a sharp razor blade.
- Hemostasis is usually obtained with aluminum chloride on a cotton-tipped applicator and/or electrocoagulation.
- The shave biopsy is described in detail step by step.
- Alternate methods of performing shave biopsies are discussed.

The shave biopsy is one of the most useful approaches for obtaining tissue for diagnostic purposes and for the removal of benign surface neoplasms. It is especially fast, easy, and effective when the lesion is raised above the skin surface. The shave biopsy and deep (scoop) shave biopsy are valuable for diagnosing many cutaneous malignancies, including basal cell carcinomas (BCCs), squamous cell carcinomas (SCCs), and melanomas. A deep shave biopsy is also called a saucerization and is one recommended method for the diagnosis of melanoma (National Comprehensive Cancer Network guidelines).[1] A shave biopsy/excision is also an effective tool for removing benign lesions such as nevi and seborrheic keratoses. After a shave biopsy, hemostasis may be obtained with aluminum chloride and/or electrocoagulation. The surface is allowed to heal by secondary intention, and no sutures are needed. The excision site usually heals well with a good cosmetic result.

Indications

The following lesions are among those that are frequently diagnosed by shave biopsy:

- BCC (Figure 9.1)
- SCC (Figure 9.2)
- Keratoacanthoma (Figure 9.3)
- Melanoma (Figure 9.4)

Shave excision can also be used to remove the following benign lesions:

- Benign melanocytic nevi
- Seborrheic keratoses (Figure 9.5)
- Sebaceous hyperplasia
- Pyogenic granulomas (Figure 9.6)
- Skin tags with a broad base
- Single wart not responding to less invasive therapies

When a pigmented lesion appears to be benign and its removal is for cosmetic reasons, it is acceptable to use a shave excision. However, it is essential to send biopsies of all lesions for review by a pathologist except typical skin tags.

Contraindications

There are no contraindications for shave biopsy based on location of the lesion.

A superficial shave biopsy is not recommended for a suspected melanoma because it runs the risk of losing important depth information used for staging and margin determination.[2] However, a saucerization that is at least the thickness of a dime (1.35 mm) is a recommended method to biopsy a suspected melanoma. If a deep shave biopsy gets below the tumor, then no depth information is lost. On the other hand, if a punch biopsy is performed of a large lesion and the punch misses the area with melanoma, this false negative result can lead to missing the diagnosis of the melanoma.[2]

Advantages of Shave Biopsy

The advantages of shave biopsy can be broken down into two categories: those that are related to the clinician and those that are related to the patient. Advantages of shave biopsy for the clinician include the following:

- Can be performed rapidly.
- Sutures are not needed.
- Procedure is relatively easy to learn.
- Multiple lesions can be easily excised at one time.
- An assistant is not required.
- Strict sterile procedure is not required.

The following advantages of shave biopsy benefit the patient:

- There are no sutures that need to be removed.
- Wound care is usually simple.
- Restriction of activities is not needed during wound healing.

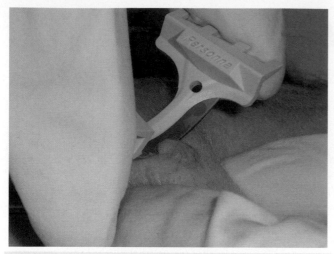

Figure 9.1 Elevated pearly lesion in the nasolabial fold with telangiectasias. A shave biopsy is to be performed to rule out a BCC. (Copyright Richard P. Usatine, MD.)

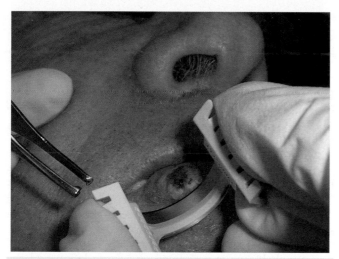

Figure 9.2 Shave biopsy of SCC on the lip. (Copyright Richard P. Usatine, MD.)

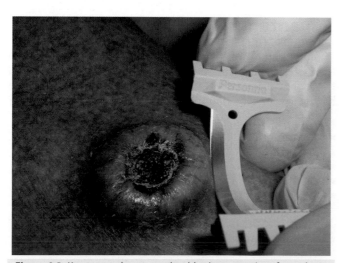

Figure 9.3 Keratoacanthoma on shoulder is appropriate for a shave biopsy. (Copyright Richard P. Usatine, MD.)

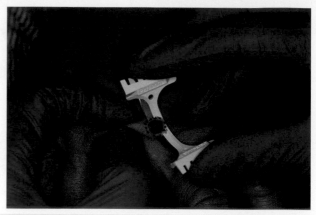

Figure 9.4 Melanoma can be shaved with a deep shave for diagnosis. (Copyright Richard P. Usatine, MD.)

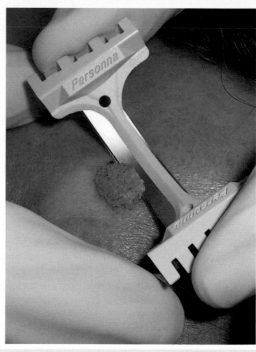

Figure 9.5 Shave excision of a verrucous appearing seborrheic keratosis on the forehead. (Copyright Richard P. Usatine, MD.)

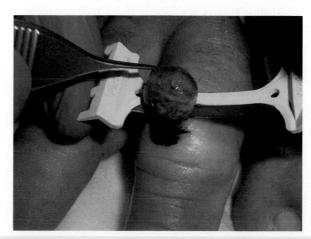

Figure 9.6 Shave biopsy of pyogenic granuloma on finger. (Copyright Richard P. Usatine, MD.)

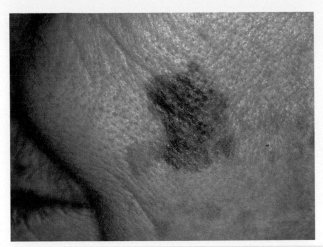

Figure 9.7 Lentigo maligna melanoma that is best diagnosed with a broad shave biopsy. (Copyright Richard P. Usatine, MD.)

- Less risks of infection and bleeding
- May give a better cosmetic result than a full-thickness excision
- Even if a change in pigmentation occurs, it is easily covered by cosmetics.
- Deep saucerization for BCC might remove the full lesion without having to perform a second procedure (especially in small nonaggressive BCC types).

A number of studies have shown the shave biopsy to produce a better cosmetic result than the punch biopsy and the fusiform diagnostic excision.[3-5] A broad scoop shave biopsy of lentigo maligna melanoma (LMM) (Figure 9.7) may give a better tissue sample than one or more punch biopsies.[1]

Disadvantages of Shave Biopsy

As with the advantages of shave biopsy, the disadvantages can also be categorized into those for the clinician and those for the patient.

Disadvantages for the clinician include the following:

- Shave biopsies of flat lesions are more challenging than elevated lesions, and a punch biopsy may be easier for an inexperienced clinician.
- Skin that is highly movable will require the clinician to keep the skin taut while performing the biopsy (e.g., pinching, stretching).

For the patient, the disadvantages of shave biopsy include the following:

- An indentation (divot) may remain.
- Hypopigmentation or hyperpigmentation may result and vary depending on skin color and sun exposure.
- Regrowth may occur (Figure 9.8).
- A second surgery may be needed if the whole lesion needs excision.
- Scarring may occur over the whole biopsy site.
- Healing on the lower legs might take longer than expected.
- Deep saucerization can be more painful and take longer time to heal.

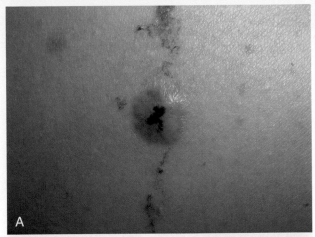

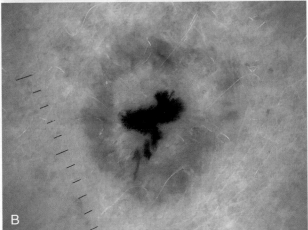

Figure 9.8 (A) Recurrent nevus that occurred within 3 months of the original shave of a benign nevus on the back of teenage girl. **(B)** Dermoscopy of the recurrent nevus showing how the pigment remains within the scar. This is a reassuring sign. Nothing needs to be done. (Copyright Richard P. Usatine, MD.)

A superficial shave biopsy should heal with little to no indentation of the skin.[6] Deep shave biopsies will more likely leave an indentation. Persistence rates of melanocytic lesions for shave biopsy range from approximately 13% to 28%.[7] Persistence does not always translate into regrowth. If regrowth does occur, it is important to have access to the original pathology report to avoid overdiagnosing a benign regrowth as a melanoma (pseudomelanoma). Methods useful to differentiate pseudomelanoma from melanoma include accurate clinical records of prior biopsy sites along with evidence of scar within the current biopsy.[7]

Dermoscopy can be used to diagnose recurrent nevi (Figure 9.8). Benign recurrent nevi tend to occur within months of the original shave biopsy, and the pigment does not go outside the scar. If the recurrence is over 1 year from excision and the lesion goes outside the scar, a new biopsy is indicated.

Equipment (Figure 9.9)

The minimum equipment necessary for a shave biopsy is:

- Sharp blade (razor blade or DermaBlade) (Figure 2.3)
- 3-mL syringe and needle for local anesthesia

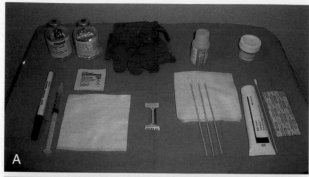

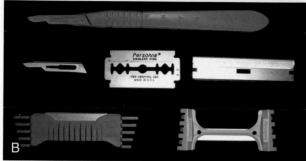

Figure 9.9 (A) Equipment and supplies used to perform a shave biopsy. **(B)** Available blades that could be used for a shave biopsy from top to bottom: #15 scalpel on disposable plastic handle, bare #15 blade, Personna double-edge blade, single-edge rigid blade, Miltex BiopBlade, DermaBlade. (Copyright Richard P. Usatine, MD.)

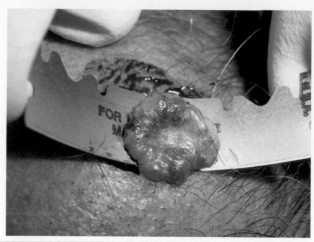

Figure 9.10 Shave biopsy with a double-edge Personna blade that was snapped in half before use. The blade easily cuts through this pigmented BCC. (Copyright Richard P. Usatine, MD.)

- Cotton-tipped applicators (CTAs) and aluminum chloride for hemostasis
- The stick end of a CTA can be used to stabilize the final cuts of the biopsy. If the lesion is pedunculated, it is handy to have a forceps to hold the lesion and to transfer the tissue into the biopsy container.
- A surgical marking pen is very useful for marking the planned biopsy with appropriate margins and is best used before administering the anesthesia.

The Personna DermaBlade is an excellent razor blade for shave biopsies. The blue plastic handle makes it easy and safe to grip the sharp razor blade and control the blade for an accurate and precise superficial or deep shave biopsy or excision. The cost of the disposable DermaBlade is about the same as a standard disposable #15 scalpel. Other options include the Personna or Wilkinson double-edge razor blades. The Personna (or Personna Plus with Teflon coating) double-edge blade is very sharp and can be broken in half for easy use (Figure 9.9B). While these do not come in sterile packaging, they can be safely used for shave biopsies without using the autoclave. They can be broken in half within their paper container to avoid cutting your hand prior to use. It might take some more time to get used to the bare blade, but once you have mastered their use, you will find them sharp and effective at a very low price (Figure 9.10).

Miltex produces a BiopBlade flexible blade for shave biopsies. Its design is similar to the DermaBlade, using a single-edge razor blade with a plastic bendable handle. It is about the same price as a DermaBlade and has no advantage over the DermaBlade. The plastic handle can snap in half if the blade is bent incorrectly, and it is more cumbersome to handle. The Personna single-edge razor blade is too rigid for

shave biopsies. All of these blades (Figure 9.9B) are available for purchase through Amazon, Delasco, and other suppliers.

Shave Biopsy: Steps and Principles

Three critical steps in the shave biopsy include *(see videos 9.1–9.6)*:

- Using 1% lidocaine with epinephrine for anesthesia and hemostasis
- Stabilizing the lesion to allow for controlled removal of the biopsy
- Dealing with any residual tissue after the initial shave

PREOPERATIVE MEASURES

- After determining that the shave technique is the best method for the patient, obtain informed consent. (*See Appendix A for a sample consent form.*)
- By visual inspection and palpation, determine the likely depth of the lesion, and plan the depth of your biopsy based on the probable diagnosis and your physical exam.
- Lightly prep the area with alcohol or another antiseptic. There is no evidence that this preparation decreases the already extremely low infection rate, but it is easy to do.
- Mark the area to be shaved with a surgical marker. It need not be a sterile marker. This is especially important in relatively flat nonpigmented lesions because after injection the margins of these lesions may not be visible (Figure 9.11).
- Inject local anesthesia. Use a 27- to 30-gauge needle with approximately 2 to 3 mL of 1% lidocaine and epinephrine (buffer the lidocaine for less pain – see Chapter 3, *Anesthesia*). Start with the needle under the lesion (greater depth is less painful), and then give the last amount of anesthesia closer to the skin surface. If the lesion is flat, consider raising the lesion some with the anesthesia (Figure 9.12A).

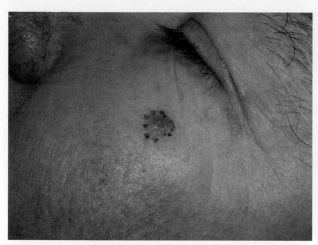

Figure 9.11 A nonpigmented growth on the cheek suspicious for a BCC. The subtle findings and lack of pigment make it a good candidate for preanesthesia marking with a surgical marker. (Copyright Richard P. Usatine, MD.)

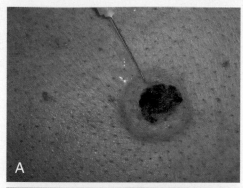

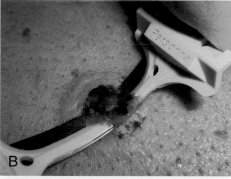

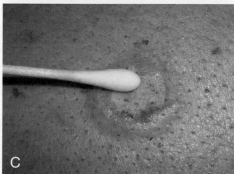

Figure 9.12 Pigmented lesion for shave biopsy to confirm clinical impression of seborrheic keratosis and rule out melanoma. **(A)** Anesthesia is given, **(B)** shave is performed, and **(C)** aluminum chloride is used to stop any bleeding. (Copyright Richard P. Usatine, MD.)

Cutting the Shave Biopsy

RAZOR BLADE (FIGURE 9.12)

- Determine how you will use your forceps or other hand to stabilize the lesion to keep it from moving during the shave. Pinching the skin on the far end of the biopsy is a very useful method; move the fingers further away as the blade gets closer.
- Grasp one end of the razor blade between the thumb and the second and third fingers of your dominant hand, creating a gentle bend in the blade (Figure 9.10 and 9.12B). Bend the blade lightly a few times before starting the procedure to make sure you are grasping it well and to determine the preferred bend of the blade. Place the blade on the skin surface, and gently advance it under the lesion while moving the blade in a side-to-side fashion. Do not bend the blade too much to avoid causing an indentation in the middle of the shave. It is ideal if the blade is mostly flat in the area of the shave. A deeper bend will give a deeper indentation, and a flatter blade will provide a larger area of excision.
- Apply gentle forward pressure during this side-to-side sawing motion and allow the blade to move through the lesion without excess pressure. With the bare razor blade you may need to put one finger against the back of the blade to push it forward when the lesion is firm. Watch each side of the blade to make sure that it is cutting along the marked area and where you intend to cut.
- On some specimens, there is a tendency for the specimen to flip over at the end of the biopsy. If needed use the stick-end of a CTA or the forceps (not fingers) to stabilize the specimen for the final cut.
- Obtain hemostasis with aluminum chloride on a CTA (Figure 9.12C). Do not make the CTA too wet with aluminum chloride, and use downward pressure with a twisting motion. Holding the CTA perpendicular to the skin against stubborn bleeders allows for maximal pressure while twisting the CTA. Occasionally a very vascular lesion will require electrocoagulation to obtain hemostasis.

SCALPEL BLADE
(See Video 9.7)

- This is only preferred when the lesion is difficult to reach with a razor blade (DermaBlade). This may occur in the folds of the pinna (Figure 9.13).
- Hold the #15 scalpel blade (on or off a blade handle) parallel to the surface of the skin.
- Move the blade through the tissue using a minimal sawing movement. The slight sawing motion helps the blade move through the tissue, but too much sawing will produce scalloped edges.
- When needed, use the stick-end of a CTA or forceps to stabilize the specimen for the final cut.

SNIP EXCISION WITH SCISSORS
(See Videos 9.9 and 9.10)

- Another variation of the shave excision for small raised lesions is the snip excision performed with sharp scissors (Figure 9.14).

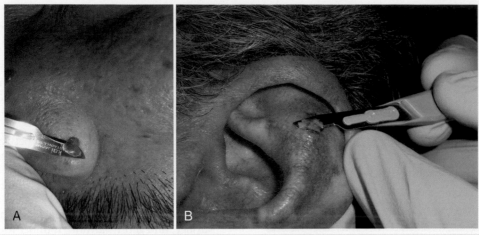

Figure 9.13 Shave biopsies with a scalpel in tight places where a small #15 scalpel blade is easier to maneuver than a larger razor blade. **(A)** Shave of pigmented lesion on nose. Path showed SK. **(B)** Shave of nonpigmented lesion in ear. Path showed an actinic keratosis. (Copyright Richard P. Usatine, MD.)

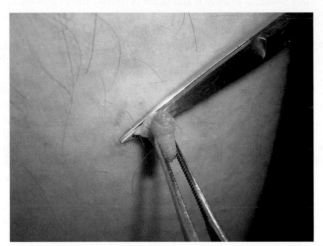

Figure 9.14 Snip excision of a skin tag. The scissor crushes the base and helps achieve quick hemostasis. (Copyright Richard P. Usatine, MD.)

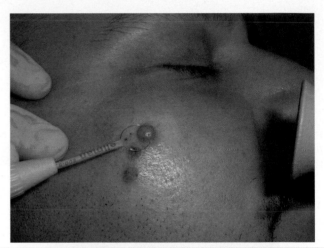

Figure 9.15 The use of a radiofrequency electrosurgical loop to perform a shave excision of a benign intradermal nevus. Note the two areas where two other nevi had been excised using this method. (Copyright Richard P. Usatine, MD.)

- Anesthesia and hemostasis are executed in the same manner as for the other types of shave excision. The only difference is that the lesion is snipped off with sharp scissors rather than shaved with a blade.
- Lesions particularly amenable to snip excision are skin tags, small warts, and polypoid nevi. We recommend using a good pair of sharp iris scissors (straight or curved). Small lesions may be snipped without anesthesia but larger lesions should be anesthetized with 1% lidocaine and epinephrine.
- The lesion is grasped with forceps and cut at the base with the scissors. The crushing effect of the scissor on the soft tissue helps to prevent bleeding. Additional hemostasis can be achieved with aluminum chloride or electrosurgery.

ELECTROSURGICAL SHAVE (SEE CHAPTER 14)

- A loop electrode may be used to perform an electrosurgical shave (Figure 9.15).
- We do not prefer this because it puts unnecessary smoke into the air, which could contain HPV or HIV particles. It also can leave burn artifact on the biopsy specimen.

- Whether the instrument is set on cut only or cut and coag, it is important to not use too much power that will result in unnecessary tissue destruction leading to increased scarring.

SAUCERIZATION (SCOOP SHAVE, DEEP SHAVE)

A saucerization technique involves the removal of the lesion using a deep shave or scoop technique with 1 to 2 mm of surrounding normal skin laterally and extending into the deep dermis.

It is easier to do a scoop shave with a DermaBlade or other razor blade than a scalpel.

A young man presents with a "dark mole" on his abdomen (Figure 9.16). Clinically and dermoscopically, it is suspicious for melanoma. Here are the steps of the saucerization biopsy (Figure 9.17), after the local anesthesia was injected.

A. Start by marking the area to be cut including the planned margin. If the lesion is suspected to be a melanoma, mark a 2 mm margin around the edge of the pigment.

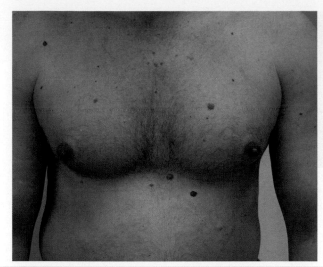

Figure 9.16 Melanoma in situ on the upper left abdomen to be biopsied in the next Figure 9.17. Note how it is the "ugly duckling" because it stands out from the other nevi due to its dark color. (Copyright Richard P. Usatine, MD)

D. To be sure that you have cut below the pigment, flip the lesion over and use some aluminum chloride to obtain adequate hemostasis to see the base of the cut. In this case the cut is below the pigment, and some fat globules are showing, indicating that the cut was deep enough to get partially through the dermis.

E. Continue the shave straight across the base and come upward, leaving another 2 mm from the edge of the pigment.

F. Use the stick end of the CTA to stabilize the specimen from flipping over, and finish the biopsy.

G. Stop any bleeding with aluminum chloride on the CTA.

H. The lesion was removed with no pigment at the base. A few small fat globules are visible at the base of the shave, and the area will still heal well by second intention. Pathology revealed melanoma in situ.

Note how the shave went completely under the pigment and the depth information was not lost. If pigment were to be found below the shave a deeper shave, punch, or full-thickness incisional biopsy could be performed of the remaining lesion.

If a full-thickness biopsy is to be performed into the subcutaneous fat, it is suggested that this is performed with an elliptical excision and closed with sutures.

When performing a deep scoop shave to remove a non-melanoma skin cancer (NMSC), it is appropriate to cut down deep enough so that small fat globules will be visible (Figure 9.18). If all the margins are clear this can serve as the definitive treatment for less aggressive NMSCs such as

B. Direct the blade downward at an angle of 30 to 45 degrees with the skin to get underneath the pigment. Stabilize the skin by pinching it on the other side of the initial cut.

C. Continue the shave straight across the base until 50% has been cut.

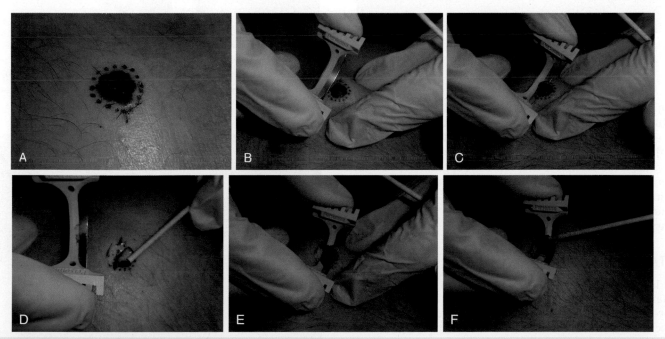

Figure 9.17 Saucerization (deep shave) step by step:

A. The area to be biopsied is marked with a surgical marker including a 2-mm margin.

B. The DermaBlade is directed downward at an angle of 30 to 45 degrees with the skin to get underneath the pigment. The skin is stabilized by pinching it.

C. The saucerization continues straight across the base until 50% has been cut.

D. To be sure to cut below the pigment, the lesion is flipped over, and aluminum chloride is used to obtain hemostasis to see the base of the cut. In this case the cut is below the pigment, and some fat globules are showing, indicating that the cut was deep enough to get partially through the dermis.

E. The deep shave continues under the lesion and comes upward following the marked margin.

F. The stick end of the CTA is used to stabilize the specimen from flipping over.

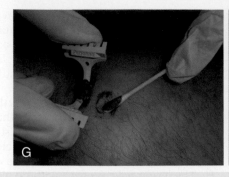

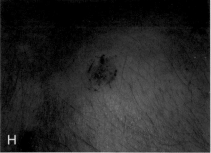

Figure 9.17, cont'd
G. Hemostasis is obtained using aluminum chloride on the CTA.
H. The lesion was removed with no pigment at the base. A few small fat globules are visible at the base of the deep shave, and the area healed well by second intention. Pathology revealed melanoma in situ. (Copyright Richard P. Usatine, MD.)

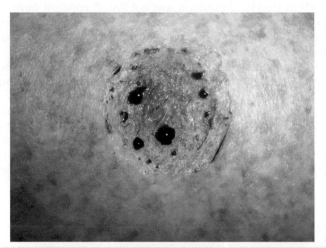

Figure 9.18 Deep shave showing a few glistening fat globules. (Copyright Richard P. Usatine, MD.)

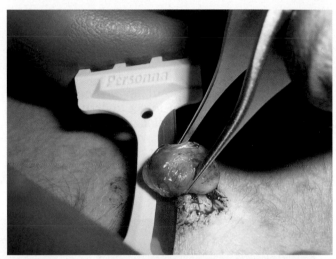

Figure 9.19 The forceps stabilize the raised lesion while the shave is performed. The lesion was confirmed to be a pyogenic granuloma by the dermatopathologist. (Copyright Richard P. Usatine, MD.)

superficial or nodular BCCs (not sclerosing) or SCC in situ. This method is not recommended for skin cancers larger than 2 cm or in danger areas around vital structures. Definitive treatment for invasive SCC and melanoma should include a full-thickness excision with appropriate margins. As with all skin cancers, regular examinations need to be done to investigate for recurrence and new cancers. A shave excision of any depth should not be the definitive surgery to treat a melanoma.

STABILIZATION TECHNIQUES

It is best to stabilize lesions during the shave biopsy to maximize the control during cutting. In Figure 9.19, forceps are used, and in Figure 9.20, the skin is pinched because the lesion is very flat. Note how the fingers of the nondominant hand are kept in the biopsy area to provide gentle countertraction and to stabilize the tissue. On certain areas of thin skin near vital structures such as the eye or hand, it may be necessary to pinch and elevate the surrounding skin with one hand while doing the biopsy with the other. The end of a CTA is useful for preventing the lesion from flipping over near the final portion of the cut (Figure 9.21). Raising a flat lesion with anesthetic just prior

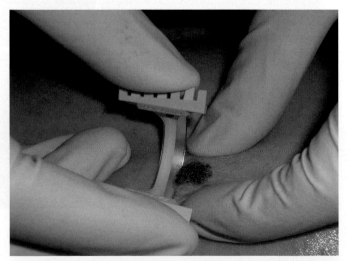

Figure 9.20 The start of this shave biopsy is stabilized by pinching the skin between the thumb and index finger of the nondominant hand. Once the shave is begun the fingers can be removed away from the blade. Care must be taken to avoid cutting oneself. (Copyright Richard P. Usatine, MD.)

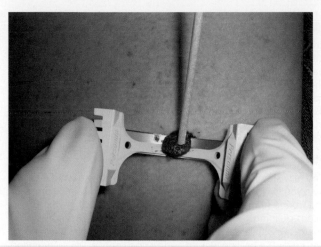

Figure 9.21 Shave biopsy with the end of a cotton tip applicator stabilizing the lesion from flipping over. (Copyright Richard P. Usatine, MD.)

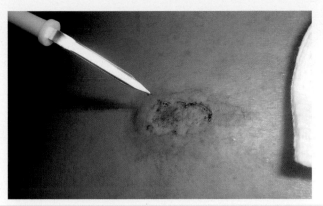

Figure 9.22 The Hyfrecator is used to destroy some remaining tissue on the edge of the excision. Note that the original hemostasis was obtained with aluminum chloride to minimize potential scarring that is more likely to occur with electrosurgery of the entire excision site. (Copyright Richard P. Usatine, MD.)

to excision can help stabilize the lesion but may increase the risk of indentation. Regardless of which method is used, it is important to not pull up on the lesion to avoid creating a deep indentation.

HEMOSTASIS

Many shave biopsies can be performed within a minute after the injection of lidocaine and epinephrine. If the lesion is very vascular (pyogenic granuloma), the patient is on anticoagulants, or the biopsy site is very vascular (such as the lip), it is best to wait 7 to 10 minutes for the epinephrine to take full effect (Figure 9.2). If enough time has elapsed between the administration of anesthesia and the start of the biopsy, the procedure can be virtually bloodless.

After the biopsy, blot the site with a dry CTA or gauze to remove any pooled blood. Then roll and twist another CTA that has been dipped in aluminum chloride back and forth over the site. Apply downward pressure with the twisting applicator to stop the bleeding (Figures 9.12C and 9.17). It is important to not leave wet blood in the field because this will dilute the aluminum chloride and minimize its effectiveness. If chemical hemostasis does not stop the bleeding or if it is desirable to destroy any remaining tissue then electrosurgery may be used (see Chapter 4, *Hemostasis*).

REMAINING TISSUE AFTER SHAVE BIOPSY

Remaining tissue is often found at the trailing edge of the lesion where the blade finished the shave. First obtain hemostasis, and then cut the remaining tissue off with your blade. If the tissue is too small to stabilize for a second cut, options to remove the remaining tissue include scraping with the blade perpendicular to the skin, using a curette, or electrodesiccation (Figure 9.22). If using electrodesiccation, the charred tissue may be left alone or wiped away with a moist gauze pad or a curette. *See video 9.8.*

Aftercare

After the procedure is complete, place a small amount of clean petrolatum and an adhesive bandage over the biopsy site, and give the patient wound care instructions. See Box 9.1 for a sample patient handout entitled "Care of Your Skin After a Shave Biopsy."

Pathology and Follow-Up

Send all pigmented lesions and any lesion suspicious for cancer to the pathologist. Skin tags may not need to be sent if these are typical and benign in their appearance. If the pathologist reports that the lesion appears benign but is incompletely excised, there is usually no need to do a further or deeper excision. However, if the pathologist recommends further excision because of suspicion for malignancy or there is a chance of malignant transformation, this recommendation must be followed.

If the lesion is premalignant (such as an actinic keratosis), it should be reexamined after it fully heals. If there is remaining scaling or evidence of the original lesion, it may be treated with cryotherapy instead of doing another excision.

If the lesion turns out to be nonmelanoma skin cancer (NMSC), definitive treatment will often be necessary unless the original biopsy was sufficiently deep and broad to excise all visible tumor and the pathologist states that there are clear margins. If you intend to remove a whole BCC or SCC in situ with a shave excision using a deeper and broader approach, and your pathologist reports clear margins, you may give the patient the choice to opt for observation or topical treatment rather than additional surgery. For high-risk lesions, based on the pathology report and the size of the lesion, it is best to perform full-thickness elliptical excisions (or Mohs surgery) for definitive treatment (see Chapter 24, *Diagnosis and Treatment of Malignant Lesions*).

Suggestion for Learning the Shave Biopsy Technique

When learning the shave biopsy technique, it may be helpful to practice on a tomato or orange. Use a razor blade and attempt to remove portions of the outer skin without encroaching on the underlying fruit (Figure 9.23). Practice performing the shave at different depths and sizes.

Box 9.1   Care of Your Skin After a Shave Biopsy

Supplies Needed

Clean petroleum jelly (a squeeze tube is cleaner than a tub) (Vaseline is one name brand) (Do not use Neosporin or Triple Antibiotic)

Dressing or gauze that is made for wound care (Band-Aid is one name brand)

Optional – cotton-tip applicators (Q-tips is one name brand)

Directions

- Keep the site clean and dry and do not remove the original dressing for 24 hours.
- After 24 hours you may shower daily. Gently wash the surgical site with soap and water in the shower or at least once daily.
- Apply petroleum jelly to the clean wound with a clean finger or CTA one to two times per day.
- Use a dressing to cover the wound. While cleansing is only needed once or twice a day, additional petroleum jelly may be added as needed to keep the wound moist.
- Tylenol (acetaminophen) or ibuprofen can be taken for pain if needed. DO NOT **start** taking any medications with aspirin or aspirin products.

REPEAT THESE INSTRUCTIONS DAILY UNTIL THE WOUND IS HEALED.

THIS MAY BE ANYWHERE FROM 5 TO 20 DAYS.

The wound will actually heal better and scar less if kept clean and covered with petroleum jelly.

Bleeding

If bleeding occurs, apply firm pressure to the site. Direct pressure should be applied to the wound. Five minutes should be adequate if the bleeding is minor and the wound is small. However, if the wound is larger and the bleeding is more severe, apply pressure for *10 minutes*, timed by looking at a clock. It is best not to discontinue pressure to see if the bleeding has stopped until 10 minutes have passed. If the bleeding continues, remove the pad and press directly with a clean gauze pad over the bleeding site. If bleeding soaks through the gauze or is not stopped by firm pressure, call and go to your doctor or an urgent care center.

Infection

If you notice pus or discharge coming from the wound this may be an infection. This is particularly worrisome if you develop a fever and the wound is red, painful, swollen, and warm. Other signs of infection could be red streaks from wound, increased pain, and painful or swollen lymph nodes (glands). A firm white coating on the wound with a light pink surrounding color is usually a normal part of the healing process and not an infection. This will go away as the new layer of normal skin is formed. If you have any suspicion of having an infection, contact your doctor/provider or an urgent care center.

Shower and Washing

You may shower daily after the first 24 hours have passed. At first, you may leave the dressing on during the shower to protect the wound from the flow of water. Alternatively, if the wound needs cleaning, the shower is helpful to remove crusts and discharge. Dry the area gently, and then apply the petroleum jelly and cover the healing wound as described above. We recommend not bathing in a tub or hot tub until the wound is completely healed over to avoid infection.

Wound Healing

After the wound looks healed over you can stop daily dressing changes. The wound may remain somewhat pink (the area cut and/or the area around the wound) and this will slowly fade over the next few weeks or months. Sometimes it can take 6 months to 1 year for the pink to fade completely.

You may experience a sensation of tightness as your wound heals. This is normal and will gradually fade. After the wound has healed, frequent, gentle massaging of the area will help to loosen the scar. Sometimes the surgery cuts small nerves, and it may take up to a year before feeling returns to normal. Only rarely will the area remain numb permanently.

Your healed wound may be sensitive to temperature changes (such as cold air). This sensitivity improves with time, but if you are experiencing a lot of discomfort, try to avoid temperature extremes. You may experience itching after your wound appears to have healed. This is due to the healing that continues underneath the skin. Petroleum jelly may help to relieve this itching. Try not to scratch the wound since this may cause it to reopen.

IF YOU HAVE ANY CONCERNS NOT ANSWERED BY THIS INFORMATION, PLEASE CALL YOUR DOCTOR/PROVIDER.

Less Than Optimal Outcomes

- Infections are rare complications of shave biopsies. The white tissue seen at the base of a healing shave biopsy and the mild surrounding erythema might concern the patient and lead them to contact your office for fear of an infection. If the patient fears an infection it is best to see them in the office for evaluation. Most of the time only reassurance is needed, but if the erythema and tenderness are more than usual and there is purulence present, then antibiotics are indicated.
- Expected but less-than-optimal outcomes that often occur after shave biopsies include the following:
  - Producing an indentation or divot in the skin. This is expected after a scoop shave. Also, this is more common in a shave done on a convex surface such as the nose (Figure 9.24).
  - Erythema that may last for months and often resolves
  - Slow healing for deeper shaves and areas such as the lower leg
  - Hypopigmentation or hyperpigmentation that can be permanent (Figure 9.25)
  - Regrowth of incompletely excised lesion. Pigment developing at the site of a nevus with a dermal component removed by shave biopsy is common (Figure 9.8). This is called a recurrent nevus, although the deeper nevus cells were not excised. On dermoscopy this appears as pigment within the original scar. If the pigment goes outside the scar or appears over a year after the original biopsy, it is best to do another biopsy.
  - Hair may regrow if the nevus had hair and is excised with a shave biopsy alone. This type of nevus may be best removed with a deeper elliptical excision. Alternatively, the hair follicles remaining after a shave biopsy may be destroyed with electrosurgery, but this is not always successful.

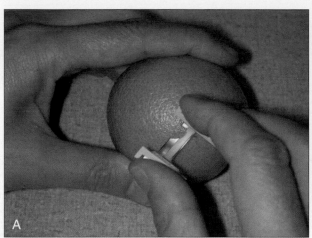
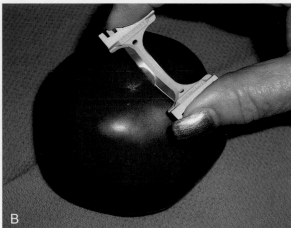

Figure 9.23 (A) The skin of an orange provides a good practice model for the shave biopsy. **(B)** We have found that the tomato is even better. (Copyright Richard P. Usatine, MD.)

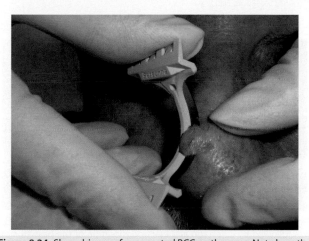

Figure 9.24 Shave biopsy of a suspected BCC on the nose. Note how the nose is held between the fingers to stabilize it for the shave biopsy. An indentation would be acceptable cosmetically because the likelihood of skin cancer was high and the patient would need a second procedure to eradicate the BCC. This patient received Mohs surgery after the biopsy proved the lesion to be a BCC. (Copyright Richard P. Usatine, MD.)

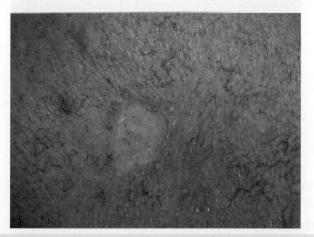

Figure 9.25 Hypopigmentation that occurred after a shave biopsy of a BCC on the face 1 year prior to this photo. The patient did not show up for treatment right after the biopsy, but no further tumor growth occurred in one year. At that visit, the patient preferred watchful waiting to additional surgery. (Copyright Richard P. Usatine, MD.)

Cosmetic Results

Gambichler et al. examined the cosmetic outcome of macular melanocytic lesions utilizing the deep shave biopsy technique with a razor blade followed by chemical hemostasis.[6] During routine skin cancer screening, 45 patients with 77 macular melanocytic nevi were prospectively recruited. Histologically 88% of the melanocytic lesions were described as completely excised, and 60% were diagnosed as atypical melanocytic nevi. At 6 months, 56 sites were available for evaluation, and mild hypopigmentation was observed in 52%, hyperpigmentation in 32%, and erythema in 23%. Recurrent nevi occurred in 13% at 6 months. In this study the evaluation of the cosmetic outcome by the patients was better than the evaluation by the physician.

In another prospective study, shave excision of 204 common acquired melanocytic nevi was performed.[8] Middermal shave biopsies were performed using a No. 15 blade followed by gentle electrocoagulation. Three months after surgery, cosmetically excellent results occurred in 33% of the patients, acceptable results in 59%, and poor results in 8%, as assessed by two dermatologists. The likelihood of having an imperceptible scar was significantly greater in lesions excised from the face. Of 192 patients surveyed, 98% stated that "the scar looked better than the original mole" and would undergo the procedure again. Clinical and dermatoscopic recurrences were observed in 19.6% of the scars.[8]

Making a Diagnosis

It helps to have a good idea of the differential diagnosis before choosing the biopsy type and location. For most shave biopsies, a clinician should excise the whole lesion or sample the portion of the lesion that appears to have the worst pathology. However, for bullous disorders such as pemphigus or pemphigoid, it is best to use a scoop shave under an intact bulla or at the border of a bulla. A punch biopsy at the border of the bulla may yield an equally good specimen. Both methods help to keep the epidermis attached to the dermis at the edge of the bulla.

Additional Examples for Shave Biopsy

BCC

In Figure 9.26, a shave biopsy is preferred on the nasal ala rather than a punch biopsy. After the diagnosis was made, this patient was referred for Mohs surgery. One study showed that specimens from punch and shave biopsies of suspected BCCs produced equivalent diagnostic accuracy rates: 80.7% and 75.9%, respectively. Either biopsy technique is appropriate for a BCC.[9] In the case presented in Figure 9.27 this woman has had multiple BCCs and has chosen to have a shave excision of a small BCC on her cheek. A previous biopsy had proven the diagnosis, and she wanted less invasive surgery than a full elliptical excision. The margins were clear, and the area healed with minimal scarring.

See video 9.5.

PYOGENIC GRANULOMA

Most pyogenic granulomas are easy to distinguish based on their clinical appearance and behavior. The rare amelanotic melanoma can appear similar to a pyogenic granuloma. Thus it is best to send all suspected pyogenic granulomas for histologic confirmation. The easiest method to do this is to do an initial shave excision before performing electrodesiccation and curettage of the base of the pyogenic granuloma (Figure 9.28). Most importantly the remaining tissue is curetted, and the base is treated with electrodesiccation. See Chapter 33, *Procedures to Treat Benign Conditions.*

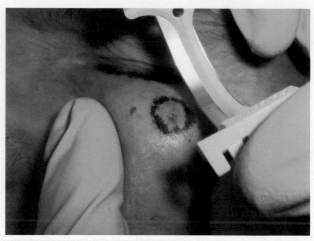

Figure 9.27 Shave excision of a small BCC on the cheek. A previous biopsy had proven the diagnosis, and the patient wanted less invasive surgery than a full elliptical excision. The margins were clear, and the area healed with minimal scarring and no recurrence. (Copyright Richard P. Usatine, MD.)

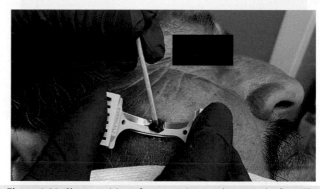

Figure 9.28 Shave excision of a pyogenic granuloma on the face. This was followed by curettage and electrodesiccation of the base to stop bleeding and prevent regrowth. (Copyright Richard P. Usatine, MD.)

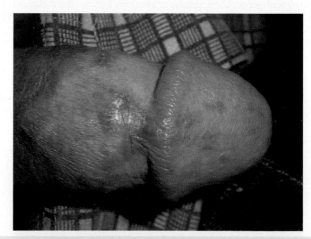

Figure 9.29 **Shave biopsy of a plaque on this penis demonstrated psoriasis.** (Copyright Richard P. Usatine, MD.)

PSORIASIS

Psoriasis is frequently a diagnosis made on clinical appearance and history only. Sometimes psoriasis presents in an atypical pattern, and a biopsy is needed to make the diagnosis. The patient in Figure 9.29 developed a rash on his penis

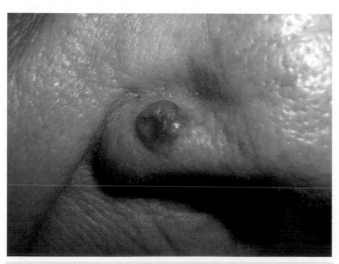

Figure 9.26 BCC on nasal ala – shave biopsy is preferred over a punch biopsy. (Copyright Richard P. Usatine, MD.)

and had no other skin findings. A shave biopsy of the lesion allowed the diagnosis of psoriasis to be made. While a punch biopsy would have provided adequate tissue, there are greater risks involved in a punch biopsy of the penis (see Chapter 20, *Working in Challenging Locations*). Having a definitive diagnosis was helpful to guide treatment of this disturbing eruption.

See *videos 9.11–9.13* for other shave examples.

Coding and Billing Pearls

The shave procedure is either used as a form of biopsy and billed under the tangential biopsy code or used to fully excise a lesion that is benign and then billed under the shave excision codes. It can be confusing sometimes to decide whether the procedure is a "biopsy" or "excision." Clearcut examples of shave biopsies include sampling a possible skin cancer or removing a piece of skin to determine the cause of an unknown rash. Shave excisions are those procedures that are used to remove a benign nevus, a seborrheic keratosis, or another benign lesion. The intent is to excise the whole lesion, and even though it is recommended to send all pigmented lesions for confirmatory pathological diagnosis, the primary reason for the procedure was not a "biopsy" but a removal of the lesion itself. Make sure that the documentation is consistent with the procedure that is billed for. If the shave is done as a biopsy, call it a shave or tangential biopsy, but if the shave is done as an excision, call it a shave excision or just an excision.

CPT codes for shave biopsies (tangential biopsy) are summarized here:

CPT Code	Description	wRVU
11102	Tangential biopsy of skin (e.g., shave, scoop, saucerize, curette), single lesion	0.66
+11103	Each additional lesion	0.38

CPT 11102, 11103 are the codes for all locations except these special locations that have site-specific skin biopsy codes. These codes are for all types of biopsies in these areas:

- Pinna (69100)
- Nail unit (11755)
- Vermilion and mucosal lip (40490)
- Penis (54100)
- Vulva (56605)

For a full list of the site-specific skin biopsy codes, see Table 28.1.

Note that the tangential biopsy codes and site-specific codes are independent of whether the lesion turns out to be benign or malignant, so there is no need to wait for the pathology result to submit the bill.

Conclusion

The shave biopsy is one of the most useful techniques in dermatologic surgery. It is widely applicable to many skin lesions and can be performed rapidly in the office setting with minimal equipment. Every clinician that performs skin surgery should master this technique.

References

1. Coit DG, Andtbacka R, Bichakjian CK, et al. Melanoma. *J Natl Compr Cancer Netw N.* 2009;7(3):250-275. doi:10.6004/jnccn. 2009.0020.
2. Ng JC, Swain S, Dowling JP, Wolfe R, Simpson P, Kelly JW. The impact of partial biopsy on histopathologic diagnosis of cutaneous melanoma: experience of an Australian tertiary referral service. *Arch Dermatol.* 2010;146(3):234-239.
3. Grabski WJ, Salasche SJ, Mulvaney MJ. Razor-blade surgery. *J Dermatol Surg Oncol.* 1990;16:1121-1126.
4. Harrison PV. Good results after shave excision of benign moles. *J Dermatol Surg Oncol.* 1985;11(668):686.
5. Hudson-Peacock MJ, Bishop J, Lawrence CM. Shave excision of benign papular naevocytic naevi. *Br J Plast Surg.* 1995;48: 318-322.
6. Gambichler T, Senger E, Rapp S, Alamouti D, Altmeyer P, Hoffmann K. Deep shave excision of macular melanocytic nevi with the razor blade biopsy technique. *Dermatol Surg.* 2000;26(7):662-666.
7. Tran KT, Wright NA, Cockrell CJ. Biopsy of the pigmented lesion – When and how. *J Am Acad Dermatol.* 2008;59:852-871.
8. Ferrandiz L, Moreno-Ramirez D, Camacho FM. Shave excision of common acquired melanocytic nevi: cosmetic outcome, recurrences, and complications. *Dermatol Surg.* 2005;31(9 Pt 1): 1112-1115.
9. Russell EB, Carrington PR, Smoller BR. Basal cell carcinoma: a comparison of shave biopsy versus punch biopsy techniques in subtype diagnosis. *J Am Acad Dermatol.* 1999;41:69-71.

10 The Punch Biopsy

RICHARD P. USATINE, MD, and ANGELA ABOUASSI, MD

SUMMARY
- A punch biopsy is a versatile method of obtaining tissue for the diagnosis of all kinds of rashes and skin tumors.
- It is often the biopsy of choice for inflammatory and infiltrative skin conditions.
- A punch biopsy can be used to remove small cysts, lipomas, and other small benign skin conditions.
- The chapter discusses the advantages and disadvantages of punch biopsies.
- When doing a punch biopsy of a bullous lesion or an ulcer, it is best to biopsy the edge.
- The chapter discusses how to choose the appropriate punch size and whether to suture the punch defect.
- A step-by-step approach is provided with illustrative photographs.
- Specific examples of punch biopsies are included.

The punch biopsy is an easy method to remove a round full-thickness skin specimen. It is often used to diagnose skin rashes and lesions of uncertain etiology. The main advantage of the punch biopsy over the shave technique is that it can yield deeper tissue with preserved architecture for pathologic evaluation. It is also easier to perform on flat lesions for clinicians that have not mastered the art of the shave biopsy for lesions that are not elevated.

Flat lesions that are amenable to punch biopsy include inflammatory skin conditions such as suspected drug eruptions, dermatoses, lichen planus, and cutaneous lupus. Infiltrative skin conditions such as sarcoidosis and granuloma annulare can be diagnosed with a punch biopsy. Also, a punch biopsy may be used to diagnose all types of skin cancers including melanoma and cutaneous lymphomas. It is not necessarily the best method for all of these conditions. See Chapter 8, *Choosing the Biopsy Type* for help in decision-making.

A punch biopsy is one option in the diagnosis of melanoma if the entire lesion is large, making it too difficult to remove the whole lesion at the time of biopsy. In this case, the diagnostic yield will generally be best if the largest punch available is used and the biopsy is performed on the darkest, most elevated, and/or most suspicious areas. Using a dermatoscope may help identify a suspicious area for the punch biopsy (see Chapter 18, *Dermoscopy*). If the suspicion for melanoma is high, excising the entire lesion is preferred, when possible, to improve the diagnostic yield. There are also times when a broad scoop shave may provide better tissue for the pathologist than a punch. The highest risk of using a punch biopsy to diagnose a melanoma is the risk of a false negative result with partial sampling when the punch is small and the lesion is large. One can reduce this risk with a 6- to 8-mm punch rather than the typical 4-mm punch. If the lesion remains suspicious for melanoma and only a punch biopsy was performed with a negative result,

the remainder of the lesion should be excised for histology (see Chapter 8, *Choosing the Biopsy Type*). *See video 10.1.*

Indications

Punch biopsy can be used to diagnose any skin condition or disease. A punch biopsy is a recommended biopsy technique for the following conditions:[1]

- Bullous diseases (Figure 10.1)
- Alopecia – both nonscarring and scarring types (Figure 10.2)
- Inflammatory skin disease such as dermatoses, psoriasis, and vasculitis (Figure 10.3). *See videos 10.2 and 10.3.*
- Infiltrative diseases such as cutaneous sarcoidosis and granuloma annulare (Figure 10.4)
- Melanoma (including nail melanoma) (Figure 10.5)
- Oral lesions such as lichen planus (Figure 10.6)
- Vulvar diseases including SCC and VIN (Figure 10.7)
- Connective tissue disorders (lupus and dermatomyositis) (Figure 10.8)

The following types of conditions may be diagnosed with a shave biopsy, but a punch biopsy can be an acceptable alternative.

- All types of nonmelanoma skin cancers and precancers
- All benign skin neoplasms

Punch biopsy can be used to remove any small skin lesion. The following lesions are often removed using this technique:

- Small nevi
- Small dermatofibromas
- Pilar cyst
- Small epidermal inclusion cysts
- Neurofibromas

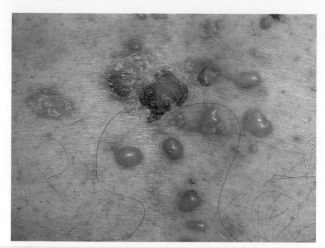

Figure 10.1 Bullous lesions on the back of a 57-year-old man suspicious for bullous pemphigoid. A 4-mm punch biopsy was performed on the edge of an intact bulla and sent for H&E staining. Another 4-mm punch biopsy was performed on perilesional skin and sent for direct immunofluorescence. The result confirmed the diagnosis of bullous pemphigoid. (Copyright Richard P. Usatine, MD.)

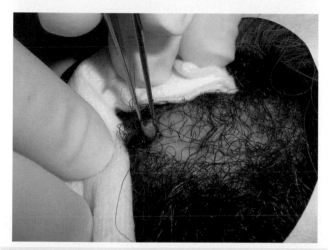

Figure 10.2 A 4-mm punch biopsy of the scalp was performed to determine the cause of the alopecia. Subcutaneous fat is visible at the base of the biopsy as it should be. The pathology was consistent with lichen planopilaris. (Copyright Richard P. Usatine, MD.)

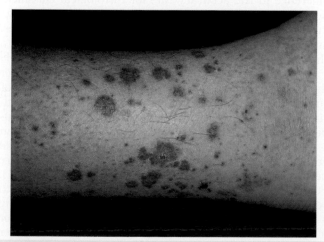

Figure 10.3 This young man developed palpable purpura on both legs. Punch biopsies were used to determine that this was an IgA-mediated leukocytoclastic vasculitis. (Copyright Richard P. Usatine, MD.)

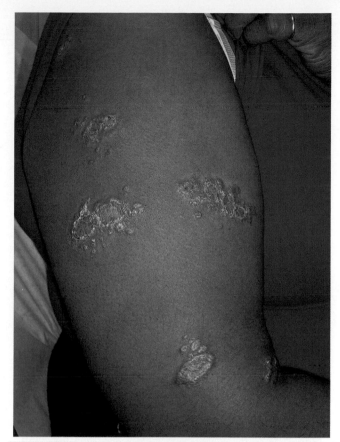

Figure 10.4 A Black woman had lesions on the face and arm suspicious for cutaneous sarcoidosis. A 4-mm punch biopsy on the arm confirmed the diagnosis. (Copyright Richard P. Usatine, MD.)

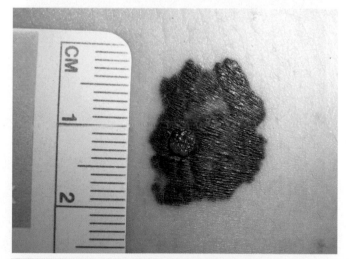

Figure 10.5 This growing pigmented lesion on the abdomen of a Hispanic woman was suspicious for melanoma. As it was nearly 2 cm in diameter, it was decided to do a 6-mm punch biopsy at the area that was most palpable. The result showed a 0.9-mm melanoma. (Copyright Richard P. Usatine, MD.)

A punch instrument can be used to create an opening in an epidermal inclusion cyst for a minimally invasive cyst removal. Some clinicians use a punch incision to remove small lipomas (see Chapter 12, *Cysts and Lipomas*).

See *video 10.4* for overview of the punch biopsy.

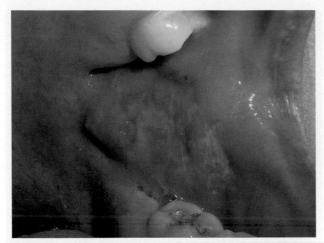

Figure 10.6 A lacy white pattern bilaterally on the buccal mucosa was suspicious for lichen planus. The presence of Wickham's striae bilaterally in the mouth makes lichen planus likely. To establish a diagnosis histologically a 4-mm punch biopsy of the buccal mucosa can be performed. Hemostasis can be achieved with aluminum chloride, hemostatic gel, or electrocoagulation. A suture is rarely needed and is generally more uncomfortable for the patient. (Copyright Richard P. Usatine, MD.)

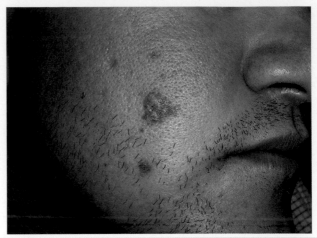

Figure 10.8 A 29-year-old man presented with lesions on the face. A 4-mm punch biopsy provided the diagnosis of discoid lupus. (Copyright Richard P. Usatine, MD.)

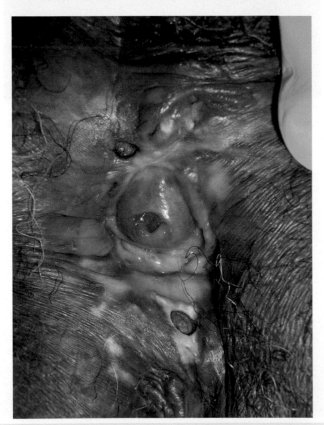

Figure 10.7 A 59-year-old woman with a long history of condyloma acuminata has suspicious areas of leukoplakia of the vulva. This photograph shows the vulva after two punch biopsies were performed. Both areas were found to have vulvar intraepithelial neoplasia 2 (VIN 2). (Copyright Richard P. Usatine, MD.)

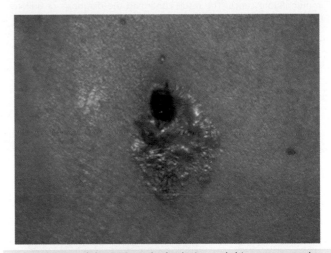

Figure 10.9 Nodular BCC on the back. A punch biopsy was used to establish the diagnosis. However, a shave biopsy would have been adequate and less invasive. (Copyright Richard P. Usatine, MD.)

Relative Contraindications and Cautions

Punch biopsy is a more time-consuming biopsy technique than needed for most BCCs or SCCs, which can be diagnosed by shave biopsy. In one study, there was no significant difference in the accuracy rate for histological classification of BCC with both the shave and the punch biopsy.[2] Punch biopsies generally bleed more than shave biopsies, and the risk of infection is somewhat higher than for a shave (Figure 10.9).

A punch biopsy does have certain risks that are greater than those of a shave biopsy, including the possibility of cutting deeper blood vessels and nerves. Therefore clinicians must be familiar with the underlying anatomy. Fortunately, most major nerves and blood vessels are deeper than a punch instrument, but digital nerves and the temporal branch of the facial nerve are more superficial, and care needs to be taken in these areas (Figure 11.2 in Chapter 11). Punch biopsies over the digits or the eyelid are generally to be avoided. When possible, it is also prudent to avoid doing a punch biopsy over superficial arteries such as digital or temporal arteries. Caution should also be exercised over areas where there is little soft tissue between the skin and the bone (over the tibia, digits, and ulna) because the punch can cut through the underlying bone.

Advantages of Punch Biopsy

The advantages of the punch biopsy for the clinician include the following:

- Can be performed rapidly (faster than a free-hand ellipse)
- It is relatively easy to learn.
- Sutures are not needed for smaller punch biopsies.
- Strict sterile procedure is not required.

The following advantages of punch biopsy benefit the patient:

- Wound care is usually simple.
- Restriction of activities is usually not needed during wound healing.
- Minimal risk of infection and bleeding

Disadvantages of Punch Biopsy

Disadvantages for the clinician include the following:

- Punch biopsies may bleed more than shave biopsies so that it may take more time to achieve hemostasis.
- Time and cost for suture placement and removal at a return visit
- Punch biopsies of a melanoma may miss the malignancy if the sampling turns out to be a nonmelanoma part of the lesion.

For the patient, the disadvantages of punch biopsy include the following:

- Possible scarring with a cross-hatch from a suture
- A second in-person visit for suture removal

MAKING A DIAGNOSIS

It helps to have a good idea of the differential diagnosis before choosing the biopsy type and location. For most punch biopsies, a clinician should choose a punch size to excise the whole lesion or sample the portion of the lesion that appears to have the worst pathology. However, for suspected immunobullous disorders such as pemphigus or bullous pemphigoid, it is best to punch the edge of the bulla to include the perilesional skin (Figure 10.10). A scoop shave under an intact bulla or at the border of a bulla may yield an equally good specimen. Both methods help to keep the epidermis attached to the dermis at the edge of the bulla.

When performing a biopsy on an ulcerative lesion of unknown origin, it is helpful to remove tissue from the edge of the ulcer rather than the center portion. For example, if pyoderma gangrenosum is suspected, the biopsy should include the edge of the lesion, with some perilesional skin (Figure 10.11).

Additionally, before starting the biopsy, the clinician should also have in mind whether the specimen will be sent for standard formalin-fixed hematoxylin and eosin (H&E) – stain, direct immunofluorescence (DIF), or tissue culture. For example, to diagnose bullous disorders, it helps to send the specimen for both H&E and DIF. The biopsy for immunofluorescence is performed on perilesional skin not including

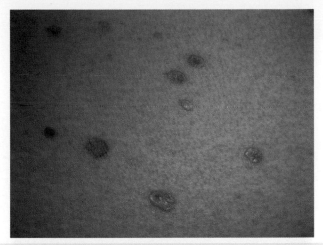

Figure 10.10 Bullous lichen planus on the back. A punch biopsy should include a whole intact bulla or the edge of a bulla. A deep shave including the edge of the bulla would also be adequate. (Copyright Richard P. Usatine, MD.)

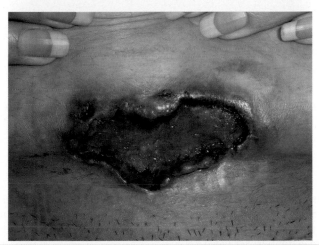

Figure 10.11 Pyoderma gangrenosum in the suprapubic region of a 19-year-old woman. The diagnosis was suspected based on the active ulcer with gun metal borders. The diagnosis was confirmed by punch biopsy of an active edge of the ulcer. (Copyright Richard P. Usatine, MD.)

the lesion itself. Suspected conditions for which a biopsy may be needed for DIF include the following:

- Pemphigus of all types (Figure 10.12)
- Bullous pemphigoid (Figure 10.1)
- Henoch-Schönlein purpura

Some of these conditions may be diagnosed with standard histology only, and the biopsy for DIF may be a second step only if needed. DIF may be helpful in predicting potential relapse in a patient with pemphigus in remission. DIF becomes positive early in the disease process of pemphigus; complement deposition shows an increase early in disease and during relapse.[3] DIF requires Michel's media for transport and should not be put into standard formalin. If two specimens are being sent simultaneously for DIF and standard pathology, two punch biopsies should be performed remembering that the DIF specimen is taken from perilesional skin. When Michel's media is not available, the DIF specimen can be placed on a sterile saline-soaked gauze pad

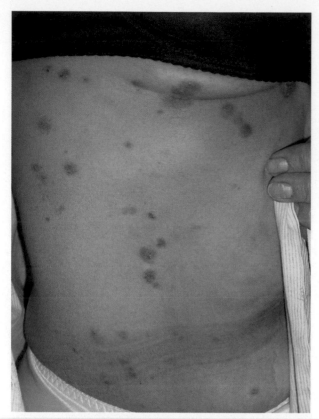

Figure 10.12 Pemphigus foliaceous on the trunk of a 50-year-old was diagnosed with two 4-mm punch biopsies – one on the edge of a bulla and the other on perilesional skin for direct immunofluorescence. (Copyright Richard P. Usatine, MD.)

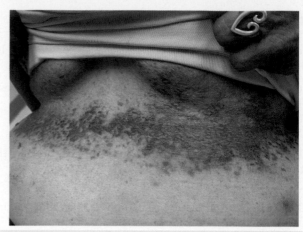

Figure 10.13 Hailey-Hailey disease (also known as familial pemphigus) was diagnosed with a 4-mm punch biopsy on the edge of the lesion and another 4-mm punch biopsy of perilesional skin for direct immunofluorescent (DIF). The biopsy on the edge was consistent with familial pemphigus, and the DIF was negative as expected in this disease. (Copyright Richard P. Usatine, MD.)

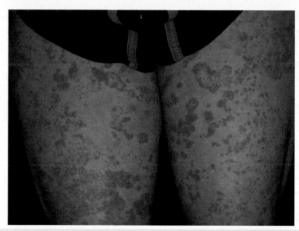

Figure 10.14 A 40-year-old woman presented with erythematous lesions on her legs and abdomen for 6 months. There were scale and small pustules, and the patient experienced pruritus. She had been given a topical steroid in the past for this. A KOH preparation was read as negative, and the patient agreed to a punch biopsy. A PAS stain on the biopsy was positive for fungal elements, and the diagnosis was tinea incognito. (Copyright Richard P. Usatine, MD.)

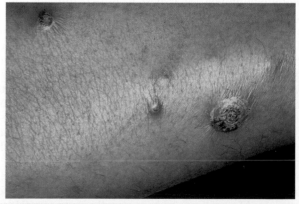

Figure 10.15 Disseminated sporotrichosis. A 4-mm punch biopsy was sent for standard histology and PAS stain. A second 4-mm punch was sent on a sterile saline gauze for fungal culture and grew out sporotrichosis. The PAS stain was also positive for fungal elements. (Copyright Richard P. Usatine, MD.)

in a sterile urine container and call the lab to have it transferred to Michel's media ASAP. Optimal biopsy site is critical when performing DIF depending on type of disease being investigated. *See video 10.5.*

- For connective tissue disease – take biopsy from established lesion that is still active, ideally older than 6 months, from sun-exposed site. Additional specimen is often taken from sun-protected area.
- Vasculitis – biopsy taken from lesion less than 24 hours old, punch biopsy or deep shave for best results
- For autoimmune bullous diseases – take a biopsy less than 1 cm away from a bulla, from normal-appearing perilesional skin.
    - Avoid lower extremities if possible as these sites can lead to false negative results.

In some instances, a negative DIF can be used to rule out an immune basis for the dermatological disease, such as in Hailey-Hailey disease (Figure 10.13), nonimmune leukocytoclastic vasculitis.[3]

If a fungal infection is suspected but KOH and culture are negative (Figure 10.14), PAS stains are useful and can be done off the specimen in the formalin. If a culture is desired for a suspected deep fungal infection such as sporotrichosis (Figure 10.15), the specimen can be sent on sterile saline-soaked gauze pad in a sterile urine container. This technique also works for all suspected bacterial infections, including atypical mycobacterial infections (Figure 10.16).

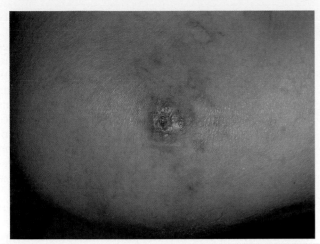

Figure 10.16 *Mycobacterium abscessus* infection on the leg diagnosed with a 4-mm punch biopsy sent for AFB stain and culture. (Copyright Richard P. Usatine, MD.)

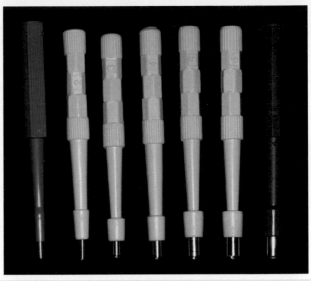

Figure 10.18 Punch biopsy tools from three different manufacturers spanning the diameters from 2 mm on the left to 6 mm on the right. (Copyright Richard P. Usatine, MD.)

Equipment

It helps to have a prepared set of sterilized instruments (Figure 10.17) ready for a punch biopsy to avoid time wasted looking for all the right equipment.

- Punch tool (2 to 10 mm available) (3 to 6 mm are preferred) – add this as needed
- Iris scissors (curved or straight)
- Adson forceps without teeth for pulling up the specimen gently
- Needle holder and sutures or hemostatic solution or absorbable gelatin sponge
- Adson forceps with teeth for suturing (optional)

Punches come in various sizes ranging from 2 to 10 mm and are available as reusable steel punches and disposable punches (Figure 10.18). Disposable punches have the advantage of being presterilized, and there is no concern for their losing their sharp edge. Reusable punches are more expensive, require sterilization between procedures, and must be maintained by proper, skilled sharpening. Disposable punches have essentially replaced reusable punches for cost, quality, and convenience.

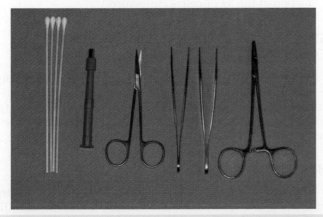

Figure 10.17 Punch biopsy instrument set. The needle holder and extra Adson forceps with teeth are useful when the punch defect is sutured. (Copyright Richard P. Usatine, MD.)

CHOOSING PUNCH SIZE

A 4-mm punch is usually adequate to obtain sufficient tissue for pathology. When the lesion is smaller than 6 mm, the punch size may be determined by the diameter required to completely excise the tissue. Punch biopsies done with punches over 6 mm may produce "dog ears" or "standing cones" when closure is attempted. If the lesion requires a punch of larger than 6 mm, it is best to do an elliptical excision. Punch biopsies between 3 and 6 mm should produce adequate tissue and be easy to close with a good cosmetic result. A minimum of a 4-mm punch is generally preferred by the pathologist to provide adequate tissue for diagnosis.

CHOOSING WHETHER TO SUTURE THE PUNCH DEFECT

- 2- or 3-mm punch defects can be left to heal by secondary intention.
- 4-mm punch defects in one study healed as well by secondary intention compared with suturing with one interrupted 4-0 nylon suture.[4] Blinded observers saw relatively little difference in the 4-mm punch results at 9 months. Note that no electrosurgery, aluminum chloride, or other hemostatic agents were applied to the biopsy sites; only gel foam was used for hemostasis in the nonsutured wounds. All wounds were dressed with petrolatum under gauze covered by an occlusive transparent dressing (Tegaderm). Dressings were left in place for 3 days, after which the gel foam was removed from the second-intention site, and both biopsy sites were cleansed with water to remove any exudate. Tegaderm was reapplied at that visit and then weekly by the patient until the biopsy sites were completely healed or reepithelialized. While these results are encouraging for the choice to leave 4 mm or less punch defects open to heal naturally, the use of gel foam and Tegaderm is not representative of standard punch aftercare. Also, this study required an

additional visit 3 days postop. Also at 2 weeks, pain was reported more commonly for the site treated by second-intention healing, and the pain lasted longer for the second-intention sites than for the primary closure sites.[4] Not surprisingly, unblinded patients preferred suture closer of the 8-mm punch biopsy sites.[4] One could inform the patient of the risks and benefits of suturing and make a joint decision keeping many factors in mind.

Punch Biopsy: Steps and Principles

Critical steps in the punch biopsy include the following:[5]

- Using 1% lidocaine with epinephrine for anesthesia and hemostasis
- Cutting the punch biopsy down to the correct depth (into subcutaneous fat)
- Not crushing the tissue while handling the specimen
- Stopping the bleeding adequately
- Avoiding dog ears in the final repair

PREOPERATIVE MEASURES

- Determine the size punch needed, and consider the pros and cons for suturing the defect if the punch size is 4 mm or less.
- Discuss with the patient the biopsy options and pros and cons for suturing the defect if the punch size is 4 mm or less. Obtain informed consent in writing or electronically. (See Appendix A for sample consent form.)
- If sutures are to be used, choose the type of suture, and set up the sterile supplies and equipment for the procedure.
- It helps to mark the area to be punched with a surgical marker. It need not be a sterile marker if the skin is prepped after marking. If the punch will be taken from a large involved area, the marking helps to make sure that the anesthesia and cut are in the same area.
- Lightly prep the area with alcohol or another antiseptic.
- Inject local anesthesia. Use a 27- or 30-gauge needle with 1% lidocaine and epinephrine (buffer the lidocaine for less pain – see Chapter 4). Start with the needle under the lesion (greater depth is less painful), and then give the last amount of anesthesia closer to the skin surface. It is important to infiltrate the skin surface and the dermis to the full depth of the planned punch (Figure 10.19B). Wait 7 minutes for maximum vasoconstriction and hemostasis if the area or lesion is very vascular. This is a good time to complete your pathology consult.

CUTTING THE PUNCH BIOPSY

- Prep the area with chlorhexidine.
- Sterile gloves are not needed. Clean your hands with hand cleanser and apply clean gloves.
- Set up your instruments so it is easy to grab the scissor with your dominant hand and the forceps with your nondominant hand. Have sterile CTAs available to stop the bleeding while getting ready to place a suture.
- Use a sterile fenestrated drape. Be prepared to handle bleeding, which may drip down the skin, by placing a gauze under the punch site in the direction that gravity will take the blood from the punch site.
- If performing a punch over 5 mm, then standing cones can be avoided by stretching the skin perpendicular to skin lines before and during the punch (Figure 10.19D). This tension should be maintained throughout the punch procedure until the dermis is fully breached. This stretching perpendicular to relaxed skin tension lines will allow the resultant wound, circular under tension, to revert to an oval or fusiform shape when the retention is relaxed. The oval defect will be aligned with the relaxed skin tension line to facilitate closure and optimize cosmesis.
- The punch is then held between the thumb and forefinger of the dominant hand (Figure 10.19).
- With downward pressure, the punch instrument is rapidly rotated back and forth between the fingers until it penetrates completely through the dermis. Feel for a sensation of getting through a firm substance and moving into the less firm subcutaneous fat. Pull up the punch and look for signs that the depth is correct. The punch specimen often raises above the surrounding tissue when the tissue has been cut to the fat layer (the dermis holds it in place if the depth is not correct) (Figure 10.20). The bleeding is often increased when the cut reaches the SQ fat, and if you pull up on the specimen you may see the yellow fat color below. If the cut was not deep enough, reinsert the punch and continue cutting until the depth is correct.
- The punch instrument is then removed, and the specimen should remain in the center of the site. Rarely the specimen may shear off and pull away with the punch. If this happens, it can be carefully removed from the punch with a needle.
- If the specimen is not elevated, apply downward compression around the punch specimen for elevation. The specimen can then be further elevated gently with a forceps (being careful not to crush the specimen) (Figure 10.19E) and cut from its base with a sharp iris scissor (Figure 10.19F).
- It is important to remember that every effort needs to be made to handle the specimen lightly and to resist the tendency to compress or crush the specimen with the teeth of the forceps. Crushed samples may result in distortion of nuclei or cell architecture.[3]

STRETCHING THE SKIN TO PREVENT STANDING CONES (DOG EARS) (FIGURE 10.21)

This is especially important when doing a punch larger than 5 mm or performing a punch on the face or other cosmetically important area. Figure 10.20 shows how stretching the skin perpendicular to skin lines will allow for a better cosmetic outcome.

HEMOSTASIS AND REPAIR

- Hemostasis should always begin with a CTA placed in the hole created by the punch biopsy (Figure 10.22). If the punch was 4 mm, then most standard CTAs are a perfect fit and can stand on their own while the clinician is loading the needle holder.

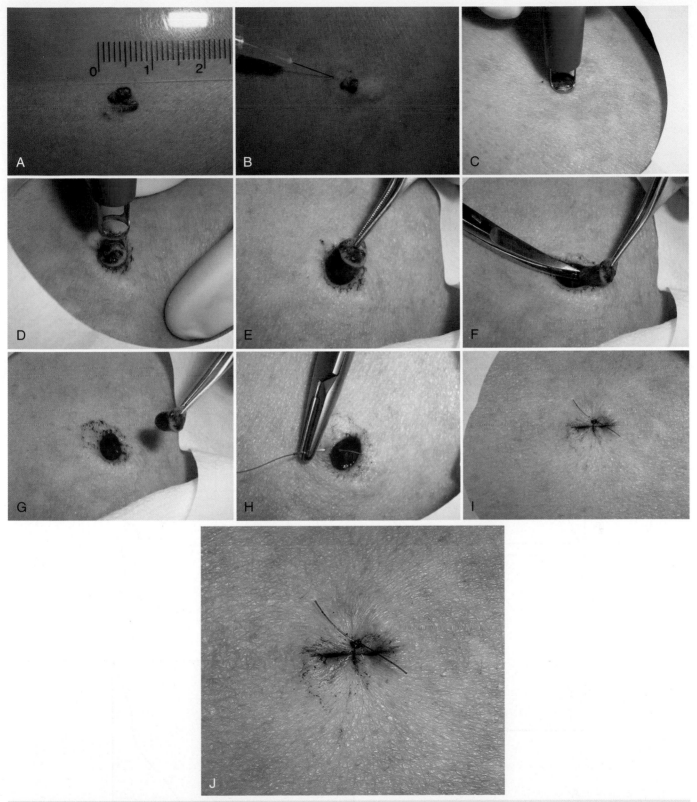

Figure 10.19 Punch sequence. **(A)** A 62-year-old woman presented with a growing lesion on her back. Dermoscopicly, it had features of a pigmented basal cell carcinoma. While we would offer a saucerization today, a punch biopsy was performed with adequate results. **(B)** Local anesthesia with 1% lidocaine and epinephrine was injected using a 30-gauge needle. The anesthesia is injected more deeply at first and then more superficially to make sure the punch biopsy site is completely anesthetized. **(C)** After sterilely prepping and draping the site, a 4-mm VisiPunch is placed on top of the lesion to make sure that it will provide an adequate biopsy. The lesion can be seen within the punch. **(D)** The skin is stretched perpendicular to skin lines and the punch biopsy instrument is twirled clockwise and counterclockwise until the blade cuts down to the subcutaneous fat. Once the fat layer is reached, the punch is lifted. **(E)** The biopsy specimen is gently lifted so that it may be snipped off with a curved sharp iris scissor. Any sharp-pointed small tissue scissor would also work. **(F)** The specimen is pulled to the side to give room for the scissor to snip the base. **(G)** The punch specimen is removed. **(H)** The punch defect is sewed. The tip of the needle is viewed in the hole before the stitch is completed. **(I)** One interrupted suture is sufficient for closure of this punch biopsy. **(J)** The punch core is raised from the skin around it once the dermis has been fully cut.

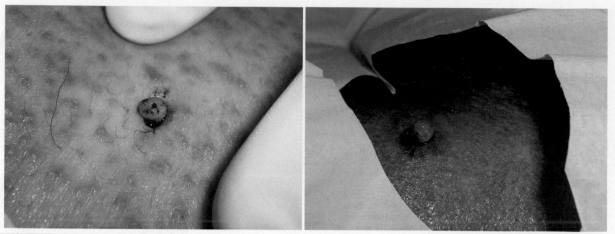

Figure 10.20 The punch specimen will raise above the surface of the skin once the punch tool cuts through the dermis into the subcutis. (Copyright Richard P. Usatine, MD.)

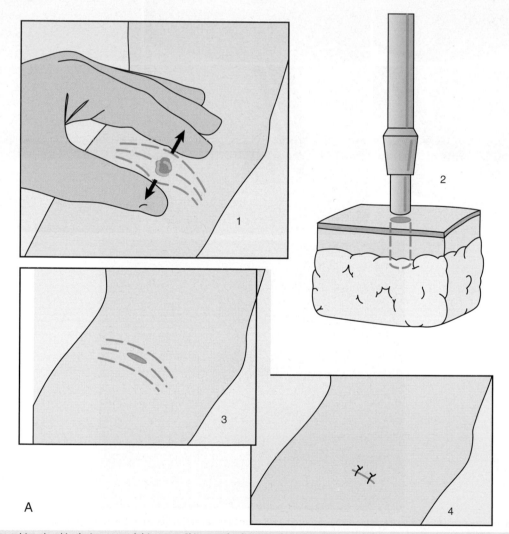

A

Figure 10.21 (A) Stretching the skin during a punch biopsy. 1, Skin stretched perpendicular to skin lines. 2, Punch to subcutaneous fat. 3, Oval defect is formed. 4, Closed defect is now linear.

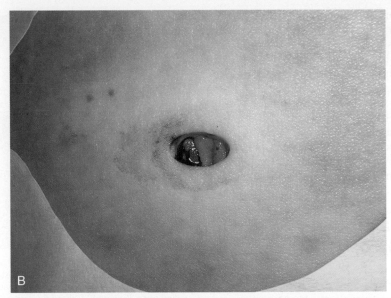

Figure 10.21, cont'd **(B)** Oval defect from a punch biopsy that was created by stretching the skin during the punch procedure. (Copyright Richard P. Usatine, MD.)

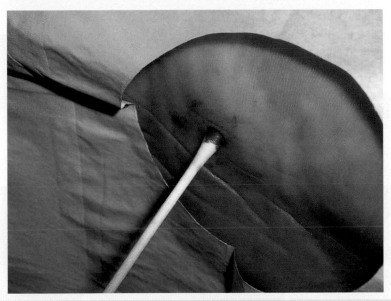

Figure 10.22 A CTA is applied to the defect produced by a 4-mm punch on the sole. It is a perfect fit to stop the bleeding. It can even stay in the hole without being held while the surgeon loads the needle holder. (Copyright Richard P. Usatine, MD.)

- If no sutures are to be placed, hemostasis can be achieved with aluminum chloride on a CTA or a hemostatic foam (see Chapter 4, *Hemostasis*). If this does not work, electrocoagulation is another option but will not work if the bleeding is brisk because the blood welling up in the small hole does not allow the current to stop the bleeding. If the aluminum chloride solution is in water, there are no concerns about using the electrocoagulation immediately as needed.
- If these methods are not working, hold pressure on the wound and place a suture.
- Preventing dog ears before suturing is rarely needed unless the punch was large in an area where there is a lot of skin tension. If dog ears seem to be likely, try gently undermining the defect with blunt dissection using the iris scissor. This often will allow the defect to elongate along skin lines. Another option has been described using two skin hooks. The skin hooks are placed on opposite ends of the wound following skin lines, and the circular defect is stretched for 1 minute. This method was found to prevent dog ears in one study.[6]
- There are many choices for suturing the punch biopsy. Nylon suture is a good and inexpensive material to use. Usually, 4-0 or 5-0 nylon is adequate. Money can be saved by purchasing sutures with a short 9-inch monofilament meant to close punch biopsies (Delasco Biopsy Suture – www.delasco.com).
- Vicryl (polyglactin 910) was compared with nylon for closure of punch biopsy sites in one study.[7] Each 3-mm punch site was closed with one simple suture. The sites were evaluated at 2 weeks and 6 months for redness, infection, dehiscence, scar hypertrophy, and patient

satisfaction. The authors found no statistically signifi-cant difference between the two suture materials in any of the above parameters.[7]

- Fast-absorbing gut can be used for closure if the area is not under tension and it is difficult for the patient to return for suture removal.
- One to two interrupted sutures are adequate for a 3- or 4-mm punch, and two to three sutures may be needed for 5- or 6-mm punch biopsies.
- The figure-of-8 suture technique (Figure 10.23) is a great method to obtain extra hemostasis if the punch site is bleeding more than usual (see Chapter 4, *Hemostasis*). *See video 10.9.*

Punch Biopsy of a Blue Nevus (Figure 10.24;

▶ *See Video 10.6*)

- In this case, a 5-mm dark lesion is likely to be a blue ne-vus but may be a nodular melanoma. The patient states

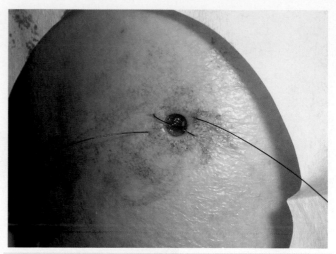

Figure 10.23 A figure of eight stitch around a punch biopsy defect prior to being tied. This suture is hemostatic and easy to perform. While the needle passes across the defect twice, the suture only needs to be tied once. (Copyright Richard P. Usatine, MD.)

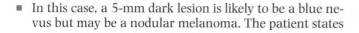
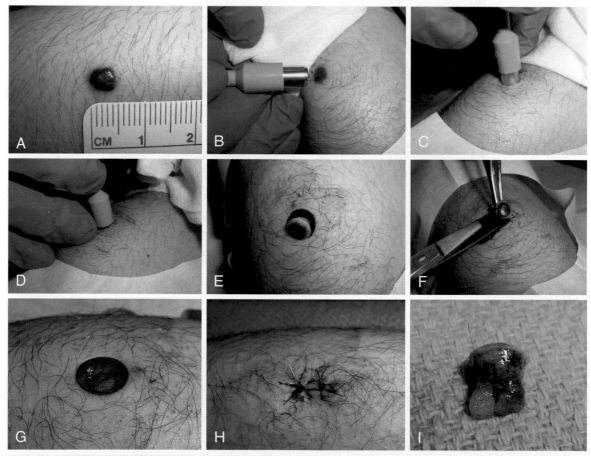

Figure 10.24 Punch sequence of a blue nevus. **(A)** A 28-year-old Hispanic woman presents with a growing 5-mm dark lesion on her arm. Dermo-scopicly, it had features of a blue nevus, but an excisional punch biopsy was performed to rule out a nodular melanoma. **(B)** After sterilely prepping and draping the site, a 6-mm punch is placed on top of the lesion to make sure that it will provide an adequate biopsy. **(C)** The punch biopsy instrument is twirled clockwise and counterclockwise. **(D)** The punch cuts down to the subcutaneous fat. Once the fat layer is reached, the punch is lifted. **(E)** The biopsy specimen is seen separated from the skin around it. Bleeding is expected. **(F)** The specimen is gently lifted so that it may be snipped off with a curved iris scissor. In this view, there is a clear margin of nonpigmented skin 360 degrees around the lesion. **(G)** The punch defect is oval as it elongates along skin tension lines. Subcutaneous fat is visible, demonstrating that the punch was performed to the correct depth. **(H)** The punch defect has been closed with two simple interrupted sutures of 4-0 Prolene. **(I)** The punch specimen is viewed showing the dark melanin in the dermis and the SQ fat below. The final diagnosis was a blue nevus. (Copyright Richard P. Usatine, MD.)

it is growing and is anxious to have it removed. It is just the right size for a 6-mm punch. The blue-black dark color of this lesion indicates that the melanin is deep in the dermis. This makes it crucial to use a punch biopsy technique for full-depth excision rather than a deep shave.

SPECIAL CONSIDERATIONS FOR HEMOSTASIS FOR PUNCH BIOPSY OF THE SCALP

- There can be significant bleeding due to the vascular nature of the scalp, and suturing can be particularly difficult because of surrounding hair.
- To shave the surrounding hair around biopsy site may be impractical and may cause increased stress and anxiety for the patient.

GELATIN FOAM INSTEAD OF SUTURING
(See Video 10.7)

- One mechanism that can help with controlling bleeding is absorbable gelatin foam sponges (Figure 4.11), which will remove the need for sutures or electrosurgery.[8]
- It is recommended that a piece of gelatin foam sponge is cut to a width that is two times the width of the biopsy site.[8]
  - Insert the sponge immediately after specific removal.
  - A wider diameter gelatin foam is preferable if bleeding is brisk or arterial in nature.
  - While waiting for foam to expand, apply gentle pressure.

- If bleeding is particularly brisk, a hemostatic mesh can be used instead of foam.
- Postprocedure care involves gentle shampooing around the site until the foam plug works its out way out of the site over a period of a few weeks.

INSTRUMENT TAMPONADE FOR SCALP PUNCH BIOPSY

- Whalen et al. have proposed a mechanism for tamponade on punch biopsy of the scalp using an instrument handle (Figure 10.25) such as blade remover, hemostat, or needle driver.[9]
- Steps to follow:
  - An assistant holds the instrument's circular handle around the area of the biopsy, which does not include any of the tissue intended for removal.
  - The assistant needs to hold firm pressure so that the entirety of the instrument handle remains in contact with the skin of the scalp to ensure appropriate tamponade of the scalp vessels.
  - At this point, perform the punch biopsy in standard manner.
  - Complete the suturing of the punch before the assistant removes the instrument handle.

DRESSING AND AFTERCARE

- Cover the final wound with clean petrolatum and a sterile adhesive bandage.

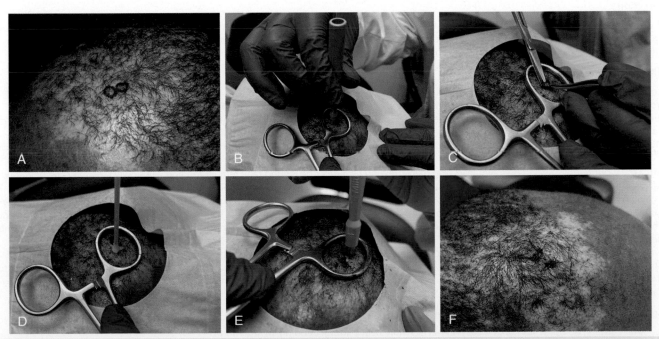

Figure 10.25 Punch sequence using an instrument for preventive tamponade. **(A)** A 34-year-old Black woman presents with hair loss and hypopigmentation of the scalp. Two adjacent punch biopsies are planned so that that dermatopathologist can view the affected hair follicles from a horizontal and vertical perspective. A surgical marker is used to mark the sites to be around hair follicles in the affected area. **(B)** After sterilely prepping and draping, an assistant holds the instrument's circular handle around the area of the biopsy site. Downward pressure is applied to the hemostat handle, and the punch biopsy instrument is twirled clockwise and counterclockwise in the first site. **(C)** The punch is lifted and snipped off at the base while pressure is still applied to the hemostat. **(D)** A CTA is placed in the punch defect, and there is little bleeding. **(E)** The first punch site was sutured, and the second punch biopsy is being performed. **(F)** The final result with both biopsy sites sutured. Even with the extra pressure of the hemostat and the anesthesia that used lidocaine with epinephrine, the physician still had to contend with significant bleeding. (Copyright Richard P. Usatine, MD.)

- If the bleeding was hard to stop or if the area is very vascular, consider applying a small pressure bandage to avoid postop bleeding. A folded 2 × 2 gauze or dental roll can be taped firmly in place or wrapped with an elastic bandage (e.g., Coban) if the site permits.
- Explain aftercare to the patient and/or their family. We usually suggest patients keep the area dry for 24 hours; then they may bathe normally. See Box 10.1 for a patient handout entitled Care of Your Skin After a Punch Biopsy.
- Sutures are generally left in place for 5 to 7 days on the face and 7 to 14 days elsewhere on the body. See Chapter 35 for further details on postoperative wound care.

Box 10.1   Care of Your Skin After a Punch Biopsy

Supplies Needed:

Clean petroleum jelly (a squeeze tube is cleaner than a tub) (Vaseline is one name brand) (Do not use Neosporin or triple antibiotic)
Dressing or gauze that is made for wound care (Band-Aids are one name brand)
Optional – cotton-tip applicators (Q-tips are one name brand)

Directions

1. Keep the site clean and dry, and do not remove the original dressing for 24 hours.
2. After 24 hours you may shower daily. Gently wash the surgical site with soap and water in the shower or at least once daily.
3. Apply petroleum jelly to the clean wound with a clean finger or cotton-tipped applicator one to two times per day.
4. Use a dressing to cover the wound, especially if the wound was not sutured. While cleansing is only needed once or twice a day, additional petroleum jelly may be added as needed to keep the wound moist. Sutured (stitched) wounds may be left uncovered without petroleum jelly after 2 days.
5. Tylenol (acetaminophen) or ibuprofen can be taken for pain if needed. DO NOT start taking any medications with aspirin or aspirin products.

For wounds that were not sutured (stitched), these will actually heal better and scar less if kept clean and covered with petroleum jelly.

Bleeding

If bleeding occurs, apply firm pressure to the site. Direct pressure should be applied to the wound. Five minutes should be adequate if the bleeding is minor and the wound is small. However, if the wound is larger and the bleeding is more severe, apply pressure for 10 minutes, timed by looking at a clock. It is best not to discontinue pressure to see if the bleeding has stopped until 10 minutes have passed. If the bleeding continues, remove the pad and press directly with a clean gauze pad over the bleeding site. If bleeding soaks through the gauze or is not stopped by firm pressure, call and go to your doctor or an urgent care center.

Infection

If you notice pus or discharge coming from the wound, this may be an infection. This is particularly worrisome if you develop a fever and the wound is red, painful, swollen, and warm. Other signs of infection could be red streaks from wound, increased pain, and painful or swollen lymph nodes (glands). If you have any suspicion of having an infection, call and go to your doctor or an urgent care center.

Shower and Washing

You may shower daily after the first 24 hours have passed. At first, you may leave the band-aid on during the shower to protect the wound from the forceful flow of water. Alternatively, if the wound needs cleaning, the shower is helpful to remove crusts and discharge. Dry the area gently and then apply petroleum jelly if the wound was not sutured. We recommend not bathing in a tub or hot tub until the wound is completely healed over to avoid infection.

Wound Healing

After the wound looks healed over, you can stop daily dressing changes. The wound may remain red and will slowly fade over the next few weeks or months. Sometimes it can take 6 months to 1 year for the redness to fade completely.

You may experience a sensation of tightness as your wound heals. This is normal and will gradually fade. After the wound has healed, frequent, gentle massaging of the area will help to loosen the scar. Sometimes the surgery cuts some small nerves resulting in local numbness. The numbness may only last a few months but may take up to a year before feeling returns to normal. Only rarely will the area remain numb permanently.

Your healed wound may be sensitive to temperature changes (such as cold air). This sensitivity improves with time, but if you are experiencing a lot of discomfort, avoid temperature extremes. You may experience itching after your wound appears to have healed. This is due to the healing that continues underneath the skin. Petroleum jelly may help to relieve this itching. Try not to scratch the wound since this may cause it to reopen.

Special Instructions for Wounds With Sutures

1. After surgery, go home and take it easy (avoid exertion, heavy lifting, bending, or straining).
2. Be very careful not to accidentally cut the sutures, especially while shaving.

Special Instructions for Wounds on the Face With Sutures

It is perfectly normal to have bruising or discoloration around the surgery site, especially if the wound is around the eye area. Do not be alarmed by this; it will eventually fade and return to normal color.

IF YOU HAVE ANY CONCERNS NOT ANSWERED BY THIS INFORMATION, PLEASE SEE US OR GO TO ANOTHER MEDICAL FACILITY IF WE ARE CLOSED.

Suggestion for Learning Punch Biopsy Technique

When learning punch biopsy technique, it may be helpful to practice on a tomato, orange, banana, synthetic skin, or pig's foot. The twirling motion to cut a core biopsy can be practiced on just about any fruit.

Complications

Complications that may arise from punch biopsy include the following:

- Cutting a vital nerve or artery (rare)
- Erythema that may last for months and often resolves
- Slow healing for a punch on the lower leg or one that is left open
- Hypopigmentation or hyperpigmentation that can be permanent
- Infection
- A punch biopsy obtained on mobile areas such as the back, which is stretched each time we bend or breathe, or the arms, which are stretched each time the muscles are flexed or pumped, may well result in some stretching of the wound. The ultimate scar, while frequently flat and flesh-colored, may become the size of the area that was removed via punch technique and not be a simple linear scar.
- Hypertrophic or keloidal scarring may rarely occur, particularly with patients predisposed to their occurrence.
- Regrowth of an incompletely excised lesion is less common than with a shave biopsy.

Specific Examples

ERYTHRODERMA

It is important to establish the cause of erythroderma quickly to initiate specific therapy. A 4-mm punch biopsy is a good start. Ask for a rapid result as erythroderma can be a life-threatening condition. This turned out to be pustular psoriasis (Figure 10.26).

PALMOPLANTAR PSORIASIS

The diagnosis of psoriasis can be made based on the clinical presentation in most cases by using clues such as the distribution, appearance, and chronicity of the lesions. A punch biopsy can be used to confirm the diagnosis in an atypical presentation when there is uncertainty. Sometimes it is difficult to determine whether hyperkeratosis on the palms and soles is from psoriasis or other conditions such as dyshidrotic eczema, keratoderma, or dermatophytosis. A punch biopsy can help direct therapy (Figure 10.27). It is especially helpful to confirm a diagnosis of palmoplantar psoriasis because these patients often need potent systemic therapy with agents that are known to have serious potential risks. Perform the punch over an area of the hand that is affected but has soft tissue below it. A shave biopsy is an option as well.

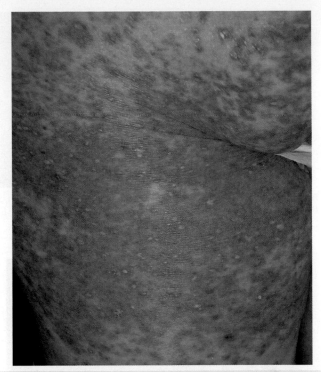

Figure 10.26 A patient with total body erythroderma and small pustules visible on the posterior thigh. While pustular psoriasis was suspected, a 4-mm punch biopsy was performed on this area and sent to pathology with a rush order. The patient was hospitalized, and the following day the diagnosis of pustular psoriasis was confirmed. Intensive treatment allowed the patient to leave the hospital improved in a few days. (Copyright Richard P. Usatine, MD.)

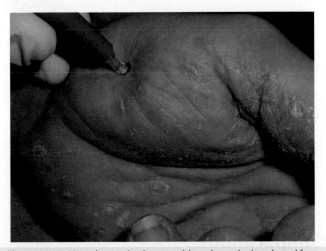

Figure 10.27 Hyperkeratotic plaques with scale on the hands and feet. A 3-mm punch biopsy of the hand confirms the diagnosis of palmar plantar psoriasis. (Copyright Richard P. Usatine, MD.)

MORPHEA (FIGURE 10.28)

Flat atrophic shiny or wrinkled patches on the skin can be morphea (localized scleroderma) or lichen sclerosis. It is difficult to tell just by looking, so a punch biopsy is very helpful. Figure 10.28A shows a 4-mm punch site from morphea on the abdomen of a young woman. In Figure 10.28B, morphea is seen on the breast of a 30-year-old woman. Diagnosis was confirmed with a 4-mm punch.

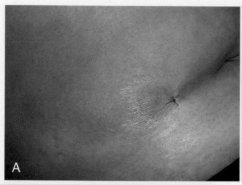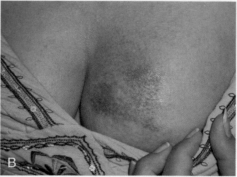

Figure 10.28 (A) Morphea or localized scleroderma on the abdomen of a young woman. Diagnosis confirmed with a 4-mm punch. **(B)** Morphea on the breast of a 30-year-old woman. (Copyright Richard P. Usatine, MD.)

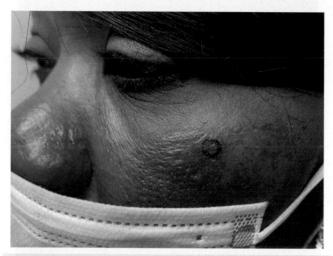

Figure 10.29 A 60-year-old Black woman presented with erythema on the left malar area for one month. A 4-mm punch biopsy provided the diagnosis of subacute cutaneous lupus erythematosus. (Copyright Richard P. Usatine, MD.)

LUPUS

A 60-year-old African American woman presents with erythema and pigmentary changes on her face for one month (Figure 10.29). A 4-mm punch biopsy is performed that demonstrates a new diagnosis of subacute cutaneous lupus erythematosus. *See video 10.09.*

Complications

Complications from a punch biopsy include the following:

- Producing a divot or indentation
- Infection
- Erythema
- Hypertrophic scar

Complications are extremely infrequent with the punch biopsy. Informed consent should be obtained so that the patient will understand the purpose of the biopsy (to help make a diagnosis) and the risks associated with it, including infection, scarring, and the need for further procedures. A complete consent form is included in Appendix A.

Coding and Billing Pearls

CPT Code	Description	Total Nonfacility RVUs
11104	Punch biopsy of skin (including simple closure, when performed), single lesion	3.52
+11105	Each additional lesion	1.73

The single punch procedure is either used as a form of biopsy and billed as CPT 11104 or used to fully excise a lesion and then billed under excision codes. Occasionally it can be confusing to decide whether the punch procedure is a "biopsy" or "excision." Clearcut examples of punch biopsies include sampling a possible skin cancer or removing a piece of skin to determine the cause of an unknown rash. Benign excision codes are used for those punch procedures that are used to remove a small benign lesion. The intent is to excise the whole lesion, and even though it is recommended to send all pigmented lesions for confirmatory pathological diagnosis, the primary reason for the procedure was not a "biopsy" but a removal of the lesion itself. Malignant excision codes are generally not used with the punch procedure because punch instruments are relatively small and not likely to provide for adequate margins around skin cancers for the definitive excision.

Make sure that the documentation is consistent with the procedure that is billed for. If the punch is done as a biopsy, call it a punch biopsy, but if the punch is done as an excision, call it a punch excision or just an excision.

Punch biopsy CPT codes are based on location only and not the size of the biopsy or lesion. CPT 11104 is the code for all locations except these special locations that have site-specific skin biopsy codes for the nail unit (11755), vermilion and mucosal lip (40490), penis (54100), and vulva (56605). The biopsy codes are also independent of whether the lesion turns out to be benign or malignant, so there is no need to wait for the pathology result to submit the bill. The codes are also independent of whether or not a suture was placed to close the punch.

CPT codes and fees for punch *excisions* are the same as for small benign excisions and are provided in Table 38.10.

These codes are based on size and location so it is crucial to measure the lesion before excising it. If the lesion is cutaneous and will be fully removed, then the punch size is the lesion size for billing. If the lesion is subcutaneous such as a lipoma or deep cyst, then the lesion size is the actual measured size before surgery and not the punch size. Don't estimate the size later because estimates are usually rounded to the nearest centimeter and the reimbursement goes up 0.1 cm above each rounded number (e.g., payment is greater for an excision of a 1.1-cm lesion than a 1.0-cm lesion). The codes are also independent of whether or not a suture was placed to close the punch, but in many cases one or more sutures will be used as the punch excisions tend to be larger than biopsies only.

Conclusion

The punch is a relatively easy and convenient procedure for getting a full-thickness biopsy. It is much easier to perform than an elliptical excision, but neither as easy nor as fast as the shave biopsy. It is preferentially used when a shave biopsy is too superficial, and a small 2- to 6-mm biopsy will provide adequate tissue sampling. While the punch biopsy is a critical skill to master, a clinician should not be performing more punch biopsies than shave biopsies (see Chapter 9, *Shave Biopsy*).

References

1. Elston DM, Stratman EJ, Miller SJ. Skin biopsy: biopsy issues in specific diseases. *J Am Acad Dermatol*. 2016;74(1):1-18. doi:10.1016/j.jaad. 2015.06.033. [Erratum in: *J Am Acad Dermatol*. 2016;75(4): 854].
2. Russell EB, Carrington PR, Smoller BR. Basal cell carcinoma: a comparison of shave biopsy versus punch biopsy techniques in subtype diagnosis. *J Am Acad Dermatol*. 1999;41:69-71.
3. Mysorekar VV, Prasad ALS, Sumathy TK. Role of direct immunofluorescence in dermatological disorders. *Indian Dermatol Online J*. 2015; 6(3):172-180.
4. Christenson LJ, Phillips PK, Weaver AL, Otley CC. Primary closure vs second-intention treatment of skin punch biopsy sites: a randomized trial. *Arch Dermatol*. 2005;141:1093-1099.
5. Tran KT, Wright NA, Cockerell CJ. Biopsy of the pigmented lesion-when and how. *J Am Acad Dermatol*. 2008;59:852-871.
6. Lo SJ, Khoo C. Improving the cosmetic acceptability of punch biopsies: a simple method to reduce dog-ear formation. *Plast Reconstr Surg*. 2006;118:295-296.
7. Gabel EA, Jimenez GP, Eaglstein WH, Kerdel FA, Falanga V. Performance comparison of nylon and an absorbable suture material (Polyglactin 910) in the closure of punch biopsy sites. *Dermatol Surg*. 2000;26:750-752.
8. Hansen LM, Wu DJ, Liu D, Aires DJ, Elston DM. Gelatin foam instead of suturing for punch biopsies on the scalp. *J Am Acad Dermatol*. 2021;84(1):e15-e16. doi:10.1016/j.jaad.2020.07.083.
9. Whalen JG, Gehris RP, Kress DW, English JC. Surgical pearl: instrument tamponade for punch biopsy of the scalp. *J Am Acad Dermatol*. 2005;52(2):347-348. doi:10.1016/j.jaad.2004.06.042.

The Elliptical Excision

DANIEL L. STULBERG, MD, NIKKI KATTALANOS, PAC, and RICHARD P. USATINE, MD

SUMMARY	

- An elliptical (also called fusiform) excision is a straightforward, effective way to remove lesions with lateral and deep surgical margins.
- Indications and contraindications are reviewed for the elliptical excision.
- A list of suggested equipment is provided.
- A step-by-step approach to the elliptical excision is discussed.
- Planning and designing the excision involves avoiding vital structures and specific motor nerves that are in various danger zones.
- The ellipse is oriented using relaxed skin tension lines and wrinkle lines.
- Surgical margins are chosen based on the diagnosis.
- Ellipse geometry is reviewed to allow for the best closure with the shortest incision.
- The most common geometry is a 3:1 ratio with 38-degree angles on the edges.
- How to cut, undermine, and repair the ellipse are reviewed.
- Standing cone repair is taught.
- Variations of the standard ellipse are covered.

An elliptical (also called fusiform) excision is a straightforward, effective way to remove lesions with lateral and deep surgical margins. The shape of the excision lends itself well to a linear repair that can be aligned for a cosmetically pleasing result.

Indications

- Removal of suspicious lesions to obtain pathology
- Removal of diagnosed malignant skin lesions for treatment
- Removal of benign lesions for cosmesis or comfort (e.g., nevi, dermatofibromas, cysts, lipomas)

Contraindications

Contraindications by lesion include the following:

- Aggressive malignant lesions with margins that are not clinically apparent should be considered for Mohs surgery (see Chapter 27, *When to Refer/Mohs Surgery*).[1] The Mohs surgeon carefully cuts and marks each specimen to be prepared for viewing under the microscope at the time of surgery. This ensures the clearest margins obtainable with the most tissue-sparing surgery.
- Recurrent basal or squamous cell cancers should be referred for Mohs surgery because Mohs surgery has the lowest statistical rate of recurrence with excisions.[2-4]
- Other factors to consider when deciding about a referral for Mohs surgery include lesion size, histology, location, cost, patient age, immunosuppression, history of transplant, availability of a Mohs surgeon, and patient preferences. (For more details, see Chapter 27.)

- There is a great app to calculate when Mohs surgery is appropriate: https://apps.apple.com/us/app/mohs-surgery-appropriate-use-criteria/id692790649

Contraindications by lesion include the following:

- In areas where there is not an adequate amount of tissue for closure, consider an alternate technique (flap, graft, electrodesiccation, cryosurgery, and topical treatments).
- For lesions involving the eyelids or in which the excision would put tension on the lid, refer to Mohs surgery, plastic surgery, oculoplastics, or another appropriate specialist.
- Cancers at the margin of the nose and ears and lips tend to have deeper involvement and should be considered for Mohs surgery.[1,5]
- Cancers in the H-zone on the face should also be considered for Mohs surgery (see Figure 27.12 in Chapter 27).

Equipment

The following equipment is required to perform an elliptical incision (also see Figure 11.1), although excision of small ellipses may not require all of the items on the list:

- Surgical marking pen
- 1% lidocaine with epinephrine
- Syringes, 5 to 12 mL
- Needles, 27- to 30-gauge 1¼ to 1½ inch for injection
- Sterile gloves
- Electrosurgical instrument for hemostasis
- No. 15 scalpel and blade handle
- Adson forceps (with and/or without teeth)
- Iris scissors (optional to have another scissor for undermining)

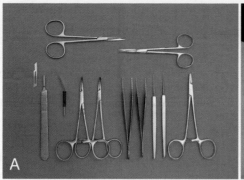
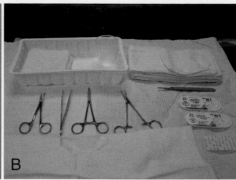

Figure 11.1 (A) Instruments for an elliptical excision from left to right: two iris scissors on top, No. 15 scalpel blade, scalpel handle, electrosurgery electrode, two mosquito hemostats, two Adson forceps, two skin hooks, needle holder. **(B)** Disposable surgical kit with sutures and adhesive strips added. (A: Copyright Richard P. Usatine, MD; B: Copyright Daniel Stulberg, MD.)

- Webster needle holder (consider gold-handled holder with carbide inserts)
- Two mosquito hemostats
- Two skin hooks (single, sharp prong)
- Sterile cotton-tipped applicators (CTAs) and gauze
- Designated suture scissors (optional)
- Small sterile metal basin (optional, used for cleaning and irrigating with sterile saline – can also be used to place sharps in during surgery to make the sterile field safer for the surgeon)
- Skin preparation solution (chlorhexidine preferred with povidone-iodine safer around the eyes)
- Sterile drapes and a single fenestrated drape
- Suture materials (see Chapter 5, *Suture Material*)
- Specimen container with formalin and label
- Dressings: 2 × 2 gauze, 4 × 4 gauze, and adhesive tape (optional nonadherent strips, wound closure strips, dental roll for pressure dressings)

Adding clean cotton gauze and CTAs (purchased in bulk) to be autoclaved in surgical sets is an efficient way to prepare for surgery. This will save time and money over individually packaged sterile gauze and CTAs and avoid wasting the paper used in the wrapping process, hence making for a greener office.

Disposable instrument setups (Figure 11.1B) may be the only option in practices that do not do regular surgeries and do not have an autoclave. Note that disposable instruments are of lower quality than nondisposables.

The Elliptical Incision: Steps and Principles

See Videos 11.1 to 11.5.
The major steps involved in the elliptical excision involve the following:

1. Planning and designing the excision
2. Anesthesia
3. Preparing the room, the patient, and the equipment
4. Incision
5. Hemostasis
6. Undermining
7. Wound closure (repair)

Perform a check of vital signs, and be aware of coexisting medical issues such as anticoagulation before starting any surgical procedure. Obtain informed consent in writing at the time of the procedure and perform a surgical time-out before starting (see Chapter 1, *Preoperative Preparation*).

PLANNING AND DESIGNING THE EXCISION

Important factors to consider when planning an excision are listed in Box 11.1.

Avoiding Vital Structures

When planning an elliptical excision, it is crucial to plan how to best avoid damaging vital structures, including sensory organs, major nerves, arteries, bones, tendons, ligaments, cartilage, and internal organs. That is not to say that such damage can always be avoided because there are areas in which the risks are higher and the surgery still needs to be performed. Complications can include but are not limited to bleeding, paresthesias, paralysis, scarring, and loss of movement or expression. Abnormal sensation at the immediate surgical site is expected and unavoidable due to damage to tiny sensory nerves. Damage to sensory nerves passing to other areas can cause more broad loss of sensation and paresthesias.

In planning the surgical excision, it is important to avoid cutting motor nerves. The temporal branch of the facial nerve is one example of a nerve at risk during facial surgery. For a superficial skin cancer in the temporal region, the clinician may choose to treat with a topical agent or scoop shave rather than an ellipse. Referring for Mohs surgery is a

---

Box 11.1 Factors to Consider When Planning an Excision

Important factors to consider when planning an excision include the following:
- Avoiding vital structures
- Placement of incision lines
- Size of the surgical margin
- Whether the closure can be accomplished with a side-to-side closure
- Whether anatomic distortion will occur

good option because the temple is part of the H-zone and Mohs surgeons are highly trained surgeons.

Danger Zones

The three following areas are not the only areas at risk but are worthy of special mention here because the motor nerves are more superficial in these areas and damage to them can cause significant problems with form and function:

- *Lateral forehead.* The temporal branch of the facial nerve (frontal branch of the facial nerve) can be damaged by any surgery of the temple area and lateral forehead. The nerve lies within the multiple fascial planes in this area; it can be difficult to see, and there is enough anatomic variation that its location can be unpredictable. The temporal branch emerges from the parotid gland, superiorly traveling in the fascial layers to the frontalis muscle (Figure 11.2A). If the temporal branch of the facial nerve is cut, the patient will have permanent drooping of the eyebrow and not be able to wrinkle the forehead on that side (Figure 11.2B). If any surgery is to be performed in this area, it is important for this risk to be discussed with the patient.[6] It also helps to check nerve function before administering anesthesia in this area because the anesthesia may cause a temporary facial nerve palsy.
- *Lateral midface.* The zygomatic branch of the facial nerve, the buccal branches, and the marginal mandibular branches emerge along the anterior portion of the parotid gland. The cervical branch emerges at the inferior aspect of the parotid gland (Figure 11.3).[6] Any of these nerves can be damaged with resultant areas of facial paralysis, so care should be used if entering the subcutaneous tissues anterior, superior, or inferior to the parotid gland and posterior to a line dropped inferiorly from the lateral canthus of the eye.
- *Lateral neck.* The spinal accessory nerve traverses under the sternocleidomastoid muscle on its way to the trapezius muscle (Figure 11.4). Within the posterior triangle between those muscles, at the level of the thyroid cartilage, it can be superficial. If this nerve is cut, the patient cannot raise the trapezius muscle. Fine hand–arm coordination can also be impaired.[6]

Placement of the Incision Line

Major factors to be considered when determining the placement of the incision line are wrinkle lines, the geometry of the tumor, and relaxed skin tension lines (RSTLs). The design of an ellipse on the face is usually done within wrinkle lines. If wrinkles are not apparent, asking the patient to smile, lift the eyebrows, or tightly close the eyes can bring out lines of facial expression (Figure 11.5A). That is because these lines run perpendicular to the muscles of facial expression (Figure 11.5B).

The RSTLs are the parallel skin lines that are seen when the skin is pinched together while the muscles are relaxed (Figure 11.5C). For example, when the skin is pinched together on the wrist, the RSTLs run horizontally from the lateral wrist to the medial wrist (Figure 11.6A). The RSTLs are one method to plan the ellipse on the trunk, extremities, and on facial areas where wrinkle lines are not apparent (Figures 11.5 and 11.6).

While the RSTLs run circumferentially around the extremities, sometimes the best direction is longitudinal such that the ellipse goes from proximal to distal in its direction. More important is often the geometry of the lesion in order to follow the long axis if the lesion is not circular or symmetric. This provides the shortest excision and scar. The critical issue is whether the tissue around the lesion is mobile enough to close the defect with sutures in the direction of the planned excision. On the forearm, a common location for skin cancers, almost any direction will work so horizontal and longitudinal are both good choices. Usually, it is best to follow wrinkle lines on the face unless the geometry of the tumor suggests otherwise.

Surgical Margin

The ellipse is designed so that the lesion is cleared with a margin. When possible, knowing the type of lesion in advance can guide the amount of tissue to be removed. The surgical margin may be 3 to 5 mm for basal cell carcinomas, 4 to 6 mm for squamous cell carcinomas, and 1 to 2 cm for invasive melanomas (Table 11.1).[1,2] When the suspicion for malignancy is low, a shave biopsy or an excision with smaller margins of 1 to 2 mm is usually adequate. For the initial biopsy of a suspected melanoma, the margin

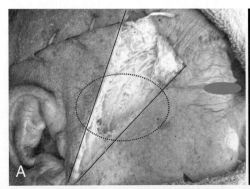
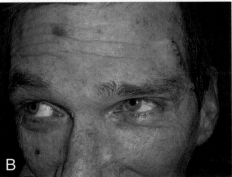

Figure 11.2 (A) The temporal branch of the facial nerve is superficial in the triangle formed by connecting the tragus to the lateral aspect of the eyebrow and the tragus to the most superior forehead crease. The temporal branch of the facial nerve is vulnerable to injury as it courses over the zygomatic arch within the zone. **(B)** This man is unable to raise his left eyebrow after receiving local anesthesia over the temporal branch of the facial nerve for the removal of a basal cell carcinoma. The effect on the nerve was temporary because the nerve was not cut. (A: From Vidimos A, Ammirati C, Poblete-Lopez C. *Dermatologic Surgery.* Saunders; 2008; B: Copyright Richard P. Usatine, MD.)

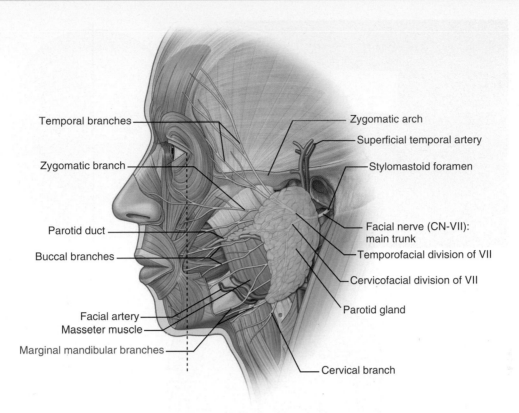

Figure 11.3 Five branches of the facial nerve exit the parotid gland (temporal, zygomatic, buccal, marginal mandibular, and cervical) and are less protected posteriorly to the line dropped from the lateral canthus. The marginal mandibular branch is vulnerable to surgical injury as it crosses the inferior edge of the mandible. (Adapted from Vidimos A, Ammirati C, Poblete-Lopez C. *Dermatologic Surgery*. Saunders; 2008.)

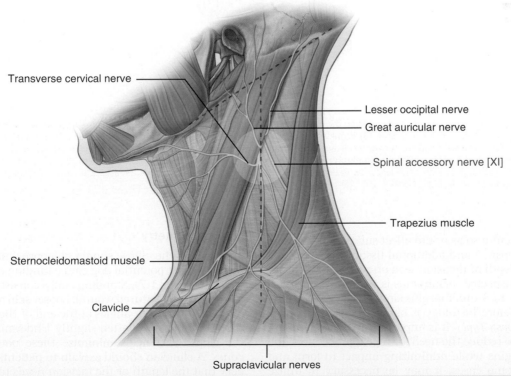

Figure 11.4 The spinal accessory nerve is vulnerable between the sternocleidomastoid and the trapezius at the level of the thyroid cartilage. (From Vidimos A, Ammirati C, Poblete-Lopez C. *Dermatologic Surgery*. Saunders; 2008.)

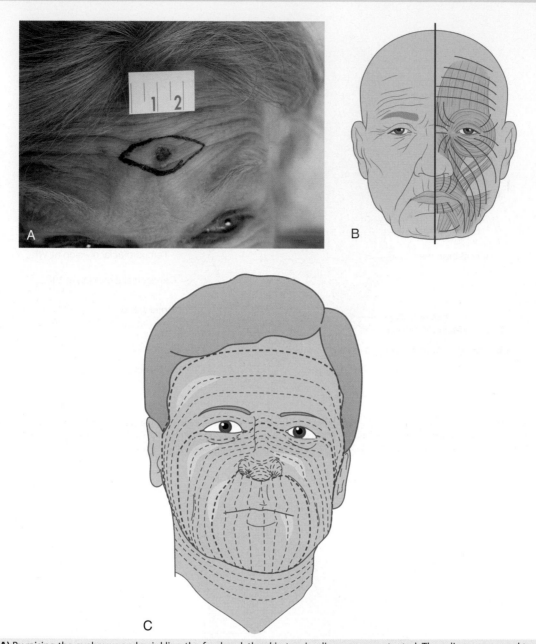

Figure 11.5 (A) By raising the eyebrows and wrinkling the forehead, the skin tension lines are accentuated. These lines were used to draw the ellipse around a biopsy-proven basal cell carcinoma. **(B)** Wrinkles, termed skin tension lines (STLs), run perpendicular to the underlying muscle fibers. For example, the STLs of the forehead are horizontal because the frontalis muscle contracts vertically. **(C)** The drawing shows relaxed STLs of the face. Examples of drawn optimal fusiform excisions (blue) run parallel to relaxed STLs. (A: Courtesy of Daniel L. Stulberg, MD; B: From Vidimos A, Ammirati C, Poblete-Lopez C. *Dermatologic Surgery.* Saunders; 2008; C: Redrawn from Hom DB, Odland RM. Prognosis for facial scarring. In Harahap M, ed. *Surgical Techniques for Cutaneous Scar Revision.* Marcel Dekker; 2000:25–37.)

should be 1 to 3 mm so as not to affect subsequent sentinel lymph node biopsy,[7,8] and additional tissue will be excised later based on depth of invasion seen on pathology. One option for some suspected melanomas is to do a scoop shave excision with 1- to 3-mm margins since a full excision may be premature before histology is obtained (see Chapter 8, *Choosing the Biopsy Type*). It is important to balance taking enough tissue to reduce the need for repeat procedures due to positive margins while minimizing impact to form and function.[9] In some cases, it may be necessary to utilize Mohs surgery or take a smaller margin if the lesion is too close to vital structures.

Ellipse Geometry

The ends of the ellipse should be approximately 38-degree angles so that potential dog ears (standing cones) are minimized (Figure 11.7). Standing cones consist of bulging skin at the ends of a sutured wound. Looser skin areas sometimes allow slightly larger angles at the end of the ellipse because the standing cones flatten slightly. Undermining the end of the ellipse also helps minimize these potential standing cones. A clinician should explain to patients before the surgery that the length of the incision needs to be about three times the diameter of the lesion. It is helpful to draw this for patients so they can see how large their incision will be.

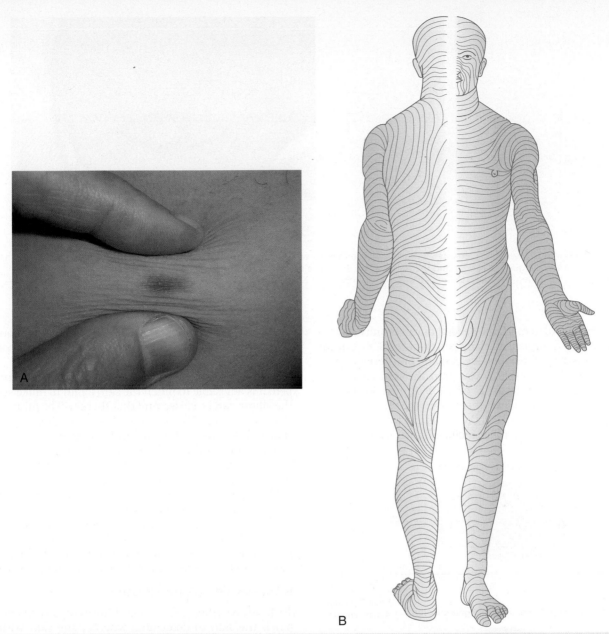

Figure 11.6 (A) Pinching the skin to determine the direction of RSTLs. **(B)** RSTLs on the body. (B: Redrawn from Fawkes JL, Cheney ML, Pollack SV. *Illustrated Atlas of Cutaneous Surgery.* Lippincott-Gower; 1992.)

Table 11.1   Surgical Margins by Lesion Type[1,2,4,5,12–15]

Lesion Type	Surgical Margin
Uncertain	Consider shave or punch biopsy to delineate prior to elliptical excision or start with 1- to 2-mm margins to avoid unnecessary tissue removal.
Benign	Visible lesion removed.
BCC	3–5 mm
SCC	4–6 mm
Initial excisional biopsy of possible melanoma	1–3 mm
Melanoma *in situ*	5 mm
Melanoma <1 mm	10 mm (discuss sentinel lymph node biopsy depending upon current recommendations)
Melanoma >= 1 mm	20 mm (refer for excision in OR with sentinel lymph node biopsy)

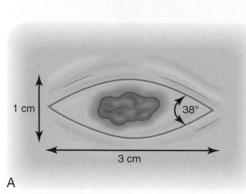

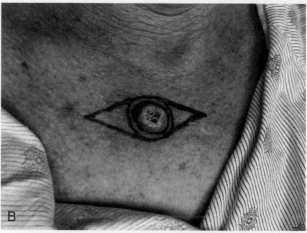

Figure 11.7 (A) Most ellipses should be three times longer than they are wide with approximately a 3:1 ratio. **(B)** In planning the excision of a keratoacanthoma, a 4-mm margin is drawn around the lesion, and a 3:1 ellipse is added along skin lines. (A: From Vidimos A, Ammirati C, Poblete-Lopez C. *Dermatologic Surgery.* Saunders; 2008; B: Courtesy of Mengyı Zha, MD.)

It is very helpful to mark the needed margins and draw the full ellipse with a surgical marking pen (Figure 11.8). Cutting free hand is a recipe for errors. A clean and nonsterile surgical marking pen is acceptable if you prep the skin again after marking the lesion. The usual ellipse is drawn so that the length of the ellipse is at least three times the width of the ellipse (Figures 11.7 and 11.8). Conditions in which a greater than 3:1 ratio may be desirable include tighter skin, skin over the joints, and curved surfaces. See Table 11.2 for conditions in which it is desirable to use a 4:1 or 2.5:1 ratio. To achieve 30° angles on the ends use 3.5:1 ratio.

Once the ellipse has been drawn with a surgical marking pen, it is advisable to pinch the skin again to make sure that the ellipse can be closed and that there will be minimal anatomic distortion. Use an alcohol wipe sparingly at the sites that will be injected with local anesthetic. Be careful to avoid removing the marking with the alcohol. Prepare the skin with chlorhexidine or povidone-iodine after injecting the anesthesia and before starting the procedure.

Show patients the planned excision before you begin the surgery. You can show the patient and any family in attendance your surgical markings before you start. Keep a handheld mirror nearby for excisions on the face so that your patient knows what you plan to do. This is a helpful method to make sure you truly have informed consent.

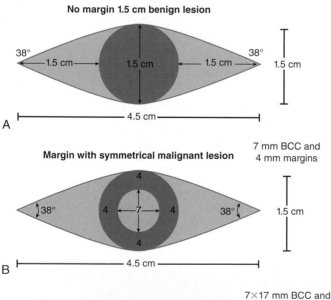

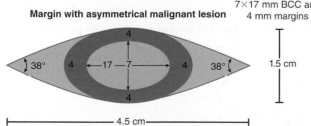

Figure 11.8 How to draw an ellipse. Start by adding margins if needed. Then use 3:1 ratio from height of the lesion. The angle comes out to about 38° rather than the often cited 30°. A 3.5:1 ratio gives a 30° angle. (Copyright Richard P. Usatine, MD.)

Is Side-to-Side Closure Possible?

To decide whether side-to-side closure can be accomplished, pinch the skin to determine whether the skin within the area is loose enough. The clinician has to predict from pinching the skin whether the two sides of the ellipse can be brought together. Areas such as the cheek, trunk, and arms are areas where an elliptical excision can be easily accomplished. Areas that are most difficult are the scalp and over the sternum and tibia.

Avoiding Distortion of Tissue

Elliptical excisions on the forehead, upper lip, and around the eye require careful planning because they can distort the eyebrow, lip, or eyelid. When possible, it is better to orient an ellipse perpendicular to the eyelid or lip margin (Figure 11.5). For facial excisions, it is important to understand cosmetic units that relate to the organs of the face. Ask the patient to perform the following maneuvers: smile, show the teeth, raise the eyebrows, and purse the lips. It is best to keep the excision within one cosmetic unit rather than crossing between two units. When planning an excision, try to avoid creating functional problems with the eyes and mouth. Avoid pulling down eyelids and causing ectropion, pulling up eyebrows, cutting significant facial nerves, or distorting the look of the lip or nasal alae.

Table 11.2 Geometry of the Elliptical Excision

Geometry	When to Use	Advantages Compared to Standard 3:1	Disadvantages Compared to Standard 3:1
3:1	Standard	–	–
4:1	Skin is tight	Less tension with closure Less likely to have dog ear	Longer incision to close Longer scar
2.5:1	Near vital organ or trying to create shorter scar	Avoid vital organ Shorter closure Shorter scar	More tension with closure More likely to have dog ear and need dog ear repair

If there is doubt about whether the ellipse can be closed or if the potential exists for anatomic distortion, creation of a flap may be necessary (see Chapter 21, *Flaps*). In some instances, the closure can be very tight. Wider undermining or thicker sutures may be required to accomplish the closure.

ANESTHESIA

The goal is to produce adequate anesthesia with minimal pain and anxiety for the patient. Local anesthesia is obtained using 1% lidocaine with epinephrine after the ellipse has been drawn. The area of anesthesia must cover the whole ellipse including the skin that will be undermined. Use of 1% lidocaine is preferable to 2% because a larger volume can be used more safely with 1%, and this volume produces greater hemostasis by distention.

Epinephrine is valuable for all elliptical excisions and is used for virtually all patients in all surgical locations. For patients with normal circulation, it is safe to use epinephrine for local anesthesia in areas such as the tip of the nose, the fingers and toes, the ears, or the penis despite old dogma. In one study, there was no evidence that buffered 0.5% lidocaine with epinephrine 1:200,000 causes ischemia or necrosis when injected into digits at the surgical site.[3] That was true despite a history of circulatory disorders, thrombosis, diabetes, smoking, anticoagulation, or significant preoperative hypertension.[3] However, in patients with severe peripheral vascular disease or Raynaud's phenomenon, one might discuss the risks and benefits with the patient.

Wait at least 7 minutes before making the incision so that the epinephrine can take effect, thus minimizing the bleeding. Maximal doses of 1% lidocaine (10 mg/mL) with epinephrine are calculated based on the formula of 7 mg/kg of body weight. For example, a 60-kg (132-pound) person could safely receive up to 42 mL at one time.

The amount of anesthesia needed depends on the location of the surgery and the thickness of subcutaneous tissue in the area. For example, the forehead and scalp have very little subcutaneous tissue because of the skull bones below, so a small amount of anesthesia will go far to distend tissue for hemostasis and numbness (Figure 11.9). However, excising an ellipse on the thigh or abdomen will require more anesthetic volume because the thicker subcutaneous tissues will soak up the volume faster. For an ellipse in the range of 1 × 3 cm to 2 × 6 cm, it is not unusual to need at least 20 to 30 mL of anesthesia. This should be safe for even the smallest adult. Plan ahead by drawing up at least one to two 10- to 12-mL syringes with anesthesia.

Add 8.4% bicarbonate in a 1:3 dilution to minimize pain and burning upon injection (see Chapter 3, *Anesthesia*).[10]

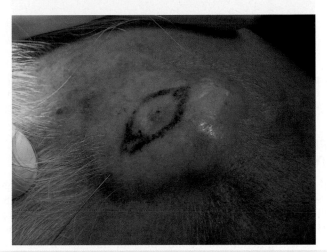

Figure 11.9 Injecting anesthesia before excising a BCC on the forehead. Note how the full ellipse with sufficient area to undermine can be anesthetized with a single injection using a 27-gauge, 1½-inch needle on the forehead. (Copyright Richard P. Usatine, MD.)

Pinch the skin at the area to be injected while injecting (based on the gate theory of pain). Use a 27-gauge needle, and inject slowly because tissue distention hurts.

There are many ways to cover the needed area with anesthesia. Small ellipses can be anesthetized by a single injection distal to one end of the ellipse (Figure 11.9). For large excisions, one method that will minimize the number of painful injection sites begins with a single injection at one end of the ellipse that is far enough out to get the area to be undermined. The anesthesia is then delivered in a fanlike fashion until adequate volume is given (Figure 11.10). The next injection can be placed within the area of anesthesia, and the anesthetic fanned out toward the other end of the ellipse. A third or fourth injection may be needed if the ellipse is large, but each of these injections may be placed within areas already numb. Injecting in the subcutaneous layer is less painful than injecting in the dermis and gives good anesthesia and reduction of blood flow via the epinephrine effect. This is a very humane method of anesthetizing a large area for surgery.

While waiting 10 minutes for the epinephrine to take effect, make sure that all of the instruments and supplies are ready. Choose your suture, and place it on the sterile tray. Consider working on charts and pathology forms while waiting. If the procedure will be time consuming, check your schedule and how many patients will be waiting while you do the surgery. To avoid feeling rushed, it often helps to do larger ellipses during designated "surgery time" and not in the middle of a busy ambulatory clinic.

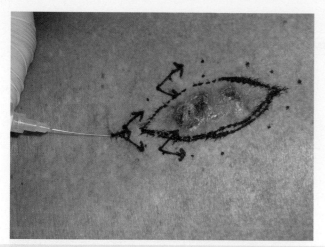

Figure 11.10 For a large ellipse, inject in a progressive fanlike manner from areas already anesthetized. Make sure the area to be undermined is numb. (Copyright Richard P. Usatine, MD.)

PREPARING THE ROOM, THE PATIENT, AND THE EQUIPMENT

If the patient is wearing clothing near the surgical site, suggest that the patient change into a gown to avoid getting bloodstains on the clothing. If hair is in the way of the surgical site, find a method to clear the field of the hair if possible using headbands, bobby pins, or hair ties. If the hair needs cutting, it is best to do this with a clean or sterile scissor and not a razor. The risk of postoperative infections increases when a razor blade is used to trim the hair at the surgical site.

Make sure the surgical table is at the right height for your work whether you choose to do the surgery sitting or standing. For those with back or feet problems, it often helps to do the surgery sitting. Once the table is in place, turn on the surgical light, and point it in the right direction.

Chlorhexidine (Hibiclens) is a very good solution for a surgical prep because it does not stain the skin, very few people are allergic to it, and it does not have to dry to be effective. Povidone-iodine is a good alternative that has the advantage of coloring the skin so it is easy to see the area that was prepped. Betadine is also safe around the eyes, and chlorhexidine can cause ocular damage. The disadvantages are that it does stain the skin, some people are allergic to iodine, and one must wait for it to dry before the field is sterile. It also needs to be removed from the skin after the surgery is complete to avoid causing skin irritation.

While your assistant is prepping the area, it is a good time to do a surgical scrub on your hands and forearms. Although skin surgery is not open-heart surgery, it is important to have clean hands before donning sterile surgical gloves. Do not wear a lab coat or tie that will contaminate the surgical site. It is a good idea to take off jewelry or watches and roll up your sleeves before starting the scrub. If you use a surgical loupe for magnification, eye goggles, or splash shields, put these on before you start scrubbing. Surgical masks are a good idea now that we are living in a time in which COVID-19 is a risk. Surgical gowns and surgical hair coverings are optional but may protect you from blood or fluid. These might reduce the risk of postoperative infections, but this has never been proven for skin surgery. Eye protection is a must to protect the surgeon, and some use a surgical mask for self-protection as well.

Once your sterile gloves are on, turn your attention to creating your sterile surgical field. Fenestrated paper fields that come in a sterilized packet are very convenient (Figure 11.11). Sterile towels may be used as an alternative. When placed on the face, patients should be able to breathe comfortably.

Now look at your equipment and make sure that you have the following:

- Scalpel blade for cutting. Attach the scalpel to the blade holder. The individual scalpel blades tend to be sharper than the scalpel blades attached to a disposable blade holder.
- Suture material including absorbable and nonabsorbable sutures on the tray (see Chapter 5, *Suture Material*).
- Electrosurgical instrument turned on and ready for use. Place the finger switch through a sterile sheath, and attach the sterile electrode.
- Instruments you expect to use. Put them in an order that makes it easy for you to reach.

If you have an assistant scrubbed in, make sure that person knows where to be and has sterile gauze in hand to help with hemostasis. It is essential to have an assistant in the room that is not scrubbed in if any additional supplies are needed.

INCISION

Check that the patient is numb and start your incision. The scalpel should be held like a pencil, with the hand holding the scalpel resting comfortably on the patient. The corner of the ellipse is incised with the tip of the blade. The sharper belly of the blade is used to cut the majority of the ellipse. Care should be taken to make the incision perpendicular to the skin surface (Figure 11.12). It may be helpful to stabilize the skin with your nondominant hand (Figures 11.12 and 11.13) to keep the ellipse from "stretching." Note how the scalpel is not

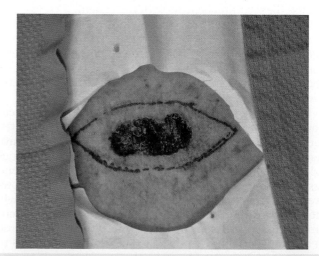

Figure 11.11 Fenestrated paper drape with surgical towels to extend sterile field and stabilize the drape. Note that the BCC was curetted to make sure that the margins were drawn adequately to achieve full clearance. (Copyright Richard P. Usatine, MD.)

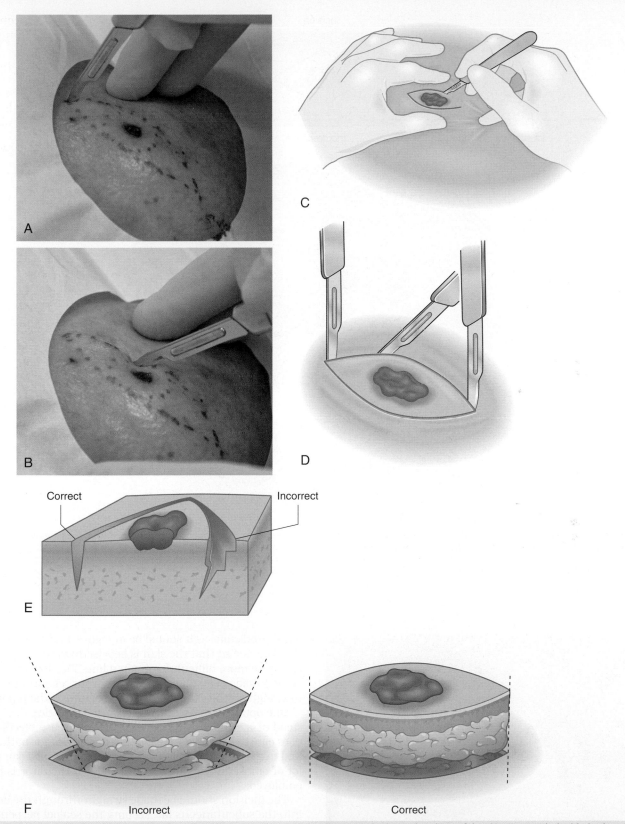

Figure 11.12 Cutting the ellipse holding the scalpel like a pencil and the blade perpendicular to the plane of the skin. Start with the blade close to 90 degrees at the tip of the ellipse **(A)**, and then decrease the angle while cutting to use more of the belly of the blade **(B)**. **(C)** The left hand is stabilizing the surrounding skin while cutting the ellipse. **(D)** Correct blade angles for cutting the ellipse. **(E)** The ellipse should be cut using one continuous cut rather than multiple cuts in a "staircasing" pattern. **(F)** The ellipse should not look like a boat but should have parallel perpendicular walls.

Incision

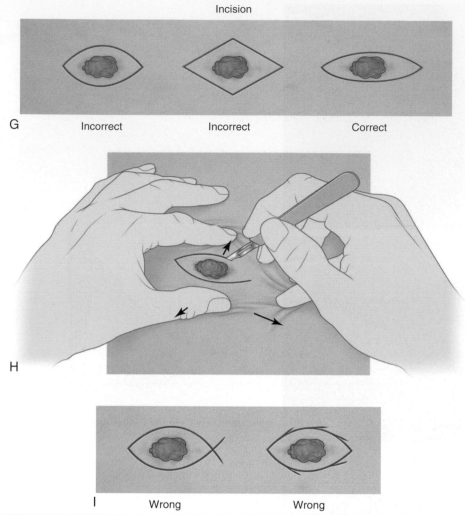

Figure 11.12, cont'd (G) When drawing the ellipse, use a smooth curved line rather than two pointed triangles together. (H) Finger pressure outward can help cut the ellipse. (I) Do not make a fish tail at the end or allow the blade to cut outside the ellipse. (A and B: Copyright Richard P. Usatine, MD; C–F: Adapted from Vidimos A, Ammirati C, Poblete-Lopez C. *Dermatologic Surgery*. Saunders; 2008; G–I: Modified from Leffell DJ, Brown M. *Manual of Skin Surgery*. Wiley-Liss; 1997:156. Copyright: John Wiley & Sons.)

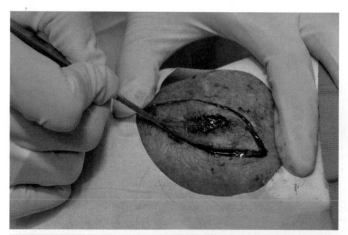

Figure 11.13 Stabilizing the surrounding skin while cutting the ellipse. While it is best to keep the scalpel perpendicular to the skin, this operator has allowed the scalpel to lean outward away from the lesion. A subsequent lack of a parallel margin can be corrected with a scissor prior to closure. (Copyright Richard P. Usatine, MD.)

as perpendicular as it should be in Figure 11.13. If the incision is made so that the skin is beveled inward or outward, it may be more difficult to obtain a fine-line closure. (If this error is made, it is still possible to use your scissors or scalpel to straighten the skin edges before beginning the repair.)

One option is to use an electrosurgical cutting device instead of a scalpel. Although this can decrease bleeding, it does cause thermal damage to the tissue sent for pathology and to the remaining tissue of the patient. It also can put a lot of smoke in the air even if a smoke evacuator is being employed.

The incision should be made straight through the dermis into the subcutaneous fat, keeping the scalpel perpendicular to the cutting axis. While making the incision, the skin can be spread open to ensure that the cut is perpendicular and the edges are vertical. When making a curved incision, there is a natural tendency to lean the scalpel to the outside of a curve. Try to avoid this.

The incision should be carried down to subcutaneous fat. With experience and confidence, this can often be performed

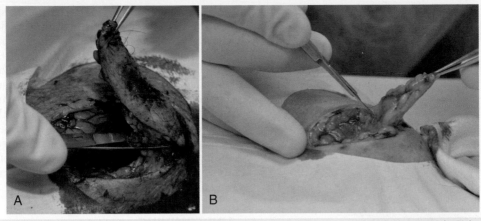

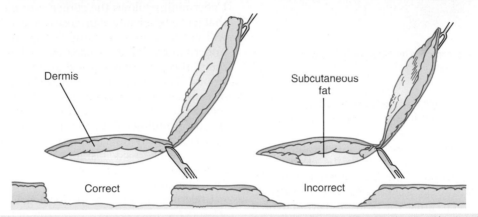

Figure 11.14 (A) Cutting horizontally under the ellipse using a sharp iris scissor. **(B)** Cutting using a scalpel. (Copyright Richard P. Usatine, MD.)

Dermis   Subcutaneous fat

Correct   Incorrect

Figure 11.15 Incision carried down to the subcutaneous fat. Correction involves parallel walls and not leaving dermis at the tips of the ellipse. (Redrawn from Fawkes JL, Cheney ML, Pollack SV. *Illustrated Atlas of Cutaneous Surgery*. Philadelphia: Lippincott-Gower; 1992.)

in one or two passes of the blade. If more passes are needed, it helps to have a surgical assistant stretch the skin perpendicular to the axis of the incision so that the incised skin will separate easily. Although the patient may experience bleeding at this point, it is best to use pressure with gauze only and not stop to electrocoagulate every bleeder.

Use caution to not cut beyond the point of the ellipse causing an overcut or fish-tail pattern at the end (Figure 11.12I). It can be helpful to reverse the scalpel so that the point of the scalpel is at the second end of the ellipse to prevent cutting beyond the point of the ellipse.

When both sides of the ellipse are in the fat layer or just above the fascia, make sure that they are of equal depth. (Invasive melanoma should be incised to the deep fat/fascia.)

Now, grasp one point of the ellipse with a toothed forceps and using the scalpel, scissor, or electrosurgical device, cut horizontally under the ellipse from that point to the other end of the ellipse (Figure 11.14). Be careful to stay at the same level in the subcutaneous fat to facilitate a good repair (Figure 11.15). Feel the specimen to make sure it does not have clinically palpable tumor. Consider marking the ellipse as demonstrated in Figure 11.16. Place the specimen in formalin.

HEMOSTASIS

After the ellipse is out, it is time to achieve good hemostasis. The use of firm pressure with gauze may be adequate. If not, proceed to electrocoagulation.

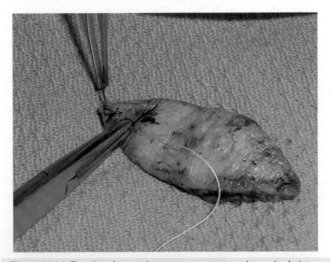

Figure 11.16 Tagging the specimen on one corner using a single interrupted suture. Make sure you record the corner marked in the chart and on the pathology requisition form. This is rarely needed but could be helpful if some of the surgical margin is positive for tumor. (Copyright Richard P. Usatine, MD.)

The major techniques to produce electrocoagulation are as follows:

1. The electrode directly contacts the bleeding site or vessel (Figure 11.17). This is the simplest approach and the usual method employed. If the bleeding is active causing

necrosis because this can increase the risk of wound infection. When a vessel is not responding to electrocoagulation, use a suture. One method is to use absorbable suture with a small figure-of-eight around the vessel (see Figure 4.5 in Chapter 4). For example, if you are already using Vicryl for your deep sutures, just use this for the hemostatic stitch.

Once hemostasis has been achieved, make sure that the whole tumor is excised. Look at and feel the base and edges of the elliptical defect and the specimen removed. If it appears that some of the tumor or cancer remains, cut it out and explain the site and orientation of this second piece to the pathologist. It is better to do this now than to wait and discover the margins were not clear.

UNDERMINING

Undermining allows the clinician to mobilize the tissue so that it can be advanced to close a defect. Most small wounds will not need undermining. Determine if and how much undermining will be needed by testing to see how mobile the skin edges are using a skin hook on either side of the wound (Figure 11.18A). When skin hooks are not available, fingers and forceps can be used (Figure 11.18B). More tension will require more undermining. Repeat this after the undermining is done to determine if there was sufficient undermining. If not, keep going until the skin is able to close in a side-to-side fashion. Minimize undermining with patients on anticoagulation because they are at higher risk for a hematoma.

Undermining may be performed by spreading the iris scissors (or other tissue scissor) under the edges of the incision (Figure 11.19). The skin hook is a very atraumatic way to hold up the skin edge for undermining. If an assistant is present, have them hold the skin up with two skin hooks giving maximal visualization for undermining. Forceps can also be used as long as these are used carefully to avoid crushing the tissue. Using blunt dissection, the undermining plane is achieved with less bleeding. However, there will be some strands of connective tissue that are better and more quickly snipped than broken with blunt dissection. Therefore the most efficient and atraumatic method of undermining involves a combination of blunt dissection and snipping (Figure 11.19). A scalpel can be used to undermine tissue more rapidly but will generally provoke more bleeding (Figure 11.20).

Do not forget to undermine at the points of the ellipse to diminish the formation of standing cones (dog ears,

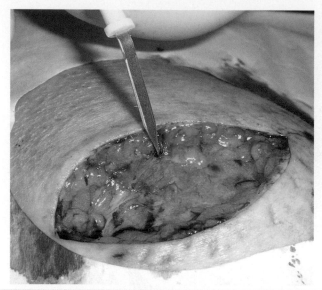

Figure 11.17 Electrosurgery is used for hemostasis. (Copyright Richard P. Usatine, MD.)

a wet field, hold pressure with gauze or a CTA, and then rapidly use electrocoagulation when the pressure is let up.

2. Clamp a rapidly bleeding vessel with a hemostat or forceps, and touch the instrument with the electrode to direct the current through the instrument to stop the bleeding. A higher wattage is often needed for this to work.

3. Special bipolar forceps grasp the tissue and are activated with a foot peddle (see Figure 4.7 in Chapter 4, *Hemostasis*). Bipolar forceps have the advantage of working in a bloody field that is not entirely dry. It is still best to dry the field as much as possible, but the current can still pass through the bleeding tissue despite the presence of blood. The bipolar forceps is the safest method in a patient with a pacemaker or implantable defibrillator.

Creating a dry surgical field is essential for good viewing of the tissues at the time of the final repair. Suturing with a dry field helps prevent hematoma formation, wound infection, and dehiscence.

The electrosurgical unit should be used just enough to stop significant bleeding so that tissue injury is minimized. Slight oozing at the wound edges can be left alone or stopped with pressure only because the suturing should stop this later. Avoid creating large areas of char and tissue

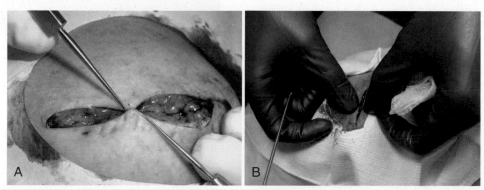

Figure 11.18 **(A)** Checking to see if the ellipse will close without too much tension using skin hooks. **(B)** Checking for closure with fingers. (A: Copyright Richard P. Usatine, MD; B: Copyright Daniel L. Stulberg, MD.)

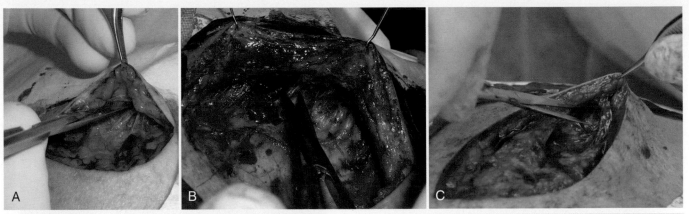

Figure 11.19 Undermining with scissors using skin hooks to elevate the skin: **(A)** using blunt dissection; **(B)** snipping fibrous fascia; **(C)** undermining the tip of the ellipse. (Copyright Richard P. Usatine, MD.)

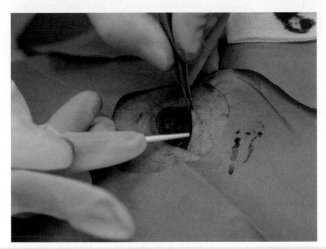

Figure 11.20 Undermining with electrosurgery can bleed less, but one must be careful to get the level correct because the electrode cuts easily at all levels. (Copyright Daniel L. Stulberg, MD.)

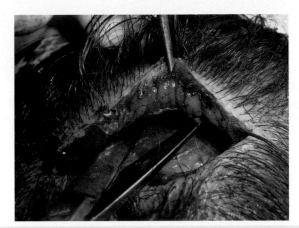

Figure 11.21 Undermining with blunt dissection is being performed below the galea to close this elliptical excision. Note the light-colored galea aponeurosis at the bottom of the cut scalp. The subgaleal plane has loose alveolar tissue like tissue paper. This avascular level is perfect for undermining. (Copyright Richard P. Usatine, MD.)

wrinkling, or bunching up of the skin) at the ends of the repair (Figure 11.19C). Finally, if new bleeding was provoked, use pressure and electrocoagulation to stop it before proceeding to suturing. CTAs are helpful to locate the bleeders under the undermined skin.

Most areas of the body are undermined within the subcutaneous fat. Some areas of the body, such as the scalp, are better undermined in a deeper plane. The scalp should be undermined in a subgaleal plane of loose alveolar tissue (below the galea and above the periosteum) because it is a bloodless, easy plane in which to widely separate the tissue. This tissue is light in color and the consistency of tissue paper. Although this may seem anxiety provoking at first, there is much less bleeding in this plane than in the subcutaneous fat, and you will not damage the skull or underlying central nervous system. See Figure 11.21 for a view of the galea.

Appropriate levels of undermining include the following (Figure 11.22):

- *Scalp:* deep to the galea aponeurotica, above the periosteum (Figure 11.22B)
- *Face:* high fat to avoid facial nerves
- *Trunk and extremities:* deep subcutaneous fat above the muscle
- *Nose:* deeper fascia or connective tissue plane

The width of undermining is determined by the size and location of the defect. Undermining is useful to loosen the surrounding skin but should not be excessive. Undermining should allow the skin edges to come together without too much tension and allow eversion of the wound edges with suturing.

WOUND CLOSURE (REPAIR)

The surgical site should be dry before initiating wound closure. If the ellipse is small and narrow and not under much tension, buried sutures may not be needed. In this case, close the wound with interrupted nonabsorbable sutures such as nylon or polypropylene (Prolene). Closure by the rule of halves is a good method in these cases (Figure 11.23).

Buried sutures (buried vertical mattress sutures, deep sutures)

Benefits:

- Take tension off wound (avoid dehiscence)
- Close dead space (avoid hematomas)
- Keep wound from dehiscing after external sutures are removed

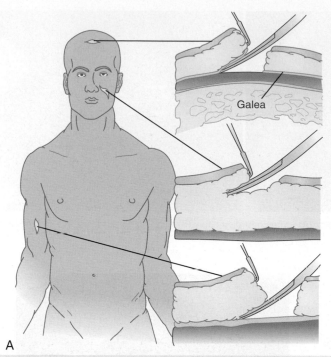

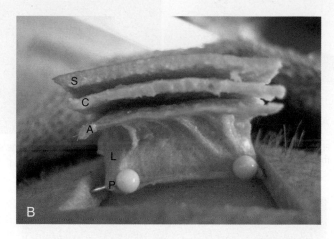

Figure 11.22 (A) Correct levels of undermining. **(B)** Levels of the scalp named using the SCALP mnemonic: S = skin, C = connective tissue, A = aponeurosis (galea), L = loose alveolar tissue (the best level for undermining as it is least vascular), P = pericranium. (A: Redrawn from Fawkes JL, Cheney ML, Pollack SV. *Illustrated Atlas of Cutaneous Surgery.* Philadelphia: Lippincott-Gower; 1992; B: From Vidimos A, Ammirati C, Poblete-Lopez C. *Dermatologic Surgery.* Saunders; 2008.)

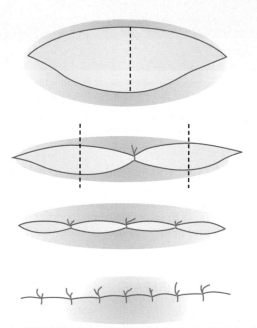

Figure 11.23 Using the rule of halves to close an ellipse not under tension. (Copyright Richard P. Usatine, MD.)

- All these benefits together decrease chance of wound dehiscence, hematoma, and spreading scar.
- Intermediate closure pays well to cover the extra time and materials needed to perform a two-layer closure.
Downside:
- Spitting sutures can occur in healing process (see Chapter 26, *Complications*).
- Extra time and materials needed (extra compensation covers this)

Most ellipses will benefit from using buried absorbable sutures to bring the skin edges together. The goal is to have the wound edges closely approximated using only buried sutures (buried vertical mattress sutures, deep sutures; see Chapter 6, *Suturing Techniques*).

The buried sutures take advantage of the undermined area. Use absorbable suture such as 4-0 polyglactin (Vicryl) on a 13- or 16-mm-long plastic needle (see Chapter 5, *Suture Material*). It is easiest to start the buried sutures at one end of the ellipse rather than the middle. The greatest tension is in the middle of an ellipse, and the skin edges tend to pull apart while you are trying to tie the deep suture. By starting at the apex furthest from you, you can begin to take tension off the wound in an area in which there is less tension to begin with. As you move the deep sutures from the apex toward the middle of the ellipse, the wound will narrow, and the sutures will be easier to tie. If a deep suture is not placed well, do not hesitate to take it out and redo it. A poorly placed deep suture can lead to uneven healing, more scarring, and more work with external suture to compensate for the error in the deep level.

The buried suture is performed in the following manner (Figure 11.24):

- Hold up the skin edge with a fine-toothed forceps, and pull it back some so you can see the bottom of the undermined area. Then place the needle from the undermined area up to the upper dermis and out near the dermal-epidermal junction (DEJ). The DEJ is not really visible so aim for about 1 mm below the surface. Use the curvature of the needle to grab a good piece of dermis.
- Hold the needle where it comes out at the DEJ with the forceps, and reload your needle holder with the needle facing the opposite direction. Then introduce the needle at

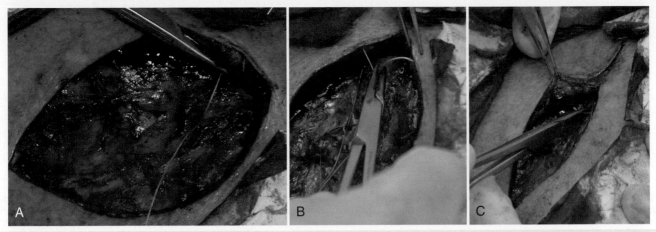

Figure 11.24 Closing the ellipse with deep vertical mattress sutures. **(A)** Start the first deep stitch at one end of the ellipse. The needle is inserted in the undermined area and is brought up to 1 to 2 mm below the dermal-epidermal junction. **(B)** Place the second half of the deep stitch starting from the same level and using the curvature of the needle to come out in the undermined area. **(C)** Continue to place deep sutures moving from one side of the ellipse toward the other. (Copyright Richard P. Usatine, MD.)

the same height with regard to the DEJ, and bring it slightly upward and outward away from the wound.

- Using the curvature of the needle, enter the undermined area, and bring it out with the suture coming toward you. In this way, both suture ends should be on the same side and easier to tie.
- Perform an instrument tie initially wrapping the suture twice around the needle holder (for surgeon's knot). Pull the two ends perpendicular to the incision, and then change direction and pull the ends parallel to the incision. Cinch the knot down so that the skin is well approximated. You may need to rock the knot back and forth to get the skin better approximated and/or crossing your hands. Put in three more knots each with a single throw. If the skin is opening between your first and second throw, try wrapping the suture three times around the needle holder. If that does not work, ask an assistant to hold the skin edges together with their fingers on both sides away of the incision and away from the edge to avoid being stuck by the needle.
- The strands of suture should be cut short but not so short as to compromise the knot below. Place the scissor above the knot, turn it 45 degrees, then cut.
- Keep repeating this process until the incision has come together to form a thin line.

If the incision is well approximated, start a running suture with 4-0 to 6-0 polypropylene (Prolene) or nylon to hold the epidermal edges together for optimal healing. A single interrupted suture is placed at one end of the wound, and only the short end is cut. The remainder of the suture is looped around the skin edges one throw at a time (Figure 11.25). This is taken to the end, and then the knot is tied to the final loop (see Chapter 6, *Suturing Techniques*). While the running suture is quick, if it does open or needs to be opened with a wound infection, it will no longer retain its strength.

If the skin is not well approximated with the deep sutures or there continues to be much tension on the wound, use interrupted sutures rather than a running suture. Simple interrupted sutures can be very useful and can be combined with a running suture. For example, a 1-2 interrupted sutures may be placed in the center of the ellipse where the

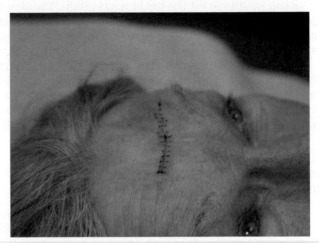

Figure 11.25 Running suture placed along natural wrinkle lines. (Copyright Daniel L. Stulberg, MD.)

tension is greatest before using running sutures from end to end. If greater wound eversion is needed and skin tension remains high, vertical mattress sutures can be beneficial (Figure 11.25). In areas where there is natural inversion such as in the creases of the forehead, vertical mattress sutures can be used for wound eversion (see Chapter 6).

Standing Cones (Dog Ear) Repair

See Video 11.6.

The best way to avoid standing cones is by planning and drawing your ellipse as described earlier. However, even with the best planning, a standing cone can still happen. Repair of a standing cone of tissue at either end of an elliptical excision is accomplished by extending the length of the excision (Figure 11.26). One method involves cutting a line through the center of the standing cone at a slight angle from the original incision. This results in one triangular overhanging edge of tissue that when trimmed will allow the skin to lie flat. This trimming is done with a No. 15 blade or scissor to neatly trim the tissue to the very end of the excision. A No. 15 blade or a sharp scissor is preferred to keep the cut perpendicular to the skin.

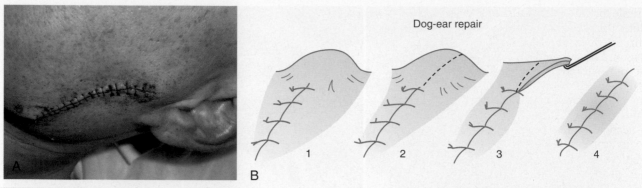

Figure 11.26 (A) Running suture after BCC removal produced standing cones (dog ears) on both ends of this ellipse. These flattened with time. **(B)** Method for standing cone removal. (1) Standing cone present. (2) Extend incision through cone along dotted line. (3) Pull over the long side and cut it off at dotted line to remove one portion of redundant skin. (4) Add one suture to flatten the cone (dog ear). (A: Courtesy of Richard P. Usatine, MD; B: Redrawn from Fawkes JL, Cheney ML, Pollack SV. *Illustrated Atlas of Cutaneous Surgery.* Philadelphia: Lippincott-Gower; 1992.)

Another method involves holding the standing cone up with a skin hook or forceps and cutting the bulging portion off as you might cut off the top of a mountain. The skin is then pushed down to see if it lies flat. Regardless of which method is used, once the skin lies flat, place a single interrupted external suture to complete the repair.

Some standing cones will flatten over time without repair. This works best when the skin is loose, as on an elderly person. Deciding when a standing cone should be surgically repaired is a judgment call that weighs the creation of a longer wound against the risk that the bulge will be forever unsightly.

CLEAN AND DRESS THE WOUND (MEDICAL ASSISTANTS AND NURSING STAFF CAN HELP WITH THIS)

- Make sure that there is no persistent bleeding before removing the drapes. Hold pressure on the wound with gauze, and see that the bleeding has come to a stop. It is desirable to press out any remaining blood before moving on because blood is a good medium for bacterial growth. If the bleeding has not stopped, hold pressure on the wound with gauze for 3 to 5 minutes by the clock. If bleeding persists, then you will need to open some sutures and look for the bleeding site.
- Clean the wound gently with sterile saline or chlorhexidine on sterile gauze.
- Apply a pressure dressing to minimize postoperative bleeding in the first 24 hours. First apply clean petrolatum from a squeeze tube using clean or sterile CTAs. A sterile 2 × 2 or 4 × 4 gauze can be folded for the first layer. A sterile nonstick pad is an alternative first layer. A dental roll makes a great second layer when extra pressure is needed. Additional gauze is added on top, and the whole dressing is tightly taped to the skin. For areas such as extremities or the scalp, a self-adherent elastic wrap that sticks only to itself (e.g., Coban) replaces tape. Of course, taping or wrapping should not be so tight as to impair circulation but needs to be firmly adherent so that the dressing does not fall off until removed in 24 hours (see Chapter 25, *Wound Care*).
- We specifically avoid using antibiotic ointments because even bacitracin ointment is a common contact allergen. Since switching to petrolatum only, we have seen no increase in postoperative wound infections.

AFTERCARE (MEDICAL ASSISTANTS AND NURSING STAFF CAN HELP WITH THIS)

- Patients may be given a handout on wound care that goes over such issues as dressing changes, pain control, bleeding complications, and wound infections (see Chapter 35). Hydrogen peroxide, alcohol, and other topical cleansers are not necessary and can be harmful to healing skin.
- The patient may shower after 24 hours, but should not soak in a bathtub, pool, lake, ocean, or other body of water until the sutures are out.
- Sutures removal times for planning follow-up:
  - Face at 5 to 7 days
  - Trunk at 7 to 10 days (up to 14 days if there was a lot of tension in the wound closure)
  - Extremities at 10 to 14 days.
  - Consider leaving the nonabsorbable sutures in longer if buried sutures were not used and other factors are present that might increase the risk of dehiscence. Factors that compromise wound healing such as smoking, older age, poor nutrition, and systemic steroids increase the risk of infection and wound dehiscence, so decisions about the timing of suture removal may be more complex in these patients.
- Because not all patients will or can read your handouts, verbally counsel the patient regarding the signs of wound infection and to contact the office or seek care if fever, erythema, purulence, or increasing pain develops.
- We often call our patients the following day after a large excision. This can put your mind at ease and makes the patient feel cared for and special. This is also the perfect opportunity to answer patient questions about wound care or potential wound complications. This 1- to 2-minute call has much value for the patient and your practice.

Complications and their prevention are described in detail in Chapter 26.

Notes on Infection

- Infection may occur regardless of the precautions taken to ensure sterility.

- Sterile technique is routinely used for full-thickness excisions that are sutured.[11,12] When wound infections occur, the most common pathogens are *Staphylococcus aureus* and *Streptococcus pyogenes*.
- Do not overlook the possibility of methicillin-resistant Staphylococcus aureus (MRSA) infections especially if the patient has a history of previous MRSA infections.
- Culture wounds that appear infected, and open sutures if needed to allow the pus to drain.
- In general, antibiotic prophylaxis is rarely indicated.
- The 2008 AAD Advisory Statement recommends antibiotic prophylaxis for subacute bacterial endocarditis in high-risk cardiac patients and high-risk patients with prosthetic joints when performing excisions that involve cutting the oral mucosa.[9] Consider antibiotic prophylaxis if significant undermining is planned (see Chapter 1, *Preoperative Preparation*).
- Consider antibiotic prophylaxis with excisions in the groin or on the lower leg in the presence of extensive inflammatory disease (see Chapter 1).

Variations

Variations in the standard ellipse include the following shapes:

1. Crescent excision
2. S-plasty
3. M-plasty
4. Partial closure

CRESCENT EXCISION

On the cheek of the face, it often looks better for the final repair to be a crescent rather than a straight line. Asking the patient to smile can show the crescentic pattern of the smile lines. See Figure 11.27 to visualize how the crescent excision is drawn and executed.

M-PLASTY

In certain situations, the ellipse should be shorter on one side to avoid having the ellipse cross into another cosmetic unit. See Figure 11.28 as an example of how the M-plasty is used on the face to shorten one side of the ellipse.

S-PLASTY

Another variation of the ellipse that works well on convex surfaces such as the cheek is the S-plasty (Figure 11.29). Each side of the ellipse is drawn in an S configuration to avoid standing cones. Use of the rule of halves is helpful when closing this type of excision. If standing cones still form, they can be excised as described previously. Cosmetically this can give a better result than a straight line over some convex surfaces.

PARTIAL CLOSURE

Some large excisions on the scalp may be very difficult to close even with extensive undermining. Although the scalp may be allowed to heal by second intention, the clinician may want to obtain a partial closure to decrease the size of the area required to heal secondarily (Figure 11.30). Temporary pulley stitches are put in as step 1 to begin the closure. The wound is then closed from the apices with interrupted sutures zippering toward the center. This leaves a smaller wound to heal by second intention, thereby reducing final healing time.

Full ellipse from start to finish (Figure 11.31).

Alternatives to an Elliptical Excision

The alternatives to an elliptical excision include the following:

- Punch excision if the lesion is small enough
- Excision with flap repair (see Chapter 21, *Flaps*)

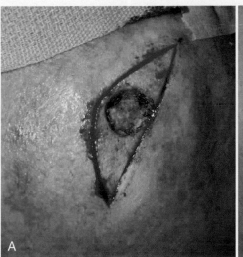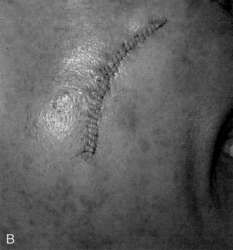

Figure 11.27 Crescent excision. **(A)** Circular defect on the cheek following removal of a basal cell carcinoma utilizing the Mohs method. The crescent excision is designed to result in a curvilinear line that follows the natural relaxed skin tension lines. Areas of use include the cheek over the malar eminence and the chin. **(B)** Crescentic repair follows smile lines. (From Robinson J, Hanke W, Sengelmann R, Siegel D. *Surgery of the Skin: Procedural Dermatology*. 2nd ed. Mosby; 2010.)

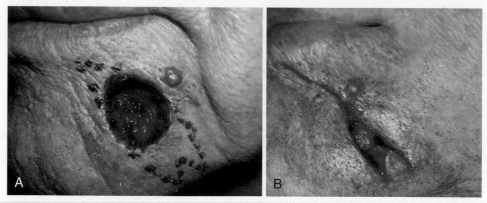

Figure 11.28 (A) M-plasty is designed to avoid crossing over into a new cosmetic unit. A tip stitch may be used to complete the M. **(B)** The final result produces a shorter scar that remains within one cosmetic unit. (From Robinson J, Hanke W, Sengelmann R, Siegel D. *Surgery of the Skin: Procedural Dermatology.* 2nd ed. Mosby; 2010.)

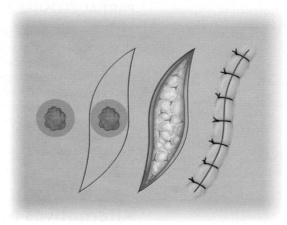

Figure 11.29 S-plasty with the lazy-S repair is designed by juxtaposing two S-shaped incisions around the defect. By approximating the center of each slightly offset S to the other, the final repair becomes a smooth serpentine line that contracts over convex surfaces with minimal buckling. It is useful when performing an excision along a convex surface such as the forearm or jaw. This minimizes the contraction and buckling seen along the length of the scar. Closing the wound with the rule of halves is helpful. (From Vidimos A, Ammirati C, Poblete-Lopez C. *Dermatologic Surgery.* Saunders; 2008.)

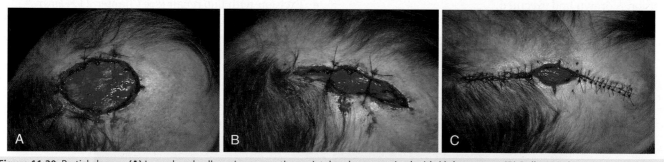

Figure 11.30 Partial closure: **(A)** Large basal cell carcinoma on the parietal scalp was excised with Mohs surgery. **(B)** Pulley stitches act as an intraoperative tissue expander. **(C)** Closing the wound from the apices and "zippering" toward the center leaves only a small wound to heal by second intention, thus reducing healing time. (From Robinson J, Hanke W, Sengelmann R, Siegel D. *Surgery of the Skin: Procedural Dermatology.* 2nd ed. Mosby; 2010.)

- Electrodesiccation and curettage for small BCCs, superficial BCCs, and SCC *in situ* (Bowen's disease) (see Chapter 14, *Electrosurgery*)
- Cryosurgical destruction with liquid nitrogen spray for superficial BCCs and SCC *in situ* (see Chapter 13, *Cryosurgery*)
- Purse string closure (see Chapter 6, *Suturing*)

Suggestions for Learning the Elliptical Excision Technique

The standard model for learning has been the pig's foot. Frozen or fresh pig's feet (not smoked) are available in many grocery stores and are good for practicing suturing and excision techniques. The skin on the pig's feet is less

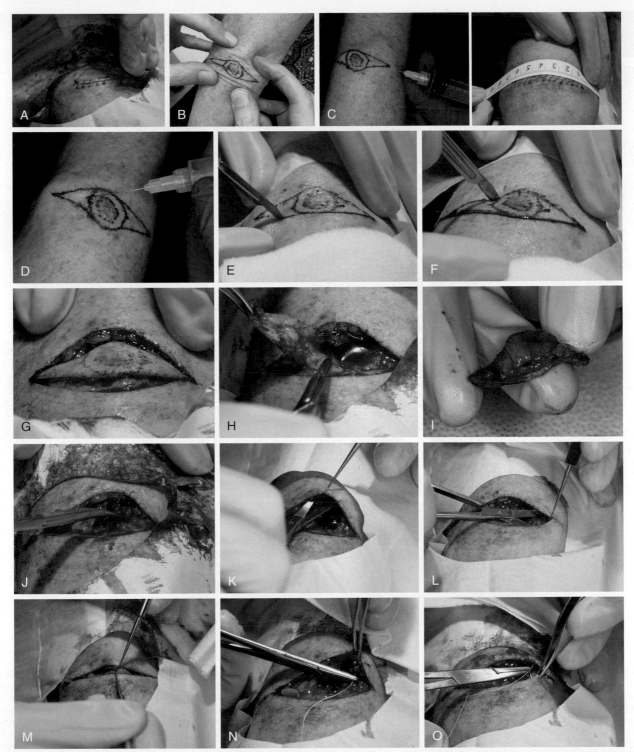

Figure 11.31 Ellipse from start to finish. **(A)** A nodular and superficial basal cell carcinoma is to be excised on the forearm of a 59-year-old woman. A circle is drawn around the biopsy site, and a 3 mm margin is added with a second circle. As the original biopsy had a 1- to 2-mm margin, an additional 3 millimeters are adequate. Pinching the skin is used to determine the best direction for the ellipse. It was determined that the best direction is circumferential, and the Burrows triangles were added to the concentric circles to create a 3:1 ellipse. **(B)** Looking at the pinched skin, you can see how there are more lines and greater mobility when the ellipse is circumferential. **(C)** Anesthesia is obtained starting at one end of the ellipse and working toward the other end. **(D)** It is especially important to make sure that there is adequate anesthesia for undermining the full ellipse including the two tips. **(E)** The ellipse is cut using the No. 15 blade, keeping the scalpel perpendicular to the surface. Tension is held on the skin with the nondominant hand to help the cutting process. **(F)** It is best to make the cuts straight down to the subcutaneous fat with as few passes as possible. **(G)** One can see that the cuts have been made into the subcutaneous fat all around. **(H)** The ellipse is cut off in the mid-fat by holding one corner of the ellipse and keeping the scalpel flat while it cuts. **(I)** Palpate the bottom and edges of the ellipse, feeling for firm cancer tissue requiring additional deeper cuts. **(J)** Hemostasis is obtained, and hemostats are useful for clamping bleeding tissue and vessels. **(K)** Undermining with blunt dissection using a skin hook to hold the skin up atraumatically. **(L)** The tips should be undermined well to avoid standing cones. **(M)** The two skin hooks can be used to determine if sufficient undermining has been performed to close the wound. **(N)** Start the closure with deep vertical mattress sutures and absorbable suture such as Vicryl. The initial needle motion is down to up. **(O)** The second part of the deep suture is placed up to down.

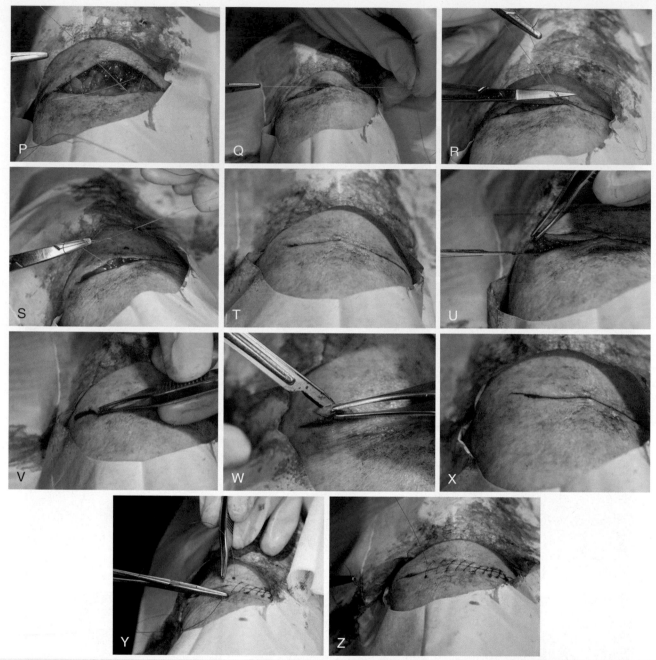

Figure 11.31, Cont'd **(P)** It helps if both strands of the Vicryl are on the same side before tying the suture. **(Q)** The suture is tied while pulling parallel to the incision. **(R)** After three knots are placed, the suture is cut close to the ties. **(S)** Additional deep sutures are placed. **(T)** The incision is nicely closed. However, there is a standing cone visible (dog ear). **(U)** The dog ear repair begins by extending the incision at an angle from the end allowing for a triangle of tissue to be formed. **(V)** The triangle is pulled over the incision to see where to cut the excess skin. **(W)** The excess skin is cut off using a scalpel or scissor. **(X)** There is no longer a standing cone or dog ear. **(Y)** As there is no further tension on the wound, the closure is completed with running Prolene. **(Z)** It is important to not pull the suture too tight as that increases the chance of scarring. **(AA)** The running suture is tied to a loop left at the end. **(BB)** The final closure is measured at 6.5 cm. It is important to make this measurement to properly code for the intermediate closure. **(CC)** The ellipse is complete. (Copyright Richard P. Usatine, MD.)

elastic than human skin, so practice with ellipses that are a 4:1 or 5:1 ratio.

Another good option is the silicone suturing pad that is available with basic surgical instruments and numerous practice sutures. These are now very affordable and easy to purchase online.

Coding and Billing Pearls

Record the location of the lesion and the width and length for coding because reimbursement varies with body location and size. Don't forget to measure the length of the final closed incision in any excision in which a two-layer closure was performed.

It is often best to know the diagnosis before excising a large lesion because this will determine the margins and whether a prior approval is needed. Also, larger lesions will be compensated at a higher rate and therefore may need prior approval. If an initial biopsy was done to determine the diagnosis, this will help to obtain prior approval for the correct procedure. If the diagnosis is unknown, hold off on billing until the pathology returns because the codes for excision of malignant lesions receive a higher reimbursement.

Tables 28.6 and 28.7 summarize the CPT codes and RVUs for excisions. Note how the RVUs go up 0.1 cm above each round centimeter. Do not round the measurements or make estimates; use exact numbers.

When calculating the size of a malignant lesion, it is important to include the necessary margins. Therefore if you are excising a 1-cm BCC with 4-mm margins, you would bill for an excision at 1.8 cm. Do not forget to make these measurements because it is crucial to getting paid for what you do.

If the repair involves significant undermining and/or deep sutures, additional codes are supplied for these types of intermediate repairs. Even the use of a single deep suture allows you to bill for an intermediate repair. The compensation for such a repair is comparable to the compensation for the rest of the excision. Therefore using deep sutures when needed not only protects the patient from risks of dehiscence and hematoma but also increases the compensation. When coding for intermediate repair, it helps to include the reason for the deep sutures in your operative note. The most common reasons are to "take tension off the wound" or "prevent dehiscence."

The CPT code for an intermediate repair is based on the length of the final closed excision. The codes for intermediate repairs encompass wide ranges of wound length, and most of the coding will be within the 2.6- to 7.5-cm range. See Table 28.9 for the CPT codes and RVUs for intermediate repairs.

Conclusion

The elliptical excision is one of the most basic and useful techniques for the excision of skin lesions. It can be aligned with skin tension lines, wrinkle lines, and other structures to give a good cosmetic result. The best results are obtained when the clinician pays close attention to the fine points of planning, designing, and executing the excision as described in this chapter.

References

1. Minton TJ. Contemporary Mohs surgery applications. *Curr Opin Otolaryngol Head Neck Surg.* 2008;16(4):376-380.
2. Thissen MR, Neumann MH, Schouten LJ. A systematic review of treatment modalities for primary basal cell carcinomas. *Arch Dermatol.* 1999;135:1177-1183.
3. Smeets NW, Krekels GA, Ostertag JU, et al. Surgical excision vs Mohs' micrographic surgery for basal-cell carcinoma of the face: randomised controlled trial. *Lancet.* 2004;364(9447):1766-1772.
4. Leibovitch I, Huilgol SC, Selva D, et al. Cutaneous squamous cell carcinoma treated with Mohs micrographic surgery in Australia I. Experience over 10 years. *J Am Acad Dermatol.* 2005;53(2):253-260.
5. Silapunt S, Peterson SR, Goldberg LH. Squamous cell carcinoma of the auricle and Mohs micrographic surgery. *Dermatol Surg.* 2005;31(11 Pt 1):1423-1427.
6. Robinson JK, Hanke CW, Sengelmann RD, et al. *Surgery of the Skin—Procedural Dermatology.* St. Louis: Elsevier/Mosby; 2010.
7. Swetter SM, Thompson JA, Albertini MR, et al. NCCN Guidelines® Insights: Melanoma: Cutaneous, Version 2.2021. *J Natl Compr Cancer Netw.* 2021;19(4):364-376. doi:10.6004/jnccn.2021.0018.
8. Tran KT, Wright, NA, Cockerell CJ. Biopsy of the pigmented lesion—when and how. *J Am Acad Dermatol.* 2008;59:852-871.
9. Kimyai-Asadi A, Alam M, Goldberg LH, et al. Efficacy of narrow-margin excision of well-demarcated primary facial basal cell carcinomas. *J Am Acad Dermatol.* 2005;53(3):464-468.
10. Vent A, Surber C, Graf Johansen NT, et al. Buffered lidocaine 1%/epinephrine 1:100,000 with sodium bicarbonate (sodium hydrogen carbonate) in a 3:1 ratio is less painful than a 9:1 ratio: a double-blind, randomized, placebo-controlled, crossover trial. *J Am Acad Dermatol.* 2020;83(1):159-165.
11. Wright TI, Baddour LM, Berbari EF, et al. Antibiotic prophylaxis in dermatologic surgery: advisory statement 2008. *J Am Acad Dermatol.* 2008;59(3):464-473.
12. Bennett R. Chapter 248: Surgical complications. In: Wolff K, Goldsmith LA, Katz SI, et al., eds. *Fitzpatrick's Dermatology in General Medicine.* 7th ed. New York: McGraw-Hill; 2007.
13. Dengel L, Turza K, Noland MM, et al. Skin mapping with punch biopsies for defining margins in melanoma: when you don't know how far to go. *Ann Surg Oncol.* 2008;15(11):3028-3035.
14. Kimyai-Asadi A, Katz T, Goldberg LH, et al. Margin involvement after the excision of melanoma in situ: the need for complete en face examination of the surgical margins. *Dermatol Surg.* 2007;33(12):1434-1441.
15. Thomas DJ, King AR, Peat BG. Excision margins for nonmelanotic skin cancer. *Plast Reconstr Surg.* 2003;112(1):57-63.
16. Bisson MA, Dunkin CS, Suvarna SK, Griffiths RW. Do plastic surgeons resect basal cell carcinomas too widely? A prospective study comparing surgical and histological margins. *Br J Plast Surg.* 2002;55(4):293-297.

12 Cysts and Lipomas

JONATHAN KARNES, MD, and RICHARD P. USATINE, MD

SUMMARY

- Patients frequently seek care for a variety of benign cysts and lipomas because of discomfort, diagnostic uncertainty, and functional or cosmetic concern.
- The chapter focuses on how to excise epidermal inclusion cysts and lipomas.
- It also covers the excision of pilar cysts, hidrocystomas, and digital mucous cysts.
- The advantages and disadvantages of various approaches to cyst removal are covered.
- Step-by-step guidance on cyst removal and lipoma excisions is provided.
- Lipomas and cysts can be removed with linear excisions, punch biopsies, and elliptical excisions.

Patients frequently seek definitive surgical care for a variety of benign cysts and lipomas because of discomfort, diagnostic uncertainty, and functional or cosmetic concern. Almost all of these can be addressed in the outpatient setting under local anesthesia when surgical therapy is indicated. Common cyst types include epidermal inclusion cysts and digital mucinous cysts. This chapter discusses characteristic features of benign cysts and lipomas with their surgical treatments.

Epidermal Inclusion Cysts (EIC) and Variants

EPIDERMAL INCLUSION CYSTS – AKA EPIDERMOID CYST

- Most common cutaneous cyst and can be removed intact
- Develops from the upper portion of a hair follicle
- Diagnosed by identifying central punctum (Figure 12.1) from which drains foul-smelling caseous or paste like material composed of sulfur-rich keratin (not sebum)
- Commonly on the face, trunk, and extremities
- Central material composed of keratin, which may have a cheesy or paste like texture
- Size may range from a couple of millimeters to several centimeters in size.
- Also called epidermoid cysts, infundibular cysts
- Pervasively misnamed sebaceous cyst by patients, clinicians, and ICD-10 codes
- Ruptured cysts enlarge, hurt, and turn intensely red due to inflammation but not infection (Figure 12.2).
- May become infected along with the inflammation
- Rare cases of malignancy forming in cyst wall

PILAR CYSTS

- Common cysts on the scalp (Figures 12.3 and 12.4)
- Also known as trichilemmal cysts or wens
- Some individuals or families have many of these over time.
- Range in size from a few millimeters to a couple of centimeters

- Cyst wall is thicker arising from the isthmus of the follicular unit.
- More firm than EICs and rarely with a punctum or drainage

MILIA

- Very small (1 to 2 mm) pearly white papule
- Often near the eyelids or mid face

Surgical Considerations for Epidermal Inclusion Cysts (EICs) and Pilar Cysts

(See Videos 12.1 to 12.5)

Common approaches to EICs and pilar cysts include the minimal excision technique, elliptical excision, and incision and drainage. Choice of technique depends on the degree of inflammation of the cyst, location and size of the cyst, and history of recurrence or scarring. For an uninflamed cyst that hasn't been operated on before, the minimal excision technique is one option involving opening the cyst to remove it through an incision smaller than the cyst itself. A more elegant approach (with less odor) involves removing the cyst intact through a larger incision or an ellipse. A markedly inflamed cyst can be treated with incision and drainage or observed until inflammation resolves, at which time the minimal excision technique may be performed. For cysts with significant scar tissue from failed surgical attempts, consider an elliptical excision around the whole cyst.

General Considerations for Epidermal Cyst or Pilar Cyst Removal

INDICATIONS

- Cyst growth
- Pain or discomfort

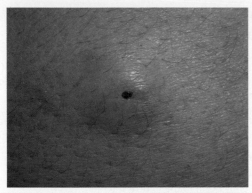

Figure 12.1 An epidermal inclusion cyst with a central punctum that looks like an open comedone. (Copyright Richard P. Usatine, MD.)

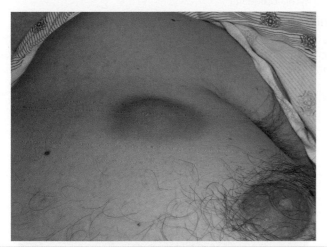

Figure 12.2 Local inflammation around an epidermal inclusion cyst can mimic cellulitis or an abscess. The best treatment is incision and drainage. (Copyright Richard P. Usatine, MD.)

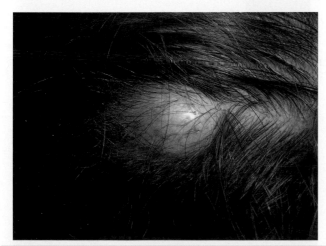

Figure 12.3 A typical presentation of a pilar cyst (trichilemmal cyst or wen) on the scalp. (Copyright Richard P. Usatine, MD.)

- Drainage
- Infection or inflammation
- Uncertain etiology
- Cosmetic appearance
- Recurrence from previous removal attempt

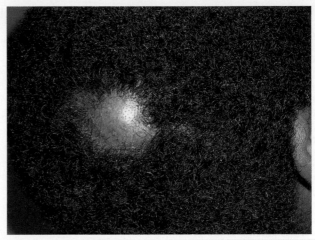

Figure 12.4 A fairly large pilar cyst with hair loss over the cyst. A simple ellipse over the cyst will remove redundant tissue. (Copyright Richard P. Usatine, MD.)

CONTRAINDICATIONS

- Avoid trying to remove cysts that are *actively inflamed* (Figure 12.2)
  - Consider instead incision and drainage, loop drainage, or observation for 3 to 4 weeks followed by minimal excision technique. This will reduce the size of the procedure and resulting scar as well as increase the rate of complete clearance.[1]
- Cysts near danger zones
  - Consider deferring or referring lesions that overlie areas such as large vascular networks, special sensory organs, or cosmetically sensitive areas. With experience, these areas may be managed in the office – but this depends on comfort, experience, and support services. Be aware of the spinal accessory nerve when neck lesions are involved since the nerve lies immediately under the skin and can be easily severed, leading to difficulty in abducting the arm (see Figure 11.4).
- Beware of the "cyst with a pulse"
  - An arteriovenous malformation or aneurysm may mimic EICs and pilar cysts. Vascular anomalies of the superficial temporal artery are particularly susceptible to being mistaken as cysts (see Figures 11.2 and 11.3). Always palpate for that pulse!
- Beware of the hard cyst/mass on the forehead or scalp
  - This may be an osteoma, and no scalpel can remove it. It is bone and should be left alone or referred out to facial plastic surgery. The skin moves over it, so don't be fooled that it is mobile. It is firmly part of the frontal bone or skull. The diagnosis can easily be confirmed with a simple radiograph (see Figure 22.2 in the ultrasound chapter).
- Diagnostic uncertainty
  - Keep the differential in mind even though the diagnosis may seem certain and routine (Box 12.1). For example, a dermoid cyst on the face can communicate with the cerebrospinal fluid in some circumstances. Consider imaging for a possible dermoid cyst if the cyst has been present on the face since early childhood and is midline (Figure 12.13). When encountering something atypical, consider imaging, perform a biopsy, or confer with a colleague before proceeding.

Box 12.1   Differential Diagnosis of Epidermal Inclusion Cysts

Bartholin's cyst (Figure 12.5)
Branchial cleft cyst (Figure 12.6)
Comedones
Dermoid cyst
Hidradenoma (Figure 12.7)
Hidrocystoma (Figure 12.8)
Milia
Mucinous cystadenoma (Figure 12.9)
Mucoid/myxoid/ganglion cyst (Figure 12.10)
Lipoma
Liposarcoma
Lymphadenopathy
Mucoceles
Neurofibromas
Osteoma (Figure 22.2)
Parotid tumor
Pilonidal cyst (Figure 12.11)
Proliferating trichilemmal cyst/malignant trichilemmal cyst
Steatocystoma
Thyroglossal duct cyst (Figure 12.12)

Dermoid cysts

- Uncommon
- Occur along congenital lines of cleavage (lingually, lateral eyes, behind the ears, and base of the nose) due to sequestration of embryonic cells (Figure 12.13)
- Most often found in children and teenagers
- Approach facial cysts in young children with caution (especially midline).

Steatocystoma multiplex

- Thin-walled, often grouped cysts 3 to 10 mm in size
- Frequently occur in the midchest (Figure 12.14)
- True sebaceous cysts with material that comes out looking like toothpaste (Figure 12.14)
- May be associated with genetic syndromes such as pachyonychia congenita

Hidrocystoma

- Occur near the eyelids and midface (Figure 12.8)
- Translucent with thin walls and fluid filled
- May be mistaken for basal cell carcinomas due to the fact they are pearly looking with visible telangiectasias in clear focus. Any nick to the thin cyst wall will clear up this dilemma as the fluid comes draining out.

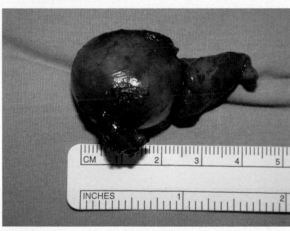

Figure 12.6 A branchial cleft cyst after removal. (Courtesy of Frank Miller, MD.)

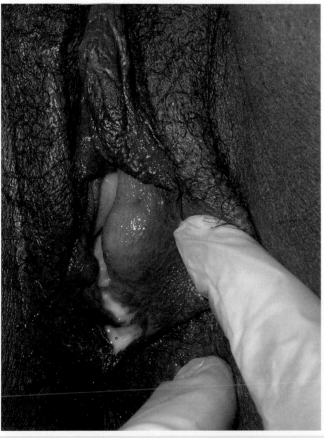

Figure 12.5 A Bartholin's duct cyst. (Copyright Richard P. Usatine, MD.)

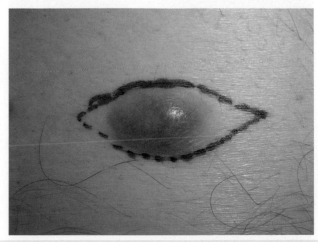

Figure 12.7 A solid cystic hidradenoma. (Copyright Richard P. Usatine, MD.)

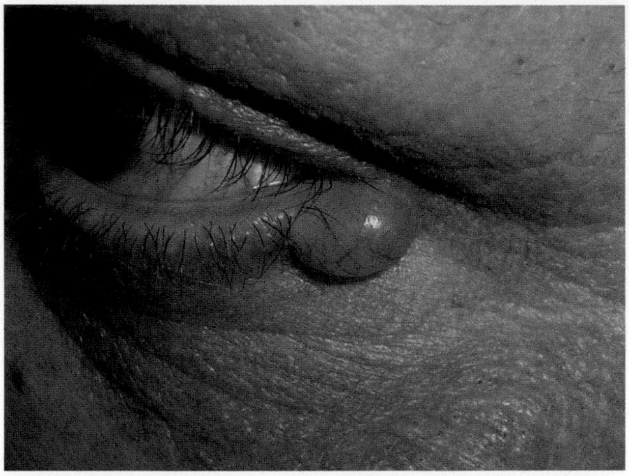

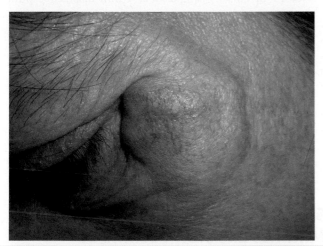

Figure 12.8 Hidrocystoma around the eye. It is benign and has a very thin wall that is easy to cut. (Copyright Richard P. Usatine, MD.)

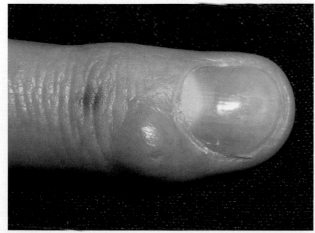

Figure 12.9 A mucinous cystadenoma near the eye. (Copyright Richard P. Usatine, MD.)

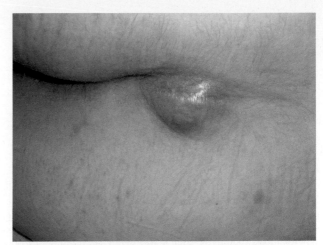

Figure 12.11 Pilonidal cyst. (Copyright Richard P. Usatine, MD.)

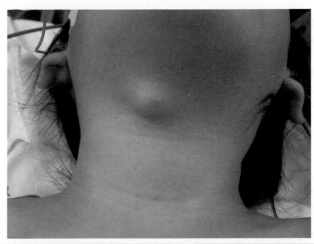

Figure 12.12 An inflamed thyroglossal duct cyst in a young girl. Note how it is midline. These will move up with swallowing. (Copyright Richard P. Usatine, MD.)

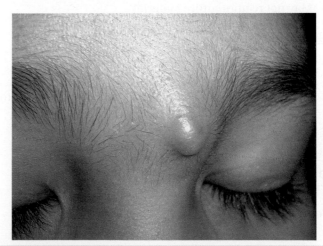

Figure 12.10 Digital mucous (myxoid) cyst on the finger. The distal to the distal interphalangeal joint is the most common location. (Copyright Richard P. Usatine, MD.)

Figure 12.13 A midline dermoid cyst on the face of a young girl. (Copyright Richard P. Usatine, MD.)

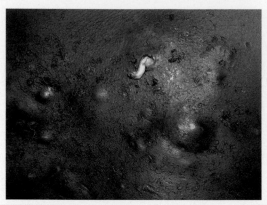

Figure 12.14 Steatocystoma multiplex on the chest of a 40-year-old Black man that started as a teenager. Note how the drainage from one cyst resembles toothpaste after it was gently squeezed. (Copyright Richard P. Usatine, MD.)

Advantages and Disadvantages of Various Approaches

Minimal Excision Technique: involves incising the cyst wall and expressing its contents to be able to remove the cyst through a smaller incision (linear opening, small ellipse, or small punch rather than a larger ellipse that surrounds the cyst). (*See video 12-4.*)

ADVANTAGES

Use of the minimal excision technique is becoming increasingly common for epidermal cyst removal. Its advantages can be subdivided into those for the physician and those for the patient.

For the physician:

- Requires only a few routine instruments
- Utilizes a small incision
- May not require suture material
- Relatively quick unless cyst wall not coming out easily
- Easy to learn

For the patient:

- Excellent cosmetic outcomes
- No need for second appointment and often no need to return for suture removal
- Faster wound healing
- Generally same-day treatment

DISADVANTAGES OF MINIMAL EXCISION TECHNIQUE

For the clinician:

- More challenging to remove the entire cyst wall compared with a larger ellipse
- Part of the procedure involves the expression of pungent cyst contents.

For the patient:

- Slightly increased recurrence

- Not all lesions can be successfully treated with this technique.

Do not use this method if:

- The lesion is inflamed (cyst wall is very tenuous, like wet tissue paper).
- It is a recurrent lesion.
- The lesion is large (over 4 cm).
- The patient has manipulated the lesion significantly, and there is likelihood of adhesions/scarring.
- Be aware that it is more difficult where the skin is very thick, such as on the back.

The Procedure

EQUIPMENT FOR THE MINIMAL EXCISION TECHNIQUE

- No. 11 or No. 15 scalpel or a 4-mm disposable punch biopsy
- Marking pen
- Syringe with a 27- to 30-gauge needle for anesthesia
- Sterile gauze
- Iris scissors
- Adson forceps with teeth
- Curved or straight hemostats are very useful.
- Needle driver and suture or skin tape
- Surgical gown and face shield – cyst contents exploding into your face or clothes can happen during the first incision or if the cyst was injected directly (and it isn't pleasant!).

Steps and Principles for the Minimal Excision Technique

(*See Video 12-4*)

PREOPERATIVE MEASURES

- Obtain informed consent. (See Appendix A for sample consent form.)
- Determine the apex of the lesion. This is sometimes around a punctum (Figure 12.1).
- Mark the apex with a line (Figure 12.14), a small ellipse, or a small circle to orient a punch or incision (include punctum), depending on which technique is chosen to enter the cyst wall. Draw a circle around the widest margins of the cyst (Figure 12.14). You may use a fenestrated drape if you plan to place a suture.
- Inject anesthetic with a 27- to 30-gauge needle around the cyst.
- Avoid injecting anesthesia directly into the cyst as this increases cyst pressure, and smelly cyst contents may squirt out the punctum. It is best to plan to inject around the cyst, performing a ring block. Anesthesia injected into the cyst is wasted and may cause pain. In Figure 12.15 the arrows show how you can start at one corner of a square and inject at the arrow ahead each time so that the new injection will be less painful from the effect of the preceding injection. A fifth injection may be added to the skin above the cyst at the site for the planned incision to ensure

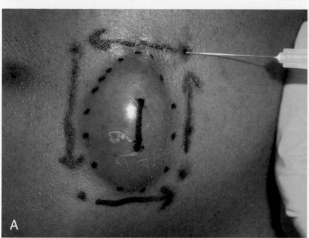 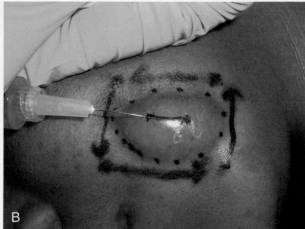

Figure 12.15 **(A)** Epidermal cyst on the face is outlined before injecting anesthesia. The solid line is drawn to match skin lines and to be about 40% of the diameter of the cyst. A ring block is marked with four arrows, and each injection starts at the end of the previous arrow. **(B)** The ring block has been performed without injecting into the cyst. The final injection is given over the cyst to make sure that the incision line is fully anesthetized. (Copyright Richard P. Usatine, MD.)

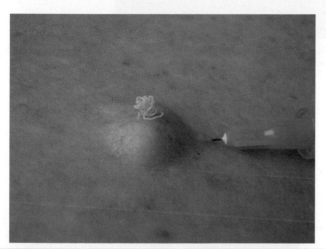

Figure 12.16 An otherwise invisible punctum is discovered when lidocaine creates pressure inside the cyst extruding keratin from the punctum. (Copyright Richard P. Usatine, MD.)

a painless surgery (Figure 12.15B). In Figure 12.16 the pressure of the anesthesia has caused some keratin to be extruded from the punctum without any harm.
- Prep the area with surgical cleanser such as chlorhexidine.

PERFORMING THE PROCEDURE
(See Videos 12.3 to 12.5)

- Stretch the skin to anchor the lesion. Incise a linear or punch opening (Figures 12.17A and B) over the cyst apex and into the cyst itself. Alternatively, cut a small ellipse around the apex, including the punctum instead of a linear or circular opening.
- Express all cyst contents with firm digital pressure on the cyst and surrounding tissue (Figure 12.17C). Keep plenty of 4 × 4 gauze on the field to mop up the contents of the cyst.
- Identify the cyst wall and dissect it from surrounding tissues using blunt dissection with an iris scissor or curved hemostat. Curved iris scissors or any curved

tissue scissors work very well. Once a small area has been dissected, you may grasp the cyst wall with forceps or hemostat (Figure 12.17D). Continue blunt dissection until the cyst wall is able to be pulled through your incision.
- Sometimes the skin incision needs to be extended or deepened to extract the entire cyst contents.
- If the cyst is attached to the fascia below, just snip this fibrous tissue with a scissor (Figure 12.18).
- Inspect the material removed. You should have extracted a nearly complete cyst wall (Figures 12.19 and 12.20). Pilar cysts have a thicker wall and are easier to extract intact (Figure 12.21).
- Inspect the cavity and verify that all the cyst wall has been removed. Note that the cyst wall may be white in light skin and may be dark in darker skin.
- Sterile cotton-tipped applicators are useful for probing the cavity and cleaning out any remaining cyst fragments.
- Consider irrigating the cavity and surrounding skin with sterile saline or water, especially if any cyst contents spilled into the incision.
- Repair the defect. With the minimal excision technique, sometimes no closure is needed. If desired, the skin may be approximated with 4-0 to 6-0 nylon or polypropylene. Skin tape may also be used.
- Some clinicians choose to not close small pilar cyst excisions and get good results. Sutures have the advantage of providing hemostasis and approximating the epidermis.[2]

Pathology

- While not strictly necessary to send benign-appearing cysts for pathological evaluation, regularly sending all surgical specimens is increasingly standard practice.
- We have cared for a few patients with squamous cell carcinoma (SCC) originally treated as a cyst without pathologic exam and have been surprised by a focal SCC in a pilar cyst sent for routine pathology.
- Possible differential diagnoses are listed in Box 12.1.

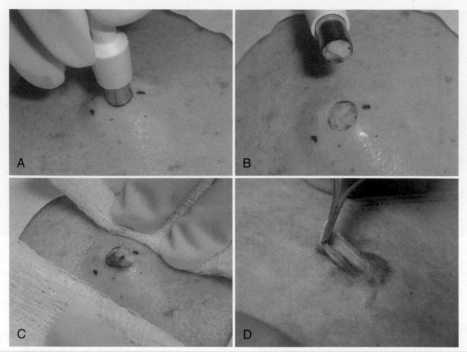

Figure 12.17 (A) A 4-mm punch creates an opening into the underlying epidermal inclusion cyst. **(B)** The punch is removed, and the keratinaceous material is seen inside the punch and in the cyst. **(C)** The cyst contents are expressed with pressure from both sides. **(D)** The cyst wall is shiny and seen being pulled through the punch incision. (Copyright Richard P. Usatine, MD.)

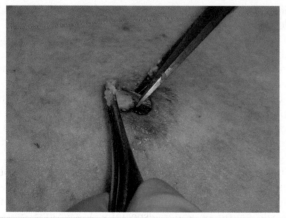

Figure 12.18 A small emptied cyst is pulled through a small punch opening and freed from underlying tissue using an iris scissor. (Copyright Richard P. Usatine, MD.)

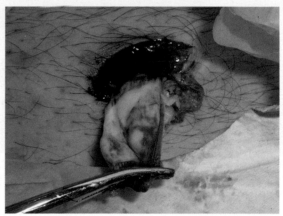

Figure 12.19 Pulling a large emptied cyst wall through the opening created by an ellipse in the abdominal wall. (Copyright Richard P. Usatine, MD.)

Major Alternatives

ELLIPTICAL EXCISION

(See Video 12.1)

- Discussed fully in Chapter 11. The preoperative measures, anesthesia, and dissection around the cyst wall are essentially the same as above.
- Best for cysts that have recurred or have scarred significantly from manipulation or repeated rupture.
- Either remove the cyst whole (en bloc) or through an ellipse larger than what you might use in the minimal excision technique.
- If a large cyst was removed, consider placing a deep layer of buried absorbable sutures to close the dead space before placing the surface sutures.

- If the cyst is large and elevated, make sure the width of the ellipse is equal to the width of the cyst to avoid dog ears (standing cones). This is especially true with large protuberant pilar cysts (Figure 12.22).
- The elliptical excision method can help large protuberant cysts with redundant skin ultimately repair flat.[3]

INCISION AND DRAINAGE (I&D) OF INFLAMED AND INFECTED CYSTS

- When patients present with an acutely inflamed or possibly infected cyst, the treatment is to incise, drain, and sometimes place a wick or packing in the incision for 2 to 3 days. (See Chapter 16, *Incision and Drainage*.)

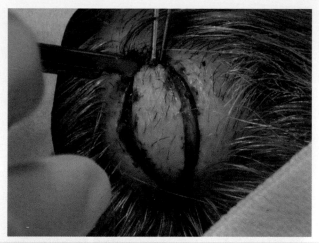

Figure 12.22 This large pilar cyst will be removed through an ellipse that extends across the full diameter of the cyst. This will allow the scalp to lie flat once the cyst is removed. If the ellipse is made shorter than this, there will be standing cones on both sides of the repaired defect. Note that the hairs were clipped with a scissor rather than shaving the scalp. Shaving increases risk of infection, but snipping with a scissor makes the surgery easier with no increased infection risks. (Copyright Richard P. Usatine, MD.)

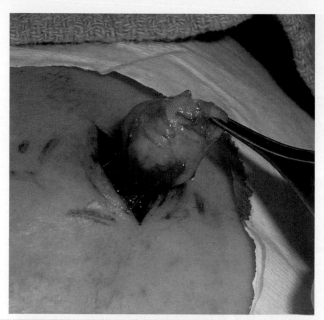

Figure 12.20 A relatively intact epidermal cyst near the shoulder is extracted through a linear incision. (Copyright Richard P. Usatine, MD.)

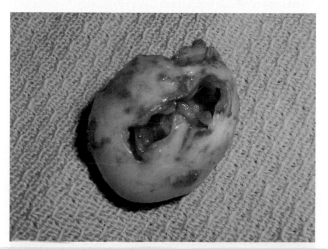

Figure 12.21 Pilar cyst has a thick wall and keeps its spherical anatomy in most cases even if it was cut and emptied. (Copyright Richard P. Usatine, MD.)

- If a follow-up visit to remove a wick or packing isn't possible, keep the packing short and fix the outside of the packing to the dressing. When the patient takes the dressing off, the wick and packing will come out simultaneously. Also, the loop drainage technique described in Chapter 16 will avoid follow-up visits for packing.
- Use a ring block for anesthesia and a No. 11 blade scalpel to incise the inflamed area. Since the incision will be packed and not closed, clean technique is adequate.
- Antibiotics are rarely beneficial since the inflammatory changes are due to a reaction to the ruptured contents rather than a true infection.

HIDROCYSTOMAS (FIGURE 12.23)

- Despite occurrence near or on the eyelids, these lesions can be excised in the office using pickups and cutting a small thin ellipse over the cyst with a sharp tissue scissor. Inject away from the eye using lidocaine and epinephrine first.
- Don't use chlorhexidine or aluminum chloride near the eye to avoid ocular damage.
- One option to make the procedure easier is to drain the fluid with the same needle used for local anesthetic (Figure 12.23). This also ensures the correct diagnosis before cutting with the scissor.
- Whether cutting directly with a scissor or aspirating with a needle, the fluid will drain out easily. For small lesions, there should be little bleeding, so pressure alone should be adequate for hemostasis. Sutures should not be needed in most cases but may help with larger cysts.
- Note that if you aspirate the fluid first and then cut the cyst at the lowest level, a suture is needed as the cut area will gape open when the patient opens the eye. If you snip a smaller portion of the cyst at the top (either full or aspirated) the smaller opening can be left open for second intention healing.
- The small ellipse of tissue can be sent to pathology confirming the diagnosis by examining the cyst wall. The pathologist can also confirm whether the cyst was of eccrine or apocrine origin. When the cost of pathology is prohibitive for the patient, a clinical diagnosis confirmed by the drainage of clear fluid should be adequate.

DERMOID CYSTS (FIGURE 12.13)

- Be aware of the precautions cited above and consider imaging. If imaging shows communication with CSF, refer to neurology.
- If a dermoid cyst is suspected and there is no communication with the CSF visible, excisional removal can be performed by sterile procedure with an ellipse as above. Always send the specimen for pathology.
- If a dermoid cyst is found on the face of a young child, refer for removal under sedation or general anesthesia.

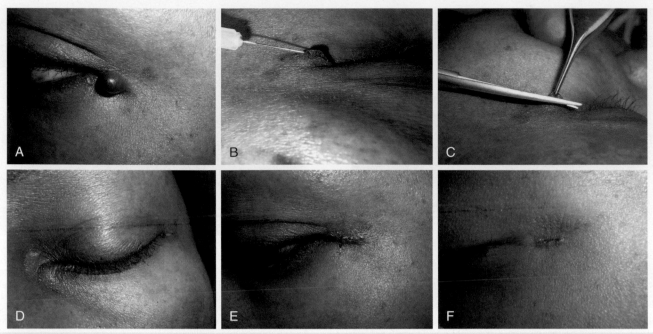

Figure 12.23 (A) Hidrocystoma at the lateral canthus. **(B)** The hidrocystoma is drained using the same local anesthesia needle. **(C)** Snipping most of the hidrocystoma wall with an iris scissor while stabilizing the cyst with Adson forceps. **(D)** The hidrocystoma is gone, and there is a small defect. **(E)** The defect was closed with a single suture. **(F)** Another example of a hidrocystoma that was snipped off and not sutured. (Copyright Richard P. Usatine, MD.)

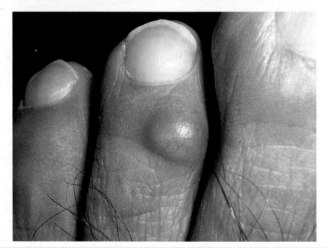

Figure 12.24 Digital mucous cyst on a toe. (Copyright Richard P. Usatine, MD.)

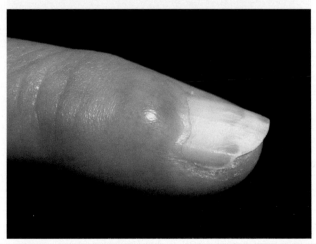

Figure 12.25 Digital mucous cyst causing nail deformity. The pressure of the cyst on the matrix typically causes a depressed trough. (Copyright Richard P. Usatine, MD.)

DIGITAL MUCOUS (MYXOID) CYSTS

(See Video 12.6)

Digital mucous cysts or myxoid cysts are ganglion cysts arising on the distal fingers or occasionally the toes (Figures 12.24 and 12.25). These are the most common cysts on the hand and are benign. The etiology is uncertain, but the cysts likely form from mucoid degeneration associated with arthritis. Cysts usually present after the 5th decade of life but can present earlier when associated with arthropathy such as rheumatoid arthritis. The most common location is the dorsal distal interphalangeal joint. Lesions can distort the nail matrix causing nail deformities and pain (Figure 12.25). When treatment is sought, options range from observation to joint surgery with

osteophyte removal and flap reconstruction. The easiest outpatient option is draining with repeat sterile needling and cryotherapy.[4,5] Alternatives include the injection of a steroid or an excision with a small flap repair. All options risk recurrence, and toes have increased recurrence compared with fingers. Radical joint surgery by an orthopedist is the most definitive and most costly option.

General Considerations in Treating Digital Mucous Cysts

INDICATIONS

- Painful digital mucous cysts
- Distortion of the nail plate (Figure 12.25)

CONTRAINDICATIONS

- An infected cyst should be managed medically with antibiotics first.

Needling and Cryotherapy of Digital Mucous Cysts

- Obtain informed consent, and discuss the small risk of scarring, nail deformities, infection in the joint space, and recurrence (10% to 15% with cryotherapy).[4]
- Local anesthesia is optional and can be done with 1% or 2% lidocaine with or without epinephrine and a 30 g needle at the site of the cyst.
- Prep the area with an alcohol swab.
- Puncture the lesion with multiple needle sticks and drain out the gelatinous fluid (Figure 12.26).
- Using a cryosurgery probe or spray nozzle, create an ice ball with a diameter 2 to 3 mm beyond the extent of the cyst (Figure 12.27). Let this thaw and repeat the cryotherapy once.

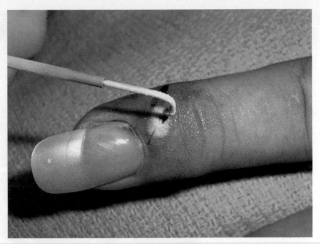

Figure 12.27 Cryotherapy of a digital mucous cyst after it was punctured with a needle and drained. Aim for a 2-mm margin of freeze around the lesion. (Copyright Richard P. Usatine, MD.)

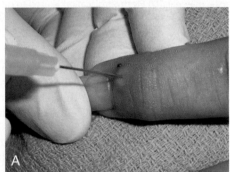
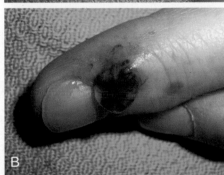
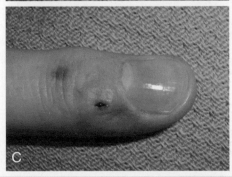

Figure 12.26 (A) Needling a digital mucus cyst. **(B)** The gelatinous material is similar to synovial fluid. **(C)** Collapsed digital mucus cyst. (Copyright Richard P. Usatine, MD.)

Alternatives

CRYOTHERAPY ALONE

- Cryotherapy is quick and effective.
- Cryotherapy alone had a 72% clearance rate in a systematic review.[4]

SERIAL NEEDLING ALONE

- Another very good alternative is serial needling without cryotherapy. This can be started and demonstrated in the office or at home by a capable patient who is given sterile needles. In an old study, the success rate was 70% with minimal expense aside from office visits.[5] More recent evaluation of needling and evacuation alone cited a 39% clearance.

EXCISION WITH SMALL FLAP REPAIR

(See Video 12.6)

- For recurrent cysts or those not amenable to conservative treatments above, excision of the cyst in the office with a small flap pinned with a few small sutures may rival the long-term cure rate of open joint surgery.[6,7]
- The easiest method for this is to create a three-sided fingertip-shaped pedicle flap around the cyst (Figure 12.28). The plane of scarring that forms under this theoretically blocks the communication from the joint space to the cyst.[6,7]

Step-by-step excision and small flap repair of the digital mucous cyst (Figure 12.28):

1. Mark the cyst for removal with the surgical marking pen, leaving the proximal side to remain uncut, allowing for maximal circulation to the flap.
2. Perform a digital block using lidocaine with epinephrine. Then perform a wing block, or add some additional local anesthetic around the cyst itself to minimize bleeding. Note how the distal finger has blanched white so that a tourniquet is not needed.

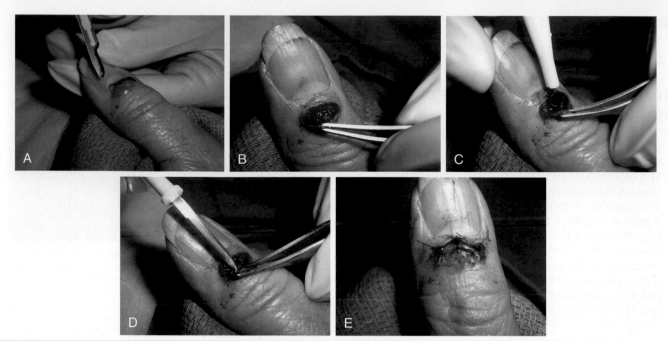

Figure 12.28 (A) Treatment of a digital mucous cyst that starts with a digital block before opening the distal end of the cyst with a No. 15 blade. **(B)** The skin is pulled back to reveal the cyst below. **(C)** 3-mm curette scrapes away the cystic material. **(D)** Electrodesiccation is used to destroy any remaining cyst while destroying any connection to the DIP joint to avoid recurrence. **(E)** The skin over this cyst is tacked down with three small 5-0 Prolene interrupted sutures. (Copyright Richard P. Usatine, MD.)

3. Cut along the marked area with a DermaBlade, razor blade, or No. 15 scalpel.
4. Lift up the flap to visualize the cyst.
5. Remove the cyst using a 3-0 curette, or dissect under it with an iris scissor.
6. Burn the base with electrodesiccation using a sharp-tipped electrode on a setting of 15 W. Be careful to not damage the skin above and around the cyst.
7. Tack down the skin flap with 5-0 or 6-0 Prolene or nylon.
8. Dress the area with petrolatum and gauze.

Complications of Any Cyst Removal Technique

- Incomplete removal may lead to localized inflammatory reactions, retained cyst material, and recurrence.
- Seromas and hematomas presenting as swelling or pain may form within the defect left by the cyst and can be treated with aspiration.
- Damage to neighboring anatomic structures including nerves can occur from deep blind probing or lack of awareness of anatomic danger zones.

Lipomas

(See Videos 12.7 to 12.10)

Lipomas are subcutaneous benign tumors composed of adipose tissue held together with connective tissue. Although they may be encapsulated, in general, they are more amorphous, lobulated masses that are either slightly lighter or darker than surrounding adipose. Lipomas typically arise after the fourth decade of life and present as single or multilobed soft tumors that are easily compressible and have a doughy consistency. Lipomas most commonly arise over the neck and trunk, though they also can be found on the extremities and face. Patients complain of lipomas when they occur on pressure-bearing areas, become painful, arise in cosmetically sensitive areas, or grow very large. In these cases or when there is diagnostic uncertainty, removal is indicated.

LIPOMA DIAGNOSIS

- Lipomas can usually be diagnosed clinically as a soft mobile subcutaneous mass.
- Differential includes many of the same entities discussed for cysts (Box 12.1).
- Also consider hematoma, panniculitis, rheumatic nodules, and metastatic cancer.
- Ultrasound can help establish an uncertain diagnosis (see Chapter 22, *Ultrasound*).

GENERAL CONSIDERATIONS FOR LIPOMA REMOVAL

There are several approaches to removing lipomas: incision and expression, elliptical excision, and liposuction.

INDICATIONS

Indications for removal of lipomas include:

- Symptomatic lesions (causing pain, discomfort, or anxiety)
- Cosmetic concerns
- Clarifying the diagnosis
- Clinical depth below the fascia
- Rapid growth and therefore concern for liposarcoma

SPECIAL CIRCUMSTANCES

- Liposarcomas can appear similar to lipomas but do not arise from lipomas.
- In the case of a worrisome lesion, consider needle aspiration or imaging.[8] However, a full excision will always provide the best tissue to the pathologist.
- Forehead lipomas are frequently under the frontalis muscle. Avoid removing these until your surgical skills and confidence in operating on the face are excellent (Figure 12.29).
- Episacral lipomas are small, tender subcutaneous nodules that are also called "back mice" and "sacroiliac lipomas." These painful lipomas occur when a portion of the dorsal fat pad herniates through a tear in the thoracodorsal fascia. They are often bilateral and movable, so they feel like little "mice" under the skin. Do not try to remove these in the office. One treatment is injection with triamcinolone and lidocaine.
- Despite these caveats, lipomas are generally straightforward to address in the outpatient setting.

PREOPERATIVE

- After obtaining informed consent, mark the borders of the lipoma with a surgical marking pen (Figure 12.29A).
- Locate the best area for the linear incision or punch, and mark it with the marking pen –taking into account skin lines and cosmetic considerations (Figure 12.29A). The incision need not be directly in the center of the lesion.

- Inject 1% lidocaine with epinephrine directly into the lipoma and the skin above it. Make sure that the skin that will be incised is well anesthetized.
- Larger lipomas can be anesthetized with very dilute ($\leq$1 g/L) tumescent lidocaine anesthesia. While this is beyond the scope of this chapter, it is worth noting that with this technique developed for outpatient liposuction, it is possible to comfortably remove even large lipomas that would otherwise require exceeding the toxic threshold of standard concentrations of lidocaine.
- Prep the area with surgical cleanser such as chlorhexidine.

LINEAR INCISION AND PRESSURE METHOD

- Draw out the linear incision so that it is approximately ⅓ to ½ the diameter of the lipoma (Figure 12.30A).
- Make a linear incision through the skin over the top of the lipoma. Hold the No. 11 blade perpendicular to the skin, and cut through the skin into the lipoma with a sawing motion.
- Very little bleeding should be encountered. If there is much bleeding reassess the diagnosis and procedure immediately (think hemangioma).
- Insert and spread the curved hemostats around the edges of the lipoma to break up the fibrous bands that attach it to the surrounding tissue.
- Do this 360 degrees, and try to get under the lipoma as well.
- Express the lipoma through the incision using digital pressure under and around the lipoma (think Dr. Pimple Popper) (Figure 12.30B).

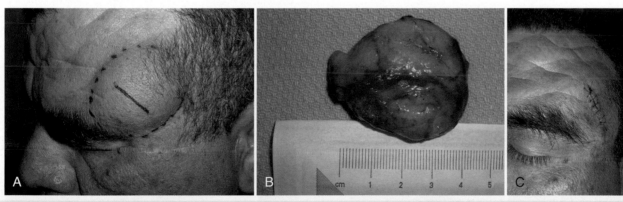

Figure 12.29 (A) Lipoma on the temple/forehead is marked with a dotted line around the circumference and a solid line to guide the incision along skin lines. **(B)** Lipoma removed without damage to the temporal branch of the facial nerve. **(C)** Linear incision closed with running sutures. (Copyright Richard P. Usatine, MD.)

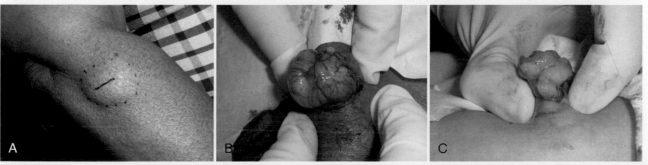

Figure 12.30 (A) Lipoma on the forearm marked for linear incision and removal. **(B)** The lipoma is extruded from the incision with the pressure from four fingers. **(C)** Firm pressure around and below the lipoma delivers it through the small opening with one hand. (Copyright Richard P. Usatine, MD.)

- Pulling the lipoma with the hemostat clamped upon it can help while squeezing the lipoma out from below with digital pressure.
- Once freed, examine that the lipoma is whole, and explore the cavity to make sure the entire lipoma has been removed.
- Bleeding should be minimal but can be stopped with electrocoagulation as needed.
- Close any dead space with deep absorbable sutures (see Chapter 6, *Suturing Techniques*).
- Close the incision with simple interrupted, running, or subcuticular sutures.
- Some clinicians use skin tape with no sutures underneath a pressure dressing.
- With experience and efficient office staff small lipomas can be removed quickly.
- Even a large lipoma can be removed using this method (Figure 12.31).

EXAMINATION AND PATHOLOGY

- Inspect the lipoma and feel it between your fingers. It should be a contiguous yellow mass without significant vascularity or calcifications (Figure 12.31E).
- Frequently, the standard of care is to send lipomas for pathological exam, but always send when significant vascularity, color variations, or tactile variations are present. In a patient with many lipomas, one may send the first lipoma but not every other typical one that follows.

- Large lipomas may require a larger container to transfer to pathology (formalin can be transferred to a sterile urine cup to make room for a larger mass).

Punch (Enucleation) Technique to Remove Lipomas

Similar to the minimal excision technique for epidermal inclusion cysts, enucleation involves entering the lipoma through a small punch through the dermis and scooping out, or enucleating, the lipoma with a small curette.

EQUIPMENT

4-to-6-mm punch biopsy tool, 3-mm skin curette, tissue scissors, and hemostat

REMOVING THE LIPOMA

- Center the punch tool over the lipoma, stretching the skin perpendicular to the skin lines. With a twisting motion, punch through the dermis and into the lipoma.
- Insert the curette through the incision, and using a finger as a guide and boundary on the surface, begin to free the lipoma by scraping it from the surrounding tissue.
- Bring a section of the lipoma through the opening and grasp it with a hemostat. Continue to curette until the entire lesion is delivered out of the small opening

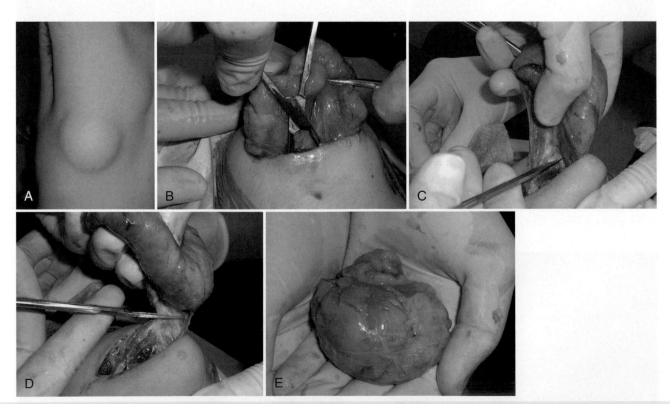

Figure 12.31 (A) Large lipoma overlying the left latissimus dorsi muscle of a young man. **(B)** Using curved hemostat to separate lipoma from surrounding tissues. **(C)** Cutting lipoma from its attachments below. **(D)** Final release of lipoma shows that it was lying directly on the chest wall muscles. **(E)** Large partially encapsulated lipoma in the hand for examination. (Copyright Richard P. Usatine, MD.)

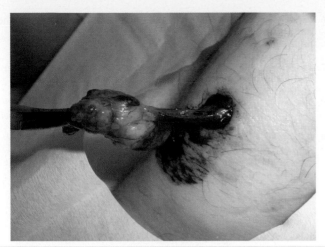

Figure 12.32 Small lipoma being extracted through a 6-mm punch incision. (Copyright Richard P. Usatine, MD.)

(Figure 12.32). Firm digital pressure around the lipoma will aid in the extraction.

- For larger lipomas some clinicians advocate multiple small incisions or punches to perform segmental extraction.[9]
- For small lipomas a punch biopsy may be used as the opening, and the lipoma can be extracted manually without a curette, similar to the method described in the linear incision technique.

ELLIPTICAL EXCISION OF A LIPOMA

- Practical for larger lipomas or those under thick skin (back of the neck, posterior trunk) and with lesions that are of uncertain diagnosis or unusually firm
- May utilize the elliptical piece of skin as a convenient handle to manipulate the underlying lipoma
- Produces a larger scar, but sometimes this is an acceptable tradeoff

COMPLICATIONS

- Scarring, formation of hematomas or seromas, infection, and recurrence
- The linear incision and enucleation methods minimize these risks.
- Seromas and hematomas may be treated with aspiration or evacuation.
- Prevent seromas and hematomas by closing dead space and applying a pressure dressing.

Coding and Billing Pearls

Epidermal cysts are skin lesions and as such, excisions are coded by size of the cyst, their location, and their benign nature. Simple excision and repair includes the anesthetic, the excision, the repair, and suture removal. The size is based on the measured size of the cyst on the skin before surgery, not the size of the incision, so a minimal cyst removal is not compensated at a lower rate because the incision was shorter. It is not expected that the excised cyst or

cyst remnants are used to measure the cyst. If a margin beyond the cyst is taken, it may be added to the size of the lesion, but this is rarely necessary. Additional repair charges may apply for an intermediate closure if deep sutures are needed to close dead space or approximate wound edges under tension. The intermediate closure charge is based on the length of the final closed wound. Make sure to document the reason for the intermediate closure.

If the cyst was infected or inflamed and the cyst was incised and drained without packing, use the code for simple I&D (10060). If multiple cysts were treated this way, or if the procedure was made more complex by the use of packing or removal of the sack, then the correct code is 10061 for "multiple or complex removal." Note that just adding some packing increases the compensation.

CODING FOR LIPOMAS

Lipoma excisions may be coded as removal of a skin lesion or as the removal of a subcutaneous tumor under the musculoskeletal codes. If the lipoma is superficial in the subcutaneous fat below the skin, the removal may be coded the same as for an excision of an epidermal cyst (excision of a benign skin lesion). Similar to epidermal cysts, the size is based on the measurement of the lipoma on the skin before surgery and not the incision. One could measure the size of an intact lipoma after surgery but the skin measurement is sufficient. Also, if a two-layered closure is performed, document the necessity for this, and bill for an intermediate closure based on the location and length of closure.

Lipomas may also be coded as excision of a subcutaneous tumor based on anatomic location and are inclusive of the excision and repair. Some coders advocate using these codes only for deep lipomas including those under fascia or under muscle. Other coders state that all lipomas should be coded with these codes. See Table 28-12 for the specific soft tissue tumor codes based on location of the lipoma.

Speak with staff and/or consultants that support coding and billing functions to help make decisions when the best coding strategy for a specific lipoma is not clear. Since the reimbursement of an excision of a benign lesion is less than the removal of a subcutaneous tumor, when in doubt the charges will less likely be challenged when billing for the former.

Conclusion

The most common "lumps and bumps" that present in an outpatient setting can be managed effectively with a combination of the techniques described above. Learning these few techniques will expand your capabilities and improve your effectiveness in treating these common problems.

Another way to improve your skills with cysts and lipomas is to use ultrasound in your office. It is very satisfying to add an ultrasound diagnosis to your clinical diagnosis and then to confirm or refute the diagnostic impression with surgery. This can also save your patients with limited resources the cost of an expensive diagnostic ultrasound (rarely needed anyway) performed by radiology. If this is of interest, please read Chapter 22 on ultrasound.

References

1. Reich D, Psomadakis CE, Buka B. Inflamed epidermal inclusion cyst. In: *Top 50 Dermatology Case Studies for Primary Care*. Springer; 2017. Available at: https://doi.org/10.1007/978-3-319-18627-6_28.
2. Chen S, Srivastava D, Nijhawan RI. Removal of large epidermoid cysts by use of a minimal-incision technique. *J Am Acad Dermatol*. 2017;77(1):e13-e14. doi:10.1016/j.jaad.2017.01.043.
3. Suliman MT. Excision of epidermoid (sebaceous) cyst: description of the operative technique. *Plast Reconstr Surg*. 2005;116:2042-2043.
4. Jabbour S, Kechichian E, Haber R, Tomb R, Nasr M. Management of digital mucous cysts: a systematic review and treatment algorithm. *Int J Dermatol*. 2017;56(7):701-708. doi:10.1111/ijd.13583.
5. Epstein E. A simple technique for managing digital mucous cysts. *Arch Dermatol*. 1979;115:1315-1316.
6. Fan Z, Chang L, Su X, Yang B, Zhu Z. Treatment of mucous cyst of the distal interphalangeal joint with osteophyte excision and joint debridement. *Front Surg*. 2022;8:767098. doi:10.3389/fsurg.2021.767098.
7. Lawrence C. Skin and osteophyte removal is not required in the surgical treatment of digital mucous cysts. *Arch Dermatol*. 2005;141:1560-1564.
8. Hornick JL. Limited biopsies of soft tissue tumors: the contemporary role of immunohistochemistry and molecular diagnostics. *Mod Pathol*. 2019;32(suppl 1):27-37. doi:10.1038/s41379-018-0139-y.
9. Park JK, Kim J, Kim JH, Eun S. Minimal One-Third Incision and Four-Step (MOTIF) excision method for lipoma. *Biomed Res Int*. 2021;2021:4331250. doi:10.1155/2021/4331250.

13 *Cryosurgery*

RICHARD P. USATINE, MD, and DANIEL L. STULBERG, MD

SUMMARY

- Cryosurgery (cryotherapy) is an easily mastered technique that is extremely useful for treating benign and premalignant lesions.
- Our preferred technique involves using liquid nitrogen with a spray gun.
- Indications and contraindications are reviewed.
- Cryosurgery is a fast procedure in which multiple lesions can be treated at the same visit.
- Cryosurgery principles and methods are discussed.
- The amount of tissue destruction can be predicted by the duration of freezing (freeze time), the amount of thaw time (time until the ice ball is defrosted), and the margin of frozen tissue around the lesion (halo diameter).
- Detailed steps and principles of liquid nitrogen spray use are reviewed.
- Other cryosurgery methods such as liquid nitrogen probes and Cryo Tweezers are taught.
- Tips for cryosurgery of specific lesions are provided.

Cryosurgery is one of the most commonly performed dermatologic procedures. We use the term *cryosurgery* here because the term *cryotherapy* is now more commonly associated with the treatment of internal malignancies and non-FDA-approved whole-body cryotherapy spas. There are many different ways to achieve cold temperatures, but clinically, the end result is to freeze the fluid in cells, which causes crystals that damage the cells, resulting in tissue destruction. Different cell types are destroyed at different temperatures (see Table 13.1). Melanocytes are relatively fragile, causing a risk for hypopigmentation with their death. Cartilage and bone are most resistant to freezing and other cells less resistant but not as fragile as melanocytes.

Cryosurgery is an easily mastered technique that is extremely useful for treating benign and premalignant lesions. In experienced hands, cryosurgery is also a valuable technique for treating small, nonaggressive nonmelanoma skin cancers (NMSCs).

Indications

Cryosurgery is most often used to treat actinic keratoses and benign conditions. Table 13.2 provides recommended freeze times and margins of freeze for benign conditions (using liquid nitrogen with an open spray technique). Table 13.3 gives recommended freeze times and margins of freeze for vascular conditions (using liquid nitrogen with a closed probe or an open spray technique). Table 13.4 lists recommendations for treating premalignant and malignant conditions (using liquid nitrogen with an open spray technique). Details on how to perform these procedures follow.

Contraindications

- Cryosurgery is almost never an appropriate treatment for melanoma except for palliation in rare cases.

- Nevi should not be treated with cryosurgery because if a nevus were to grow back, it might appear malignant, and a biopsy could be suspicious for melanoma (pseudomelanoma).
- Cryosurgery should not be used for NMSCs that are aggressive. This includes recurrent basal cell carcinoma (BCC) or squamous cell carcinoma (SCC), any large BCC or SCC, sclerosing BCC, micronodular BCC, poorly differentiated SCC, and any skin cancer with perineural spread. Avoid cryosurgery for cancers on the ala of the nose, the lip, and the ear. If Mohs surgery is indicated, cryosurgery is usually not.

Contraindications for cryosurgery are listed in Table 13.5.

Advantages of Cryosurgery

The advantages of cryosurgery can be categorized into those for the clinician and those for the patient. Advantages for the clinician include the following:

- Ease of procedure
- Speed of procedure
- Multiple lesions may be treated at the same visit
- No need for injection of anesthetic (unless treating skin cancers for which the freeze times are longer)
- Clean procedure with no contamination or need for antiseptics
- Relatively low supply cost after initial investment
- Has an 83% to 88% cure rate for actinic keratoses[1-3]
Advantages for the patient include:
- Ease of procedure
- Speed of procedure
- No injections (in noncancerous lesions)
- Pain is tolerable (for adults and many children over age 8).
- No sutures

Table 13.1 Key Events During Freezing Including Cell Death

Temperature (°C)	Event
+11 to +3	65% of capillaries and 35% to 40% of arterioles and venules develop thrombosis.
−0.6	Freezing begins to occur in tissue.
−4 to −7	Melanocytes die.
−15 to −20	100% of blood vessels develop thrombosis.
−20	Cells in sebaceous glands and hair follicles die.
−21.8	Ice crystals theoretically form in the tissue (the eutectic temperature of sodium chloride solution).
−20 to −30	Keratinocytes and malignant cells die.
−30 to −35	Fibroblasts die.
−50 to −60	All cells die including cartilage cells.

Source: Adapted from Vidimos A, Ammirati C, Poblete-Lopez C. *Dermatologic Surgery.* Saunders; 2008; Table 8.3.

Table 13.2 Cryosurgery of Benign Lesions

Name of Skin Lesion	Freeze Time* Total (seconds)	Freeze-Thaw Cycles	Halo Diameter (mm)	Open Spray (OS) Probe (P) Forceps (F) or Tweezer Cotton-Tipped Applicator (CTA) Intralesional Steroid (IS)
Acne cysts	5–10[†]	1	0	OS
Acrochordon – skin tags	5	1–2	0	OS or F
Angiofibromas (adenoma sebaceum)	10	1	0	P or OS
Angiomas (cherry and spider angiomas)[††]	5–10	1	0	P or OS
Benign lichenoid keratosis	5–10	1	2	OS
Chondrodermatitis nodularis	5–10	2	1–2	OS
Dermatofibromas	10	2	2 mm	OS
Dermatosis papulosa nigra	5	1	0–1	OS
Digital mucous cyst	10	2	0	OS after needling
Granulation tissue	5–10	2	0	OS
Granuloma annulare	5–10	1–2	0	OS
Keloids and hypertrophic scars	5–10	1	1	OS (with IS)
Lymphangioma circumscriptum	10	1–2	1	P
Molluscum	5	1–2	0	OS
Mucocele	10	1	0	P or OS
Pearly penile papules	5	2	0	OS
Porokeratosis	5–10	1	1	OS
Prurigo nodularis	10	1	1	OS (consider IS)
Pyogenic granuloma	10–15	2	1	F or P
Sebaceous hyperplasia	5–10	1	0	OS or P
Seborrheic keratoses	5–15	1–2	2	OS
Solar lentigo	3–5	1	0	OS or CTA
Syringoma	3	2	0	P or OS, F
Tattoos	15	2	1	OS
Venous lake	5–10	2	1–1.5	P
Viral warts (common, flat, plantar)	5–10	1–2	1–2	OS
Filiform wart	5	1–2	1	F or OS
Anogenital wart	5	2	1	OS
Xanthelasma	3	1–2	0	P or F

Disclaimer: All times are based on the available studies and author experience.

*The freeze time is a good starting time for an initial treatment. It is based on times for smaller to medium-sized lesions that have not been treated before.

[†]The freeze time range includes a range of times based on the variable sizes and locations of lesions. Smaller lesions on thinner, more delicate skin should receive treatments at the lower end of the range. The appropriate freeze time varies depending upon the aperture and configuration of the spray tip and whether or not a continuous or pulsatile spray is applied.

[††]Many vascular conditions are best treated with electrosurgery or lasers except for a venous lake, in which cryosurgery is a preferred treatment. Cryosurgery for the other vascular conditions is an option. Regardless of the vascular lesion being treated, the closed probe technique with applied pressure is recommended.

Source: Adapted from Usatine R, Stulberg DL, Colver G, Jackson A. *Cutaneous Cryosurgery: Principles and Clinical Practice.* 4th ed. CRC Press, Taylor & Francis Group; 2015.

Table 13.3   Recommendations for Treating Premalignant Conditions* (Using Liquid Nitrogen With an Open Spray Technique)

Premalignant and Malignant	Freeze Time (seconds)†	Freeze-Thaw Cycles	Halo Diameter (mm)
Actinic keratosis	5–10	1–2	1
Actinic cheilitis	5	2	0
Bowen's disease (skin)	20–30	1–2	2
Bowen's disease (genitalia)	15–20	1	2

*Cryosurgery is a preferred treatment based on good evidence for actinic keratoses. It is also preferred for actinic cheilitis. Treatments for actinic keratoses and actinic cheilitis may be followed by topical treatments for better field treatment. Cryosurgery for Bowen's disease (SCC in situ) is one option among many choices including surgery, electrodesiccation, and curettage based on the lesion, location, and patient preference.

†Freeze times – includes a range of times based on the variable sizes and locations of lesions. Smaller lesions on thinner, more delicate skin should receive treatments at the lower end of the range. Patients receiving treatments of 20 seconds or more should be offered local anesthetic first. All times are based on the available studies and author experience.

Source: Adapted from Usatine R, Stulberg DL, Colver G, Jackson A. *Cutaneous Cryosurgery: Principles and Clinical Practice*. 4th ed. CRC Press, Taylor & Francis Group; 2015.

Table 13.4   Recommendations for Treating Malignant Conditions* (Using Liquid Nitrogen With an Open Spray Technique)

Type of Lesion	Freeze Time Average (seconds)†	Freeze-Thaw Cycles	Halo Diameter (mm)
Superficial BCC (not on face)	25–30	1	3–5
Nodular BCC (not on face)	30	2	3–5
BCC (face)	30	2	3–5
Keratoacanthoma	30	2	4–5
SCC in situ (Bowen's disease)	30	2	4–5
SCC	30	2	4–5

*Cryosurgery for in situ and malignant conditions is only one treatment option, and the others including surgery, electrodesiccation and curettage, and Mohs surgery should be discussed with the patient. Cryosurgery should not be used for large (>2 cm) and/or aggressive BCC or SCC and any cancer with perineural invasion.

†Freeze times – includes a range of times based on the variable sizes and locations of lesions. Smaller lesions on thinner, more delicate skin should receive treatments at the lower end of the range. Patients receiving treatments of 20 seconds or more should be offered local anesthetic first. All times are based on the available studies and author experience.

Source: Adapted from Usatine R, Stulberg DL, Colver G, Jackson A. *Cutaneous Cryosurgery: Principles and Clinical Practice*. 4th ed. CRC Press, Taylor & Francis Group; 2015.

Table 13.5   Contraindications for Cryosurgery

Contraindications	Category
BY LESION	
Melanoma	A
Recurrent basal cell carcinoma (BCC) or SCC	A
Histologically aggressive BCC, SCC (defined in Chapter 24)	A
BCC or SCC >2 cm or in high-risk areas (H zone on face – see Chapter 24)	A
Nevus	A
Any undiagnosed lesion suspicious for nonmelanoma malignancy (tissue should be sent for pathology first)	R
BY AREA	
Skin cancer on ala nasi and nasolabial fold	R
Neoplasm of upper lip near vermillion border	R
Neoplasm over the shins	R
BY PATIENT	
Previous adverse reaction to cryotherapy (e.g., cold anaphylaxis)	A
Cryoglobulinemia	R
Myeloma, lymphoma	R
Autoimmune disorders (including pyoderma gangrenosum)	R
Raynaud's disease, especially when lesion is on fingers, toes, nose, ears, penis	R

A, Absolute; R, relative.

Disadvantages of Cryosurgery

As with the advantages of cryosurgery, the disadvantages can also be categorized into those for the clinician and those for the patient. Disadvantages for the clinician include the following:

- Liquid nitrogen needs to be delivered and stored in a secure ventilated area (generally inexpensive but may be more difficult to obtain in a remote rural area).
- The clinician must be confident of the diagnosis because no tissue will be sent for pathology.
- Cryosurgery is not as accurate as a scalpel or laser in cosmetic work.
  Disadvantages for the patient include:
- Erythema and swelling are the norm. Blistering is common.
- Pain, especially throbbing pain around the nail folds
- Pain with walking if plantar warts are treated
- May require multiple visits
- Hypopigmentation (see the *Complications* section later in this chapter for more risks)

Equipment for Liquid Nitrogen

- Dewar (holding container) and dispensing device (Figure 13.1)
- Spray guns (Figure 13.2)

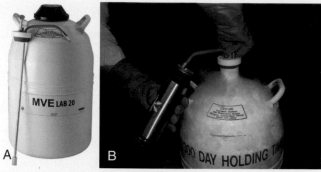

Figure 13.1 (A) Dewar tank and liquid nitrogen dispenser. **(B)** When the dispenser is placed within the tank and a seal is obtained, the liquid nitrogen rises through the metal tube and comes out through the filter at the end of the blue tube to fill the cryosurgical spray gun. (A, Copyright Brymill, Inc; B, Copyright Richard P. Usatine, MD.)

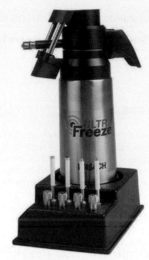

Figure 13.3 Wallach liquid nitrogen spray gun and tips. (Copyright Wallach, Inc.)

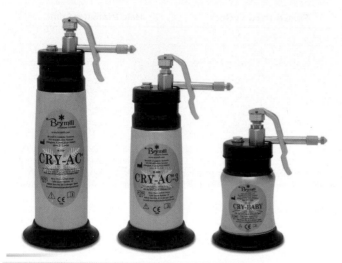

Figure 13.2 Three types of cryosurgical spray guns from Brymill. (Copyright Brymill, Inc.)

- Cryo Tweezers (for skin tags) (Figure 13.3)
- Various tips and probes (Figure 13.4)
- Styrofoam cups for use with Cryo Tweezers.

While we suggest liquid nitrogen as the gold standard, other methods involve the following equipment:

- Compressed gas in tanks or cartridges with appropriate gun or spray tips (nitrous oxide or carbon dioxide)
- Refrigeration – mechanically cooled probe
- Refrigerant liquids that evaporate with associated cones and swabs.

Cryosurgery: Principles and Getting Started

- Factors that affect the freezing of tissue are listed and explained in Table 13.6.
- If you do not know the diagnosis, do not use cryosurgery. Lesions well suited to treatment with cryosurgery are listed in Tables 13.2 to 13.4.
- Advise the patient regarding treatment options and expected results.

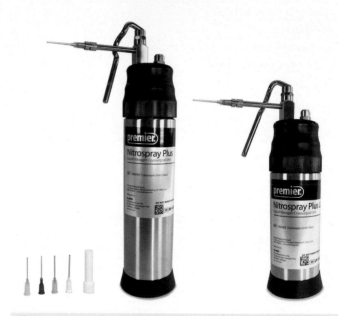

Figure 13.4 Premier Nitrospray gun with needle tips. (Copyright Premier, Inc.)

- Obtain informed consent at the time of the procedure based on the risks and benefits as laid out in this chapter. Most of the time, verbal consent should be adequate. If the procedure could result in hypopigmentation on the face, it may be a good idea to get written consent.

Cryosurgery Methods

Many different techniques are used to perform cryosurgery. The most common ones are listed in Table 13.7, which explains how the cryogen is applied and its temperature.

LIQUID NITROGEN *(See Video 13.1)*

Most dermatologists and many primary care providers have access to liquid nitrogen. It is the gold standard for

Table 13.6 Factors That Affect the Freezing of Tissue

Factor	Key Principles
Rate of tissue freezing	Rapid freezing causes more cell death. In the open spray technique, this is influenced by the rate of liquid nitrogen spray to the skin (aperture and configuration of the spray conduit).
Rate of intermittent spraying	A faster rate for an intermittent spray results in a deeper but narrower depth of freeze. A slower rate for an intermittent spray results in a more superficial but wider depth of freeze.
Halo diameter	The wider the halo, the deeper the freeze at the periphery of the lesion.
Distance of spray tip to tissue	The closer the tip is to the tissue, the colder the tissue may become because air is not as good a conductor as tissue.
Tissue temperature	Final tissue temperature of less than $-30°C$ will kill malignant cells.
Duration of freezing	Having the tissue remain adequately frozen for a longer period of time causes more tissue injury. Maximum cell death rate occurs at 100 seconds.
Rate of thawing	Slow thawing causes more cell death.
Repetition of freeze-thaw cycles	More freeze-thaw cycles cause more cell death. Malignant tumors require multiple freeze-thaw cycles. All cellular structures show damage by electron microscopy after two cycles below $-30°C$.

Source: Adapted from Vidimos A, Ammirati C, Poblete-Lopez C. *Dermatologic Surgery.* Saunders; 2008; Table 8.2.

Table 13.7 Forms of Various Cryogens and Temperatures

Cryogens	Form	Temperatures (°C)
Liquid nitrogen	Open spray, closed probes, and CTA Tissue temperature is less cold if delivered with CTA.	-196
Nitrous oxide in tank	Closed probes on special gun	-89
CO_2 in tank	Closed probes on special gun	-79
CryoPen	Refrigerated closed probes	-75
Verruca-Freeze (chlorodifluoromethane and propane)	Chemical spray into cones or disposable buds with evaporation producing the cold	-70
Wartner (dimethyl ether and propane)	OTC foam applicator for warts only	-57
Histofreezer (dimethyl ether and propane)	Application is via disposable 2- and 5-mm buds	-55

cryosurgery. Various cryoguns are available that efficiently and effectively deliver the liquid nitrogen to the skin at the coldest temperatures.

Liquid nitrogen is stored in dewar containers ranging in size from 5 to 50 L. The nitrogen may be withdrawn using a ladle, a valve system, or a withdrawal tube (Figure 13.1). The withdrawal tube is the most simple and efficient way to extract liquid nitrogen from the storage container. *See video 13.2.*

For those clinicians who are still working with cotton-tipped applicators (CTAs) and liquid nitrogen in a cup, it is possible to do cryosurgery on benign and premalignant conditions. This method does not get cold enough for treating cancer or most vascular lesions. Dip the CTA into the liquid nitrogen and then touch the CTA to the lesion to be treated. The CTA can be unwound a bit and rewound to make a smaller point, or loose cotton from a cotton ball can be wrapped around the CTA for larger lesions to maintain the freezing temperature longer. The increased amount of cotton will hold more liquid N_2 to extend the freezing time.

A more time-effective and more efficacious approach is to use a *cryogun* (Figures 13.21, 3.3, and 13.4). Once filled, the unit can be used to treat many lesions rapidly. The spray method allows the clinician to reach tissue temperatures of up to $-62°C$ (based on our measurements with a thermocouple), while the CTA is not likely to get below $-20°C$. Although there

is a cost involved in the purchase of a cryogun, these units can last a clinician's full career and pay for themselves very quickly. The reimbursement for cryosurgery is excellent for only a few minutes of your time.

Michael D. Bryne developed the first commercially available handheld spray device using liquid nitrogen for medical use in 1968. His family continues to run the Brymill Corporation, which sells the most widely used cryoguns. The variety of cryoguns available from Brymill include (Figure 13.2):

- CRY-AC®, standard 500-mL capacity – the main workhorse unit
- CRY-AC®-3, smaller capacity of 300 mL – easy handling with shorter holding time
- CRYBABY® smallest capacity of 150 mL – very portable with shortest holding time

Wallach, Premier, and other companies also make various liquid N_2 (LN_2) sprayers (Figures 13.3 and 13.4). Whichever LN_2 sprayer you use, it helps to have an assortment of apertures and tips. The tips that are available for the Brymill cryoguns include:

- Four spray tips with round apertures from 0.04 to 0.016 inches, with A being the largest and D the smallest (Figure 13.5). The C tip is a good all-purpose tip.

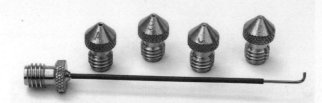

Figure 13.5 Spray tips A through D are arranged in order of largest aperture to the smallest aperture. One extended bent spray tip in front. (Copyright Brymill, Inc.)

- Long 20-gauge bent directional spray tip with blue cover. This longer tube (3 inches) with an 80-degree angle attenuates the flow of the LN$_2$ so that the spray is less shocking to the patient (Figure 13.5). This is good for children and adults who fear this therapy. It also allows for pinpoint accuracy on smaller lesions. It can be helpful for treating anogenital condylomas because it allows the clinician to be further from the lesions being treated with a tight freeze diameter to avoid overspray and damage to surrounding sensitive tissues.
- Shorter straight metallic color tips have similar benefits to the long blue tube but with less attenuation of flow. This is a good all-purpose tip. Figure 13.6 shows a comparison of the open aperture tips.
- Closed probes are useful on vascular lesions to compress the lesion and freeze it simultaneously (Figure 13.7). Closed probes come in many sizes and shapes, ranging from 1 mm to 2.5 cm in diameter. The probes are available in round flat shapes, conical and spherical shapes,

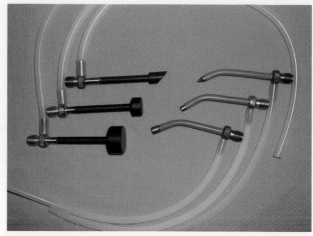

Figure 13.7 Closed cryoprobes with different shapes and sizes apply simultaneous pressure and freezing. These are especially helpful when treating vascular lesions. The liquid nitrogen is vented out of the white plastic tube. (Copyright Richard P. Usatine, MD.)

and shapes for use on the cervix. The liquid nitrogen is vented out of a plastic tube so that no spray touches the patient. The spray freezes the probe tip for direct application to a lesion. One method to avoid the probe sticking to the skin is to freeze the probe before applying it to the patient. The closed probes have a "low" infection risk since there is no breach of the patient's skin. Cleaning of the closed probes can be done with an alcohol wipe or antiviral antibacterial wipe after and prior to use.

A *cryoplate* is a transparent plate with four conical openings of various diameters (3, 5, 8, and 10 mm) (Figure 13.8). Used with A–D apertures, the cryoplate provides localization of freezing and protection of sensitive areas such as the eyes. It is good for the novice but is limited by the fact that each opening is round and includes a preset diameter.

Cryocones come as a set of six Neoprene cones of various sizes used to concentrate spray within a limited area. These can be used for irregularly shaped lesions because they can be shaped to the lesion. Sizes are 6, 11, 16, 25, 30, and

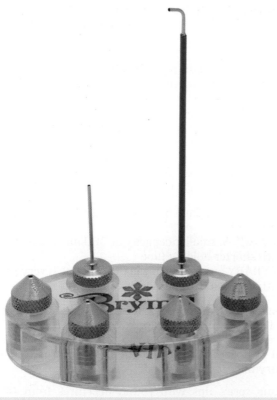

Figure 13.6 Spray tips with different apertures. One extended blue bent spray tip and one straight spray tip. (Copyright Brymill, Inc.)

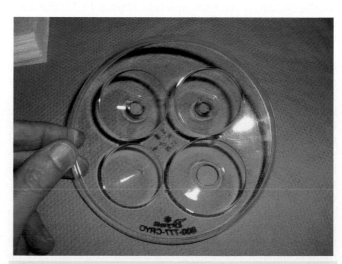

Figure 13.8 A cryoplate with four different size apertures for controlled freezing diameters. (Copyright Richard P. Usatine, MD.)

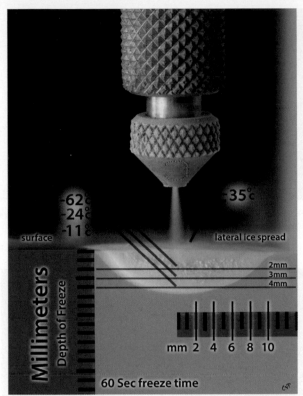

Figure 13.9 The liquid nitrogen sprays from the tip at −196°C, and the cold dissipates in the tissues farther from the direct spray. An ice ball was produced by a spot freeze for 60 seconds using liquid nitrogen sprayed through a C-tip onto an agar plate. The ice ball spreads out in a hemispherical pattern. Temperatures were measured using a thermocouple below the surface and infrared sensors from a Cry-Ac® TrackerCam on the surface. The ice ball is coldest at the center just below the surface. While the surface is receiving the cold spray it also is warmed by the ambient air above the agar, and the measured temperatures are somewhat colder just below the surface. In living tissue, circulating blood warms the deeper parts so that the gradients are somewhat different. The coldest points of the ice ball are at the center, no matter the depth or model. (Copyright Richard P. Usatine, MD and Craig LaPlante.)

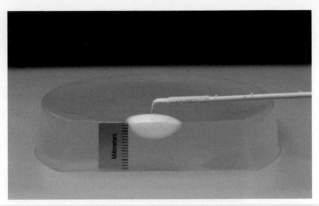

Figure 13.10 A real-life demonstration of the shape of the ice ball produced when liquid nitrogen is sprayed at a single point of agar. The ice ball spreads out in a hemispherical pattern. The coldest point of the ice ball is the center just below the surface. (Copyright Richard P. Usatine, MD.)

Cryosurgery With Liquid Nitrogen Spray: Steps and Principles

See Videos 13.3–13.7

1. Hold the cryogun relatively upright to avoid having the LN$_2$ suddenly come out of the pressure relief valve and scare everyone in the room. This release from the pressure valve usually does not happen unless the cryogun is tilted to the horizontal position.
2. Make sure that the patient is in a stable position and not a moving target. If the lesion is on the hand, see that the hand is resting on the exam table or patient's leg so as not to move.
3. Hold the tip 1 to 2 cm from the lesion, making sure that the spray is perpendicular to the skin (Figure 13.11A). If using a bent spray probe, adjust the position of the cryogun and tip to achieve a 90-degree angle to the skin (Figure 13.11B). Stabilize your hands and body so that your aim will be accurate and consistent.
4. Compress the trigger to start the spray. The pattern of spray should be determined by the size, elevation, and depth of the lesion. The following techniques are options:
   - Steady continuous spray will produce a wider and shallower freeze zone. This may be sufficient for actinic keratoses and seborrheic keratoses.
   - Pulsing the spray intermittently in one spot will cause the freeze to stay localized (less lateral spread) and deepen with the duration of spray. This is good for thicker lesions such as common warts, molluscum, dermatofibromas, and keloids.
   - Using a paintbrush technique moving the spray in a spiral or back-and-forth motion will give a more superficial freeze for larger superficial lesions including solar lentigines. Moving the spray back and forth across the lip may be more tolerable for diffuse actinic cheilitis than freezing one portion at a time as the lip is very sensitive (Figure 13.12).
5. Make sure that the freeze reaches all edges of the lesion with the desired halo diameter (see Tables 13.2 to 13.4). The halo is the area of normal skin around the lesion that is frozen (Figure 13.13). It should be symmetrical around the lesion. When the lesion is not

38 mm. Some people use plastic ear specula to control their freeze diameters.

When working around sensitive structures including the eyes, a tongue depressor can be used to shield the eye from the overspray.

Freezing Times, Thaw Times, and Halo Diameters

The amount of tissue destruction can be estimated by the duration of active freezing (freeze time), the amount of thaw time (time until the ice ball is defrosted and is no longer white), and the margin of frozen tissue around the lesion (halo diameter). Factors that affect the freezing of tissue are summarized in Table 13.6.

Figure 13.9 shows how the temperature of the freeze is lowest in the middle of a continuous stationary freeze and why a halo diameter is helpful. Figure 13.10 shows the typical geometry of the hemispherical freeze that occurs in the tissues. Intermittent (pulsatile) spraying can increase the duration and depth of freeze with minimal increase in freeze diameter.

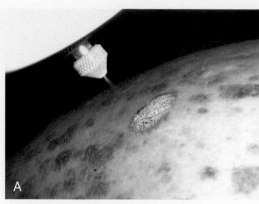
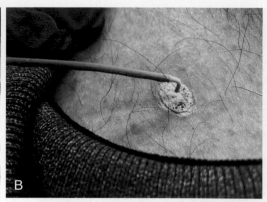

Figure 13.11 (A) Cryosurgery performed using liquid nitrogen sprayed at 90 degrees to the surface with a C-tip at a height of 1 to 2 cm from a seborrheic keratosis. **(B)** Cryosurgery of another seborrheic keratosis using a bent tip spray aligned at 90 degrees to the surface. (Copyright Richard P. Usatine, MD.)

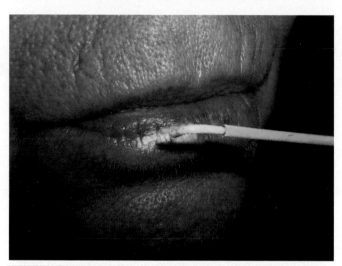

Figure 13.12 Actinic cheilitis is being frozen using a bent spray tip and a paintbrush-type motion back and forth to minimize the pain and keep the freeze from going too deep. (Copyright Richard P. Usatine, MD.)

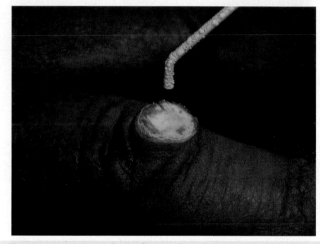

Figure 13.14 A wart is being frozen after excessive keratin was pared down with a sharp sterile razor. (Copyright Richard P. Usatine, MD.)

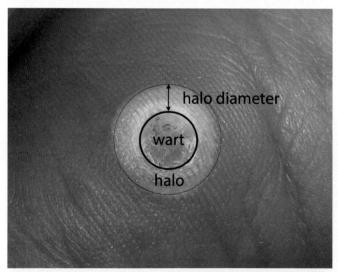

Figure 13.13 Halo diameter around a common wart to ensure a lethal freeze at the edge of the wart. One should attempt to create a halo that is symmetrical 360 degrees around the wart. (Copyright Richard P. Usatine, MD.)

circular, it may be necessary to move the spray slightly back and forth to achieve an oval or linear pattern instead of a circle.

6. Freeze to the time suggested in Tables 13.2 to 13.4. Smaller lesions on thinner, more delicate skin should receive treatments at the lower end of the time range.

7. Watch the thawing. If the area thaws asymmetrically, one area might not have received sufficient freeze time. You can add some freezing to that area. If the whole area thaws faster than expected, consider a second freeze-thaw cycle.

8. If the lesion is very thick (especially with warts) consider paring it down with a scalpel or razor blade so that the base can be more effectively treated (Figure 13.14).

9. If you will be treating a lesion for more than 20 seconds, give the patient a choice to have a local anesthetic first. In particular, if you are treating a malignancy with two 30-second freezes, local anesthesia with lidocaine is necessary. While epinephrine is not needed for hemostasis, it does slow systemic absorption of the lidocaine. Lidocaine without epinephrine is also acceptable.

10. Most unanesthetized patients become very uncomfortable with freeze times over 10 seconds (watch their

body language and facial expressions) and consider stopping when this discomfort occurs. Then use a second freeze time to reach the desired total freeze time.

Cryosurgery With Liquid Nitrogen Probes: Steps and Principles

1. If you do not have a probe equal to the size of the lesion, you should choose a probe smaller than the lesion, and freeze the area until the desired freeze margin is achieved. A probe larger than the lesion would unnecessarily destroy normal surrounding tissue.
2. Make sure the spray hose vent is facing away from the patient and provider to avoid unwanted freezing (Figure 13.15).
3. Freeze the end of the probe before applying it to the patient to prevent the probe from sticking to the patient.
4. If the probe sticks to the patient, do not pull it off because significant tissue damage may occur. If the probe is taking longer than expected to detach from the patient, use your fingers or warm water to rewarm the adherent probe.

LIQUID NITROGEN: CRYO TWEEZERS

See Videos 13.8–13.9

Cryo Tweezers are designed to freeze skin tags and other small raised lesions without the overspray and inaccuracy inherent in spraying a small raised target. The Cryo Tweezers have a Teflon-coated brass tweezer end that holds the cold temperature after dipping them in liquid nitrogen. They have a thin "necked" portion between the heavy tweezer ends and the handle to minimize the cold spread up the handle (Figure 13.16). The tweezers should be dipped into a Styrofoam cup with LN_2 so that the tips are covered, but not the handles. The initial dip should be long enough that the LN_2 has stopped boiling away from the originally warm tweezer tips (about 20 seconds). Avoid leaving the tweezers in the liquid nitrogen after the bubbling settles as the handles will get unnecessarily cold. Expect the handle to get cold, so it helps to wrap them in one to two 4 × 4 gauzes or paper towel to protect the clinician's fingers. Alternatively,

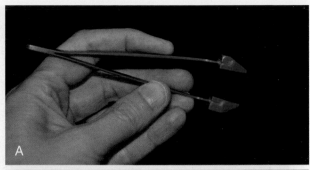
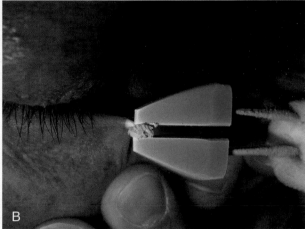

Figure 13.16 (A) The Cryo Tweezer at room temperature. **(B)** Cryo Tweezer being used to freeze a filiform wart on the lower eyelid. Note how the freeze reaches the normal tissue. 4 × 4 Cotton gauze is used to protect the clinician's hand. (Copyright Richard P. Usatine, MD.)

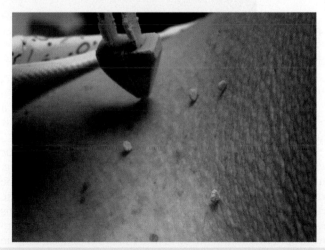

Figure 13.17 The Cryo Tweezer is an ideal instrument for quickly freezing small to medium skin tags with minimal pain and no bleeding. (Copyright Daniel L. Stulberg, MD.)

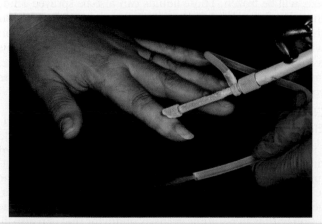

Figure 13.15 A cryoprobe can be used to treat a pyogenic granuloma over the finger joint to avoid the scarring that might occur with surgery or electrosurgery. The cryoprobe was made cold before applying to the lesion, and the vent was pointed away from the patient. The physician did not continue to hold the vent once it began to freeze. (Copyright Richard P. Usatine, MD.)

an insulated glove can be used to handle the Cryo Tweezers. The skin tags are then grasped and held with the Cryo Tweezers until the freeze margin reaches normal tissue at the skin surface (Figure 13.16). The tweezers can be used to treat many skin tags before they warm up. When treating more than 10 skin tags (Figure 13.17) you may need to redip the tweezers when you note that the freeze time is lengthening.

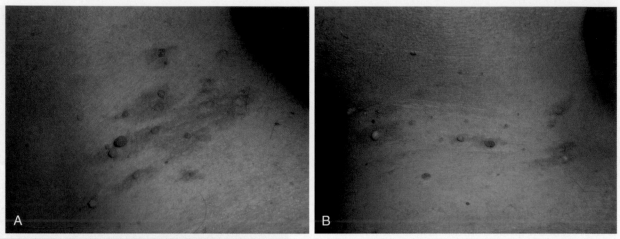

Figure 13.18 Two methods of treating skin tags with cryosurgery. **(A)** Cryo spray was applied to one side of the neck and showing the erythema caused by the overspray. **(B)** Cryo Tweezers applied to the skin tags of the other side of the neck in the same patient show much less collateral damage to the surrounding skin. (Copyright Richard P. Usatine, MD.)

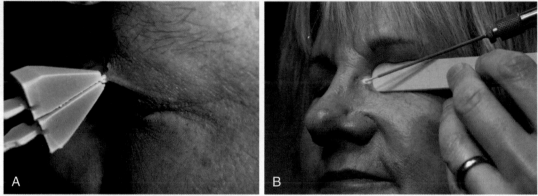

Figure 13.19 (A) The Cryo Tweezer can safely treat skin tags or warts on the eyelids. The lesion is grasped carefully and pulled away from the eye; the cold will not be transmitted to the eye itself. **(B)** A tongue depressor can be used to protect the eye while freezing a small benign lesion next to the eye. (Copyright Richard P. Usatine, MD.)

When patients are treated with Cryo Tweezers and a cryogun, most will state that the Cryo Tweezer hurts less. It causes less damage to surrounding tissue (Figure 13.18).

The Cryo Tweezers are particularly good for skin tags or warts on the eyelids. After grasping the elevated papule, pull the whole lid away from the eye to protect the globe from cryodamage (Figure 13.19A). Then continue the freeze until the whole tag or wart is white to the base. This avoids any spray that may enter the eye. Another method to avoid spraying liquid nitrogen into the eye is to use a tongue depressor as a protective shield (Figure 13.19B).

Cryo Tweezers can be cleaned between patients with an alcohol wipe or other antiviral antibacterial wipe. The LN$_2$ itself does not kill viruses even though it kills human cells invaded by viruses.

ALTERNATIVES TO LIQUID NITROGEN

Evaporative Liquids

Volatile liquids produce cold temperatures when they evaporate. They are commercially available compressed in various spray cans. These can be directly applied to a lesion by spraying into a cone placed firmly against the patient's skin to prevent the liquid from running out. After the evaporation, the lesion and a surrounding margin, based on the cone size, will be frozen. These liquids can also be sprayed on or through (depending on the brand) a foam-tipped applicator that comes with the product and then applied to the lesion with a CTA and liquid nitrogen (see earlier discussion). This technique has a lower initial cost for equipment but is not as fast and versatile in its use. Also, the temperatures are not as cold (see Table 13.6).

Closed Probes (Nitrous Oxide, Carbon Dioxide, or Electrical Refrigeration)

Closed probes can be chilled by guns that release compressed nitrous oxide or carbon dioxide or by an electrical refrigerating device (CryoPen). The CryoPen can be touched to the lesion, with varying size tips, similar to applying liquid nitrogen with a CTA. Other closed probes are placed against the lesion with water-soluble gel as a conductor that can also fill in gaps in the tissues. Dip the tip into a dab of water-soluble gel on a paper towel, and then touch the tip to the lesion. For efficiency, touch the tip with the gel onto a number of lesions before starting the cryosurgery. After the tip is in contact with the lesion, activate the cryogun and hold in place until the desired freeze is obtained. Lifting the device and the skin after the skin has adhered due to the contact freeze may spare deeper tissues from freezing.

Complications

Complications of cryosurgery are listed in Box 13.1. Careful and thoughtful application of the principles in this chapter will prevent most complications.

Box 13.1 Pitfalls in Cryosurgery

Expected (More Often With Longer, Deeper Freezes)

- Pain during freezing, thawing, and healing
- Blister formation – sometimes hemorrhagic (Figure 13.20)
- Intradermal hemorrhage
- Edema around treatment site
- Weeping of fluid (especially after treating cancer)

Immediate and Less Common

- Headache affecting forehead, temples, and scalp
- Syncope

Delayed and Rare

- Infection of the wound site
- Hemorrhage from the wound site
- Pyogenic granuloma

Prolonged and Rare

- Milia
- Hypertrophic scars
- Neuropathic pain at cryosurgery site

Occasional Permanent Unintended Consequences

- Hypopigmentation (most common and most visible in persons of color)
- Nail dystrophy (when treating periungual warts)
- Ectropion and notching of eyelids
- Tenting or notching of the vermilion border of the lip, ear, or ala of nose
- Atrophic or depressed scar
- Alopecia

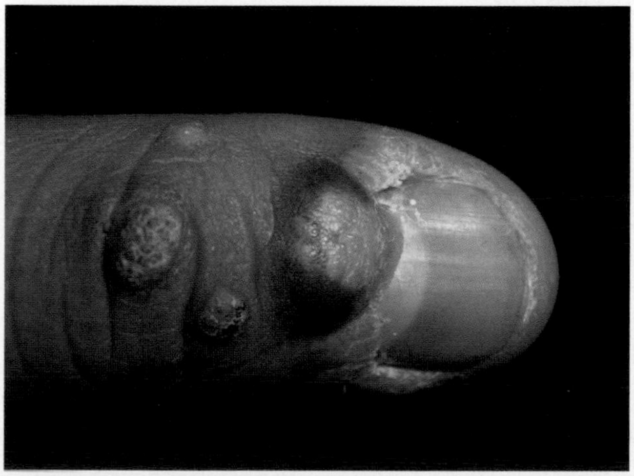

Treating Specific Lesions

CONDYLOMA

Condyloma acuminata are generally very responsive to cryosurgery. Many lesions can be treated rapidly without local anesthetic. Consider offering topical or local anesthetic to patients who have larger lesions. The bent spray tips are particularly useful for genital and perianal condyloma because the spray volume and speed are somewhat attenuated (Figure 13.21). While this may require slightly longer freeze times, it improves patient comfort during the procedure. The end of the spray tip should be held within 1 cm of the lesion so it freezes (Figure 13.22). The Cryo Tweezers are also excellent for small raised or flat condyloma. With the thin, flexible skin of the penile shaft, even relatively flat lesions can be pinched, elevated, and treated with the tweezers with less discomfort than standard cryo spray. The patient may be given a prescription for a topical medication such as podofilox or imiquimod to start 2 weeks

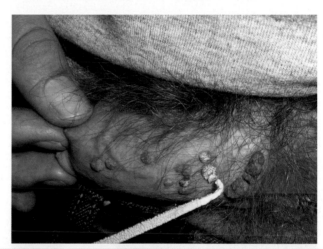

Figure 13.21 An open spray technique is being used to treat condyloma on the penis. The bent spray tip is held close to the condyloma so that the freeze can be carefully controlled. (Copyright Richard P. Usatine, MD.)

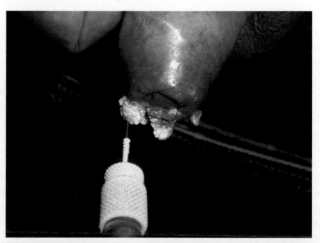

Figure 13.22 Condyloma acuminata on the foreskin has caused a phimosis and is now being treated with cryosurgery to the offending lesions with a straight-tip aperture. (Copyright Richard P. Usatine, MD.)

Figure 13.20 Hemorrhagic blisters formed after a vigorous freeze of periungual warts. This is not an uncommon reaction to cryosurgery and will resolve with no treatment and no harm. (Copyright Richard P. Usatine, MD.)

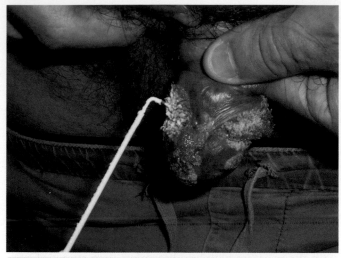

Figure 13.23 Cryosurgery to these large condyloma acuminata is much less painful now that EMLA cream is being applied to the lesions 10 minutes before treatment in the clinic. (Copyright Richard P. Usatine, MD.)

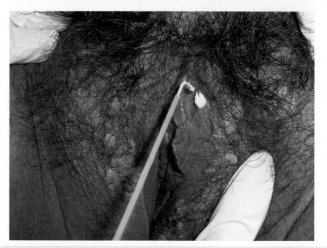

Figure 13.24 Condyloma acuminata on the vulva is being treated with cryosurgery using the bent tip spray after the patient applied EMLA cream at home. (Copyright Richard P. Usatine, MD.)

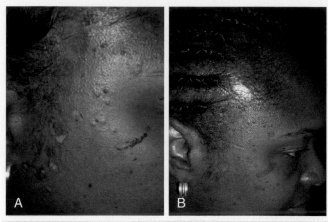

Figure 13.25 Dermatosis papulosis nigra that was treated with liquid nitrogen using an open spray technique. **(A)** Hypopigmentation occurred around many of the treated lesions within the first month. **(B)** The hypopigmentation was temporary, and the patient was delighted with the final result of treatment. (Copyright Richard P. Usatine, MD.)

DERMATOSIS PAPULOSIS NIGRA

The many small seborrheic keratoses that make up dermatosis papulosis nigra (DPN) can be treated with cryosurgery. Because DPN is more frequently found on the face of women of color, it is important to avoid causing permanent hypopigmentation. This risk should be clearly spelled out and accepted by the patient before starting therapy. This is one time when we suggest getting a written consent signed. It also is prudent to test the cryosurgery out on a few lesions away from the midface to see how the patient will respond before treating many central lesions. The patient in Figure 13.25 was very pleased with her results. She was willing to accept some temporary or permanent hypopigmentation just to make sure that her seborrheic keratoses were flattened so that they would not show under makeup. For patients with dark skin, it is good to offer simple electrodestruction as an alternative, since that method may be less likely to cause permanent hypopigmentation (see Chapter 14).

KELOIDS AND HYPERTROPHIC SCARS
(See Video 13.7)

Keloids and hypertrophic scars can be a frustrating and cosmetically disfiguring complication of injury or irritation to the skin. Treatments have included steroid injections, applying silicone sheeting, and excising and injecting the margins with steroids and cryotherapy alone or in conjunction with steroid injection. The data on the use of cryotherapy is nicely summarized in Table 13.8. Cryosurgery as mentioned can lead to hypopigmentation and occasionally postinflammatory hyperpigmentation as in Figure 13.22.[1]

MOLLUSCUM CONTAGIOSUM

Cryosurgery is an excellent treatment method for molluscum. The greatest limiting factor is the age and maturity of the patient. This technique should not be used with young and fearful children unless they are willing to cooperate with treatment. For older children and adults, molluscum can be treated using the open spray technique. Because molluscum can be so small, the bent spray tips are particularly

after cryosurgery. If the patient cannot afford one of these topical medications, cryosurgery may be repeated every 2 to 3 weeks until the lesions are gone.

Topical anesthetics such as lidocaine/prilocaine 2.5%/2.5% are effective especially for HPV on moist mucosal surfaces rather than fully keratinized skin. Cauliflower-like condyloma on moist mucosal surfaces such as under the foreskin of an uncircumcised man may achieve significant numbing within 5 minutes allowing for in-office application of lidocaine/prilocaine 2.5%/2.5% (Figure 13.23). Use of this lidocaine/prilocaine 2.5%/2.5% on the shaft of the penis or the keratinized vulva may require 1 to 2 hours for significant numbing and may be best applied at home after the patient has been given a prescription to use (Figure 13.24).

Make sure you use site-specific billing codes for cryosurgery of the penis, vulva, or perianal area. These do pay at a higher rate (see Table 28.3 in Chapter 28).

Table 13.8   Cryosurgery of Keloids and Hypertrophic Scars: Clinical Results

Study	Total Number of Patients	Significant to Complete Remission		Recurrences	
		Number	%	Number	%
CRYOSURGERY AS MONOTHERAPY					
Keloids					
Mende[9]	7	5	71		
Zouboulis et al.[10]	55	28	51	–	
Rusciani et al.[11]	40	34	85	–	
Ernst and Hundeiker[12]	234	158	68	9	4
Zouboulis et al.[13]	20	16	80	–	
Total	**356**	**241**	**68**	**9**	**3**
Hypertrophic Scars					
Zouboulis et al.[10]	38	29	76	–	
Ernst and Hundeiker[12]	51	43	84	2	4
Total	**89**	**72**	**81**	**2**	**2**
CRYOSURGERY COMBINED WITH INTRALESIONAL CORTICOSTEROIDS					
Keloids					
Hirshowitz[14]	58	41	71	9	16
Ernst and Hundeiker[12]	56	38	68	2	4
Zouboulis et al.[13]	20	19	95	–	
Banfalvi et al.[15]	25	21	84	–	
Total	**159**	**119**	**75**	**11**	**7**

Source: From Robinson J, Hanke W, Sengelmann R, Siegel D. *Surgery of the Skin: Procedural Dermatology.* 2nd ed. Mosby; 2010; Table 10.3.

nice. These are also easier for younger children to tolerate (Figure 13.26). Usually a 3- to 5-second freeze time to the edge of the lesion is adequate.

SEBORRHEIC KERATOSIS

See Videos 13.3 and 13.4

Seborrheic keratoses are frequently treated with cryosurgery. Very good cosmetic results can be obtained with cryosurgery of seborrheic keratoses from the scalp down to the legs. The open spray technique is a very fast and easy method of treating one or many seborrheic keratoses. The freeze time should be determined by the thickness and location of the seborrheic keratosis. It is better to underfreeze and have to do a second freeze than to overfreeze and cause permanent hypopigmentation, scarring, or atrophy (Figure 13.27). In many cases, Medicare and insurance companies will consider this cosmetic and will not pay for this procedure. If the seborrheic keratosis (SK) is inflamed, use that ICD-10 code, and the chance that it will be covered is greater.

SOLAR LENTIGINES

Solar lentigines may be quite responsive to depigmentation with cryosurgery. However, there is a risk of hypopigmentation or postinflammatory hyperpigmentation. It may be best to try this treatment on the dorsum of the hand before performing it on the face. Make sure you are certain of the diagnosis before proceeding as it is not good to freeze a lentigo maligna melanoma (LMM) that appears like a large solar lentigo. Visual diagnosis may be adequate in some cases; however, it is best to

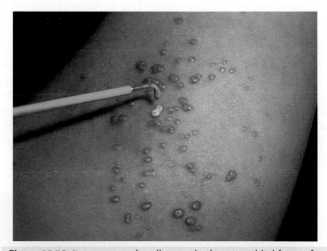

Figure 13.26 Cryosurgery of molluscum in the antecubital fossa of a child with atopic dermatitis. The bent tip spray allowed for precise treatment with minimal discomfort. (Copyright Richard P. Usatine, MD.)

examine the lesion with a dermatoscope first before applying cryotherapy. LMM often shows polygonal lines, rhomboidal patterns, circle-in-circle patterns, and destruction of the pilosebaceous unit (see Chapter 18, *Dermoscopy*). Because solar lentigines can be large and superficial, a paintbrush method with an open spray technique is useful.

WARTS

Warts are covered in detail in Chapter 23, *Procedures to Treat Benign Conditions.*

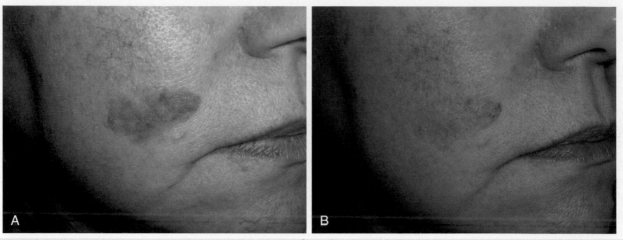

Figure 13.27 (A) Large seborrheic keratosis on the face. **(B)** Some seborrheic keratosis remains on the edge after cryosurgery using a spray paint technique. Note that there is no hypopigmentation or scarring and a second treatment provided a full resolution with a great cosmetic result. It is better to undertreat than overtreat especially in cosmetically sensitive areas. (Copyright Richard P. Usatine, MD.)

VASCULAR LESIONS

Pyogenic Granuloma

While the success rate for treating a pyogenic granuloma should be higher with a shave excision and electrosurgical destruction, some children will allow you to freeze their lesion but will not permit you to inject local anesthetic for the preferred surgical method. A Cryo Tweezer is a good choice if the PG is small (Figure 13.28). It is much less scary than a spray or probe. Another option is to perform cryosurgery with a closed probe (Figure 13.29).

Venous Lakes

Venous lakes are vascular tumors that appear most commonly on the lower lip. They can be compressed with an adherent cryoprobe and then frozen, destroying the venous lake.[4] Freeze the cryoprobe with liquid nitrogen first before applying (Figure 13.30) so that the probe does not stick to the lip when the freeze is complete.

Dr. Kuflik, a pioneer in cryosurgery, published one case study of a venous lake being treated with cryosurgery and provides these recommendations: use of freeze time of 5 to 15 seconds (depending upon the size of the lesion) with a cryoprobe pressed against it to compress the blood within. He recommends a 1- to 1.5-mm halo diameter.[4] This treatment may need repeating multiple times every 3 weeks for a full cure. Data on success rates are not published, and our experience shows mixed results with venous lakes. Current studies focus on using lasers for treatment.

PREMALIGNANT LESIONS

Actinic Keratoses
(See Video 13.6)

Primary treatment recommended for isolated actinic keratoses (AKs) is cryosurgery with liquid nitrogen.[5] Any of the open spray techniques can be used with the cryogun. The smaller lesions can be treated for 5 to 10 seconds, whereas

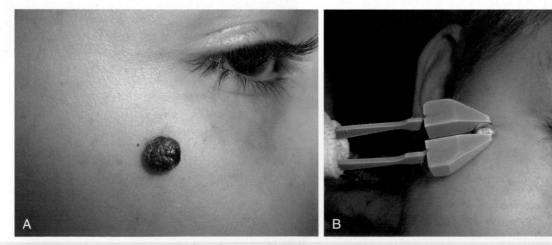

Figure 13.28 (A) Pyogenic granuloma on the face of a young girl. **(B)** The Cryo Tweezer is freezing and compressing the pyogenic granuloma laterally. Note the end of the 4 × 4 gauze wrapped around the handle of the Cryo Tweezer to prevent a freezing injury to the clinician's hand. (Copyright Richard P. Usatine, MD.)

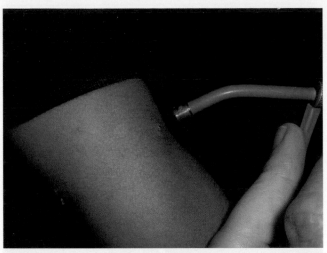

Figure 13.29 A closed probe is about to be applied to a pyogenic granuloma in a 7-year-old boy. While he was unwilling to allow an injection of local lidocaine for electrosurgical treatment, he was able to tolerate a cryosurgery with no anesthesia. The closed probe was chosen to compress the vascular tissue of this lobulated hemangioma. (Copyright Richard P. Usatine, MD.)

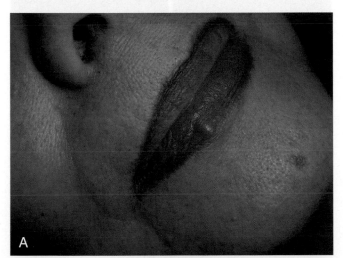

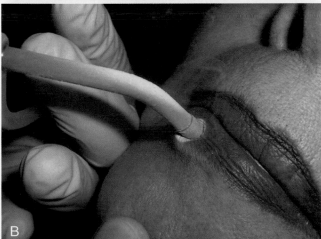

Figure 13.30 (A) Venous lake on the lip. **(B)** Venous lake being frozen with liquid nitrogen and a closed probe. This avoids the uncomfortable overspray that occurs when using a spray tip. (Copyright Richard P. Usatine, MD.)

Table 13.9 Actinic Keratoses of the Face and Scalp Larger Than 5 mm – Cure Rates With a Single Freeze[3]

Single Freeze Time (seconds)	Cure Rate (%)
<5	39
5–20	69
>20	83

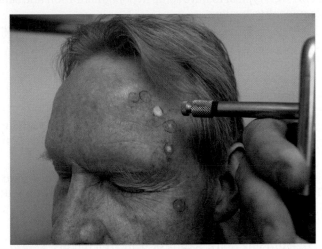

Figure 13.31 Multiple actinic keratoses being treated with a "C" aperture tip. The AKs were marked first prior to treatment. (Copyright Daniel L. Stulberg, MD.)

the thicker, more hypertrophic lesions should be treated for 10 to 20 seconds. A single freeze cycle should be adequate unless the thaw time appears too short. Table 13.9 shows the percentage cure of actinic keratoses with a single freeze-thaw cycle. Tissue destruction increases if longer freeze times or repeated freeze-thaw cycles are performed.[3]

The most efficient method of treating many AKs is to have your cryogun with you in the exam room when examining a patient known to have many AKs. Once you and the patient determine that cryosurgery is to be done, freeze each AK as you find it. Another option is to mark the location of AKs because they are often more easily palpated than seen (Figure 13.31). For suspected pigmented AKs, it is best to use the dermatoscope to make sure that you are not freezing a lentigo maligna. Sometimes, you will see that the borders of the AK become more visible as the freezing is occurring.

Count your AKs as you go because you are paid individually for each AK until you reach 15. Then one global CPT code is used for 15 AKs and above.

Malignant Lesions

After developing proficiency with multiple benign lesions, it is reasonable to consider using cryosurgery for the least aggressive NMSCs. Studies have shown that cryosurgery has similar effectiveness to electrodesiccation and curettage for correctly chosen BCCs. The most commonly recommended regimen is to maintain a freeze for 30 seconds, allow full thawing, and then repeat the 30-second freeze.[6] Keep in mind that the recommended surgical margin for excision of BCC is 3 to 5 mm, so the freeze margin around the BCC should be 3 to 5 mm. Clinical cure rates are approximately 90%, so appropriate follow-up is important.[6] If the lesion recurs after treatment, surgical excision or Mohs surgery may be indicated. These longer freeze times can be painful and difficult to tolerate, so inject with lidocaine for anesthesia prior to treatment. Efficacy and appearance are not as highly rated as surgical management, and after treatment there will likely be a prolonged period (weeks) of erythema, exudate, and healing, so judgment should be used in presenting the option of cryotherapy with surgical management.[6] It is typical to have some hypopigmentation and skin atrophy after healing.

When cryosurgery is usually not the treatment of choice:

- Skin cancers >2 cm diameter
- Skin cancers with margins that are not clear
- Recurrent cancers
- Tumors in areas of high risk for recurrence
- Tumors on lower limbs, where healing is poor
- Higher risk BCCs – sclerosing, infiltrating, and micronodular
- Most invasive SCC (especially if there is perineural invasion)
- All melanomas and all Merkel cell carcinomas[7]

Patient selection – consider the following factors for individual patients that may favor this approach to treatment:

- Poor risk for surgery
- Elderly and not wanting surgery
- In a nursing home setting or dementia (Figure 13.32)
- Small superficial BCC
- SCC in situ

One or two freeze-thaw cycles for BCC[7]:

In a study of cryosurgery for BCC, a 95.3% cure rate was achieved in the treatment of facial basal cell carcinomas with a double freeze-thaw cycle.[6] This is compared with a cure rate of only 79.4% when facial lesions were treated with a single freeze-thaw cycle. Treatment of superficial truncal basal cell carcinomas with a single freeze-thaw cycle achieved a cure rate of 95.5%. One 30-second freeze-thaw cycle to superficial truncal BCCs appears adequate.[6] Note that nodular truncal BCCs were not studied, so it might be best to use a double 30-second freeze-thaw cycle for these thicker tumors.[6]

Method for nonmelanoma skin cancers amenable to cryosurgery:

- Use a surgical marker and circle the full skin cancer.
- Measure 3 to 5 mm around the border and draw the desired halo diameter (Figure 13.33).
- Use lidocaine with or without epinephrine for local anesthesia.
- Good spray tip choices for the Brymill Cry-Ac systems include the C-tip and the short straight tip. Do not use a bent spray tip for treating skin cancer because the flow rate of liquid nitrogen is slower.
- Start the freeze and a stopwatch simultaneously – do not just estimate the 30-second freeze time. It helps to have a second person in the room to watch the time on a watch or smartphone.
- In most cases the spray trigger can be fully pressed and held, and intermittent pulsing only needs to be initiated if the freeze ball extends beyond the halo diameter.
- If a second freeze cycle will be used, allow the area to thaw until the white is no longer visible. Then perform a second 30-second freeze.

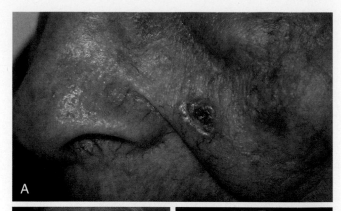
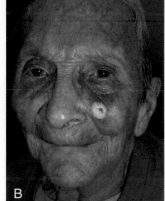
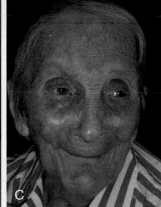

Figure 13.32 (A) BCC on the cheek of a 94-year-old woman with Alzheimer's disease. The patient was nonverbal and unable to understand her diagnosis or the treatment options. The family was adamant about treating the patient right away. **(B)** Given the options they chose cryosurgery. The patient's head had to be held for the injection of local anesthetic. However, she did remain still for the cryosurgery which did not hurt. A double 30 second freeze-thaw cycle was used. **(C)** 7 months later at a follow-up visit there was no evidence of recurrence clinically, and the patient was happy. There was hypopigmentation and slight scarring that was very acceptable to the family. (Copyright Richard P. Usatine, MD.)

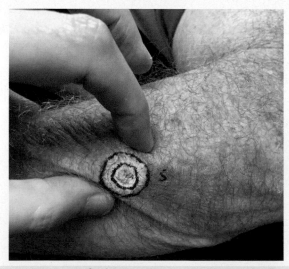

Figure 13.33 A superficial BCC on the arm is being treated with cryosurgery. A 5-mm halo was drawn around the BCC biopsy site, and local anesthesia was injected. Then liquid nitrogen was applied for 30 seconds. The freeze ball is palpable, demonstrating the depth of freezing. (Copyright Richard P. Usatine, MD.)

- Explain to the patient once again about the likelihood of some pain, swelling, and liquid drainage for a few days. However, most patients tolerate this well by our experience and have no more side effects than the other treatments available.

CRYOSURGERY COMPARED WITH CURETTAGE FOR SUPERFICIAL BCC

One clinical trial compared cryosurgery to curettage alone for nonfacial superficial BCC (sBCCs) with a diameter of 5 to 20 mm. These patients were randomized to either cryosurgery using one freeze-thaw cycle with a 4-mm halo versus curettage. In total, 228 sBCCs in 97 patients were included in the analysis. At 3 to 6 months, no residual tumors were seen in any of the treated areas. After 1 year, the clinical clearance rates for curettage and cryosurgery were 95.7% and 100%, respectively ($P = .060$). Wound healing times were shorter for curettage (4 weeks) compared to cryosurgery (5 weeks; $P < .0001$). Overall, patient satisfaction at 1 year was high. Both treatment methods showed high clinical clearance rates after 1 year, while curettage reduced the wound healing time.[8]

Palliation

As our population ages we see more and more patients who are frail and elderly with NMSCs. Some of these patients will do well with surgical excisions for the cancers. For those patients who may not be able to tolerate excisional surgery, cryosurgery may be used to shrink a skin cancer for palliation.

Learning the Techniques

See Videos 13.10–13.15

Bananas and agar plates (Figure 13.10) provide the best models for practicing cryosurgery. Agar plates are useful for observing the pattern of the freeze ball that develops based on the aperture used, the rate of flow, and the intermittent spray technique used. If you use a banana, you may cut open the frozen area quickly to see the depth and geometry of the freeze. That may not be needed, and the banana can be left intact during practice. The banana peel will darken, allowing you to see the pattern and extent of your cryosurgical technique (Figure 13.34). Try rotary or back-and-forth spray motions to cover broader areas for more superficial freezes.

Aftercare

Advise the patient that swelling, erythema, and blistering are the norm with cryosurgery and that the treated skin will subsequently slough off in the coming 1 to 2 weeks. Elevating an extremity post procedure can reduce throbbing in cryosurgery of the digits. Adhesive bandages may be used to protect the area if blistering develops. If the blister pops, some clean petrolatum covered by a bandage allows for moist comfortable healing. If it is very painful, a thin hydrocolloid dressing can be used.

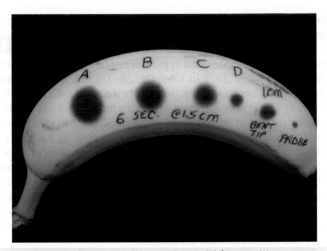

Figure 13.34 A banana makes a great model for practicing cryosurgery. Moving from left to right the first four brown spots were created using a Brymill cryogun with aperture tips A through D spraying 1.5 cm from the banana for 6 seconds each. The next brown spot was created using a bent tip spray 1 cm from the banana. And the final small brown spot was made using a probe tip applied directly to the banana. (Copyright Daniel L. Stulberg, MD.)

Coding and Billing Pearls

When cryosurgery is used for tissue destruction, coding is based on the skin destruction codes detailed in Chapter 28, Coding and Billing for Dermatologic Procedures. Benign and premalignant tissue destruction has essentially been divided into three types of CPT codes based on these diagnoses and generally independent of the means of destruction:

1. Skin tags: 11200, 11201
2. Benign other than skin tags or cutaneous vascular lesions (includes warts and seborrheic keratoses): 17110, 17111
3. Premalignant (actinic keratoses): 17000, 17003, 17004.

(Note that laser destruction of cutaneous vascular lesions has separate codes.)

The general destruction codes shown in Box 13.2 are usually independent of the method of destruction and the

---

Box 13.2 CPT General Destruction Codes for Cryosurgery

11200 Removal of skin tags by cryosurgery or any other destructive technique, any area, up to and including 15 (billed once only)

11201 Removal for each additional 10 skin tags or portion thereof (may be billed more than once)

17110 Destruction by any means including cryosurgery for warts/benign lesions other than skin tags up to 14 lesions (this is a single code used once only regardless if 1 or 14 lesions are treated)

17111 15 or more lesions (stand-alone code, not per lesion)

17000 Destruction by any means including cryosurgery for all premalignant lesions (AKs), first lesion

17003 Second through 14th lesion (this code is billed for each lesion from 2 to 14) (charge each lesion)

17004 15 or more lesions (stand-alone code, not per lesion)

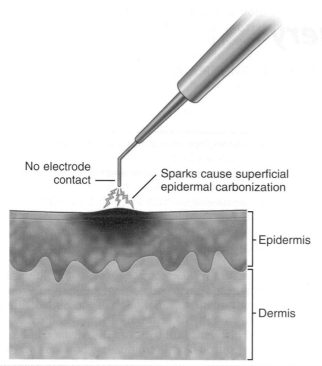

Figure 14.1 In *fulguration*, the electrode is held away from the skin so that there is a sparking to the surface (such as happens with *fulgur*, "lightning"). Fulguration produces a high intensity but more shallow level of tissue destruction that may reach the upper dermis. *(Adapted from Sebben JE. Electrosurgery. In Ratz JL, ed., Textbook of Dermatologic Surgery. Philadelphia: Lippincott-Raven; 1998.)*

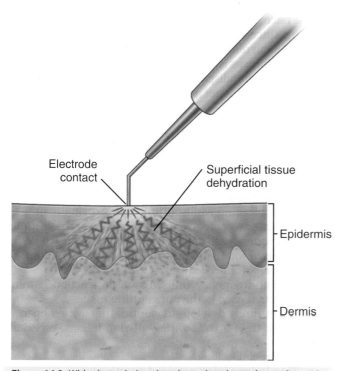

Figure 14.2 With *electrodesiccation*, the active electrode touches or is inserted into the skin to produce tissue destruction deeper into the dermis. *(Adapted from Sebben JE. Electrosurgery. In Ratz JL, ed., Textbook of Dermatologic Surgery. Philadelphia: Lippincott-Raven; 1998.)*

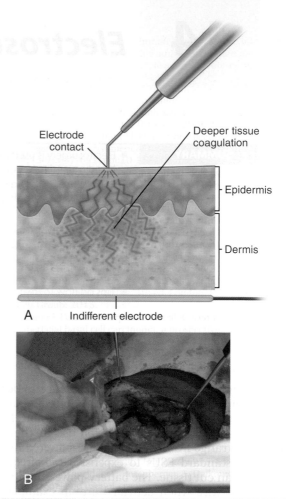

Figure 14.3 (A) *Electrocoagulation* is used to stop bleeding in deep and superficial surgery. In this image an indifferent electrode is being used to produce deeper tissue coagulation. Electrocoagulation can also be performed without an indifferent electrode. **(B)** Electrocoagulation is being performed in the undermined area of an ellipse using a Hyfrecator while the surgical assistant holds up the tissue with skin hooks. *(A: Adapted from Sebben JE. Electrosurgery. In Ratz JL, ed., Textbook of Dermatologic Surgery. Philadelphia: Lippincott-Raven; 1998.)*

Disadvantages of Electrosurgery

- Safety risks exist but these events are rare (electrical shocks, burns, fires, or interference with pacemakers).
- May cause hypertrophic scars and keloids
- Smoke may carry viral particles, which have the potential to transmit infections (e.g., HPV, HIV).
- Odor of smoke plume is like a bad BBQ.
- Excessive smoke may exacerbate asthma.
- Delayed hemorrhage
- Unsightly wound
- Slow healing, especially if a large area is treated (healing can be slower than scalpel shave excision)
- Small lesions are obliterated, resulting in no specimen being available for histology unless a biopsy was performed first.
- Electrosurgical artifacts can occur at margins if used for excisional biopsy or removal (e.g., radiofrequency cutting).

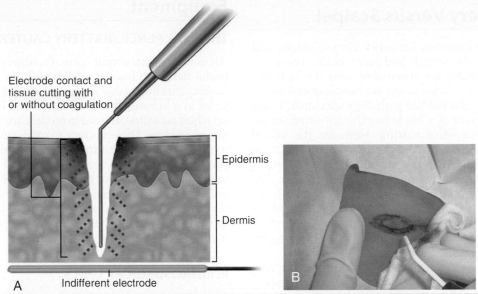

Figure 14.4 (A) In *electrosection*, the unit is set so the electrode cuts tissue. This mode requires an indifferent electrode. (B) Electrosection is being performed with a Vary-Tip electrode attached to a Surgitron. An indifferent electrode is placed under the patient near the surgical site. *(Copyright Richard P. Usatine, MD.)*

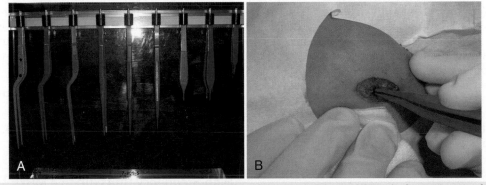

Figure 14.5 (A) Selection of bipolar forceps that could be used on a number of electrosurgical units. (B) Bipolar forceps in action for electrocoagulation while doing an elliptical biopsy. Note that a small gap is preserved between the ends of the bipolar forceps around the bleeding site. *(Copyright Richard P. Usatine, MD.)*

Electrosurgery Versus Cryosurgery

Cryosurgery is often the treatment of choice for seborrheic and actinic keratoses as well as simple warts. It is faster and easier to perform than electrosurgery for these indications because it does not require anesthesia. Cryosurgery also tends to cause less scarring than electrosurgery, especially if the lesions are very superficial. However, cryosurgery may be more likely to cause hypopigmentation because the cold preferentially destroys melanocytes. This is especially important in darker skin tones. Electrosurgery can be quicker than cryosurgery for extensive condyloma, especially if a cutting current is used.

There is a risk of developing human papilloma virus (HPV) in the respiratory tract from inhaling the plume (smoke) from an HPV lesion as it is being treated.[1-3] Intact HPV DNA has been isolated from the plume of verrucae that were treated with electrosurgery and lasers. In Loop electrosurgical excision procedure (LEEP) procedures, 30% of the time, HPV DNA was recovered from the smoke of the procedure.[4] Another study showed 10% of gynecologists performing LEEP were found to have HPV present in their nasal epithelium.[5] Fortunately the use of an N-95 mask reduced the incidence, and all of the cases of nasal carriage resolved. Therefore, it is prudent for clinicians to use a smoke evacuator while performing laser and electrosurgical treatment of verrucae and other viral lesions (see section "Safety Measures With Electrosurgery"). These personal risks, and the need for additional equipment and safeguards, may be one factor used to determine the physician's choice of therapy for viral lesions.

One disadvantage of cryotherapy over electrosurgery is that with cryosurgery the final result cannot be seen immediately, and there is more subjective judgment involved in performing the treatment. However, the degree of damage can be estimated accurately. Cryosurgery also causes more postoperative swelling, which may be uncomfortable for the patient but is only a transient phenomenon.

Electrosurgery Versus Scalpel

The traditional instruments for performing excisions and shave biopsies are the scalpel and razor blade. These are inexpensive, the blades are disposable, and the cuts are clean. The cold steel blades cause no heat-induced tissue damage that could obscure the pathology specimen. Using electrosurgery in place of a blade has the advantage of facilitating hemostasis while cutting. However, the lateral heat produced by the electrosurgical instrument can cause residual tissue damage that might result in slow healing as well as artifact on the edges of the biopsy specimen. The higher the frequency, the less residual damage on both the specimen removed and on the viable tissue remaining. Also, the cutting is very quick and it may go more deeply than desired, excising excessive amounts of tissue or damaging deeper nerves and vessels.

High-frequency electrosurgery on the pure cutting current will approach but not match the scalpel for producing a specimen free of burn artifact. Therefore, if a malignancy (especially melanoma) is suspected, unless wide margins are being obtained, it may be best to obtain a biopsy with a razor or scalpel (cold steel).

For excising benign lesions, the small amount of lateral heat may not interfere with wound healing when used carefully on a low-power cutting setting. A shave excision using a blade followed by electrosurgery with a loop electrode can lead to a nearly scar free result and combines the best of both techniques to optimize the results. The mode can be set for either cutting/coagulation (blend) or preferably pure cutting only. Ideally then, the lesion (commonly a nevus or seborrheic keratosis [SK]) is shaved off with a blade, and then the loop of the radiofrequency (RF) unit removes the residual tissue and controls any bleeding. If the loop will be used to perform the shave, pure cutting will make a smooth cut and usually control bleeding with less damage to the remaining tissue and to the biopsy specimen. The coagulation function is then used if needed to control bleeding.

The Ellman Surgitron models are high-frequency units (often termed *radiofrequency* unit because it operates at 4.0 MHz, which is in the range of a radio). They employ a Vari-Tip fine-wire electrode that is adjustable in length for cutting through the skin for elliptical and other full-thickness excisions. On the pure cutting setting, the Vari-Tip electrode can cut with less lateral heat and can allow the physician to do quick and bloodless excision of benign lesions. A combined cold steel (blade) and electrosurgical procedure can also be used here. While the scalpel cuts through the skin to provide better depth control, deeper dissection/undermining, and excision with cutting or blended cutting and coagulation can control bleeding.

In summary, no instrument can beat the scalpel (or razor blade) for cost, quality of pathologic specimen, and minimization of tissue damage. The high-frequency electrosurgery units are more expensive to purchase and operate. A radiosurgery unit can be used to perform several kinds of surgery that have been traditionally performed with a scalpel. This may be beneficial if the lesion is benign and very vascular, but even standard electrosurgery is sufficient for these lesions.

Equipment

THERMAL PENCIL/BATTERY CAUTERY

An inexpensive thermal "pencil" cautery (Figure 14.6) is a useful device to have in offices without an electrosurgical device. This disposable device consists of two penlight batteries in a housing connected to a wire filament that heats up when activated. Reusable models are also available with disposable tips. These battery cautery units can be a useful tool for treatment around the eyes and on patients with pacemakers, and the disposable units are packaged sterilely to drop onto a surgical tray. Thermal pencil cautery units are excellent for opening a subungual hematoma. When the hot electrode perforates the nail, the heated tip is cooled by the blood from the hematoma, preventing damage to the nail bed.

ELECTROSURGICAL UNITS

There are a number of companies that make ESUs including Aaron, ConMed, Delasco, Ellman, and Valleylab. Standard noncutting units are the workhorse devices that most dermatologists and primary care providers use in their offices. High-frequency (radiofrequency) units are high-priced and cut tissue instead of a razor blade or scalpel. These radiofrequency units are heavily marketed to PCPs but are rarely used by dermatologists in their offices because they prefer blades to cut tissue with scalpels and other blades.

Standard Electrosurgical Units (Noncutting, Lower Frequency)

- Hyfrecator 2000 (ConMed) (Figure 14.7); *See Video 14.2*
- Electricator (Delasco)
- Bovie DERM 942 (Figure 14.8A)

High-Frequency Units (up to 4 MHz)

- Bovie Bantam PRO (Figure 14.8B)
- Cameron-Miller (various models)
- Ellman Surgitron
- Force FX (Valleylab)

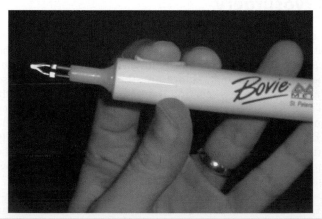

Figure 14.6 Note the red-hot tip of this handheld disposable electrocautery unit. This unit performs true hot electrocautery. *(Copyright Richard P. Usatine, MD.)*

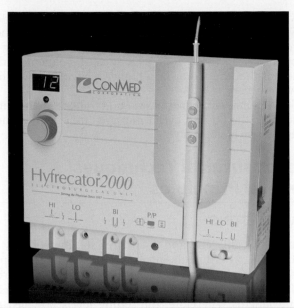

Figure 14.7 The Hyfrecator 2000 from the ConMed Corporation is a commonly used electrosurgical unit in the office. *(Copyright ConMed Corporation.)*

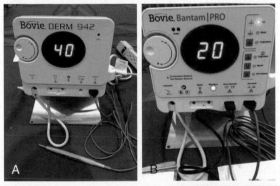

Figure 14.8 **(A)** The Bovie DERM 942 electrosurgical unit is similar to the Hyfrecator 2000. **(B)** The Bovie Bantam PRO electrosurgical unit can be used for cutting in addition to bipolar and other typical electrosurgical applications. *(Copyright Richard P. Usatine, MD.)*

- LEEP (CooperSurgical)
- Quantum 2000 (Wallach Surgical)

With high-frequency cutting units, accessories are disposable, including grounding pads and standard handpieces. This adds a significant cost per procedure just for tips in addition to increasing waste.

Hyfrecator [Hyfrecator 2000 (ConMed) Figure 14.7] is the most commonly used ESU in the office setting, so information provided here will be specific to this instrument, but it can be readily adapted to others. This is not meant as an endorsement of this unit. However, their features will be used to provide practical advice for performing electrosurgery.

Accessories

HYFRECATOR

- Electrolase blunt and sharp tips (Figure 14.9)
- Sterile sleeves for handle (Figure 14.10) (a sterile glove will work if a sterile sleeve is not available)

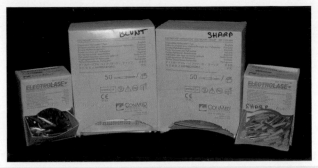

Figure 14.9 Commonly used disposable electrodes for the Hyfrecator 2000. These are available in blunt or sharp versions and may be purchased sterilely packaged or as nonsterile clean electrodes. The sterile sharp versions are what we use in excisional surgeries so that the sterile blunt tips are not needed. *(Copyright Richard P. Usatine, MD.)*

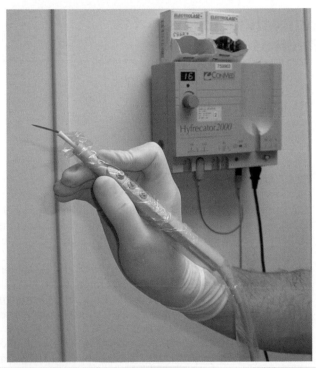

Figure 14.10 A sterile sheath has been applied over the Hyfrecator handle so that it can be used in a sterile surgical procedure. *(Copyright Richard P. Usatine, MD.)*

- Nondisposable bipolar forceps (optional) (Figure 14.5) and foot switch

SMOKE EVACUATORS

- Electrosurgery creates a smoke (plume) with a bad smell. The smoke may contain viral particles. With the standard use of masks in the office, the clinician, patients, and staff are better protected than before the COVID-19 epidemic. Cutting with electrosurgery creates the most smoke. In this case, it is best to use a smoke evacuator to remove the plume. Multiple companies manufacture stand-alone smoke evacuators (Figure 14.11). These can be even more expensive than the ESU. Another reason is to cut with a scalpel and minimize adding smoke

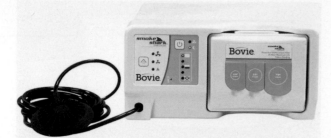

Figure 14.11 An example of a smoke evacuator by Bovie. *(Courtesy Bovie.)*

into the office environment. When constructing or remodeling an office, consider installing an exhaust fan (a typical bathroom fan works) to help remove the smoke during electrosurgery.

Indications for Use of Electrosurgery

- Controlling bleeding (coagulation)
- Destruction of tissue
- Nail matrixectomy
- Excising tissue
- Vaporization of tissue fragments

Precautions

- Pacemakers (see section "Pacemaker Problems," p. 14-9).
- Electrosurgery is not indicated as a treatment modality for obtaining a biopsy of pigmented lesions suspicious for melanoma.
- Electrodesiccation and curettage (ED&C) should generally be avoided in the following circumstances:
  - Aggressive (micronodular, infiltrating, morpheaform, sclerotic), large nodular (greater than 1 cm), or recurrent basal cell carcinoma (BCC)
  - Superficial BCC larger than 2 cm will also have a higher recurrence rate with ED&C (see Chapter 24, *Diagnosis and Treatment of Malignant and Premalignant Lesions*).
  - Aggressive and large squamous cell carcinomas (SCCs) should be excised. SCC *in situ* and well-differentiated small superficially invasive SCCs may be treated with ED&C.
  - Immune-suppressed patients, especially those who have had organ transplants, may be best served by excising the lesions to ensure complete removal in all but the smaller lesions (less than 7–8 mm).
  - Patients with slow healing (diabetes, peripheral vascular disease) may do better with excisional rather than destructive methods.

Location is also an important consideration when using destructive techniques for nonmelanoma skin cancers (NMSCs). Higher recurrence rates are associated with NMSC in the following areas:

- Alar groove, preauricular and periocular
- H-zone on the face. Associated with higher recurrence rates for recurrent BCC treated with surgery rather than

Mohs surgery (see Chapter 27, *When to Refer/Mohs Surgery*). This was not true for primary BCC in these regions treated with surgical excision. ED&C may be performed in the H-zone as long as the patient understands that there may be a higher recurrence rate than with surgery.[6]
- SCC on non–sun-exposed skin and mucous membranes such as the lip and eyelid margins (may also be more aggressive biologically)

Electrosurgical Techniques: General Principles

POWER SETTING

Every ESU is different, and the desired setting will vary for each model, procedure, lesion, or patient. Even two supposedly identical electrosurgical models may require different settings or minor adjustments on different days or with different patients. Therefore, the setting levels provided are only starting points (Table 14.1 and Box 14.1). The basic principle for setting the correct power output is to start low and increase the power until the desired outcome (destruction, coagulation, or cutting) is achieved. For ablation/destruction, the tissue should bubble or turn gray. Keep in mind that destruction of tissue below the visible area of treatment can occur. The power setting for coagulation is generally higher than the setting needed for tissue destruction. A rule of thumb is to use the lowest power setting that accomplishes a given result so as to achieve cosmetically acceptable outcomes.

Radiofrequency modes are:

- Pure cutting current (that still has 10% coagulation)
- Blended cutting and coagulation (approximately 50% of each)
- Coagulation (hemo)
- Fulguration (similar to the Hyfrecator)
- Bipolar coagulation

ANESTHESIA

Local anesthesia will be needed for virtually all electrosurgery with the exception of the treatment for telangiectasias, small skin tags, and fine angiomas where either no or topical anesthesia is adequate. Injecting 1% to 2% lidocaine with epinephrine before the procedure will provide painless electrosurgery. However, short bursts of low current can be less uncomfortable than needle anesthesia in some individuals. Topical anesthesia with ethyl chloride is contraindicated because ethyl chloride is flammable. Anesthetic creams (see Chapter 3, *Anesthesia*) can be used for anesthesia before treatment of facial telangiectasias and eliminates the effects of distortion from injectable anesthesia.

PRACTICAL PEARLS FOR ANY ELECTROSURGERY

1. It helps to stabilize the physician's operating hand against the patient's body part so that if the patient moves, the hand with the electrode moves with the patient, avoiding burning tissue outside of the target area.

Table 14.1   Range of Power Settings with the Hyfrecator 2000

Lesions	Power Setting (Watts on Low)	Type of Electrode
Benign		
Angiomas (cherry)	2–2.5	Sharp or blunt
Angiomas (spider)	2–2.5	Sharp or needle
Condyloma acuminata	12–18	Blunt
Dermatosis papulosa nigra	2–2.5	Blunt or sharp
Pyogenic granulomas	18–20 or switch to high	Blunt
Sebaceous hyperplasia	2–2.5	Blunt
Seborrheic keratosis	10–14	Blunt
Skin tags (acrochordons)	2–2.5	Sharp
Telangiectasias	2–2.5	Sharp or needle
Verrucae vulgaris	12–18	Blunt
Verrucae plana	12–18	Sharp or Blunt
Malignant		
Basal cell carcinoma	16–20	Blunt
Squamous cell carcinoma	16–20	Blunt

Disclaimer: Every patient and every electrosurgical unit is different. These numbers are just suggestions, and each clinician must find the best settings based on experience with their patients and unit.

Box 14.1   Electrosurgical Settings

Suggested Settings for Hyfrecator 2000 or Bovie A942

Cosmetic destruction of angiomas, telangiectasias, sebaceous hyperplasia, and skin tags without anesthesia: 2–2.5 W on low
ED&C: 14–18 on low
Coagulation after shave: 12–14 on low
Coagulation after removing a pyogenic granuloma: 18–20 on low, sometimes >20 on high is needed.
Coagulation during full-depth excision (ellipse): 12–20 on low
Consider switching to high if coagulation on low at 20 is not working. However, it may be best to find and tie off a bleeding vessel or wait while applying pressure with gauze.

Disclaimer: Every patient and every electrosurgical unit is different. These numbers are just suggestions and each clinician must find the best settings based on experience with their patients and unit.

2. *Electrode contact time.* Keep this to a minimum as the longer the duration of electrosurgery, the more likely the patient will feel some pain even if adequately anesthetized.
3. *Intensity of power.* Use the minimum wattage needed to get the job done. If the power is too high, it will cause unintended tissue damage.

Practical Pearls Specific to Radiofrequency Electrosurgery (*See Video 14.3*)

1. Activate the electrode with the foot or hand switch before touching the skin/lesion with the electrode. Touching the lesion dissipates energy into the tissues instead of vaporizing the tissue in the path of the electrode.
2. It helps to stabilize the physician's operating hand against the patient's body part so that if the patient moves, the hand with the electrode moves with the patient avoiding cutting outside the intended area.
3. While cutting, move the electrode using a smooth uninterrupted movement. The intensity should be adjusted until the electrode moves through the tissue like a hot knife through butter.
4. Always use a neutral plate ("antenna") or grounding plate as specified by the manufacturer. The neutral plate should be under the patient and not far from the operative site. The neutral plate does not have to touch the skin and will allow the use of lower power settings if closer to the operative site. A true grounding plate must be in direct contact with the skin, and proximity to the operative site is of less importance.
5. *Intensity of power.* If the intensity of the power is too high, it will cause sparking and increased tissue destruction. If too low, it will cause tissue drag, which can increase lateral heat and increase the risk of bleeding as well as a less desirable cosmetic outcome.
6. *Electrode size.* Smaller electrodes with finer wire cause less lateral heat and require less power to operate than larger ones.
7. Tissue must be moist to obtain the desired effect. The moisture allows for the water molecules to vaporize and cause the desired effect. It will be almost impossible to obtain any effect whatsoever on highly keratinized (dry) tissue. Wipe over dry lesions with a moist 4 × 4 to provide the moisture needed.
8. Reusable electrodes must be clean and free of carbon to work well. Use fine sand paper to keep them shiny and clean and then sterilize.

Safety Measures With Electrosurgery

POTENTIAL HAZARDS OF ELECTROSURGERY (TO PATIENT AND PHYSICIAN)

- Fire and burns
- Electric shock

- Transmission of infection through electrode, smoke plume, or spattering blood
- Pacemaker interference

SAFETY PRECAUTIONS TO AVOID POTENTIAL HAZARDS

Fire and Burns

- Be sure the alcohol has dried if used to prepare the skin. Do not leave alcohol swabs anywhere near active electrodes.
- Do not use ethyl chloride as the local anesthetic.
- Keep oxygen and other flammable material away from electrosurgical equipment.
- Make sure a fire extinguisher is available.
- Be careful of bowel gas, which contains methane in perirectal procedures. This is more of a problem with patients under general anesthesia who lack control. The gas can explode.

Electric Shock

- Keep electrosurgical equipment functioning properly; if there are signs of malfunction, have the equipment fixed before use.
- Use a three-pronged plug connected to an outlet that is not overloaded.
- Do not use the outlet in the treatment table.
- Make sure the patient is not grasping or touching metal portions of the treatment table. In our treatment rooms the tables have metal foot rests. Patients wearing sandals have been shocked when their bare feet touch this footrest. The effect has been shocking, but no harmful effects have been seen. We have learned to look at the feet before starting electrosurgery to avoid this complication. (Figure 14.12)

Transmission of Infection Through Electrode

- Always wear disposable gloves.
- When using reusable electrodes, clean them after each use by removing the char and follow by sterilizing them in an autoclave or liquid solution. The char can be

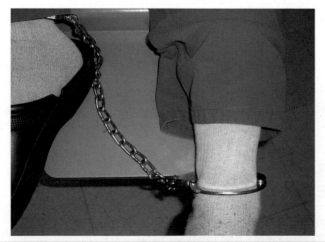

Figure 14.12 Make sure the patient's bare skin is not touching metal on your exam table/chair before using electrosurgery. *(Copyright Richard P. Usatine, MD.)*

removed using fine sand paper, an ultrasonic cleaner, or by activating the electrode in a moist 4 × 4 gauze folded over the tip.

- Disposable electrodes are standard for the Hyfrecator 2000.

During sterile procedures options include the following:

- Use a sterilized handle and cord (reusable is preferred as a greener option).
- Place a nonsterile handle into a sterile sheath so that it covers the hand switch and a good portion of the cord. Another option is to use a sterile glove held open while an assistant places the nonsterile handpiece into a finger of the glove by holding the attached wire and lowering it. A sterile electrode tip can then be used to pierce a finger of the glove as it is plugged into the hand piece so it can be secured in place. The physician can then hold the handpiece, which is now within a sterile glove.
- For short procedures in which minimal electrocoagulation is needed, an assistant who is not part of the sterile field can apply the electrosurgery tip to a hemostat or to pickups that are grasping a bleeder as needed.

TRANSMISSION OF INFECTION THROUGH SMOKE PLUME OR SPATTERING BLOOD

Transmission of infection through a smoke plume or spattering blood is a potential risk when treating lesions of viral origin. This is especially true when treating HPV infection in all types of warts. Intact HPV DNA has been recovered in the smoke plume of verrucae treated with electrosurgery and the carbon dioxide laser.[1-3] One case report suggests that a physician acquired an HPV infection of the larynx (laryngeal papillomatosis) while performing laser therapy on HPV-infected lesions.[1] This has not been reported with electrosurgery.

A publication of the National Institute for Occupational Safety and Health (NIOSH) states that research studies have confirmed that smoke plume can contain toxic gases and vapors such as benzene, hydrogen cyanide, and formaldehyde, bioaerosols, dead and live cellular material (including blood fragments), and viruses.[7] At high concentrations the smoke causes ocular and upper respiratory tract irritation in health care personnel. Smoke evacuators should be used whenever possible, and the various filters and absorbers used in smoke evacuators should be replaced on a regular basis. These materials should be disposed of with other biohazardous waste.[7]

Although there may also be a potential risk of transmission of hepatitis, herpes, or HIV through blood splatter or smoke plume, there is no scientific evidence showing such transmission. Nevertheless, it is best to follow certain safety measures (especially if the lesion is of viral origin or the patient is known to be infected with HIV or hepatitis).

1. Avoid cutting with electrosurgery when a scalpel or other blade will do the job just as well.
2. Use a smoke evacuator with the intake nozzle held within 2 inches of the operative area. It is essential to use the evacuator when treating any viral lesion.
3. The physician and treatment team should wear surgical masks and eye protection. N95 surgical masks that filter

down to 0.5 micron are available and should be used for extensive cases.

4. Consider using a different treatment modality based on evaluation of the risks and benefits of treatment.

IMPLANTED ELECTRICAL DEVICES AND PACEMAKER PROBLEMS

With advances in medicine, there are now implanted electrical devices (IEDs) to assist patient with many issues. These include cochlear implants, nerve stimulators, deep brain stimulators and vagal nerve stimulators, and others in addition to implantable cardiac defibrillators and pacemakers. Electrosurgery should be considered carefully in these individuals. Electrical current, especially in the cutting mode, using higher power devices in the operating room and using electrosurgery in close proximity to the device or its electrodes may activate, inactivate, or damage these devices. Although newer devices have electrical filters and are supposedly "shielded" from these effects, if an alternative method of treatment is acceptable, it should be considered. Electrodesiccation with low power units was not found to interfere with cardiac devices in a retrospective study of 46 patients.[8] An in vitro study found no interference using Hyfrecators with ICDs and no interference with pacemakers until used at maximal settings at 3 cm from the pacemaker or 1 cm from the pacemaker at usual settings.[9]

- Battery-operated heat-generating cautery can be used safely but is not as versatile as the ESUs.
- Low power units like the Hyfrecator appear safe as long as used further than 3 cm from cardiac devices.
- Avoid cutting with electrosurgery when a scalpel or other blade will do the job just as well.
- If a cutting unit is still to be used, place the antenna/ground plate next to the lesion, away from the device.
- Arrange the arc of current between the device and ground so it does not pass through the heart, IED, or electrodes.
- Use only short bursts of power.
- Do not perform electrosurgery in proximity to the heart.
- Use bipolar forceps if available.

In clinical practice, the use of bipolar forceps or true electrocautery (with heated wire) are the preferred options of experienced cutaneous surgeons when electrosurgery is required in a patient with a pacemaker or an implantable cardioverter-defibrillator (ICD).[10] In this study, the clinicians used routine precautions including utilizing short bursts of less than 5 seconds (71%), use of minimal power (61%), and avoiding use around the pacemaker or ICD (57%).[10] One hundred sixty cutaneous surgeons reported the following complications: reprogramming of a pacemaker (six patients), firing of an ICD (four patients), asystole (three patients), bradycardia (two patients), depleted battery life of a pacemaker (one patient), and an unspecified tachyarrhythmia (one patient). Overall this was a low rate of complications (0.8 case/100 years of surgical practice), with no reported significant morbidity or mortality.[10] Bipolar forceps were utilized by 19% of respondents and were not associated with any incidences of interference.[10]

Treating Specific Lesions

GENERAL APPROACH

Consider the risks and benefits of the relevant treatments. Once the decision has been made to use electrosurgery:

- Gather all of the necessary surgical supplies, staff, and confirmation of the procedure.
- Plug the electrosurgery device directly into the wall socket, not the exam table/chair.
- Turn on the unit and choose the appropriate settings including mode and power. Some ESUs require a few moments to "warm up."
- Place the antenna or grounding plate/pad in the proper position if using a cutting device.
- If using a foot pedal, place it within easy reach.
- Choose the tip to be used for the particular application, and place it in the handpiece.
- Check to see that when the foot pedal or the finger control is pressed, the unit activates.

When used in the fulguration or coagulation mode, be sure to leave space between the electrode tip and the tissue to produce a "spark gap." Gently bring the tip to the tissue until the spark jumps the gap or tap the lesion to obtain the desired effect. If the tip is applied firmly to the tissue in a continuous fashion, desiccation instead of fulguration will occur and cause deeper tissue destruction and more scarring. Ideally, the power will be set just high enough to cause graying or light charring of the tissue and cessation of bleeding. When treating areas that are bleeding, such as the base of a BCC that has been coagulated, slight amounts of blood will provide excellent conduction to desiccate/destroy the tissue. Too much blood, however, can disperse the energy and prevent the desired effect. Apply pressure to the base of the lesion with gauze or a cotton-tipped applicator to reduce bleeding and remove blood before proceeding. It can be helpful to keep the gauze pressed on the lesion and slowly expose a portion for treatment/electrocoagulation and then expose more tissue to treat, keeping a drier field to work with.

When used in the cutting mode, the electrode will cut continuously. When set properly, it will move through tissue smoothly without catching or "stalling." If the cutting is not smooth, try the following: make sure the mode selected is pure cutting; moisten the tissue; move slower; check to be sure the electrode tip is shiny and clean; confirm that the grounding pad/antenna is plugged in and placed properly; turn up the power. Excessive sparking and smoke means the power (wattage) is set too high, and the tissue will often appear black. When adjusted properly, the newly cut tissue will appear almost normal but will not be bleeding.

BENIGN LESIONS

Angiomas (Cherry)
(See Video 14.3)

Cherry (also called capillary or senile) angiomas are usually asymptomatic and have no malignant potential. Reasons to remove them include cosmetic concerns, growth, recurrent trauma (e.g., cutting them while shaving), or bleeding. Electrosurgery is probably the most effective, inexpensive treatment.

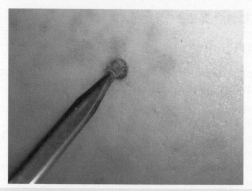

Figure 14.13 A blunt Hyfrecator electrode is being used for electrodesiccation of this small cherry angioma. More than one pass was needed here as the setting was low to accommodate the absence of anesthesia. *(Copyright Richard P. Usatine, MD.)*

Topical or local anesthesia with epinephrine is often used if the lesions are greater than 4 mm. Larger cherry angiomas should be anesthetized and shaved off first before lightly electrodesiccating the base. Smaller cherry angiomas do not require anesthesia and can be lightly touched with the electrode on a low setting. The Hyfrecator is used on low at 2 to 2.5 W (Figure 14.13) using the sharp tip for smaller lesions and the blunt tip for larger lesions. The char can be left alone or wiped off with moist gauze. If red tissue remains, gently and briefly tap the electrode tip on the area again.

Angiomas (Spider)

Spider angiomas can be treated with the same power settings as cherry angiomas. As opposed to telangiectasias, they have a more papular or central feeding vessel with small fine vessels extending from the central area. Spider angiomas can be effectively treated with laser therapy, intense pulsed light (IPL), or electrocoagulation. Injecting lidocaine with epinephrine may obscure the lesion due to vasoconstriction. Thus, it is more common to use topical anesthetic or to treat without any anesthesia after explaining this to the patient.

Electrodesiccation of the central feeding vessel should eradicate the entire angioma. This can be done with a sharp tip electrode, an epilation needle, or a metal-hubbed

33 gauge needle with an adapter. The sharp tip electrode on the Hyfrecator works well. Treat the central feeding vessel first, and then if the surrounding vessels are still visible, treat those separately at various points along the radial vessels (Figure 14.14)

If using a needle inserted into the central vessel, it often bleeds preventing a good coagulation effect. A blunt tip can then be used to coagulate the central vessel. If bleeding is still a problem, apply pressure to the base of the lesion to decrease blood flow. Use caution to avoid over-coagulation leading to excessive scarring. No curettage is needed afterward. The very lowest setting that causes blanching of the vessel should be used. Using excessive energy that can cause permanent indentations should be avoided. It is normal to see skin flushing around the treatment site in the office. No special aftercare is needed. However, the patient should not scrub the treatment site vigorously while in the healing stage.

Should the lesion recur, a more aggressive approach or laser can be tried. Although scarring is minimal, it is not uncommon to have a very small residual hypopigmented area at the electrosurgery site. It is important to counsel the patient about this and documentation it in the chart, since this is usually done for cosmetic purposes. If a patient is concerned regarding this, laser or IPL can destroy these tiny blood vessels without harming the skin although at more expense.

Condyloma Acuminata

If there are multiple, small condyloma, it may be prudent to initiate cryosurgery or topical treatments such as trichloroacetic acid. The patient may also be sent home with a prescription for podofilox, a purified podophyllin preparation (Condylox), or imiquimod (Aldara). Cryosurgery is an excellent alternative especially with the use of Cryo Tweezers for very accurate treatment without overspray (see Chapter 13, *Cryosurgery*). Condyloma acuminata may also be treated with electrosurgery using either a cutting or a desiccation method. The cutting mode and large loop are especially beneficial for extensive and/or large lesions.

A local anesthetic should always be used before using electrosurgery in the genital area. Electrosurgery can remove condyloma with a single treatment, and sites heal in 7 to 14 days usually with minimal scarring. This may be

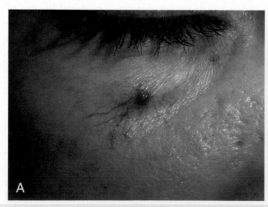
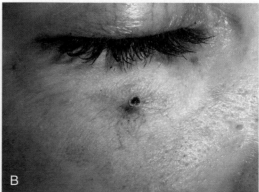

Figure 14.14 (A) Large spider angioma. **(B)** After electrosurgical destruction of the center papule and treatment of the peripheral vessels. *(Copyright Richard P. Usatine, MD.)*

particularly appealing to the patient who has failed multiple treatments with various chemicals and/or cryosurgery. Do counsel the patient regarding the risk of recurrence as the viral infection may remain present even though the skin lesions are removed.

There are two electrosurgery options. One is to use light electrofulguration or electrodesiccation with a ball/blunt electrode (coagulation or fulguration settings). This is ideal for multiple small lesions. The other is to perform radiosurgery with a loop electrode (usually not as large as the LEEP electrodes) using a pure cutting current. Using "pure cutting" generally provides enough hemostasis while also reducing the likelihood of scarring. The goal is to destroy the lesion with minimal effect on the surrounding normal skin. Note that with spray or adherent probe cryotherapy, a 1- to 2-mm halo of frozen normal tissue around the lesion is needed, but with electrosurgery, only the abnormal tissue is removed.

If there are only a few small lesions, therapy can be accomplished without magnification. However, when lesions are large or extensive, removing them under magnification (magnification loupes or the colposcope) helps complete removal, limits excessive tissue removal, and identifies lesions that are too small to be seen with the naked eye.

The unit should be set for pure cutting with the power set based on the ESU and the loop size. The condyloma should be "debulked" on the first pass, and then the edges should be lightly "feathered" to ensure there is no remaining tissue and to blend the treated skin into the surrounding normal tissue. *A common error is to go too deeply with the loop.* **Use caution**. The penile skin is extremely thin, and the RF loops cut very fast. Going too deeply will not only increase bleeding but also secondary scarring. The same can happen with the vulvar and perianal tissues. Alternatively, if one attempts to perform a flat shave with a surgical blade, it is difficult to cut the mobile skin, and bleeding obscures the operating field. That is the beauty of high-frequency electrosurgical removal: limited if any bleeding, controllable depth, minimal tissue destruction, and little scarring even with larger lesions. Using magnification during removal enhances all of these benefits even more.

The sequence for removal of a condyloma using high-frequency electrosurgery is as follows:

- Soak the area with acetic acid (moistened 4 × 4 gauze or spray bottle of vinegar). (optional).
- Examine under magnification (if colposcope or dermatoscope is available).
- Anesthetize as needed with 1% lidocaine and epinephrine using a 30-gauge needle. If extensive warts are to be treated on the penis, consider performing a penile block with 1% lidocaine only.
- Turn on the smoke evacuator, and have an assistant hold the tip within 2 inches of the lesions as they are treated.
- Turn on the unit and select pure cutting mode at the appropriate level. Test the setting on the top portion of the largest condyloma until it is just right (staying away from the base of the lesion until the setting is correct).
- With magnification assistance, remove the lesion using a loop electrode in a superficial sweep, gradually going deeper until all visible abnormal tissue has been removed (Figure 14.15).

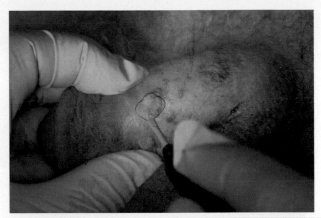

Figure 14.15 Removal of condyloma using radiofrequency shaving. A large dermatologic loop using a pure cutting mode is employed. Caution is needed lest the loop cut too deeply. *(Copyright John L. Pfenninger, MD.)*

- Wipe treated area with a 4 × 4 gauze moistened with acetic acid and reinspect area.
- Treat any bleeding with light electrofulguration or apply aluminum chloride for hemostasis (ferric subsulfate tends to leave an iron deposit stain especially in the genital area, and silver nitrate can leave gray marks/tattooing).
- When all lesions have been removed, apply petrolatum ointment to hasten healing and to prevent treated tissue from adhering to undergarments. Lidocaine ointment 5% can also be used to provide an anesthetic effect.
- All tissue removed should be sent to pathology since it is difficult to discern Bowenoid papulosis from benign condylomas with the naked eye.
- Because persistence of some viruses and growth of small, grossly undetectable lesions is common, a follow-up exam is generally done in 4 to 6 weeks to check for recurrences.
- With the association of HPV and cervical cancer, be sure you have addressed all issues regarding pap smear screening, immunizations, and safe sex practices.

Nevi – Benign

See Video 14.4.

One method for removal of benign nevi is high-frequency (radiofrequency) electrosurgery. Patients may ask for a nevus to be removed for cosmetic concerns or because of repeated trauma to them (e.g., under a bra strap, where routine shaving cuts them on the face or legs). There is no real advantage to this over using a DermaBlade or razor blade but some clinicians with RF units prefer this method. *All excised pigmented lesions regardless of method used for removal should be sent to the pathologist.*

The technique described here is for benign-appearing nevi rather than concerning nevi. The best way to discern this is by using a dermatoscope in addition to the clinical exam and history.

The following electrosurgical technique is for the removal of presumed benign nevi with RF (Figure 14.16):

- Anesthetize with 1% or 2% lidocaine with epinephrine. Be careful not to distort the lesion any more than necessary.

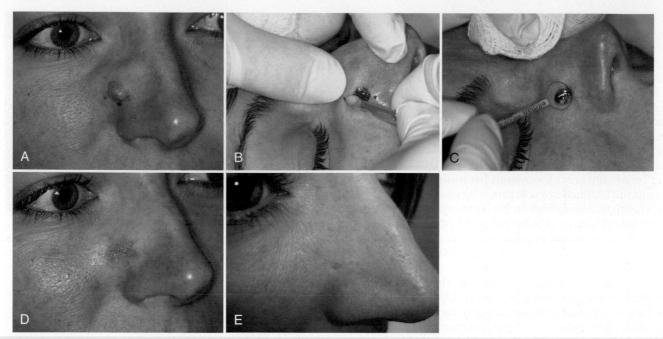

Figure 14.16 **(A)** A benign intradermal nevus on the face has been anesthetized prior to shave excision. **(B)** The nevus is excised with a No. 15 scalpel blade. **(C)** The remaining tissue is feathered with RF surgery using a loop electrode. **(D)** Immediate result. **(E)** Cosmetic result 1 year later. *(Copyright John L. Pfenninger, MD.)*

- Use a No. 15 scalpel blade or razor blade to shave off the lesion. If the lesion has no worrisome features, shave flat to avoid any depression of the scar.
- Using an RF unit and a wire loop electrode, "smooth out" the lesion to eliminate any residual tissue as well as to stop the bleeding using a light "feathering," sweeping motion. Blend in the edges of the shave with the surrounding skin. Keep the tissue moist with a dampened 4 × 4 gauze to make this step easier.
- Send the tissue to pathology.
- Dress the wound with petrolatum and an adhesive strip and give the patient wound and follow-up instructions.

Although radiosurgery is used to *finish the shave*, using the loop to remove the lesion primarily, instead of using a blade, is discouraged (due to burn artifact and the chances of the excision going too deeply). A well-done shave biopsy with a blade can also be completed with nothing more than aluminum chloride for hemostasis. This is less expensive, faster, and does not put smoke in the air. Either way, this is billed as a shave excision rather than a shave biopsy because the intent was to remove a benign lesion rather than biopsy for diagnosis.

Pyogenic Granuloma
(See Video 14.5)

Pyogenic granulomas are very vascular benign tumors also known as lobulated capillary hemangiomas (Figure 14.17). They occur most commonly on the fingers, face, lips, and gingiva but can be found anywhere from head to toe. Pyogenic granulomas often occur at the site of minor trauma and are more common in pregnancy. These vascular lesions are ideal for electrosurgical treatment.

In a randomized controlled study (RCT) comparing cryotherapy with liquid nitrogen versus curettage and electrodesiccation of patients with pyogenic granuloma, the curettage and electrodesiccation had the advantage of requiring fewer treatment sessions to achieve resolution and better cosmetic results.[11]

Before treatment, inject 1% lidocaine with epinephrine to cause blanching of the skin at the base of the lesion. Epinephrine is needed because of the extreme vascularity of these lesions. If the pyogenic granuloma is on a finger, start with a digital block with lidocaine and epinephrine. Some physicians place a temporary tourniquet around the base of the finger to control bleeding during the procedure. If choosing this approach, the tourniquet may be left on for up to 30 minutes safely.

Wait 10 minutes after the injection to gain the benefit of the epinephrine. Lab slips and forms can be filled out and equipment gathered during this time. The elevated portion of the lesion is then shaved off with a blade or a loop electrode using a cutting/coagulation current. Send the specimen for histology to rule out the remote possibility that the lesion is an amelanotic melanoma. The base of the wound is curetted with a 3- to 5-mm dermal curette to remove the remaining tissue. Before electrocoagulating the base, compress the tissue with gauze to control bleeding. Pooled blood or active bleeding will diminish the effectiveness of electrosurgery. In Figure 14.17, after blotting the blood away, the base is treated with electrodesiccation. (It may be necessary to use your ESU on a high wattage for these vascular lesions.) Further curettage and desiccation may be required a number of times to destroy the whole pyogenic granuloma and to stop the bleeding. If some tissue remains, the pyogenic granuloma will often regrow.

SEBACEOUS HYPERPLASIA

Sebaceous gland hyperplasia of the face is a common condition as people age. It is asymptomatic and not dangerous, but patients often ask for treatment for cosmetic reasons.

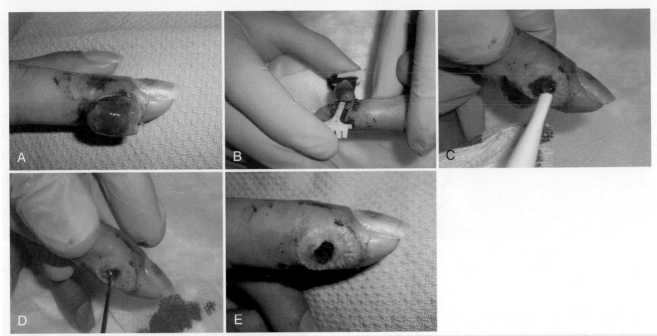

Figure 14.17 **(A)** Pyogenic granuloma that started during pregnancy. **(B)** Shave excision after pregnancy. **(C)** Curettage. **(D)** Electrofulguration with visible spark to the remaining vascular tissue. **(E)** Final result. More than one cycle of curettage and electrodestruction may be needed to stop the bleeding and prevent recurrence. *(Copyright Richard P. Usatine, MD.)*

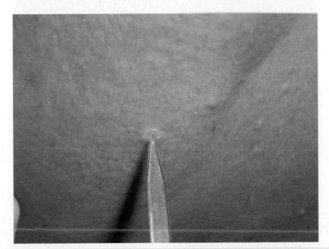

Figure 14.18 The blunt electrode is being used to treat sebaceous hyperplasia of the face without local anesthesia. The Hyfrecator is set at 2.1 watts. The tip is passed across the lesion or around the annular component while the Hyfrecator is actuated. *(Copyright Richard P. Usatine, MD.)*

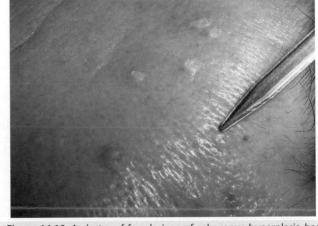

Figure 14.19 A cluster of four lesions of sebaceous hyperplasia has been treated with electrosurgery, leaving melted lesions with surrounding temporary erythema. *(Copyright Richard P. Usatine, MD.)*

Occasionally it may be unclear whether what appears to be sebaceous hyperplasia may actually be a BCC. Dermoscopy is a great method to resolve this issue. If the diagnosis is still uncertain, a biopsy is indicated. It is easiest to do a shave biopsy with a DermaBlade or scalpel. The base can then be treated lightly with electrosurgery.

When the diagnosis is certain, electrodesiccation is an option. Since it is cosmetic, let the patient know that treatment may not be covered by insurance. No anesthesia is needed. The treatment method with the Hyfrecator involves moving the blunt electrode (low-power 2.1–2.5 watts) around the somewhat annular tissue (Figure 14.18) and watching the lesion melt like butter (Figure 14.19) (the

lipids in the sebum do actually melt and give further confirmation of the diagnosis). Patient satisfaction is usually high despite the fact that tiny scars and recurrences are not uncommon.

Seborrheic Keratosis

If there is any question about whether a presumed SK is malignant, perform a shave biopsy with a razor blade to obtain a good specimen for pathology. However, a dermoscopic exam can most often help you distinguish between a benign SK and a lesion suspicious for melanoma. When dealing with a benign-appearing SK, another technique for removal is to lightly fulgurate the lesion and then wipe it off with a wet gauze or curette. Because this does not provide

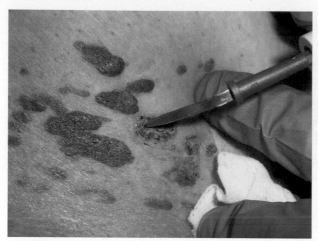

Figure 14.20 Electrosurgery can be used in conjunction with a curette or wet gauze to superficially remove seborrheic keratoses. (*Copyright Richard P. Usatine, MD.*)

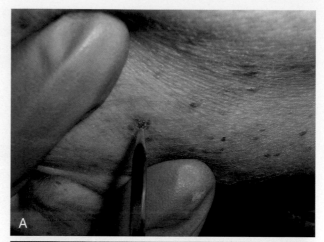

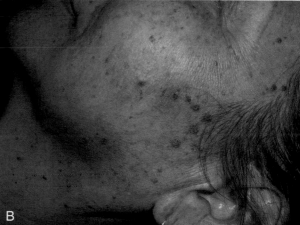

Figure 14.21 (A) Dermatosis papulosa nigra on the face of a Hispanic woman being treated with electrosurgery using a hyfrecator and a blunt electrode on a setting of 2.5 watts with no anesthesia. **(B)** The patient tolerated the procedure well, and the lesions can be seen with temporary surrounding erythema. The result was cosmetically excellent with no unwanted hypopigmentation. (*Copyright Richard P. Usatine, MD.*)

tissue for pathology, this approach should not be used if the lesion has suspicious features (i.e., may be a melanoma). The advantage of this technique is that the desiccated SK is easily removed from the skin below, without going deeper than necessary (Figure 14.20). This allows for good control of the depth of removal and can minimize scarring. However, these lesions are very hyperkeratotic and thus quite dry, often making any electrosurgical attempts at removal more difficult unless they are hydrated first using water-moistened 4 × 4 gauze.

When using radiosurgery to shave these lesions, it may help to outline the lesion with a surgical pen. A large round loop electrode can be used to shave off the lesion with a single initial pass using a pure cutting setting. The skin can be smoothed, using the loop like an artist painting with a brush, while keeping the electrode at a 90-degree angle to the skin surface. Gentle strokes are used to feather the edges of the lesion into the normal skin. A moist 4 × 4 gauze is used between passes of the electrode to remove tissue and moisten the skin. Because the electrical current kills potential infectious organisms, there is no need to use sterile water or saline to moisten the gauze; tap water is fine. Remember that radiosurgery, if set at too high of a power or with any coagulation setting, may still cause more tissue destruction than just a surgical blade, so that the chance of hypopigmentation or scarring may be greater. However, using a combined technique like that described above for a nevus optimizes ease of removal while limiting complications.

■ Dermatosis papulosa nigra is a condition with multiple small SKs on the face usually found in darker skin types. It can be treated with light electrodesiccation using a blunt electrode on a Hyfrecator setting of 2.3 to 2.8. (Figure 14.21) Note how there is a pink blush that normally occurs immediately after treatment.

SKIN TAGS (ACROCHORDONS)

There is no absolute cutoff for differentiating between large, medium, and small skin tags. We define the *smallest* skin tags as those lesions that are too small to be grasped easily with forceps and therefore are difficult to shave or snip off.

The *largest* wide-based lesions are those that would be difficult to remove with a single snip of a sharp iris scissor. These are best shaved off with a razor blade after injecting lidocaine and epinephrine.

To treat a small or medium skin tag with electrosurgery, light electrodesiccation or fulguration (blunt or sharp electrode) should be used (Figure 14.22A). This is done without anesthesia with a setting of 2.1 to 2.5 on the Hyfrecator. After the lesion is charred to a gray color, the char can be removed with a gauze, or it can be allowed to fall off on its own.

The eyelid is a location where it is important to be very careful when using chemicals for hemostasis. It is also important to be careful with electrosurgery near the eyes. Before activating, light electrodesiccation shifts the skin so that it does not overlie the globe, which allows for hemostasis without endangering the eye. For radiosurgery of a skin tag, a loop electrode with a cut and coagulation setting of 4 to 6 W should be used after lidocaine and epinephrine are injected first. The skin tag should be shaved off with the loop alone or grasped with the forceps in the loop first (Figure 14.22B). Cryosurgery with the Cryo Tweezers is an excellent alternative that is safer and easier to perform (see Chapter 13, *Cryosurgery*).

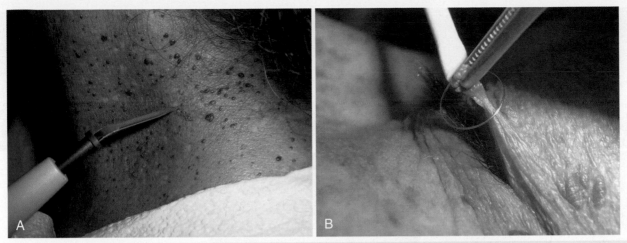

Figure 14.22 **(A)** Skin tags on the neck of a Hispanic woman being treated with electrosurgery using a Hyfrecator and a blunt electrode in a setting of 2.5 watts with no anesthesia. **(B)** An electrosurgical loop on a cutting instrument is about to transect an eyelid skin tag. Local anesthetic was injected prior to cutting with RF current. This method allows for cutting and coagulation simultaneously, thereby avoiding getting blood or hemostatic chemicals into the eye. *(Copyright Richard P. Usatine, MD.)*

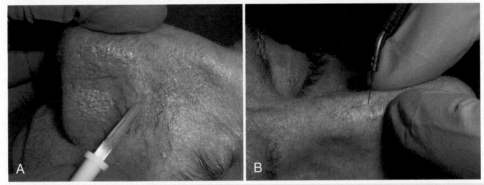

Figure 14.23 **(A)** Electrosurgical treatment of facial telangiectasias using a sharp disposable electrode with approximately 2 W of energy and no local anesthetic. **(B)** Electrocoagulation of nasal telangiectasias using a specialized epilation needle. The tip of the needle is inserted into the telangiectasia, and the current is actuated for approximately 1 second. *(Copyright Richard P. Usatine, MD.)*

TELANGIECTASIAS

Telangiectasias (Figure 14.23) are fine veins that occur commonly on the face and legs. Electrosurgery works best for fine telangiectasias on the face and not for these veins on the legs. Any telangiectasia over 1 mm in diameter is likely to bleed and persist. Treatment of these lesions is for cosmetic reasons, so it is important to review the various options (laser) and the possible complications including small dot scars or failure to improve.

Before treating telangiectasias discuss with the patient the pros and cons of using topical anesthesia.

1. It is possible to treat without topical anesthesia in most cases. Areas around the nose, however, are especially sensitive. If a topical anesthetic (e.g., EMLA) is used, allow it to remain in place for at least 15 minutes. Injecting the area with a local anesthetic can obscure the lesion.
2. Choose the sharp tip electrode for the Hyfrecator or a fine-needle (33-gauge) electrode. The Ellman company provides fine-needle electrodes for the Surgitron that are specially coated with Teflon for treating telangiectasias. This limits burning of the overlying skin. Only the very tip is active while the rest of the needle is shielded.

ConMed also provides fine-needle electrodes for use with the Hyfrecator as an alternative to the disposable sharp tip electrode.

3. Magnification loupes are very helpful since the smaller telangiectasias respond best and will be more easily identified.
4. Use a low-power coagulation/hemostasis setting. Use 2 to 2.5 W for the Hyfrecator. For the Ellman, 2 W works well.
5. Wipe off the topical anesthetic if used. With the patient in a supine position to limit movement, begin treatment by warning the patient that you will start. The hand holding the handpiece should rest on the patient so that it moves with the patient should the patient suddenly jerk or pull away. Touch the sharp tip electrode of the Hyfrecator to the telangiectasia, and press the button for a short burst only. If using a fine needle, insert it into the vein superficially, enough to penetrate into the lumen. Then activate the instrument. This can transmit the energy further in contrast to fulguration which is intended to be superficial. The needle may even pass through the small diameter vessel but remain as close to the surface as possible to limit tissue damage. Do not cannulate the vein; instead, place the needle in a perpendicular position

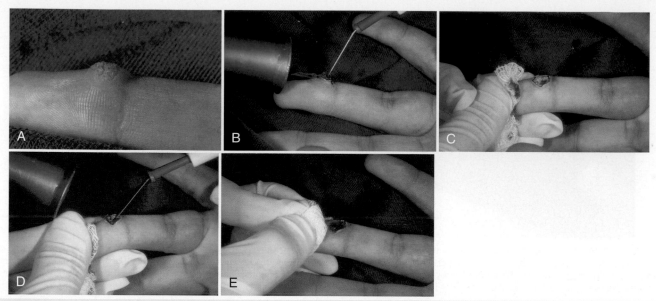

Figure 14.24 (A) Common wart not responding to cryosurgery. **(B)** Electrodesiccation with the Hyfrecator and smoke evacuator. **(C)** Charred tissue removed with gauze. **(D)** Repeat electrodesiccation. **(E)** Immediate result. *(Copyright Richard P. Usatine, MD.)*

to it. Generally, it is not helpful to find the "feeding trunk" since the entire vein will need to be treated anyway or they will recur. If the "feeder" is treated first, the vessel may go into spasm, making the remainder of the vein hard to find. With this in mind, start distally with the smallest part of the vein and march toward the central (larger portion) of the vessel. One technique is to keep the electrode activated and just "tap" into the vein every 3 mm along the entire path.

6. Bleeding is not uncommon, especially as the vessels become larger. Cautiously turn up the power slightly. If this does not help, apply pressure. If the vessel continues to bleed, it is likely that it is not occluded and chances for recurrence are higher.

Complications include the discomfort while doing the procedure, bleeding (controlled with pressure), recurrence, and persistent red or brown marks. The discoloration generally clears but takes time and is more common if the power is set too high or if sensitive skin is treated. If the vessels are extensive and very fine or, very "large" such as those seen with rhinophyma and rosacea, it is best to go with a laser treatment.

WARTS (VERRUCA VULGARIS)

Patients seek treatment for warts (lesions caused by the HPV) because warts can cause pain, can be unsightly, and can spread to other parts of the body or to other individuals. HPV can infect many parts of the body. In this section, we will only address these HPV infections of the skin: verruca vulgaris, plantar warts, and planar (flat) warts.

Most warts can be treated easily with cryotherapy as described in Chapter 13 or with intralesional injection as discussed in Chapter 15. Patients may use topical agents at home. However, some warts are refractory to all treatments. Also, if the warts are small (a few millimeters) and there are only a few lesions, electrosurgery has the advantage of

providing a single in-office treatment with visible removal of the wart at the time of treatment. Cryotherapy and intralesional injection methods are more likely to require multiple visits for treatment.

Electrosurgery of warts always requires local anesthesia. If treating the digits (Figure 14.24), use a digital block with lidocaine and epinephrine (see Chapter 3, *Anesthesia*). Fulguration or electrodesiccation/coagulation/hemostasis settings are used to destroy the wart (Figure 14.24B). Refer to Table 14.1 for power settings. The sharp tip electrode is generally used. With smaller lesions, desiccated tissue is then wiped away with a moist gauze or a curette (Figure 14.24C). If any wart tissue remains, the remaining tissue should receive additional electrosurgery and be wiped away until the final deep layer shows a uniform clear dermis (Figure 14.24D and E). The base of the lesion, however, is often charred by the treatment, obscuring the underlying tissue so this needs to be wiped off to inspect the base. Warts are an epidermal lesion so care should be used not to penetrate through the dermis.

If the wart is large and protuberant, the tissue can be shaved off first ("debulked") with a razor blade or scalpel. A dermal curette can be used to catch the edge of the wart tissue and pop it out like a pea to debulk further. Also, warts are very hyperkeratotic and dry, so the electrosurgical application may not work well. Soaking with a moistened 4 × 4 gauze or with surgical jelly beforehand will help. Care should be taken not to burn surrounding tissue excessively, which can cause painful permanent scarring. In the fingers, use care to avoid the digital nerves and arteries on the sides of the digits. There is no benefit to using RF methods in the destruction of warts.

Possible *complications* include significant pain, recurrence, hypopigmentation, and scarring. Caution must be used on the plantar surfaces because scarring can cause long-term problems of pain with ambulation. Treatment around the nails may lead to deformities of the nail if the matrix is injured. In some instances, before resolving, treatment can induce a paradoxical reaction where the wart may grow or multiply.

MALIGNANT LESIONS

ED&C is a useful method of treating NMSCs. It should never be used for a melanoma. If a malignancy is suspected, it is often best to biopsy it before definitive treatment. Even experienced clinicians with the aid of a dermatoscope can be mistaken about the diagnosis at times, and sometimes even with a correct diagnosis, a high-risk type NMSC may be found on pathology, which is more appropriately treated with surgery and not a destructive method. Shave biopsies are adequate for most NMSCs. If the lesion is either a pigmented BCC or a melanoma, a deep shave excision (saucerization) may be performed. (See Chapter 8, *Choosing the Biopsy Type*).

Electrodesiccation and Curettage

▶ *See Videos 14.6 and 14.7.*

"Electrodesiccation and curettage" has many names including "curettage and desiccation" and "curettage and cautery." In fact, the names that start with curettage are more accurate as the procedure begins with curettage. Start with a curette size to match the lesion size (usually 5 mm – typical range between 3 and 7 mm). The curette allows the clinician to scrape away the soft malignant tissue until reaching the characteristic gritty feel of healthy dermis. The electrodesiccation/fulguration may be performed with the Hyfrecator (or similar unit) and a blunt tip electrode. The high-frequency units also have a fulguration mode.

There are *contraindications* for using electrosurgery to treat BCC or SCC based on the histology and location. Sclerosing (morpheaform), micronodular, "aggressive" BCCs as well as SCCs in non–sun-exposed areas over 7 to 8 mm can be more aggressive and are best treated with excision. The superficial type of BCC or an SCC *in situ* may be successfully treated with ED&C.

One study compared recurrence rates of 268 consecutive primary nonmelanoma tumors (BCCs and SCCs) treated by surgical excision or ED&C. The recurrence rates between the two types of treatment were not found to be significantly different.[12] A meta-analysis of all studies reporting recurrence rates of BCC between 1947 and 1987 reported a 5-year recurrence rate of approximately 8% for ED&C.[13]

An analysis of recurrence rates of 2314 previously untreated BCCs removed by ED&C showed that increasing lesion diameter, high-risk, and middle-risk anatomic sites were independent risk factors for high recurrence rates.[14] Risk stratification by anatomic site on the face is depicted in (Figure 14.25). From 1973 to 1982 the following recurrence rates were found:

- *Low-risk sites (neck, trunk, and four extremities)*. BCCs of all diameters responded well to curettage electrodesiccation with an overall 5-year recurrence rate of 3.3%.
- *Middle-risk sites (scalp, forehead, preauricular and postauricular, and malar areas)*. BCCs less than 10 mm in diameter had a recurrence rate of 5.3%.

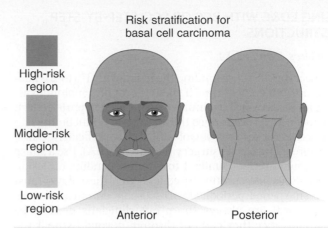

Figure 14.25 Risk stratification for basal cell carcinoma on the face and head. *(From Robinson J, Hanke W, Sengelmann R, Siegel D.* Surgery of the Skin: Procedural Dermatology, *2nd ed. Philadelphia: Mosby; 2010.)*

- *High-risk sites (nose, paranasal, nasal-labial groove, ear, chin, mandibular, perioral, and periocular areas)*. Lesions less than 6 mm in diameter had a recurrence rate of 4.5%.[14]

The authors concluded that BCCs less than 6 mm in diameter, regardless of anatomic site, as well as selected larger BCCs depending on their anatomic site, are effectively treated by ED&C.[14]

One caveat is that the American Association of Dermatology 2006 guidelines recommend avoiding ED&C for the treatment of BCC on the scalp, beard, and other areas with terminal hair growth as BCC may spread down the hair follicles and missed with treatment.[15] Recurrence rates of primary NMSCs treated by excision versus ED&C ×3 were studied in a private dermatology practice. Tumors up to 2 cm in size were included. One percent of excised tumors recurred, whereas 3% treated with ED&C did. This study found the recurrence rates to be essentially the same in spite of the fact that they used electrosurgery to treat tumors larger than generally recommended. ED&C was quicker, less costly, had fewer complications, and the scars were often less.[12] A more recent 2018 systematic review of the literature and metanalysis reported a 6.9% recurrence rate for BCC treated with ED&C.[16]

The American Academy of Dermatology 2016 guidelines for the treatment of SCC indicate that ED&C can be considered for small low-risk SCCs although they noted limited comparisons with other treatments and potential variability in success between clinicians.[17] Organ transplant recipients frequently develop multiple SCCs. In one study, appropriately selected low-risk SCCs in 48 organ transplant recipients were treated by ED&C. Only histologically confirmed SCCs were considered in this study.[18] The mean follow-up time was 50 months, and 13 residual or recurrent SCCs were observed in 10 patients. The overall rate of residual or recurrent SCCs was 6%, with 7% for SCCs on the dorsum of the hands or fingers, 11% for SCCs on the head and neck, 0% for the forearms, and 5% for the remaining non–sun-exposed areas (shoulder, legs). In organ transplant recipients with many SCCs, ED&C can be a safe therapy for appropriately selected low-risk SCCs, with an acceptable cure rate.[18]

USING ED&C WITH BCC OR SCC: STEP-BY-STEP INSTRUCTIONS

See Videos 14.6 and 14.7.

- Inject the skin surrounding the lesion with 1% to 2% lidocaine with epinephrine. If there is a lot of remaining vascular tissue wait 10 minutes for the full epinephrine effect. Otherwise, proceed once the anesthesia is functioning.
- Curette the softer tissue of a BCC or superficial SCC first before using electrosurgery (Figure 14.26A). Use a sharp dermal curette, usually 3 to 5 mm depending on lesion size. Reusable curettes (used less often these days) must be sharpened periodically. Disposable curettes (current standard) are always sharp but clinicians need to be careful since they can cut through normal tissue if too much pressure is applied. Curettage is effective because the BCC or SCC is softer than the surrounding normal skin and it also has a characteristic friable or sometimes gelatinous appearance. The abnormal tissue is removed by scraping with the curette in all directions. It can be helpful to mentally picture scraping across the lesion toward all of the numbers on a clockface sequentially.
- Scrape across the surface of the lesion instead of digging down into normal dermis. NMSC arises at the interface of the epidermis and dermis so unless very advanced, there should be some intact dermis. Once the dermis is reached there will be a gritty feel to scraping over normal dermis and often an audible scratching sound.
- Fulgurate the base of the lesion of the surrounding normal tissue (Figure 14.26B). The general rule for a BCC is that a margin of 3 to 5 mm of normal tissue should be removed with an excision. ED&C provides this margin.
- One additional cycle is performed for a total of two cycles. Treatment time is 5 minutes or less. The original studies were done with less sharp reusable curettes and recommended three cycles. Two cycles should be adequate with the new sharp disposable curettes, but three cycles is an option when starting to learn this procedure.
- After the 2 to 3 cycles are performed, burn the border one final time by going around the circumference with the electrosurgical device (Figure 14.26C).
- Dress the wound with petrolatum and an adhesive strip or gauze. Wound care is as simple as covering the area with clean petrolatum and a clean dressing daily after washing.

- The wound may take 3 to 4 weeks to heal, usually with some hypopigmentation. It is essential that the patient understand the principles of moist healing and adheres to them.

Treating SCC *in situ* with ED&C follows the same steps (Figure 14.27).

One caveat is that should the curettage penetrate into the subcutaneous fat, it indicates either that the tumor has invaded deeply, or that the curettage was overzealous. It is best to perform a full excision in those situations. The same can happen if a punch was performed recently for the diagnosis, and this is one reason that a shave biopsy is usually superior to a punch for the diagnosis of NMSC.

Learning the Techniques

See Videos 14.8–14.11.
Regardless of the unit used, it is possible to practice the electrosurgery techniques with a piece of uncooked beef steak or pig's or beef feet, which are frequently available in local grocery stores or can be found at butcher shops. The steak should be a fresh, inexpensive cut of steak that is not too fatty and without many tendinous attachments. Pig's feet with their attached skin are excellent for practicing ED&C. It is not necessary to use a smoke evacuator while practicing on meat, but there will be significant odor if not working in a well-ventilated area.

PRACTICING ED&C WITH THE HYFRECATOR

- The pig's foot should be touched broadly with the gloved nonoperating hand to create a ground (this is necessary since the sample has small mass in contrast to a real patient and will not absorb the energy enough to get effective electrodesiccation. This will not shock the clinician as long as one does not initiate or break contact with the sample during use).
- Begin with the handpiece plugged into the low setting.
- Practice activating the handpiece and coming close to the steak until the sparks of fulguration appear.
- Turn up the current to see how the sparking and tissue destruction (cooking of the steak) increase.
- Try the same exercise with the electrode touching the meat to produce electrodesiccation.

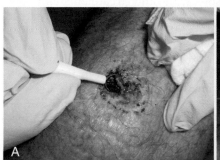 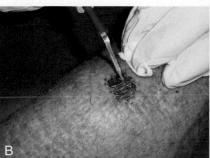 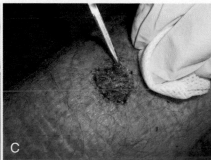

Figure 14.26 Electrodesiccation and curettage. **(A)** Curettage of a nodular basal cell carcinoma on the arm showing how the soft malignant tissue is easily scraped from the normal surrounding skin. **(B)** Electrodesiccation after curettage of the BCC. The blunt electrode is moved back and forth across the treated area. **(C)** A small margin of normal tissue is treated using a circular motion around the periphery. *(Copyright Richard P. Usatine, MD.)*

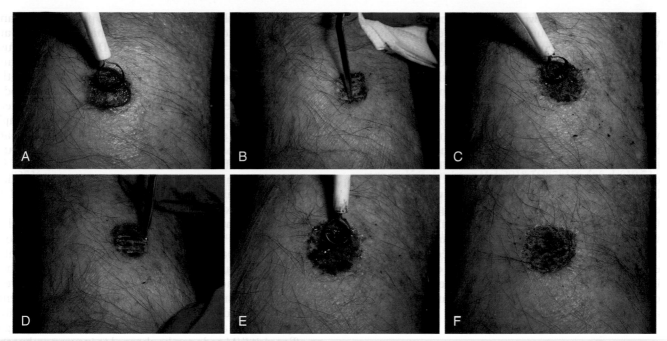

Figure 14.27 Electrodesiccation and curettage. **(A)** Curettage of a squamous cell carcinoma *in situ* on the arm. **(B)** Electrodesiccation after curettage. The blunt electrode is moved back and forth across the treated area. **(C)** Curettage is repeated for this second cycle. **(D)** Electrodesiccation is repeated. The electric spark is visible in this image. **(E)** Curettage is repeated for this third cycle and much less tissue is obtained. **(F)** The final electrodesiccation was performed as before, and a small margin of normal tissue was treated using a circular motion around the periphery. (*Copyright Richard P. Usatine, MD.*)

- Then plug the handpiece into the high setting as a learning exercise. Observe the increased destruction of tissue without turning up the digital number (the destructive power of 20 on high is higher than 20 on low). Note that most ED&C for NMSC works well with settings of about 16 to 17 watts on low.
- For ED&C practice, electrodesiccate a 1-cm circle on the pig's skin until it is thoroughly darkened. As there is no real lesion here, we start with electrodesiccation and end with curettage (opposite to real ED&C for NMSC).
- Using a dermal curette, scrape off the dark charred material, which should easily scrape off.
- Curette until you feel the gritty sensation when you reach the dermis.
- Scrape across the defect in all of the directions of the numbers on a clock face.
- Repeat a cycle of ED&C.

PRACTICING RADIOSURGERY

Follow these guidelines for practicing with the Ellman Surgitron and other high-frequency units:

- Wear exam gloves to avoid inadvertent shocks from the device, and be extremely careful what the tips contact. **These instruments cut very quickly and effectively!**
- To practice cutting, place the steak on a paper towel or blue pad sitting on top of the "antenna" plate. Begin with a round wire electrode (either small or large, with the latter requiring slightly more power but providing a flatter excision) in the handpiece, and set the unit to "cut" on a mid-range setting. Be sure the meat is moist and not dried out on top. Perform the usual sequence, and activate the electrode *before* touching the meat to provide a smooth cut with minimal tissue damage. Cut through the meat, keeping the loop at a right angle to the tissue. Compare how this looks and feels to activating the electrode *after* touching the meat. Note that when doing it this way, the electrode will often not cut at all.
- Repeat this exercise after turning the power up to a much higher setting and observe more spark and smoke. The tissue will also have more char (damage). The ideal setting will provide enough power to cut smoothly through the meat without catching ("stalling") and yet leave little tissue damage behind.
- Now turn the power to a low setting. Note how the electrode drags. Determine which setting will allow the electrode to move through the meat without either sparking or a drag.
- To simulate cutting off a benign lesion place the electrosurgical loop near an edge of the steak. Reach through the loop with the forceps and grasp an edge of the steak and lift it up. Activate the unit and slice cleanly underneath the raised tissue.
- Practice making true vertical incisions in the meat using the Vari-Tip electrode, again on the "pure cut" setting. It is ok to hold the handpiece in your fingers like a pen/pencil, but instead of holding it at an angle as taught in school, rotate the handpiece to cut vertically instead of at an acute angle to the skin.
- Change the length of the electrode by pulling or pushing the very fine wire to the desired length in the insulating portion of the tip to see how the depth of the cut can be varied as needed for the depth of the skin or tissues. Increase and decrease the power as above to see effects.
- Remove the antenna plate (neutral electrode) from under the meat, and try cutting with a loop on a setting that is optimal. Note that it is almost impossible to cut at

15 *Intralesional Injections*

RICHARD P. USATINE, MD, and JIMENA CERVANTES, MD

> **SUMMARY**
> - Intralesional injections of steroids are used to decrease inflammation in lesions such as hidradenitis, cystic acne, and granuloma annulare, to flatten keloids and hypertrophic scars, and to increase hair regrowth in alopecia areata.
> - Indications and contraindications are reviewed.
> - Recommendations for steroid strength and needle size are listed by diagnosis.
> - How to dilute triamcinolone to the proper concentration is discussed.
> - Tips on how to treat specific lesions are covered.
> - Intralesional injections for warts using candida antigen and other options are discussed.

Intralesional injections of steroids are used to decrease inflammation in lesions such as hidradenitis, cystic acne, and granuloma annulare, to flatten keloids and hypertrophic scars, and to increase hair regrowth in alopecia areata. The standard injectable steroid in dermatology is triamcinolone acetonide (Kenalog). Diluting the steroid when needed and injecting the steroid into the correct location are the most crucial aspects of this process. This chapter focuses on injectable steroids but will also address injectable Candida antigen and other agents for the intralesional treatment of verrucae.

Indications

Indications for the use of intralesional steroid injections in dermatology include the following:

- Acne cysts
- Acne keloidalis nuchae
- Alopecia areata
- Discoid lupus
- Granuloma annulare
- Hidradenitis suppurativa
- Hypertrophic scars
- Keloids
- Lichen simplex chronicus
- Prurigo nodularis
- Psoriasis
- Sarcoidosis

Contraindications

Intralesional injection of steroids should be avoided in these situations:

- When lesions are too extensive
- When there is a local infection
- When the patient is unwilling to accept the potential of skin atrophy and hypopigmentation as side effects.

Equipment

The equipment used for intralesional injections is listed here:

- Injectable steroids (triamcinolone acetonide 10 mg/mL and 40 mg/mL) (Figure 15.1)
- Needles (25, 27, and 30 gauge)
- Syringes (1, 3, 5, or 6 mL) (Luer-Lok is preferable)
- Vials of sterile saline or 1% or 2% lidocaine without epinephrine (for dilution)

Eye and face protection – a face shield is preferable even in clinicians who wear glasses.

Informed Consent

Patients should be informed of the risks of skin atrophy, incomplete resolution of the lesion, and hypopigmentation. Have the patient sign a consent form, especially if the lesion is on the face. Special care should be taken when treating lesions on the face in darkly pigmented individuals because hypopigmentation can be a particularly unacceptable side effect. As with all informed consent, the patient should be made aware of alternative therapies. Alternative therapies for keloids are listed in Table 15.1.

Steroid Strength

Once the appropriate-strength steroid for the injection has been chosen, the standard-strength preparations may need to be diluted to produce the desired strength. Recommendations for steroid strength and needle size are listed in Table 15.2. Triamcinolone acetonide suspension is available in two strengths: 10 and 40 mg/mL. It is essential to dilute the steroid, especially for injections of cystic acne of the face. Dilution can be performed quickly and safely for each patient using simple math or Table 15.3.

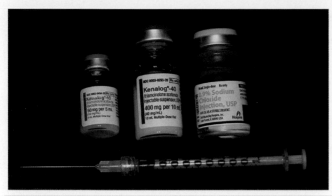

Figure 15.1 Injectable triamcinolone acetonide with sterile saline for injection and a Luer-Lok 1-mL syringe (with 27 gauge needle) used for intralesional injections. *(Copyright Richard P. Usatine, MD.)*

Table 15.1   Therapies for Keloids

Topical	
	Corticosteroids
	Retinoids
	Imiquimod
	Mederma
	Vitamin E
Injectable	
	Corticosteroids
	Interferons
	5-Fluorouracil
	Verapamil
	Bleomycin
Surgical	
	Surgical debulking or excision
	Laser debulking or excision
	Radio-frequency electrosurgery planing
Physical	
	Laser therapy
	Radiation therapy
	Compression therapy
	Silicone sheeting
	Cryotherapy
	Fractional laser ablation

Source: Adapted from Baldwin H. Keloid management (Chapter 44). *In:* Robinson JK et al., eds., *Surgery of the Skin: Procedural Dermatology.* Philadelphia: Elsevier; 2005.

Triamcinolone is most often diluted with sterile normal saline for injection. Alternatives include 1% or 2% lidocaine (without epinephrine). The isotonicity and neutral pH of sterile saline makes it the preferred solution for dilution. The use of lidocaine can increase chance of atrophy of the skin due to the increased risk of flocculation of the steroid.

A 1-mL Luer-Lok or tuberculin syringe is useful for making a single dilution before injection. To create a 2 mg/mL concentration, draw 0.4 mL of sterile saline into a 1-mL syringe and add 0.1 mL of 10 mg/mL triamcinolone. Other dilutions are listed in Table 15.3. Turn the syringe upside down a number of times to mix the new suspension. Recommended needle sizes by lesion are listed in Table 15.2.

Treating Specific Lesions

See Video 15.1.

ACNE NODULES AND CYSTS

Patients with tender large nodulocystic lesions can expect to get symptomatic relief within 24 hours of an intralesional injection. The lesion will flatten within 2 to 3 days with an effective injection.[1] Although this should not be the primary treatment of acne, it can provide short-term relief while employing more long-term treatment regimens.

One small study evaluated the effectiveness of intralesional injections of steroids in the therapy of nodulocystic acne.[1] They found that 0.63 mg/mL of triamcinolone was as effective as 2.5 mg/mL.[1] Betamethasone injections were no better than saline controls.[1] One review article states that concentrations of 3.3 and 5 mg/mL of triamcinolone are standard dilutions for intralesional acne injections.[2]

We recommend using 2 to 3.3 mg/mL of triamcinolone for nodulocystic acne depending on the location of the lesions and the experience of the clinician and patient. Triamcinolone can be injected with minimal pain using a 30-gauge needle on a 1-mL syringe at a 45- to 90-degree angle with the skin (Figure 15.2).

For acne cysts on the face, it is safer to use 2 mg/mL to make sure that atrophy does not occur. On the trunk consider using 2.5 to 3.3 mg/mL of triamcinolone. Enough suspension should be injected to see and feel the cyst become distended, but no more than 0.1 mL is needed for any one cyst. One injection site per acne cyst should be adequate. If the cyst is large and soft, do not inject more volume because that can lead to atrophy. If there is a lot of purulent material inside the cyst, a quick incision and drainage (with lidocaine and a No. 11 scalpel) before injecting the steroid may be helpful.

ACNE KELOIDALIS NUCHAE

Acne keloidalis (Figures 15.3 and 15.4) occurs on the posterior neck most commonly in men with dark skin tones. It is an inflammatory condition that is exacerbated by shaving the back of the neck. It has features of acne, folliculitis, and scarring alopecia. Over time keloidal-type scars occur and can become very large. Treatment and prevention include not cutting the hair too short and using topical steroids and topical retinoids. Tender and painful keloidal nodules can be injected with triamcinolone for some relief. Concentrations of 10 to 40 mg/mL may be used. The heavier the fibrosis and scarring, the larger the needle needed to inject the lesion. These lesions are usually very tough and fibrotic so do not expect to get much steroid

Table 15.2   Guide to Intralesional Injections (Always Use Face Shield)

Diagnosis	Triamcinolone(mg/mL)[a]	Needle Size (gauge)	Amount per Lesion *Rough Guide (mL)
Acne cysts (face and neck)	2	30	0.1
Acne cysts (trunk)	2–5	27–30	0.1
Acne keloidalis nuchae	10–40	25–27	0.2–0.5
Alopecia areata	5	27	Varies by size
Discoid lupus	5	27	0.3–0.5
Granuloma annulare	5	27	0.4–0.5
Hidradenitis suppurativa	10	27	0.5
Hypertrophic scars	10–20	25–27	Varies by size
Keloids	10–40	25–27	Varies by size
Lichen simplex chronicus	5	27	Varies by size
Prurigo nodularis	5	27	0.1–0.2
Psoriasis	5	27	Varies by size
Sarcoidosis	5	27–30	0.2–0.5

*Rough guide as lesion size varies and steroid amount and strength should be lower for the face. Keep the total amount of triamcinolone to a maximum of 40 mg in one visit.
Acne dilution for 2 mg/mL: 0.1 mL of 10 mg/mL triamcinolone with 0.4 mL of normal saline in 1 mL syringe
Use 10 mg/mL triamcinolone in all cases except for refractory keloids.
[a]For lesions on the face, always start with lower concentrations.

Table 15.3   Common Triamcinolone Dilutions in a 1-mL Syringe

Concentration (mg/mL)	mL of Triamcinolone 10 mg/mL	mL of Sterile Saline for Injection
2	0.1	0.4
2.5	0.2	0.6
3.3	0.2	0.4
5	0.3	0.3

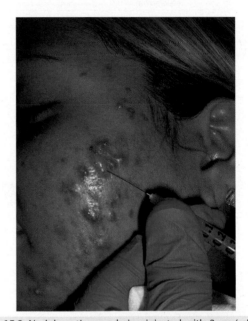

Figure 15.2 Nodulocystic acne being injected with 2 mg/mL triamcinolone before starting isotretinoin. *(Copyright Richard P. Usatine, MD.)*

volume into the area, which is one reason that high concentrations are recommended. Other types of scarring alopecia such as lichen planopilaris can be injected with steroid - see video 15.2.

ALOPECIA AREATA (FIGURE 15.5)

Considering the possibility of spontaneous remission in the early stages of the disease, it is reasonable to reassure the patient and recommend tincture of time. However, many patients are seeking an active treatment. Intralesional steroid for alopecia areata is a well-accepted standard treatment and often gives patients hope that they will regain their hair. Using the intralesional steroid injection method over other treatment options allows for better penetration of the epidermal barrier to decrease inflammation of small, isolated patches (<3 cm) of AA. There are no randomized clinical studies confirming this as the most effective therapeutic choice; however, 60% to 75% of patients with AA who undergo treatment experience hair regrowth approximately within 6 weeks of treatment.[3] Recommended concentrations of triamcinolone range from 2.5 mg/mL to 10 mg/mL for the scalp, but the higher concentrations often cause scalp atrophy.

Therefore we recommend using 5 mg/mL of triamcinolone for the scalp. AA can affect the eyebrows and the beard. It is recommended to be an experienced injector prior to attempting these aesthetic locations. For those regions it is safer to stick with a lower concentration of triamcinolone such as 2.5 mg/mL.[3] A long 27-gauge needle (1.25–1.5 inches) will allow for treatment of larger areas with fewer injections per site; a spacing of 0.5–1 cm between punctures is recommended. In children or highly sensitive adults, one can consider the use of a topical anesthetic, vibratory techniques, or local

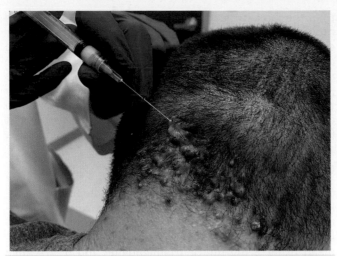

Figure 15.3 Acne keloidalis nuchae injected with 40 mg/mL triamcinolone using a 25 gauge needle as the lower concentration injections were not effective. *(Copyright Richard P. Usatine, MD.)*

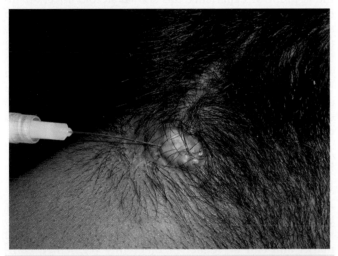

Figure 15.4 Acne keloidalis nuchae injected with 10mg/mL triamcinolone using a 27 gauge needle. Note the blanching of the affected tissue as the injection is intralesional. *(Copyright Richard P. Usatine, MD.)*

cooling of the affected area prior to injecting to help minimize the discomfort.[3]

A systematic review of concentrations of intralesional triamcinolone acetonide used in the treatment of alopecia areata for hair regrowth found pooled rates of hair regrowth to be[4]:

- 62.3% with less than 5 mg/mL
- 80.9% with 5 mg/mL
- 76.4% with 10 mg/mL

Skin atrophy was described in a subset of studies and occurred in 4 of 120 subjects (3.33%) treated with a concentration of 5 mg/mL and 12 of 59 (20%) treated with a concentration of 10 mg/mL.[4]

Our experience is such that we use 5 mg/mL for the best effectiveness with the least skin atrophy.

We use a long 27-gauge needle (1.25–1.5 inches) to allow for treatment of larger areas with fewer injections per site (Figures 15.5 and 15.6).[4]

Alopecia areata can affect the eyebrows and the beard. For those regions it is safer to stick with a lower concentration of triamcinolone such as 2.5 to 3.3 mg/mL.[3]

CUTANEOUS LUPUS

Intralesional steroids have been used for decades to treat patients with all types of localized cutaneous lupus (Figure 15.7).[5,6] Widespread cutaneous lupus is best treated with topical steroids and systemic agents when indicated. For specific local lesions that are not responding well, discuss the option of intralesional steroids with the patient. Our recommendation is to use from 2.5 to 5 mg/mL depending on the site. Special care should be taken when treating lupus on the face in an individual with dark skin tones because hypopigmentation can be a particularly unacceptable adverse effect. Patients should also be made aware that the lupus itself can cause hypopigmentation.

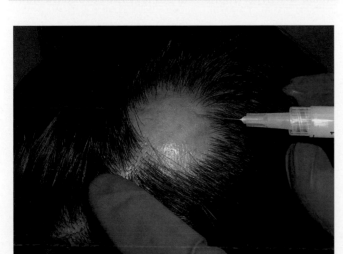

Figure 15.5 Alopecia areata being injected with 5 mg/mL triamcinolone. Note how the affected area is blanching and swelling with the injection at the follicular level.

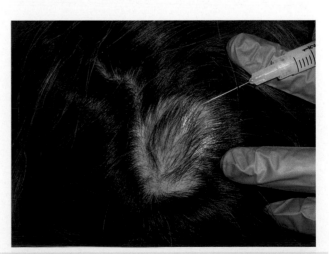

Figure 15.6 Reinjection of alopecia areata at a site where regrowth of hair has occurred after previously being injected with triamcinolone. While the regrowth is dark sometimes the new hair is white. *(Copyright Richard P. Usatine, MD.)*

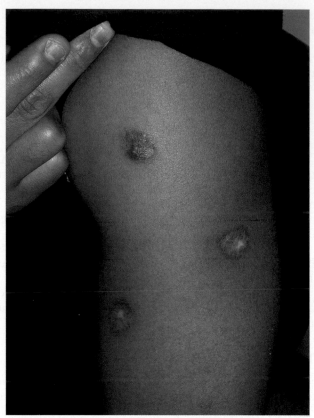

Figure 15.7 Discoid lupus on the arm. The top lesion is inflamed and can benefit from intralesional steroid. *(Copyright Richard P. Usatine, MD.)*

than the face. It may be best to use the lower end of this range when injecting hidradenitis around the breasts because this area is of more cosmetic concern. Because the cysts are often larger than acne, a 3- to 6-mL syringe may be needed to provide more volume for injection. Asking the patient to point out and count the number of lesions to be injected is very helpful in planning how much steroid to draw up. We usually use 10 mg/mL undiluted with about 0.5 mL for each lesion (with a maximum of 40 mg in 1 day).

GRANULOMA ANNULARE

Granuloma annulare (Figure 15.9) is an idiopathic granulomatous disease that typically appears in ringlike formations. Treatments for localized disease include high-potency topical steroids and injections of triamcinolone. We recommend using 5 mg/mL of triamcinolone and a 27-gauge needle. Four injection sites are usually needed to cover one annular lesion, so a syringe larger than 1 mL is often needed. Inject into the granulomatous lesion and not below the lesion. Our experience has shown steroid injections to be more effective than topical steroids, and studies also show that 70% of patients have improvement compared to those noninjected with steroids. It is also thought that the mechanical trauma in the act of injection itself, can help involute GA lesions. With this theory cryosurgery can also be considered for a destructive method of treatment; one cycle of 10 to 60 s can have improved outcomes.[7] If the condition is disseminated, there are other treatments to consider.

HIDRADENITIS SUPPURATIVA

See Video 15.4.

Injecting painful acute hidradenitis suppurativa cysts (Figure 15.8) is similar to injecting acne cysts, but a higher concentration of triamcinolone (5–10 mg/mL) is acceptable because these lesions are usually in the axilla, chest, neck, groin, and buttocks, and less prone to atrophy. Also, a little skin atrophy is generally more acceptable in these locations

HYPERTROPHIC SCARS AND KELOIDS

See Video 15.2.

A *hypertrophic scar* (Figure 15.10) is one in which the scar tissue is raised and prominent over the area that was cut, burned, or traumatized. It may show prominent suture marks and can be redder or differently pigmented compared with the surrounding tissue. Hypertrophic scars frequently regress over a few years. A *keloid* (Figure 15.11) is similar to a hypertrophic scar but it grows beyond the limits

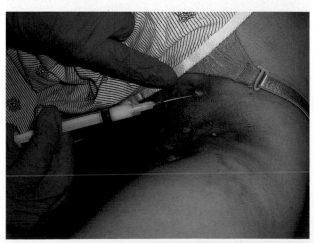

Figure 15.8 Severe hidradenitis suppurativa being injected with 10 mg/mL triamcinolone for pain relief that usually starts within 1 day. *(Copyright Richard P. Usatine, MD.)*

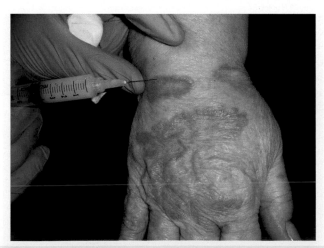

Figure 15.9 Granuloma annulare being injected with 5 mg/mL triamcinolone. While the patient has disseminated GA, she has requested injections of the lesions that are most symptomatic. *(Copyright Richard P. Usatine, MD.)*

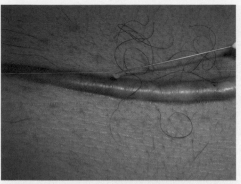

Figure 15.10 Hypertrophic scar after a knife wound being injected with 10 mg/mL triamcinolone. *(Copyright Richard P. Usatine, MD.)*

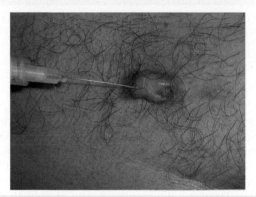

Figure 15.11 A keloid from acne on the chest being injected with 40 mg/mL triamcinolone. Note the blanching. *(Copyright Richard P. Usatine, MD.)*

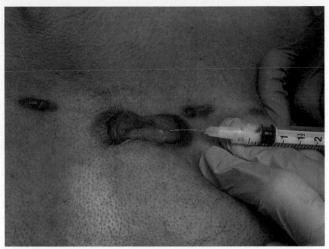

Figure 15.12 A keloid on the chest in skin of color being injected with 40 mg/mL triamcinolone. *(Copyright Richard P. Usatine, MD.)*

of the original injury/surgery and does not regress. Keloid is derived from Greek to describe its clinical description; it means "crab's claw."[7] Keloids tend to become quite raised and enlarged. There are histologic differences between hypertrophic scars and keloids. For the purpose of intralesional injection, however, they are treated identically.

Individuals with darker skin tones are at higher risk of developing keloids. Keloids most commonly occur on the ears after piercings and on the chest and shoulders after surgery or trauma but can occur anywhere on the skin. Keloids frequently occur after skin piercings and acne scarring. Table 15.1 provides a list of possible treatments for keloids. Surgical excision frequently induces more scarring exacerbating the original problem. If excision is deemed necessary, scarring can be limited by injecting steroids into the surgical site after surgery, using minimal tissue pressure techniques, and postoperative occlusion with silicone sheets for several months.

Initially start with 10 mg/mL of triamcinolone for the first treatment of a keloid or hypertrophic scar. The needle should be introduced into the body of the keloid at a 20- to 30-degree angle with the skin (Figure 15.12). It is important that the tip of the needle is *within* the keloid and not below it. Proper needle position should result in significant pressure while injecting and blanching of the keloid as the suspension is injected into the area. If the solution flows in easily, the needle is most likely too deep. If the needle is too deep, reposition it and restart the injection. Inject firmly while advancing the needle and observing the keloid blanch.

Large keloids may need multiple injections at one time to adequately infiltrate the lesion. Sometimes the needle can be pulled back and reoriented for the next injection from the same puncture site. The quantity injected should be just enough to blanch the entire keloid white. Hypertrophic scars are injected using the same technique. A 3-mL Luer-Lok syringe facilitates the injection into these firm structures. Without the Luer-Lok it is easy for the needle to come off and spray the clinician in the eyes. Even with a Luer-Lok syringe it is important to wear eye protection when injecting lesions under pressure. Most patients have 50% to 100% resolution of keloids after intralesional steroid as monotherapy. There is a 33% recurrence rate after 1 year and 50% after 5 years. We recommend starting at a lower dose (10 mg/mL) due to the side effects of hypopigmentation and skin atrophy and reevaluate every 6 weeks for possible reinjection into the mid-dermis with a stronger concentration. For example, treating a keloid on the chest, injections can start at 10 mg/mL and increase by 10 mg/mL (with a maximum of 40 mg/mL) pending clinical evaluation for scar resolution.[8]

Keloids can be treated with cryosurgery alone or in combination with intralesional steroids. Comprehensive review of eight studies found acceptable results using cryotherapy in combination with intralesional steroid to decrease pruritus, pain, and reduce scar volume. However, caution must be used in darker skin tones, as persistent hypopigmentation was observed in some cases. These two therapies whether used alone or in combination are widely available, useful for most anatomic locations, and cost-effective methods of treatment.[9]

In one small controlled study, 10 patients with keloids were treated with intralesional steroid and cryosurgery vs. intralesional steroid or cryosurgery alone.[10] Patients were treated at least three times 4 weeks apart. In terms of keloid thickness, the keloids responded significantly better to combined cryosurgery and triamcinolone vs. triamcinolone alone or cryotherapy alone. Pain intensity was significantly lowered with all treatment modalities. Pruritus was lowered only with the combined treatment and intralesional corticosteroid alone.[10]

In another study 20 patients with hypertrophic and keloidal scars received two 15-second cycles (total 30 seconds) of cryosurgery treatments once monthly for 12 months with intralesional injections of 10 to 40 mg/mL triamcinolone once monthly for 3 months.[11] Topical application of silicone gel was added three times daily for 12 months. The control group included 10 patients who received treatment with silicone sheeting only. After 1 year, improvement was seen in all parameters, especially in terms of symptoms, cosmetic appearance, and associated signs compared to baseline and compared to the control group.[11]

Layton et al. reported that the intralesional injection of a steroid is helpful, but cryotherapy is more effective (85% improvement in terms of flattening) for recent acne keloids located on the back.[12] Treatment with intralesional triamcinolone was beneficial, but the response to cryosurgery was significantly better in early, vascular lesions.[1]

If the keloid is older and/or firmer, it may not respond to injection therapy as well as softer and newer lesions. In such cases, it may help to pretreat the keloid with cryotherapy. It is not necessary to freeze a margin of normal tissue. After liquid nitrogen or another freezing modality is applied to the keloid, it is allowed to thaw and develop edema. This generally takes 1 to 2 minutes, which allows for easier introduction of intralesional steroids into the lesions.

In one double-blind clinical trial, 40 patients were randomized to receive intralesional triamcinolone (TAC) or a combination of TAC and 5-fluorouracil (5-FU).[9] Both groups received injections at weekly intervals for 8 weeks and lesions were assessed for erythema, pruritus, pliability, height, length, and width. Both groups showed an acceptable improvement in nearly all parameters, but there was more significant improvement in the TAC + 5-FU group ($P < 0.05$ for all except pruritus and percentage of itch reduction). Good to excellent improvement was reported by 20% of the patients receiving TAC alone and 55% of the patients in the group receiving TAC and 5-FU.[13] A randomized control trial study supports this finding with showing recurrence rates of 17.5% in 3 months when TAC is used with intralesional 5-FU. Combination does show superior results and less recurrence rate compared to TAC monotherapy. It is of note that patients may require anesthetic prior to injection to 5-FU to decrease discomfort.[9,10]

According to one article, simple excision of earlobe keloids can result in recurrence rates approaching 80%.[9] Earlobe keloids may be excised with a shave excision and injection of the base with steroid; these have a recurrence rate of 15.4% with an average 12- to 25-month follow up. This is quick, simple, requires fewer treatment sessions and is effective treatment with high patient satisfaction[9] (Figure 15.13). It is hard to get much volume of steroid into the base of these keloids, so 40 mg/mL triamcinolone is preferred as the concentration for injection. Surgical excision plus pressure therapy is minimally invasive, inexpensive, and had lower rates than surgical excision plus intralesional steroid injection and/or excision and cryotherapy for auricular keloids. Pressure therapy can be achieved with clip-on earrings. After 18 months it had 10.6% average recurrence rate. Excision with cryotherapy can work well for larger auricular keloids with a recurrence rate of 15%, 43 months postprocedure date.[9]

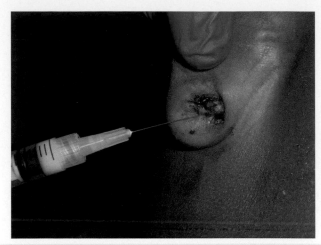

Figure 15.13 A keloid was shaved from the posterior ear lobe and the bleeding stopped using electrocoagulation. The base is being injected with 40 mg/mL triamcinolone to prevent regrowth. *(Copyright Richard P. Usatine, MD.)*

According to one article, simple excision of earlobe keloids can result in recurrence rates approaching 80%.[11] A randomized prospective trial comparing steroid injections versus radiation therapy found that 2 of 15 keloids (12.5%) recurred after surgery and radiation therapy, whereas 4 of 12 (33%) recurred after surgery and steroid injections. These results did not produce a statistically significant difference. No alteration of skin pigmentation, wound dehiscence, or chronic dermatitis was observed in any patient in either group.[11] While radiation therapy was considered easy to obtain in this study, it is reasonable to use steroid injections in office practice.

LOCALIZED DERMATITIS (LICHEN SIMPLEX CHRONICUS, PRURIGO NODULARIS)

One paper describes using 2.5 mg/mL triamcinolone for localized dermatitis (such as lichen simplex chronicus, prurigo nodularis, and nonspecific eczema).[14] We recommend using 2.5 to 5.0 mg/mL triamcinolone with a 27-gauge needle for the treatment of localized dermatitis. Because prurigo nodularis (Figure 15.14) can be particularly difficult to treat, a higher concentration may be needed. In our experience, we have found intralesional steroids to be more effective and better tolerated than cryosurgery for PN. Also, we have seen less hypopigmentation from IL steroid than cryosurgery.

PSORIASIS

See Video 15.5.

Our experience and those of others have found that 2.5 to 5 mg/mL IL triamcinolone is highly effective for small plaques of psoriasis on the trunk and limbs.[14] In one small series, five patients with chronic intermittent palmoplantar pustulosis were treated with intralesional injections of 3.3 to 5.0 mg/mL of triamcinolone acetonide.[15] Prompt clearing of symptoms and lesions occurred and lasted 3 to 6 months. Side effects included hypopigmentation, cutaneous

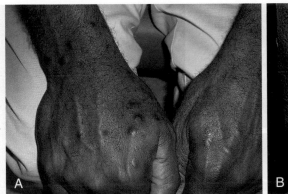
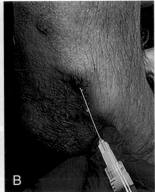

Figure 15.14 (A) Prurigo nodularis about to be injected with triamcinolone. The patient preferred this to previous cryotherapy. **(B)** Prurigo nodularis being injected with 5 mg/mL triamcinolone. *(Copyright Richard P. Usatine, MD.)*

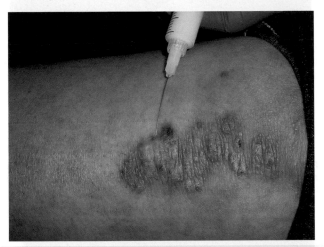

Figure 15.15 Stubborn area of plaque psoriasis over the knee being injected with 5 mg/mL triamcinolone. *(Copyright Richard P. Usatine, MD.)*

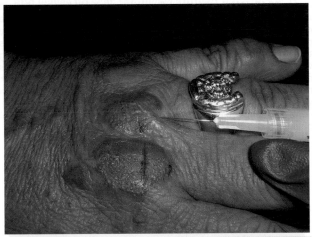

Figure 15.16 Plaque psoriasis over the MCP joints being injected with 5 mg/mL triamcinolone using a 30 gauge needle. *(Copyright Richard P. Usatine, MD.)*

atrophy, and, in one patient, exacerbation of a latent dermatophyte infection.[15]

We typically use 5.0 mg/mL triamcinolone with a 27-gauge needle for intralesional injections of localized psoriasis. (Figure 15.15). The risk of atrophy and hypopigmentation to the skin is lower when compared to injection in other areas of the skin with intralesional steroid injections.[16] These injections can be particularly useful for stubborn plaques over the MCP joints that may evade treatment even for those on biologic agents. (Figure 15.16)

PSORIATIC NAIL DISEASE

There is little to no data to guide the injection of nail psoriasis. The literature suggests using triamcinolone 2.5 to 10 mg/mL, and we have found 5 mg/mL to be effective. To minimize pain, we use a 30 gauge needle. A 1 mL syringe allows for more precise injections of small amounts of steroid (typically 0.1–0.2 mL per nail).

At a minimum we use topical anesthesia such as prilocaine/lidocaine (EMLA). Many patients prefer a digital block for initial injections as this appears to be a scary proposition. Over time, we have noticed that patients are fine with the topical anesthetic only. This can reduce the number of injections in one finger from 4 to 1.

We have found no studies that compare the effectiveness of the site of nail unit injections. The nail pathology stems from the inflammation of the matrix, so our injections go straight for the matrix and not into the nail bed or nail folds. While we have tried bilateral injections with success, we have concluded that a single injection into the center of the matrix is best and least painful. It also is easier to get the needle into the matrix while avoiding the lateral horns of the nail. We inject until we see the lunula turn white and prefer if the nail bed turns white too (Figure 15.17)

LICHEN PLANUS

See Video 15.6.

Lichen planus, another papulosquamous condition, also can respond well to intralesional triamcinolone (Figure 15.18). Just as in psoriasis, it is not used for extensive disease. It helps with local areas not responding to topical or systemic treatment.

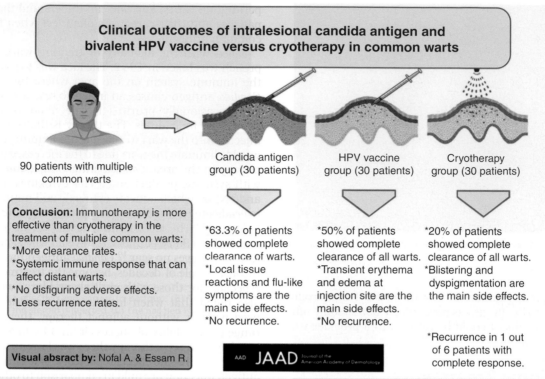

Figure 15.22 Visual abstract of *Candida* study by Nofal A and Essam R. (Graphic courtesy of Nofal A and Essam R.) Previously published in JAAD.[19]

The recurrence rate in immunotherapy groups was 0% versus 16.7 % in the cryotherapy group.[19]

Group (A) included 30 patients who were treated with intralesional *Candida* antigen injection (0.3 mL of 1/1000 solution of *Candida* antigen into the largest wart; Allergy Laboratories, Inc. Oklahoma City, USA). Another takeaway message from this study is that if *Candida* antigen is not available, the HPV vaccine is an acceptable alternative. We have no explanation for the low effectiveness of the cryosurgery group, but would not use this data to discourage cryosurgery as an optional treatment for warts (see Chapter 14).

Candida antigen has been used as a test antigen for anergy in tuberculosis testing for over 60 years but does not have FDA approval for the treatment of warts. Because it is approved for human use, malpractice policies will cover its administration should any unforeseen problems arise. The only contraindication is a history of allergy to *Candida*, which is rare. Because the *Candida* antigen is not live, it can be used in immunocompromised persons as well.

Candida Protocol: Steps and Principles[20,21]

1. Obtain the *Candida* antigen (generic 1:1000 or proprietary Candin 1:500). Avoid getting allergy extracts from HollisterStier, as the concentration is very high and will need some strong dilution.

4. Inject 0.1 mL into the largest 1 or 2 warts *intralesionally or intradermally*. (see Box 15.1).
   - The injection should take some force. If it goes in too easily, the needle is subdermal, and the needed response will not occur. Inject as if you were trying to obtain a wheal, although it will not happen due to the fibrous nature of the wart tissue (Figure 15.23).

Box 15.1   Candida injection for Warts

- Use undiluted Candida antigen and draw up 0.1–0.2 mL with a 25–27 gauge needle.
- A small needle is used to avoid losing this precious solution inside a large needle.
- Inject the 1–2 largest lesions with 0.1 mL per lesion using 27–30 gauge needle.
- The injections may be repeated every 2–4 weeks. We typically repeat every 4 weeks.

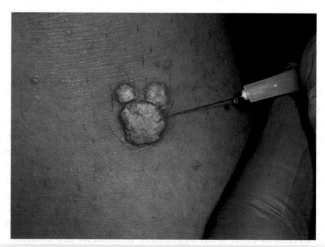

Figure 15.23 *Candida* antigen injection of a wart on the leg using a 30 gauge needle. *(Copyright Richard P. Usatine, MD.)*

- Wear protective face shield since the solution often "squirts out" of the wart.
- Use a Luer-Lok syringe since the needle may pop off with the pressure applied unless it is locked in place. A 30-gauge needle limits the pain of injection and allows the injection of sensitive areas including the end of the finger (Figure 15.24).

6. Establish a return visit for 2-4 weeks. Should the warts resolve, the visit can be canceled. If the warts persist, another treatment can be given. A third visit should be set up after the second if needed.

7. If after three injections at monthly intervals the warts persist, consider these 2 options:
   - If the verrucae are smaller, continue with the *Candida* antigen if so desired.
   - Consider intralesional injections with MMR or HPV vaccine.[19]

9. Expect tenderness for a few days, erythema, peeling, and occasionally some pruritus (Figure 15.25). Occasionally there can be a vigorous immune response with erythema and tenderness (as also occurs with too concentrated or too much volume of solution). There will be no scarring, hypo- or hyperpigmentation, or open wounds.

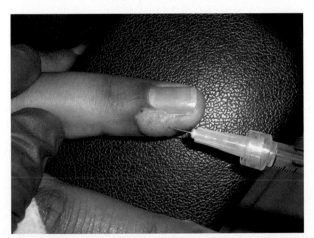

Figure 15.24 Candida antigen injection of periungual warts in a child using a 30 gauge needle. (Copyright Richard P. Usatine, MD.)

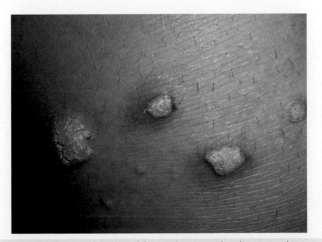

Figure 15.25 It is not unusual for erythema to develop around warts injected with *Candida* antigen. These warts on the leg were injected the day before this photo was taken. (Copyright Richard P. Usatine, MD.)

10. Patients may resume normal activities including bathing and group sports immediately after injection being limited by pain only.

Aftercare for All Intralesional Injections

No special aftercare is needed other than follow-up for inspection of the results and consideration of additional treatments.

Coding and Billing Pearls

Intralesional injections have two CPT codes for giving the injections (see Box 15.2). These should be simple to use since there is one code for up to and including seven lesions (not separate injections) and one code for eight lesions and above. If it takes three injections to inject one large plaque of psoriasis, this is still counted as one lesion.

J-codes are used to bill for the injectable material:

J3301 Injection, triamcinolone acetonide, not otherwise specified, per 10 mg
J9040 Injection, bleomycin sulfate, 15 units

Box 15.2 CPT Codes and Their Medicare Reimbursement Amounts

11900 Intralesional Injection (up to 7) $51
11901 Intralesional Injection (more than 7) $66

References

1. Levine RM, Rasmussen JE. Intralesional corticosteroids in the treatment of nodulocystic acne. *Arch Dermatol.* 1983;119:480-481.
2. Taub AF. Procedural treatments for acne vulgaris. *Dermatol Surg.* 2007;33:1005-1026.
3. Ramos PM, Anzai A, Duque-Estrada B, et al. Consensus on the treatment of alopecia areata – Brazilian Society of Dermatology. *An Bras Dermatol.* 2020;95 Suppl 1(Suppl 1):39-52. doi:10.1016/j.abd.2020.05.006.
4. Yee BE, Tong Y, Goldenberg A, Hata T. Efficacy of different concentrations of intralesional triamcinolone acetonide for alopecia areata: a systematic review and meta-analysis. *J Am Acad Dermatol.* 2020;82(4):1018-1021. doi:10.1016/j.jaad.2019.11.066.
5. Verbov J. The place of intralesional steroid therapy in dermatology. *Br J Dermatol.* 1976;94(suppl 12):51-58.
6. Callen JP. Treatment of cutaneous lesions in patients with lupus erythematosus. *Dermatol Clin.* 1994;12:201-206.
7. Wang J, Khachemoune A. Granuloma annulare: a focused review of therapeutic options. *Am J Clin Dermatol.* 2018;19(3):333-344. doi:10.1007/s40257-017-0334-5.
8. Ekstein SF, Wyles SP, Moran SL, Meves A. Keloids: a review of therapeutic management. *Int J Dermatol.* 2021;60(6):661-671. doi:10.1111/ijd.15159.
9. Thornton NJ, Garcia BA, Hoyer P, Wilkerson MG. Keloid scars: an updated review of combination therapies. *Cureus.* 2021;13(1):e12999. doi:10.7759/cureus.12999.
10. Yosipovitch G, Widijanti SM, Goon A, et al. A comparison of the combined effect of cryotherapy and corticosteroid injections versus corticosteroids and cryotherapy alone on keloids: a controlled study. *J Dermatolog Treat.* 2001;12:87-90.
11. Boutli-Kasapidou F, Tsakiri A, Anagnostou E, Mourellou O. Hypertrophic and keloidal scars: an approach to polytherapy. *Int J Dermatol.* 2005;44:324-327.

12. Layton AM, Yip J, Cunliffe WJ. A comparison of intralesional triamcinolone and cryosurgery in the treatment of acne keloids. *Br J Dermatol.* 1994;130:498-501.

13. Darougheh A, Asilian A, Shariati F. Intralesional triamcinolone alone or in combination with 5-fluorouracil for the treatment of keloid and hypertrophic scars. *Clin Exp Dermatol.* 2009;34:219-223.

14. Richards RN. Update on intralesional steroid: focus on dermatoses. *J Cutan Med Surg.* 2010;14:19-23.

15. Goette DK, Morgan AM, Fox BJ, Horn RT. Treatment of palmoplantar pustulosis with intralesional triamcinolone injections. *Arch Dermatol.* 1984;120:319-323.

16. de Berker DA, Lawrence CM. A simplified protocol of steroid injection for psoriatic nail dystrophy. *Br J Dermatol.* 1998;138(1):90-95. doi:10.1046/j.1365-2133.1998.02031.x.

17. Salman S, Ahmed MS, Ibrahim AM, et al. Intralesional immunotherapy for the treatment of warts: A network meta-analysis. *J Am Acad Dermatol.* 2019;80(4):922-930.e4. doi:10.1016/j.jaad.2018.07.003.

18. Nofal A, Marei A, Amer A, Amen H. Significance of interferon gamma in the prediction of successful therapy of common warts by intralesional injection of Candida antigen. *Int J Dermatol.* 2017;56(10):1003-1009.

19. Nassar A, Nofal A, Bakr, NM, Essam R, Alakad R. Comparative efficacy of intralesional Candida antigen, intralesional bivalent HPV vaccine, and cryotherapy in the treatment of common warts. *J Am Acad Dermatol.* 2022;87(2):419-421. doi:10.1016/j.jaad.2021.08.040.

20. Phillips RC, Rhul TS, Pfenninger JL, Garber MR. Treatment of warts with Candida antigen injection. *Arch Dermatol.* 2000:136:1247-1275.

21. Attwa E, Elawady R, Salah E. "Cryo-immuno-therapy" is superior to intralesional Candida antigen monotherapy in the treatment of multiple common warts. *J Dermatolog Treat.* 2021;32(8):1018-1025. doi:10.1080/09546634.2020.1720585.

16 *Incision and Drainage*

DANIEL L. STULBERG, MD, BERNADATTE G. GILBERT, MD, PATRICK MORAN, DO
and RICHARD P. USATINE, MD

SUMMARY

- Uncomplicated skin abscesses are commonly encountered in the primary care and emergency department settings.
- It is important for clinicians to be well-versed in performing incision and drainage of uncomplicated skin abscesses.

Incision and drainage (I&D) is an essential in-office procedure for skin abscesses and related infections. Commonly, patients will present with the acute onset of localized pain, swelling, and erythema indicating abscess formation (Figure 16.1). These can be the result of trauma, insect stings or bites, a secondary infection or inflammation of an epidermoid cyst, paronychia from nail-biting or manipulation, or may arise without a clear inciting event. The most common pathogens are *Staphylococcus aureus* and *Streptococcus* bacteria. Classic physical exam findings include an erythematous, tender to palpation, fluctuant, indurated lesion often with "pointing." Pointing is visible thinning or stretching of the overlying skin where if untreated the lesion may completely erode through the skin and rupture. The finding of fluctuance is key in the diagnosis of an abscess. When the diagnosis is in question, needle aspiration (Figure 16.2) and/or ultrasonography may be useful in the detection of an abscess (see Chapter 22, *Ultrasound in Dermatology*).

Recommendations for the use of systemic antibiotics for patients undergoing I&D for a skin abscess vary. The 2014 Update by the Infectious Diseases Society of America regarding the diagnosis and management of skin and soft tissue infections stated that antibiotics should only be given in immunocompromised patients or those with signs and symptoms of systemic infection.[1] In addition, the guidelines stated that antibiotics should be considered in patients with multiple abscesses, at the extremes of age, and when there was lack of response to I&D alone.

In 2016, a landmark article on this issue was published in the *NEJM* by Talan et al. They found in a large multicenter study that trimethoprim-sulfamethoxazole treatment resulted in a higher cure rate among patients with a drained cutaneous abscess than placebo in settings in which Methicillin-resistant Staphylococcus aureus (MRSA) was prevalent.[2] Subsequently, the 2018 *BMJ* Rapid Recommendation on the use of antibiotics after I&D for uncomplicated skin abscesses recommended shared decision-making in the choice of whether to initiate antibiotics, making a weak recommendation favoring Trimethoprim-sulfamethoxazole (TMP-SMX) or clindamycin in addition to I&D over I&D alone.[3] TMP-SMX was weakly recommended over clindamycin due to its lower risk of diarrhea. Benefits

of antibiotics in addition to I&D included a decreased risk of treatment failure at one month and a decreased risk of recurrence at three months.[2]

Other indications for the use of antibiotics in treating an abscess include the presence of surrounding cellulitis (Figure 16.1) or other signs or symptoms of further infection. Some patients may be colonized with MRSA and develop recurrent abscesses. In this situation they are often treated with systemic antibiotics including TMP-SMX, clindamycin, or others based on local sensitivity patterns. Mupirocin is applied inside the nares twice daily for 5 days, and topical chlorhexidine skin washing is commonly used to try to clear the carrier state, although the literature does not clearly support these practices.[4,5]

Indications for Procedure

The following lesions should be treated with I&D:

- Abscess (small abscesses that are spontaneously draining may be observed and treated with warm compresses)
- Abscessed epidermoid cyst
- Furuncle – abscess related to the hair follicle
- Carbuncle – coalescence of furuncles
- Paronychia – abscess at the nail margin

Contraindications and Cautions

- This chapter deals with superficial abscesses seen in routine office practice. Deep abscesses and those of body compartments including the palm of the hand require more interventional radiology or extensive surgical intervention.
- Perirectal abscesses should be approached cautiously. They may be associated with deep disease or underlying inflammatory bowel disease, and care should be taken not to damage the anal sphincter, which can cause incontinence.[6]
- I&D of abscesses of the face can lead to scarring, so choose the line of incision along skin tension lines, wrinkles, or other structures to minimize the prominence of the scar. Needle aspiration and antibiotics can

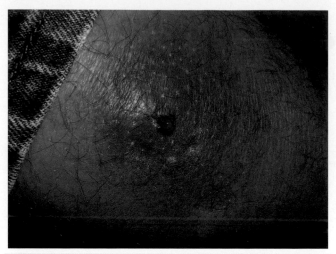

Figure 16.1 An abscess with surrounding cellulitis on the leg caused by MRSA. (Copyright Richard P. Usatine, MD.)

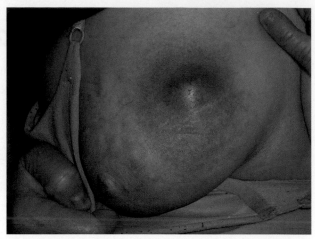

Figure 16.3 A breast abscess that started with an inflamed epidermoid cyst. An abscess with surrounding cellulitis developed. Any abscess in the breast should lead to consideration of breast cancer. (Copyright Richard P. Usatine, MD.)

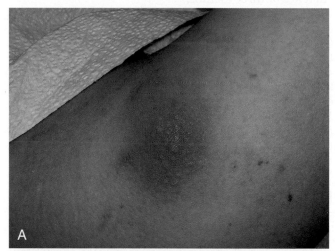

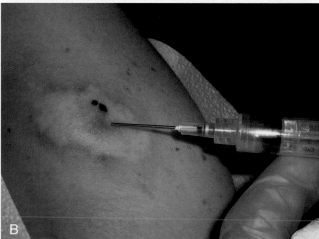

Figure 16.2 (A) An area of erythema and swelling on the arm of a woman with a history of injecting drugs. **(B)** As the diagnosis was not clear between an abscess and cellulitis, the area was anesthetized, and an 18-gauge needle was used to aspirate the lesion demonstrating pus and confirming a diagnosis of abscess. (Copyright Richard P. Usatine, MD.)

be tried as initial treatment with close follow-up and an informed patient understanding that I&D may ultimately be necessary.

- Be cautious to avoid damage to underlying structures including nerves and blood vessels.
- Abscesses and infections in closed spaces including the hand, foot, orbits, etc., require additional intervention and consultation.
- Crepitus or gas seen on imaging connotate more serious infection, e.g., necrotizing fasciitis, which is a surgical emergency and should be promptly treated by the appropriate colleague.
- Breast abscesses (Figure 16.3) in a nonlactating woman should prompt evaluation for possible cancer. Periareolar abscess has a high potential for complications and warrants evaluation by a surgical colleague.
- Abscesses of the central face in the "danger triangle" between the bridge of the nose and the angles of the mouth may lead to further complications and may be best treated with antibiotics and warm compresses if possible. On rare occasion these infections may lead to cavernous sinus thrombosis and septic phlebitis.[7]

Advantages of Incision and Drainage

CLINICIAN

- Curative
- Simple to perform
- In-office

PATIENT

- Curative
- Reduction in pain after the immediate surgical discomfort
- In-office, avoids higher emergency room or surgical center cost and copay
- Family member or friend can be instructed to do the repacking

Disadvantages of Incision and Drainage

CLINICIAN

- Time for collecting supplies, anesthesia, and the procedure
- Expense of stocking supplies
- Possibility of body fluid exposure

PATIENT

- Pain of procedure
- Scarring
- Bleeding
- Recurrence

Equipment

- Antiseptic agent (e.g., alcohol, povidone-iodine, or chlorhexidine)
- Local injectable anesthetic (e.g., 1% or 2% lidocaine with or without epinephrine – epinephrine can reduce bleeding, give an extra hour of anesthesia and if needed allow larger volume to be used)
- Topical anesthetic (e.g., ethyl chloride, prilocaine-lidocaine, tetracaine mix used for paronychia or prior to anesthetic injection)
- Clean gloves, gown, and face shield for eye and face protection
- Drapes
- 3 to 12 mL syringe
- 18 gauge or fill needle
- 25-, 27-, or 30-gauge 1.5-inch needle to inject anesthesia
- Number 11 or 15 disposable scalpel or blade and scalpel handle
- Instruments – hemostat, Adson forceps, scissors
- 4 × 4-inch clean gauze pads
- Cotton-tipped applicators (CTA)
- Packing material (plain gauze packing tape)
- Culture swab and transport media if recurrence or needed for complicated or high-risk patient, otherwise usually not indicated[1]
- Irrigation materials (normal saline solution, large syringe with 19 gauge IV catheter or needleless irrigation device, splash protection, basin) if desired, but literature does not support change in clinical outcomes
- Dressing 4 × 4 gauze or nonadherent dressing and tape, or large adhesive dressing
- Scissors

Procedure: Steps and Principles

- Counsel the patient regarding the diagnosis of abscess and that the recommended treatment is I&D. Obtain informed consent verbally or in writing.
- Abscesses may be more difficult to anesthetize than routine lesions if not injected broadly around the abscess and given more time than for simple excisions. It is thought that the acidic environment of the infection makes the lidocaine less effective.

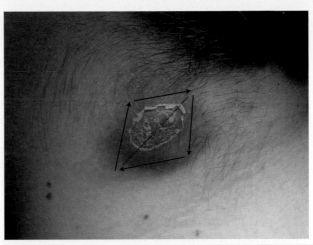

Figure 16.4 The arrows show one method of providing anesthesia to an abscess by injecting laterally and deep to the abscess. The dotted arrows indicate injections done below the abscess. It is best to avoid injecting directly into the abscess cavity. (Copyright Richard P. Usatine, MD.)

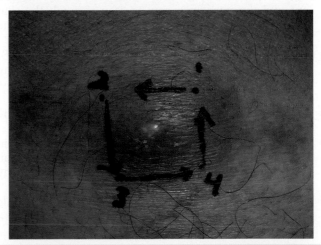

Figure 16.5 Planning a ring block around an abscess. Each subsequent injection should be in an area that was at least partially anesthetized. (Copyright Richard P. Usatine, MD.)

- After antiseptic prep and the use of a topical anesthetic if desired, inject the local anesthetic through uninfected skin immediately lateral to each side of the abscess in a fanning pattern around and underneath the abscess (Figure 16.4).
- Inject the anesthetic while advancing the needle or by initially inserting it to the desired depth and injecting as the needle is withdrawn.
- Unless the abscess is very small, inject from the other side in the same fashion.
- Another alternative approach is to use a ring block (Figure 16.5), which involves injecting around the abscess to make a ring with each subsequent injection to be initiated in an area with some previous anesthesia (see Chapter 3, *Anesthesia*).
- Avoid injecting into the abscess itself, as that will increase pressure and pain, and may cause the abscess to spontaneously rupture under pressure, increasing the risk of exposure to the clinician. For this reason, proper eye and barrier protection is recommended.

- While the anesthetic is taking effect, set up the rest of the instruments.
- Clean gloves and clean technique are used.
- If packing is indicated (for larger abscesses), open the bottle of plain gauze packing tape, and use the forceps to pick up the end and extract a length of the gauze that will be more than enough to pack into the abscess cavity. Cut the strip with the scissors just above the bottle, and the end will fall back cleanly into the bottle.
- Some clinicians use iodoform gauze to pack abscesses. The authors use plain gauze as it seems to cause less burning discomfort. Iodine, even in dilute concentrations, is toxic to new tissue growth.
- In cosmetically sensitive areas, and whenever possible, align the incision along the normal skin tension lines or along structures where the scar will be less visible after healing.
- Once adequate analgesia is achieved, use the #11 (or #15) scalpel blade perpendicular to the skin, and incise in a linear fashion into the lesion at the area of "pointing" if present where the skin has already thinned out and the purulence can be seen through the skin (Figure 16.6A). Extend the incision to allow adequate exploration, drainage, and packing.
- The pus will usually spontaneously drain (Figure 16.6B) or may spray out under pressure. Express the remaining purulent material by compressing toward the abscess from both sides.
- Use the hemostats to explore the cavity and break up any loculations (Figure 16.6C).
- If the abscess is from an inflamed or infected epidermoid cyst, use the hemostat to pull out as much of the cyst wall as possible to help prevent recurrence. Then express any remaining purulence.
- Some practitioners will irrigate at this stage with sterile saline (Figure 16.6D). This is a common practice, but a literature review found no concrete evidence to support the practice or that it improves clinical outcomes.[8,9]
- CTAs can be used to clean out remaining pus and keratinaceous material while determining the size and depth of the abscess cavity.
- Wound packing is recommended when the abscess is >5 cm in diameter or in the setting of a pilonidal abscess or an abscess in an immunocompromised or diabetic patient.[10]
- When it is indicated, use the Adson forceps to grasp the plain gauze packing tape and start packing it into the deepest portion of the abscess cavity (Figure 16.6E). The stick end of a CTA also works well for packing an abscess (Figure 16.7).
- Continue to pack the gauze filling the cavity. Do not pack the cavity too tightly as that may lead to tissue necrosis. Leave a 2- to 3-cm tail outside of the wound to facilitate later removal.
- Cover the gauze tail with 4 × 4 gauze or nonadherent dressing with tape or an adhesive bandage. If desired give the closed bottle of plain gauze packing tape to the patient labeled with their name for the follow-up repacking if indicated.
- If repacking, return in 2 days and take off the dressing.
- Grasp the tail of the packing tape and in one long swift movement remove the entire strip of gauze. This is quicker and preferable to prolonging the discomfort of tugging out the gauze inch by inch.
- Repack the abscess if indicated.

Aftercare and Packing of Abscesses

- The patient should keep the area clean and dry and follow up in 2 days for a recheck and repacking if indicated.

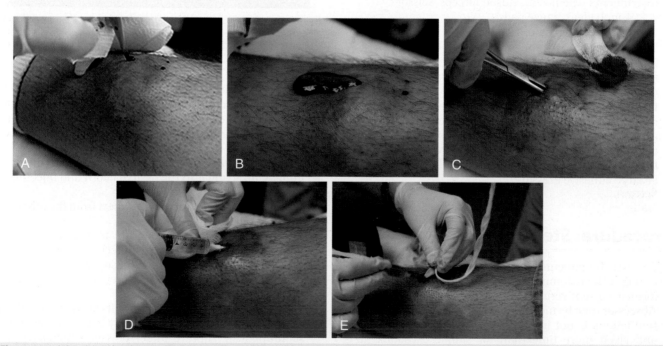

Figure 16.6 (A) Incising the abscess. **(B)** Release of pus. **(C)** Breaking up loculations. **(D)** Irrigating the abscess cavity. **(E)** Packing the abscess cavity with strip gauze. (Copyright Daniel L. Stulberg, MD.)

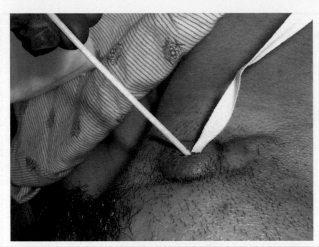

Figure 16.7 Packing an infected cyst with strip gauze using the stick end of a cotton-tipped applicator (CTA) to introduce the gauze into the space that was evacuated. The CTA works even better than the forceps and can reach the far end of a deep defect. (Copyright Richard P. Usatine, MD.)

Repacking can be done at office visits, or if there is a reliable friend or family member, this can be done at home. Repacking is uncomfortable, but usually tolerable without anesthetic. Hard evidence is lacking regarding the frequency and length of time to repack abscesses.[11] The length of time should allow for the wound to contract and enough epithelialization to occur to allow healing from the inside out and prevent the abscess pocket from sealing up and reforming as an abscess again. There is wide variation in packing recommendations as there is little to no evidence to guide this practice.

- One option is to remove the gauze and repack every 2 days until not able to repack, or until the usual number of days that one would leave sutures in for that body location for a routine excision, whichever is sooner. For example, 1 week after I&D of facial abscesses, 10 days for abscesses of the trunk, and 2 weeks on the extremities.
- For a small to medium abscess that was packed in the office, it may be adequate to just ask the patient to pull out the packing in the shower in 2 days and not repack at all.
- Another option is to pull 1 to 2 cm of the gauze out each day until the gauze is out. This may be less painful but may allow purulent packing material to stay inside the wound for a prolonged time.
- Some authors conclude that the value of packing is not statistically better than no packing.[9]

Loop Drainage Technique

The loop drainage technique is an alternate, less-invasive approach to abscess management. This technique involves making two punctures in the abscess, breaking up loculations, and irrigating as above.[12,13] Instead of packing, a surgical loop is passed through the two punctures and tied outside of the wound to allow drainage during healing (Figure 16.8).

This technique is described in several papers,[14-16] and Aprahamian in 2016 recommended it as the "definitive treatment of choice for subcutaneous abscesses in children."

Performing the loop drainage technique:

- Using palpation, or if necessary ultrasound, clinically identify the borders of the abscess.
- Make a 4- to 5-mm incision into the abscess cavity at one end of the abscess.
- Insert a hemostat or similar instrument through the incision, and break up any loculations within the abscess cavity.
- Determine the extent of the cavity with the hemostat while breaking up adhesions.
- If the abscess is large, make additional 4- to 5-mm incisions at 4-cm intervals as needed to further break up loculations and at least one incision at the opposite side of the abscess from the first incision to allow the loop placement.
- Compress the abscess and express the purulent material.
- Irrigation via the incision(s) may help remove debris.
- Using a hemostat or needle holder, pass a vessel loop, narrow drain, or sterile rubber band into and through the incisions at opposite ends of the abscess.
- Keeping the loop loose, tie the free ends of the loop together making sure not to cinch the loop down on the skin during tying. Start with a friction knot, and then secure with square knot throws. See Chapter 6, *Suturing Techniques*, as needed for details on knot tying.
- Cover the area with gauze or similar dressing to absorb the expected drainage.
- Instruct the patient that it is ok to bathe and redress the area.
- Once the drainage stops and the erythema resolves, typically at 7 to 10 days, the patient or their caregiver should cut and pull out the loop.
- No follow-up visits are required unless the patient has questions or is experiencing difficulties.
- Use code 10061 for complicated I&Ds since the procedure is complicated by the need for a drain wick (i.e. the loop).

There is a device called Quickloop (Figure 16.9) that incorporates many of these steps into a single device. The unit combines a suture needle mounted on an irrigating tube with an in-line blade to make the 4- to 5-mm incisions. The needle and blade portion of the instrument are cut off from the tubing, and the abscess is irrigated after clipping the tube back to itself to form the loop (Figure 16.9). The process is similar to the steps above. See https://emdevicelab.com/ for additional information.

The basic loop technique can be practiced on a lemon or orange (Figure 16.10).

Paronychia

See Video 16.1.
Paronychia is a local infection of the nail fold (Figure 16.11). It may be started by nail biting or manipulating the nail or nail margins. A #11 blade scalpel can be used to incise the abscess (Figure 16.11). Packing is not needed. Counsel the patient to use warm soaks three times a day and to open the abscess manually if it closes and express any purulence until it heals.

Vessel Loop Method of Incision and Drainage

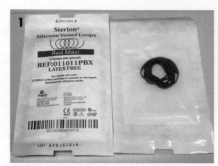

1 Instead of traditional gauze packing, a sterile silicone loop is used. This is commonly referred to simply as a "vessel loop" and is readily available from the operating room (this device is used by vascular surgeons).

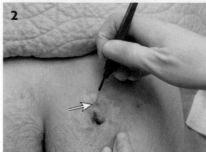

2 After sterile preparation and anesthetic infiltration, make a small (5–10 mm) incision at the periphery of the abscess. If possible, make the incision where the abscess is already pointing, noted by the *white arrow*.

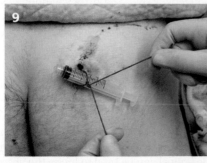

3 Express as much pus as possible from the incision. Obtain cultures if clinically indicated.

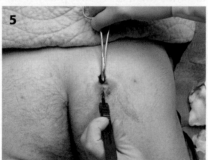

4 Use a hemostat to probe the abscess cavity and break up loculations.

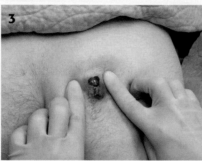

5 Probe with the hemostat to find the opposite edge of the abscess cavity. Position the tip of the hemostat underneath the area of the second incision, tent the skin, and make another stab incision over the hemostat tip.

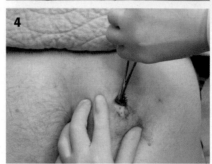

6 Optionally irrigate the cavity with a syringe and plastic intravenous catheter.

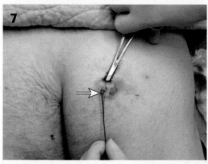

7 Place the hemostat through the cavity so that it exits the second incision. Grab the end of the vessel loop *(arrow)*.

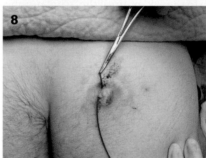

8 Pull the vessel loop through the abscess cavity so that it exits through the first incision.

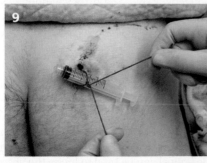

9 Tie the two ends of the vessel loop together. To avoid excessive skin tension, tie the loops over a syringe. Tie at least five knots, as the loop material is slippery. Tie the last two knots tightly, by stretching the loop almost to the breaking point.

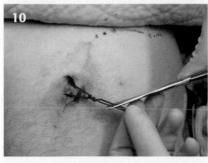

10 Remove the syringe, and then trim the ends of the vessel loop. Note that it is not tied tightly against the skin. Refer to the text for information on discharge instructions and loop removal.

Figure 16.8 Using a vessel loop for a loop drainage procedure. (For more details, refer to: McNamara WF: An alternative to open incision and drainage for community-acquired soft tissue abscesses in children, *J Pediatr Surg* 46:502–506, 2011; Ladd AP: Minimally invasive technique in treatment of complex, subcutaneous abscesses in children, *J Pediatr Surg* 45:1562–1566, 2010; and Tsoraides SS, Pearl RH, Stanfill AB, et al: Incision and loop drainage: a minimally invasive technique for subcutaneous abscess management in children, *J Pediatr Surg* 45:606–609, 2010.)

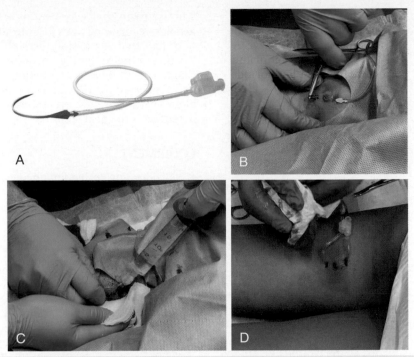

Figure 16.9 (A) A Quickloop device designed for easy abscess treatment. **(B)** Quickloop in action. **(C)** Irrigation with Quickloop in place. **(D)** Final appearance after the procedure is completed. (Copyright EM Device Lab, Inc.)

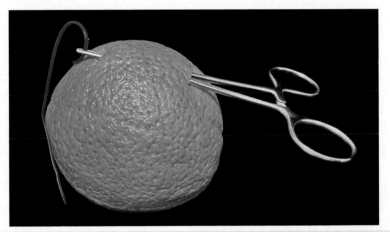

Figure 16.10 Showing how you can use an orange to teach the loop drainage technique. (Copyright Richard P. Usatine, MD)

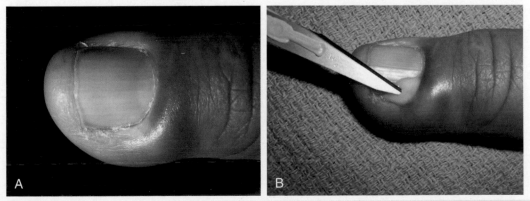

Figure 16.11 (A) Acute paronychia. **(B)** Incision of paronychia with #11 blade at cuticle. (Copyright Richard P. Usatine, MD.)

Incision and Drainage:

- Numb the area with local anesthesia. The options include a digital block and spraying the area to be incised with ethyl chloride.
- If the abscess involves the proximal nailfold then the #11 blade can be inserted between nail plate and the cuticle to avoid creating a scar.

Felon (Abscess of the Pulp of the Distal Digit)

A felon can be extremely painful. Perform a digital block and incise the abscess with a scalpel (Figure 16.12).

Complications of an Abscess

- Scarring will occur from an abscess rupturing and thinning the skin. A well-placed incision can lessen the scar or its prominence, but a scar will be present nonetheless.
- Recurrence is not unusual due to the wound closing too early, an undiagnosed loculation, or underlying deeper infection, e.g., osteomyelitis.
- Septicemia, or advancing infection, e.g., necrotizing fasciitis, may occur in association with an abscess.
- Bleeding may occur from damage to blood vessels during the course of I&D or as a result of infection eroding into adjacent vessels.
- Damage to other adjacent structures may also occur as a result of infection eroding into adjacent structures or causing inflammation of nearby structures.

Unroofing/Deroofing Hidradenitis Suppurativa

See Video 16.2.

Deroofing/unroofing is a procedure used for hidradenitis suppurativa (HS) in which the "roof" of an abscess, cyst, or sinus tract is surgically removed and the lesion is allowed to heal by secondary intention. The terms *deroofing* and *unroofing* are used interchangeably in the literature, and we will use them that way here as well. In one review of 55 articles, recurrence rates for unroofing (14.5%) were found to be half that of excision (30%).[17]

Often it helps to try intralesional triamcinolone (see Chapter 15, *Intralesional Injections*) in the inflamed, painful, and tender active HS lesion as the first step of treatment along with systemic treatments. When this fails, then deroofing is the next step.

EQUIPMENT

- 1% lidocaine with epinephrine
- #15 scalpel
- Instruments – Adson forceps, iris scissors, or any sharp tissue scissors
- 4×4-inch clean gauze pads
- CTA
- Probe (helpful but optional as probing can be performed with CTA)
- Disposable skin curette (helpful but optional as curettage/clearing of gelatinous material can be performed with CTA and 4 × 4 gauze)
- Electrosurgical instrument for hemostasis (hemostatic gel or foam may be used as an alternative)

STEP-BY-STEP DEROOFING PROCEDURE

See Video 16.2

- Palpate the lesion to determine where to draw the boundaries of the likely deroofing (Figure 16.13A).
- Anesthetize the involved area with 1% lidocaine and epinephrine.
- Open the most involved area by cutting with the #15 scalpel (Figure 16.13B).
- Use the skin curette and or gauze to scrape away any gelatinous or purulent material (Figure 16.13C).
- Determine the extent of the sinus track using a probe, curette, or CTA (Figure 16.13D).
- Extend the incision over the involved area using the scissors or scalpel.
- Using the forceps and the scissor, cut away the skin on top of the involved area to unroof the whole lesion (Figure 16.13E). (While the scalpel could be used here, the scissor gives better control of the unroofing.)

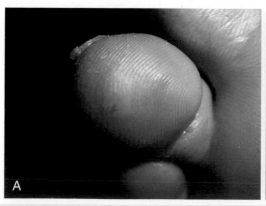
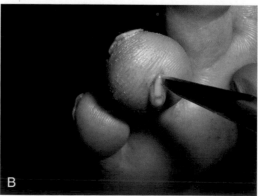

Figure 16.12 **(A)** A felon is an abscess of the pulp of the distal digit. **(B)** After a digital block the #11 blade scalpel treats the felon by draining the pus. (Copyright Richard P. Usatine, MD.)

- Once better visualization is obtained (Figure 16.13F), use the probe, curette, or CTA to find any additional sinus tracks (Figure 16.13G). Gauze may also be helpful to wipe away material that can block visualization of the whole lesion.
- Use electrosurgery or hemostatic gel/foam to stop any bleeding (Figure 16.13H).
- The final deroofed lesion should have a clean base with no active bleeding (Figure 16.13I). Cover the area with petrolatum and final dressing.
- Wound care instructions – remove the dressing in 24 hours and shower and reapply petrolatum and nonstick pad/gauze. Continue this daily until follow-up visit or full healing.
- Follow up in 2 to 6 weeks (Figure 16.13J).

Notes on Specific Lesions

- Some facial abscesses in cosmetically sensitive areas may initially be managed with needle aspiration, antibiotics, and close follow-up. However, if an I&D is indicated, this should be performed without delay or referred out for management.
- Perirectal abscesses occur in close proximity to the anal sphincter and care should be taken to avoid cutting across the sphincter. If incising, proceed as superficial as possible and parallel to the muscle fibers. As with facial abscesses, they may sometimes be initially managed cautiously with needle aspiration and antibiotics and close follow-up, but have a higher risk of deeper infection and fistula tracking especially with inflammatory bowel disease and may require surgical consultation. Perirectal abscesses more commonly involve anaerobic and gram-negative bacteria.

Special Populations

- Immune compromised patients may be particularly susceptible to infections and may present with an abscess or skin infection. Evaluation should consider the patient's history, current symptoms, and physical findings. Laboratory testing, imaging studies, and systemic antibiotics may be needed and should be determined based on the overall clinical picture. In contrast to routine superficial abscesses where culture of the abscess fluid or cavity is not usually required, cultures may be helpful in these patients to guide antibiotic therapy of atypical organisms, including fungi that may be present.

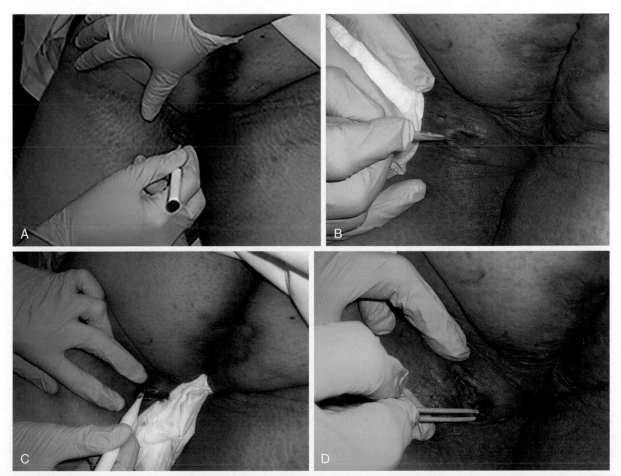

Figure 16.13 (A) Deroofing procedure on the upper thigh near the buttocks of a woman suffering with hidradenitis. After palpating the lesion not responding to intralesional injections and systemic therapy, the area is marked with a surgical marker. **(B)** After local anesthesia with 1% lidocaine and epinephrine, the involved area is opened with a #15 blade scalpel. **(C)** A 5-0 curette is used to scrape out the gelatinous inflammatory material and to probe the tunnel (sinus tract) within the lesion. **(D)** Cotton-tip applicators make great probes and can also be used to clean out the tunnel.

Continued

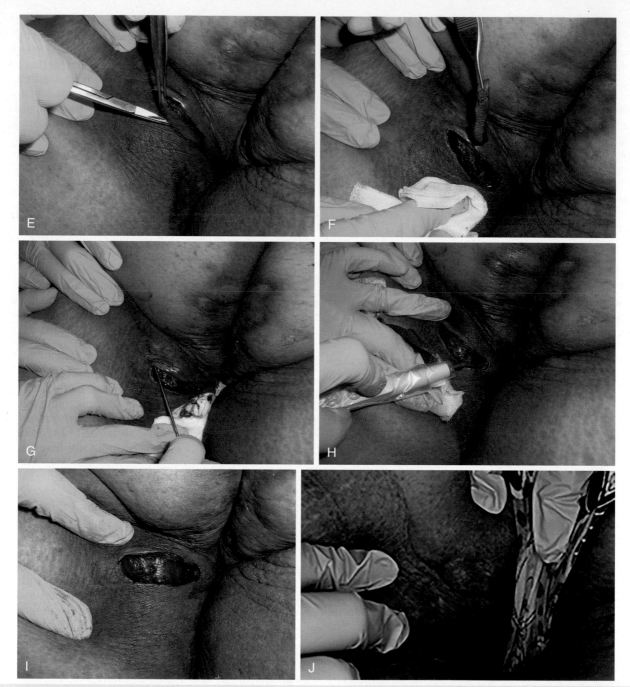

Figure 16.13, cont'd.   (E) An iris scissor is used to cut off the roof of the tunnel. **(F)** The roof is held up with the Adson forceps. **(G)** A metal probe is used to determine if there is additional area that needs treatment. This can also be done with a CTA or curette. **(H)** The Hyfrecator is used to obtain hemostasis in the few areas where bleeding has occurred. **(I)** Fully deroofed tunnel. **(J)** At a six-week follow-up the second intention healing is complete with minimal scarring. (Copyright Richard P. Usatine, MD.)

Coding and Billing Pearls

- I&D of abscess (e.g., carbuncle, HS, cutaneous or subcutaneous abscess, cyst, furuncle, or paronychia); simple or single – CPT code 10060.
- I&D of abscess (e.g., carbuncle, HS, cutaneous or subcutaneous abscess, cyst, furuncle, or paronychia); complicated or multiple – CPT code 10061.
- Use code 10061 when multiple I&Ds are performed or if the **procedure** is complicated by the need for a drain, wick, or heavy material evacuation.

Conclusion

Skin abscesses are common and I&D will be the definitive treatment for most patients. It is important for clinicians to be skilled in performing I&D in the treatment of skin abscesses. Data suggest that the loop drainage method has some advantages for children and adults, so we suggest attempting this procedure to broaden your skillset. As the incidence of hidradenitis is on the rise, it is important to learn how to unroof a hidradenitis lesion. Following the steps in this chapter and watching the accompanying videos can facilitate learning these skills.

References

1. Stevens DL, Bisno AL, Chambers HF, et al. Infectious Diseases Society of America. Practice guidelines for the diagnosis and management of skin and soft tissue infections: 2014 update by the Infectious Diseases Society of America. *Clin Infect Dis.* 2014;59(2):e10-e52. [Erratum in: Clin Infect Dis. 2015 May 1;60(9):1448]. doi: 10.1093/cid/ciu444.

2. Talan DA, Mower WR, Krishnadasan A, et al. Trimethoprim-sulfamethoxazole versus placebo for uncomplicated skin abscess. *N Engl J Med.* 2016;374(9):823-832. doi:10.1056/NEJMoa1507476.

3. Vermandere M, Aertgeerts B, Agoritsas T, et al. Antibiotics after incision and drainage for uncomplicated skin abscesses: a clinical practice guideline. *BMJ.* 2018;360:1-8. doi:10.1136/bmj.k243.

4. Loeb M, Main C, Walker-Dilks C, et al. Antimicrobial drugs for treating methicillin-resistant *Staphylococcus aureus* colonization. *Cochrane Database Syst Rev.* 2003;(4):CD003340.

5. Wendt C, Schinke S, Württemberger M, Oberdorfer K, Bock-Hensley O, von Baum H. Value of whole-body washing with chlorhexidine for the eradication of methicillin-resistant *Staphylococcus aureus*: a randomized, placebo-controlled, double-blind clinical trial. *Infect Control Hosp Epidemiol.* 2007;28(9):1036-1043.

6. Ho YH, Tan M, Chui CH, Leong A, Eu KW, Seow-Choen F. Randomized controlled trial of primary fistulotomy with drainage alone for perianal abscesses. *Dis Colon Rectum.* 1997;40(12):1435-1438.

7. Puymirat E, Biais M, Camou F, Lefèvre J, Guisset O, Gabinski C. A Lemierre syndrome variant caused by *Staphylococcus aureus. Am J Emerg Med.* 2008;26(3):380.e5-380.e7.

8. Chinnock B, Hendey GW. Irrigation of cutaneous abscesses does not improve treatment success. *Ann Emerg Med.* 2016;67(3):379-383.

9. Badour J, Singh M, Jones J. BET 1: Is routine irrigation of a cutaneous abscess necessary? *Emerg Med J.* 2018;35(2):126-127. doi:10.1136/emermed-2017-207424.2.

10. List M, Headlee D, Kondratuk K. Treatment of skin abscesses: a review of wound packing and post-procedural antibiotics. *S D Med.* 2016;69(3):113-119.

11. Pastorino A, Tavarez MM. Incision and drainage. [Updated Jul 31, 2021]. In: *StatPearls [Internet].* Treasure Island, FL: StatPearls Publishing; 2022. Available at: https://www.ncbi.nlm.nih.gov/books/NBK556072/.

12. Gottlieb M, Schmitz G, Peksa GD. Comparison of the loop technique with incision and drainage for skin and soft tissue abscesses: a systematic review and meta-analysis. *Acad Emerg Med.* 2021;28(3):346-354. doi:10.1111/acem.14151.

13. Gaszynski R, Punch G, Verschuer K. Loop and drain technique for subcutaneous abscess: a safe minimally invasive procedure in an adult population. *ANZ J Surg.* 2018;88(1-2):87-90. doi:10.1111/ans.13709.

14. Aprahamian CJ, Nashad HH, DiSomma NM, et al. Treatment of subcutaneous abscesses in children with incision and loop drainage: a simplified method of care. *J Pediatr Surg.* 2017;52(9):1438-1441. doi:10.1016/j.jpedsurg.2016.12.018.

15. Ladde J, Baker S, Lilburn N, Wan M, Papa L. A Randomized Controlled Trial of Novel Loop Drainage Technique Versus Standard Incision and Drainage in the Treatment of Skin Abscesses. *Acad Emerg Med.* 2020;27(12):1229-1240. doi:10.1111/acem.14106.

16. Tsoraides SS, Pearl RH, Stanfill AB, Wallace LJ, Vegunta RK. Incision and loop drainage: a minimally invasive technique for subcutaneous abscess management in children. *J Pediatr Surg.* 2010;45(3):606-609. doi:10.1016/j.jpedsurg.2009.06.013.

17. Saylor DK, Brownstone ND, Naik HB. Office-based surgical intervention for hidradenitis suppurativa (HS): a focused review for dermatologists. *Dermatol Ther.* 2020;10(4):529-549. doi:10.1007/s13555-020-00391-x.

17 Nail Procedures

RICHARD P. USATINE, MD, ARIADNA PEREZ SANCHEZ, MD, and ROBERT GILSON, MD

SUMMARY

- Equipment for nail procedures reviewed.
- It is safe to use lidocaine with epinephrine for digital blocks.
- A tourniquet can be created from a glove and can be used safely for at least 30 minutes.
- Procedures such as the partial nail plate removal with destruction of nail matrix are described.
- Biopsy techniques to diagnose nail unit melanoma and other nail unit tumors are discussed in detail.
- Treatment of pincer nails and onychomatricomas are described.
- Guidance on how to evacuate a subungual hematoma is provided.

Overview

Nails serve an important function to protect the end of our fingers and toes, to increase mechanical traction, and to enhance fine touch. Nails also serve important personal and social functions, such as scratching and grooming and to be used as aesthetic adornments (Figure 17.1).

Nails can be traumatized, infected, or become dysmorphic secondary to cutaneous or systemic disease. Skin cancers can form under or around nails. This chapter will cover the various types of specialized surgical procedures and biopsies performed on the nail unit.

Anatomy of the Nail Unit

What we call the "nail" is actually the nail plate that sits on the nail bed and is surrounded by the nail folds. The nail plate is made of keratin and is produced by the nail matrix found below the proximal nail fold. See Figure 17.2 for detailed nail anatomy.

Nail Procedures

1. Digital and wing blocks
2. Partial nail removal – ingrown nail and pincer nail
3. Matrixectomy – chemical and physical
4. Nail removal (nail avulsion)
5. Biopsies to diagnose skin cancers – punch, shave, longitudinal excision
6. Subungual hematoma evacuation
7. Surgical removal of benign tumors

EQUIPMENT (FIGURE 17.3)

Needed for nail plate removals:

- One nail elevator (periosteal elevator, septum elevator, or Freer elevator)

- One nail splitter (English anvil type)
- One straight or curved hemostat (not small Mosquito type)

Additionally needed for other nail surgeries:

- One sharp iris scissor, Gradle scissor, or other fine-tipped scissor
- Needle holder
- Adson forceps (no teeth or fine teeth only)
- Skin hooks (single or double pronged)

Common nail conditions requiring nail procedures:

- Ingrown nail requiring partial nail excision
- Deformed and painful nail requiring full nail plate avulsion
- Pincer nail when painful
- Longitudinal melanonychia (LM) requiring biopsy of the nail matrix
- Growing mass with partial or full destruction of the nail plate requiring biopsy
- Subungual hematoma requiring drainage

STEPS COMMON TO MANY NAIL PROCEDURES

Local anesthesia is most effective with a digital block or wing block or both (Figure 17.4). These blocks are explained fully in Chapter 3, *Anesthesia*. Both are not difficult to perform. The digital block is somewhat less painful than the wing block. The wing block has the benefit of producing local hemostasis because it distends the tissues near the area of surgery, and the epinephrine helps hemostasis. The best anesthesia and hemostasis for nail matrix biopsies is obtained with the digital block followed by the wing block.

Alternatively, transthecal anesthesia (Figure 17.5) is a less commonly used digital block for the second, third, and fourth digits. Its advantage is that the neurovascular structures are avoided; however, it does go through the tendon sheath. Two mL of 1% to 2% lidocaine with or without epinephrine is injected into the flexor digitorum tendon sheath at the webspace through the palmar side of the metacarpophalangeal joint crease.[1] One method involves

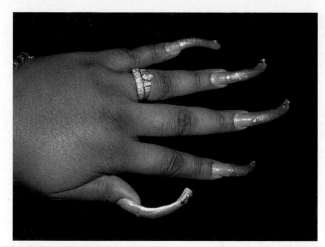

Figure 17.1 Nails serve important social functions including being aesthetic adornments. (Copyright Richard P. Usatine, MD.)

duration (3–6 hours), easing the postoperative pain after nail surgery.[1,8] The anesthesia may be given at the base of the digit or in the web space (Figure 17.4).

Additionally, a wing block can be added to the digital block to ensure complete anesthesia using lidocaine and epinephrine too. The onset of anesthesia is fast, and it provides better hemostasis at the site of surgery (Figure 17.4C). As always, make sure that good anesthesia has been obtained before starting the procedure.

Chlorhexidine (Hibiclens) or chlorhexidine-alcohol may be used to clean the surgical site for all procedures that follow. Data on surgical scrubs indicates that chlorhexidine-based scrubs are most effective in decreasing postop infection rates.[9]

USE OF GLOVE FOR TOURNIQUET AND STERILE FIELD

A tourniquet is not always needed for nail plate removal surgeries (partial or complete) especially when epinephrine is used in the digital block. It is worth using a tourniquet for nail matrix biopsies to allow for better visualization during the biopsy. A tourniquet may also help when doing a

fanning out the lidocaine to add an additional 1 mL of lidocaine to each side of the finger (Figure 17.5). Transthecal anesthesia can be done for the toes as well.

A digital block may be performed with 1% or 2% lidocaine and epinephrine. Multiple studies have confirmed the safety of using epinephrine on the digits and for digital blocks.[2-7]

Using 2% lidocaine has the advantage of delivering more anesthetic in less volume but 1% is adequate as well. Usually 3 to 5 mL is sufficient. Ideally, no more than 5 mL total is used to avoid pressure-induced/fluid tourniquet effect. That is injected perpendicular to the digital side on both sides of the middle phalanx and a few millimeters below the DIP joint. Further ways to reduce the pain from anesthesia include buffering the lidocaine, warming to room temperature, using the finest point 30 gauge needle, and distractions such as pinching or tapping the skin. Another alternative is bupivacaine 0.25% to 0.50% or ropivacaine 1%, both anesthetics have a rapid onset of action (2–10 minutes) and long

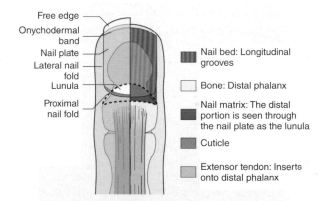

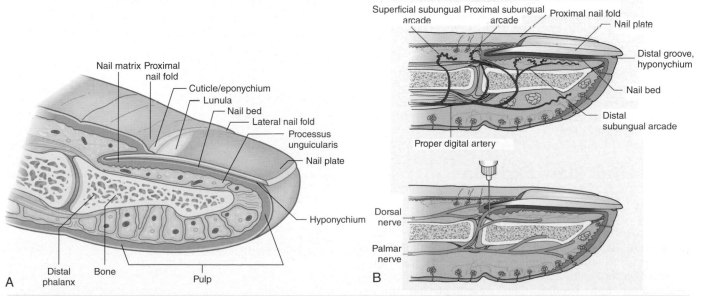

Figure 17.2 **(A)** Detailed anatomy of the nail unit. (*Modified from Vidimos A, Ammirati C, Poblete-Lopez C. Dermatologic Surgery. London: Saunders; 2008.*) **(B)** Surgical anatomy of the nail unit. (From Bolognia: *Dermatology Fourth Edition.* © 2018, Elsevier Limited. All rights reserved.)

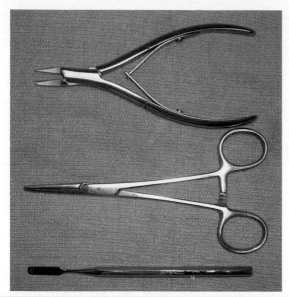

Figure 17.3 Instruments for nail surgery – nail splitter, straight hemostat, and nail elevator. (Copyright Richard P. Usatine, MD.)

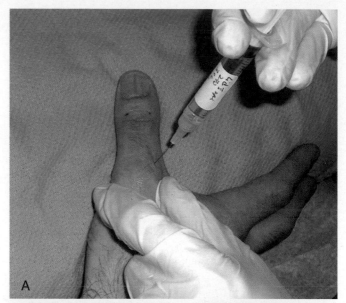

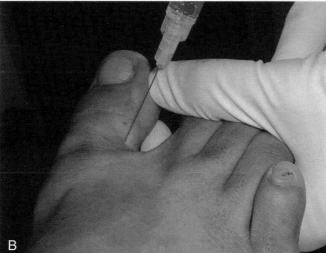

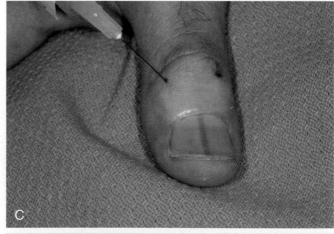

Figure 17.4 (A) Digital block of the thumb using 2% lidocaine without epinephrine. **(B)** Digital block of the large toe with needle pointed toward the web space. **(C)** Wing block using lidocaine with epinephrine. (Copyright Richard P. Usatine, MD.)

chemical or electrosurgical matrix ablation as a dry matrix field increases the effectiveness of this procedure.

- For finger or toenail matrix biopsies: A finger of a sterile glove can be used to make a sterile tourniquet. Along with a hemostat (Figure 17.6A–C), cut off the end of a glove finger, then cut a line at the tip. This can be rolled back over a finger or toe to create a tourniquet. Nail plate removal surgery does not need to be sterile, but the sterile gloves tend to work better for creating tourniquets. You can also use a large sterile glove on the foot to help with sterility.
- To increase the pressure of the tourniquet, use a hemostat to twist the glove material tighter around the digit as needed during the surgery (Figure 17.6C).
- Time limit recommendations for tourniquets in the literature vary from 30 minutes to over 2 hours. In a large study of tourniquet use in hand surgery, even those 60 patients whose tourniquet time exceeded 2 hours showed no postoperative complications.[10]
- A whole sterile glove can also be placed on the hand to create a sterile environment for finger and nail surgery.
- Then carefully cut a slit in the glove finger with a sterile scissor to be able to roll back the glove over the involved finger. You can also use a large sterile glove on the foot to help with sterility.

Partial Nail Plate Excision

See Videos 17.1–17.3.

The most common indication for partial nail plate excision is an ingrown nail (especially the large toenail). An ingrown nail (onychocryptosis) occurs when the nail plate is too large for the nail bed (Figure 17.7). The nail plate puts pressure on the lateral nail fold and does not fit properly in the lateral nail groove. The treatment for this is to make the nail plate less wide on the involved side. The best way to prevent this from recurring is to ablate the nail

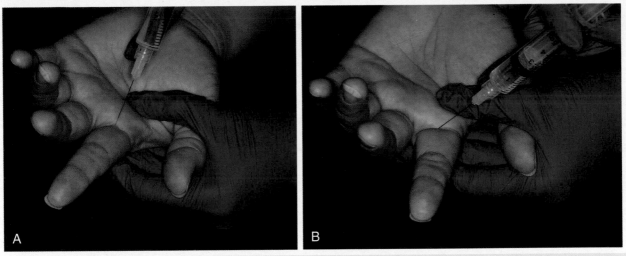

Figure 17.5 **(A)** Transthecal anesthesia for a digital block goes through the tendon sheath on the palmar (or plantar) side. Two mL of 1% to 2% lido-caine with or without epinephrine is injected into the flexor digitorum tendon sheath at the webspace through the palmar side of the metacarpopha-langeal joint crease. **(B)** One method involves fanning out the lidocaine to add an additional 1 mL of lidocaine to each side of the finger. (Copyright Richard P. Usatine, MD.)

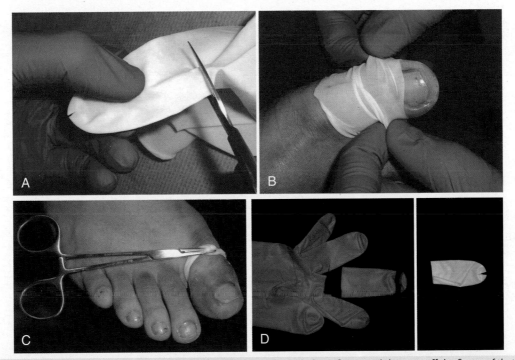

Figure 17.6 Creating a tourniquet from a sterile glove. **(A)** Make a small snip at the end of one finger and then cut off the finger of that glove. **(B)** Roll the finger onto the digit allowing the digit to expand the small hole at the end of the "finger." This should fit snugly. **(C)** Grasp the glove material with a hemostat, and turn it around to tighten the tourniquet as needed. **(D)** Alternate method of making a tourniquet is to snip the tip of the finger off rather than snipping the tip vertically. (Copyright Richard P. Usatine, MD.)

matrix on the involved side using chemical or electrosurgi-cal destruction.

Steps to follow:

1. Anesthetize, sterilize, and drape the affected digit as de-scribed above.
2. Use nail elevator (Freer elevator or periosteal elevator) to free the nail plate from the cuticle and proximal nail fold. *The Freer elevator isn't named for its function, but after American ENT surgeon Otto "Tiger" Freer (1868–1939).*

3. Insert elevator under the nail plate in the area where the nail plate will be removed. Insert it all the way to the nail matrix (Figure 17.8A). Be careful to avoid damaging the underlying nail bed by keeping the elevator close to the bottom of the nail plate (Figure 17.8B).
4. Insert hemostat under the free portion of the nail and clamp down on this nail segment (Figure 17.8C). Rotate the nail segment from lateral to medial until the lateral horn is released and the portion of the nail is fully

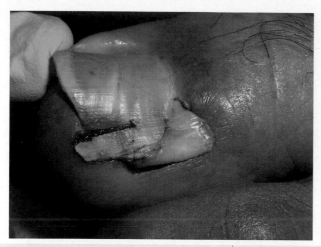

Figure 17.7 Ingrown toenail (onychocryptosis) in the middle of a partial nail avulsion. The oversized nail plate can be seen prior to cutting it off. (Copyright Richard P. Usatine, MD.)

removed (Figure 17.8D). This makes it easier to cut off the lateral portion of the nail without leaving the proximal lateral horn in place.

5. Use the nail splitter to cut the lateral portion of the nail to be removed (Figure 17.8E).
6. Bleeding can usually be stopped with direct pressure alone, but electrocoagulation or chemical hemostatic agents such as aluminum chloride can be used if necessary. If a tourniquet is used, there should be little to no bleeding until it is removed (Figure 17.8F).
7. If the lateral corner of the matrix is to be destroyed to prevent recurrence, use phenol, trichloroacetic acid (TCA), or electrosurgery (Figure 17.8G). See exact instructions below.
8. Granulation tissue or swelling of the lateral nail fold can be ignored, as it will resolve in the healing process (Figure 17.8H).
9. Release the tourniquet, and dress the digit with petrolatum and sterile gauze.

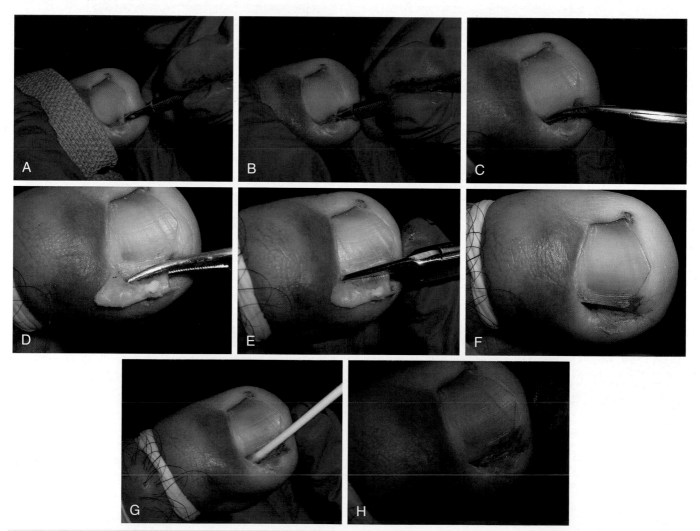

Figure 17.8 Partial nail plate excision to treat an ingrown toenail. **(A)** Nail elevator is inserted under the offending nail. **(B)** It is inserted all the way to the matrix. **(C)** A curved or straight hemostat is clamped on the nail. **(D)** Hemostat still clamped on the nail after the lateral horn is turned out. **(E)** Nail splitter cutting off the offending lateral nail portion. **(F)** The new nail plate is no longer too large. **(G)** Phenol is being used to kill the lateral matrix and prevent a recurrent ingrown nail. **(H)** The whitening of the skin is where the phenol came in contact with the skin. (Copyright Richard P. Usatine, MD.)

10. Encourage the patient to remove the dressing 24 hours after the procedure and soak the foot with lukewarm water and a small amount of soap, chlorhexidine, or povidone-iodine soap.[1]
11. Encourage the patient or soak the foot once or twice daily with a small amount of soap or chlorhexidine in water to prevent infection and accelerate healing.
12. Optional method: Reverse the order of steps 4 and 5, and start by cutting edge first. Then clamp the hemostat on the lateral nail plate edge, and rotate the nail from lateral to medial until the lateral horn is released. Make sure you get the full proximal lateral horn out.

Destruction of Nail Matrix

▶ See Videos 17.2 and 17.3.

In a 2020 metaanalysis, the authors compared phenol, sodium hydroxide (NaOH), and TCA 90%, with the primary outcome of reduced recurrence after partial nail avulsion. Phenol and TCA showed significantly lower recurrence compared to placebo. NaOH didn't show any significant difference in comparison with placebo. Phenol is contraindicated in pregnant patients and pregnant clinicians. The study concluded that TCA is comparable to phenol with the added benefit that TCA can be used on the pregnant population.[11] Another study evaluated the use of NaOH, TCA 90%, and phenol 88%, and assigned five patients to each group (n = 15). They concluded that TCA is an effective agent with the advantage of reduced postoperative pain and faster re-epithelization of the wound compared with phenol and NaOH.[12]

Phenol or TCA application:

- Bleeding is stopped by applying a tourniquet.
- The matrix area must be bloodless before the phenol or TCA is applied, or it will not work as well.
- Cover the surrounding nail fold with petrolatum (Figure 17.9) to protect the normal tissue from the caustic effects of either chemical.

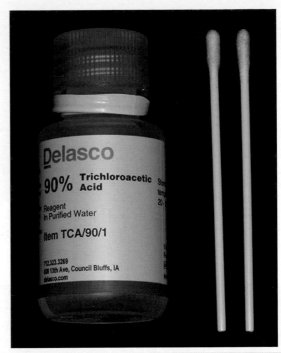

Figure 17.10 90% Trichloroacetic acid in water with small applicators to destroy one portion of the nail matrix. (Copyright Richard P. Usatine, MD.)

- The application is best performed with a cotton-tip applicator with a small cotton tip (Figure 17.10).
- The phenol or TCA is vigorously rubbed into the exposed matrix for 1 to 2 minutes total (Figure 17.11). This can be divided up into 30-60 second applications.
- During each 1-minute application the cotton tip should be rotated over the matrix.
- For each new application application a new cotton-tipped applicator should be chosen.
- We suggest neutralizing the phenol or TCA after application with any available noncaustic liquid such as saline, water, alcohol or chlorhexidine solution. The goal is to clean the phenol or TCA off the surrounding tissues to avoid collateral damage.

One study found that partial nail avulsion with phenolization gave better results than partial avulsion with matrix excision.[6] Local antibiotics applied to the surgical site did not reduce signs of infection or recurrence. Of note, use of Neosporin or bacitracin may be associated with contact dermatitis. The use of phenol did not produce more signs of infection than matrix excision.[6]

One way to purchase phenol now is "Phenol EZ SWABS." This comes as a package with phenol in a sealed ampule and dedicated cotton swab sticks (Figure 17.12). It is more expensive per patient but does reduce the possibility of a phenol spill from an open bottle. See Box 17.1 for cost considerations with chemical matrixectomy.

PHYSICAL MATRIXECTOMY (ELECTRODESTRUCTION)

Another method involves the use of electrical destruction (electrofulguration). This can be performed with a standard electrode or a special matrixectomy electrode that has a Teflon-coated top and a metallic bottom (Figure 17.13).

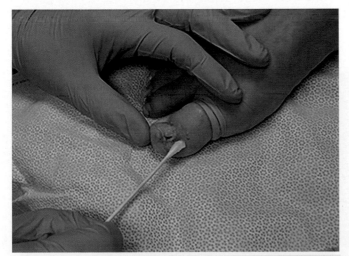

Figure 17.9 Applying petrolatum on the normal skin after a partial nail avulsion prior to applying the caustic agent such as phenol or TCA to kill the lateral matrix (during treatment of an ingrown nail). (Copyright Richard P. Usatine, MD.)

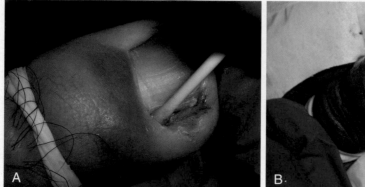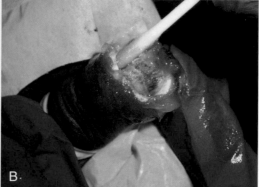

Figure 17.11 **(A)** Applying phenol with a cotton-tip applicator to destroy a portion of the nail matrix to prevent a recurrent ingrown toenail. **(B)** Applying trichloroacetic acid to the nail matrix of an extremely dysmorphic toenail after petrolatum was used to protect the surrounding skin. (Copyright Richard P. Usatine, MD.)

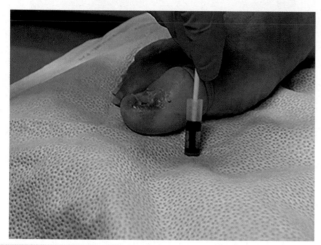

Figure 17.12 "Phenol EZ SWABS" in a sealed ampule with a dedicated cotton swab stick. (Copyright Richard P. Usatine, MD.)

The Teflon prevents damage to the upper nail fold. This matrixectomy electrode is produced by Ellman Cynosure to be used with their radiofrequency electrosurgical units. However, a standard electrosurgery disposable electrode may be used with a Hyfrecator or similar electrosurgical unit, and the tip may be placed close to the matrix so that most of the electrical energy reaches the matrix but not the upper nail fold. The best method for electrodestruction in this procedure is fulguration in which the electrical energy sparks to the matrix. The specific matrixectomy electrode should be used with an electrocoagulation setting (16–20 on hemo using the dual frequency Surgitron). The electrode should be kept slightly above the matrix so that the spark of electricity can be seen and heard. Some authors recommend curetting the nail matrix before using

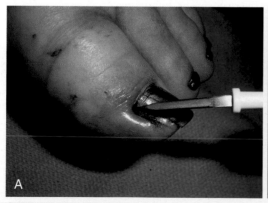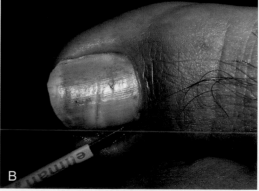

Figure 17.13 Two electrosurgical methods to perform a physical matrixectomy. **(A)** Using the sharp-tipped disposable electrode for the Hyfrecator. **(B)** Using a special Ellman electrode with a Teflon-coated top and a metallic bottom. The Teflon prevents damage to the upper nail fold while the metal bottom conducts the radiofrequency to destroy the matrix in that region. (Copyright Richard P. Usatine, MD.)

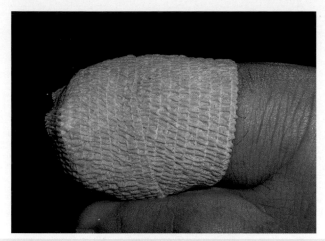

Figure 17.14 Light pressure dressing after partial avulsion of nail with ingrown toenail. (Copyright Richard P. Usatine, MD.)

electrosurgery (a 3-mm round skin curette or a special nail curette can be used).[3] The data is limited for physical matrixectomy. In one study, they compared phenolization versus electrocautery application after partial nail extraction, and they found a significant difference between the two groups, indicating the phenolization has a faster healing time, up 4.5 times in comparison with the electrocautery group.[13]

WOUND DRESSINGS

Place a dab of petrolatum on the site, and cover with sterile gauze. A light pressure dressing may be applied with self-adhesive bandages, especially if there was a significant amount of bleeding (Figure 17.14). Self-adhesive bandages are made by Coban, Medique, and Dynarex.

Full Nail Plate Removal (Nail Avulsion)

Patients with severely hyperkeratotic nails that cannot be easily clipped may request a full nail plate removal. While a warm bath or the application of 40% urea may make it easier to clip such nails some patients will want them removed completely. The nail matrix should be permanently destroyed if the patient does not want the nail to regrow. This may be performed with phenol, TCA, or electrodestruction.

TOTAL NAIL AVULSION (FIGURE 17.15)

1. The procedure is performed in an identical manner to the partial nail removal except that the full nail is removed.
2. Use a nail elevator to free the nail plate from the cuticle and proximal nail fold.
3. Insert elevator under the lateral nail plate in the area where the hemostat will be clamped. Insert it all the way to the nail matrix. Be careful to avoid damaging the underlying nail bed by keeping the elevator close to the bottom of the nail plate.
4. Insert the hemostat under the free portion of the nail, and clamp down hard. Rotate the nail from lateral to medial until the lateral horn is released, and then keep

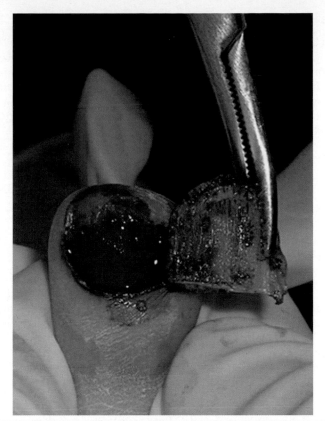

Figure 17.15 A painful dysmorphic nail is being avulsed using the distal approach and the lateral curl technique. Note the ridges on the underside of the nail plate that normally keep the nail plate attached to the nail bed. (Copyright Richard P. Usatine, MD.)

rotating until the nail is fully removed. (It is often easier to start on the left side for right-handed clinicians and the right side for those persons who are left handed.)
5. Use chemical and/or electrocoagulation to stop any significant bleeding.
6. Matrix destruction should only be performed when the goal is to prevent the nail from growing back. Use phenol, TCA, or electrodestruction.

Biopsies to Diagnose Pigmented Nail Changes (Acral Melanoma Versus Benign Longitudinal Melanonychia)

We will describe four biopsy techniques to be used to diagnose nail melanoma and other malignancies that can occur in the nail unit. The easiest biopsy to perform is a 3-mm punch biopsy of the nail matrix at the origin of the pigmented band. Occasionally a shave biopsy is preferred if the pigmented band is wide. The advantage of a shave biopsy is that it may reduce or limit matrix scarring and subsequent nail dystrophy. The disadvantages include that a full or partial nail avulsion is required, and this can result in nail splitting, paronychia, and dorsal pterygium.[14,15] When melanoma is suspected a full-thickness ellipse in the matrix is another option. When the pigment is in the lateral nail and nail fold, a lateral longitudinal excision may be needed.[7]

WHETHER TO BIOPSY?

There are many rules and algorithms that have been developed to diagnose subungual melanoma early. They have similar criteria, and none are without their flaws and limitations. Most have evidence based on small numbers and few studies as subungual melanoma is not a common diagnosis. We will present the clinical ones first and then one based on dermoscopy.

The ABCDEF mnemonic system was developed to detect nail melanoma (see Box 17.2).[16]

Lee et al. performed a study of Korean patients with subungual melanoma *in situ* to develop a strategy for early diagnosis.[17] This was their ABCD rule:

"A" stands for adult age (age >18 years);
"B" for brown bands in brown background;
"C" for color in periungual skin; "Hutchinson sign"
"D" for one digit.

The sensitivity and specificity for their ABCD rule applied to their Korean patients with subungual melanoma *in situ* and nail melanocytic nevi were 100% and 96.6%, respectively.[17]

Other strategies include the recommendation to biopsy pigmented nails when:

1. The pigment is >3 mm wide (Figure 17.16).
2. It is the only nail with a dark and significant color variation (Figure 17.16).
3. It is associated with nail dystrophy or deformity (Figure 17.17).
4. There is a positive Hutchinson or micro-Hutchinson sign. Hutchinson sign is the extension of pigmentation to the skin adjacent to the nail plate involving the nail folds or the tip of the digit (Figure 17.18A). Micro-Hutchinson sign is when the extension of the pigmentation to the skin adjacent to the nail plate is detected by dermoscopy alone (Figure 17.18B). A pseudo-Hutchinson sign occurs in ethnic melanonychia or when nail pigmentation is viewed through a clear cuticle and is not a sign of melanoma (Figure 17.18C).

Longitudinal melanonychia (LM) is a pigmented band that occurs in the nail plate from the proximal to the distal aspect. In patients with LM, clinical features that may suggest early

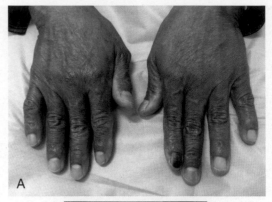

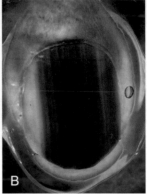

Figure 17.16 (A) Melanoma *in situ* in an African American man with one solitary dark nail. The pigment is >3 mm wide and >2/3 the width of the nail. **(B)** Dermoscopy shows a micro-Hutchinson sign along with atypical pigmented lines. (Courtesy of Ash Marghoob, MD.)

nail melanoma and warrant a biopsy of the nail matrix include:[18-20]

- Melanonychia that develops during adulthood, involves a single digit (in particular, the thumb, index finger, or great toe), and enlarges rapidly
- LM >3 mm in width with variegated pigmentation or proximal widening (triangular shape) (Figure 17.19)
- Preexisting LM that becomes darker or wider or demonstrates blurred, lateral borders
- LM associated with nail plate fissuring, splitting, or dystrophy
- Melanonychia extending to the nail folds (Hutchinson sign)

These clinical rules/algorithms do not include the use of dermoscopic evaluation but are helpful to determine when LM should be biopsied. The biopsy itself should not be of the skin showing the Hutchinson sign but the matrix where the melanoma originates. In one study, dermoscopic features of nail melanoma were significantly associated with a brown coloration of the background and the presence of irregular longitudinal lines (in their color, spacing, thickness, and parallelism).[21]

Benign causes of hyperpigmentation of the nail plate include ethnic melanonychia (aka racial melanonychia) (Figure 17.20) and melanocytic activation. Ethnic melanonychia is the most common cause of LM (especially in patients with darker skin tones) and more likely if multiple nails are involved (Figure 17.20). Other common benign

---

Box 17.2   The ABCDEF mnemonic system was developed to detect nail melanoma.[16]

"A" stands for ages 40 to 70 years (peak incidence being between the 5th and 7th decades) and African Americans, Asians, and Native Americans in whom acral lentiginous melanoma accounts for approximately one-third of melanoma cases.

"B" stands for *b*and with "*b*rown to *b*lack" and with "*b*readth" of 3 mm or more, and *b*lurred borders.

"C" stands for *c*hange in size or *c*olor or lack of *c*hange after adequate treatment.

"D" stands for the *d*igit most commonly involved (thumb, hallux (big toe), or index finger).

"E" stands for *e*xtension of the pigment onto the proximal and/or lateral nail fold (Hutchinson sign).

"F" stands for *f*amily or personal history of dysplastic nevus or melanoma.[16]

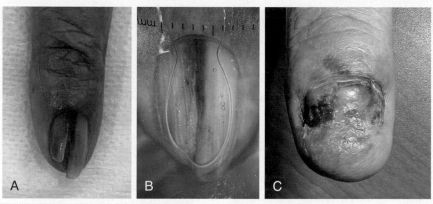

Figure 17.17 (A) Melanoma *in situ* in an African American woman with nail dystrophy and widening of pigment proximally. **(B)** Dermoscopy shows irregular pigmented granules. **(C)** Another acral lentiginous melanoma showing nail destruction and a positive Hutchinson sign. (C, Courtesy of Dr. Dubin at http://www.skinatlas.com; and Color Atlas of Family Medicine.)

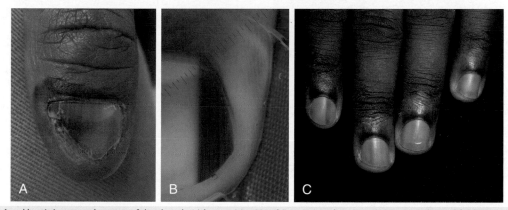

Figure 17.18 (A) Acral lentiginous melanoma of the thumb with a positive Hutchinson sign showing pigment on the nail fold. *(Reproduced with permission from Robert T. Gilson, MD.)* **(B)** Dermoscopy of a melanoma *in situ* shows a micro-Hutchinson sign along with atypical pigmented lines. *(Courtesy of Ash Marghoob, MD.)* **(C)** Ethnic melanonychia with multiple nails showing hyperpigmented lines and pseudo-Hutchinson sign (dark pigmentation on the proximal nail folds without a diagnosis of melanoma). (Copyright Richard P. Usatine, MD.)

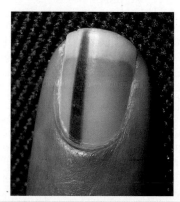

Figure 17.19 Melanonychia with widening of the pigmented band as the nail grows. This is a worrisome sign, and biopsy was performed only showing a growing benign nevus. (Copyright Richard P. Usatine, MD.)

causes are benign melanocytic hyperplasia, nevi, trauma, fungal, and medications. Squamous cell carcinomas (Figure 17.21) may also involve the nail unit and be hyperpigmented.

DERMOSCOPY

In a retrospective observational dermoscopic study, nail melanoma cases were significantly associated with a pigmented band involving greater than 2/3 the width of the nail plate, grey and black colors, irregularly pigmented lines, Hutchinson and micro-Hutchinson signs, and nail dystrophy. Granular pigmentation (seen best with dermoscopy) was found in 40% of melanomas (Figure 17.17) and only in 3.5% of benign lesions.[22] Other dermoscopic features of nail melanoma are longitudinal brown to black lines with irregular color, spacing, and thickness. Lines usually show loss of parallelism and may vary within single lines.

Other reasons to be concerned for nail melanoma include abrupt onset of LM after middle age, personal or family history of melanoma, rapid growth, darkening of a melanonychia band, pigment variegation, blurry lateral borders, irregular elevation of the surface, a bandwidth >3 mm, proximal widening of the pigmented band (Figure 17.19), associated nail plate dystrophy, and single rather than multiple digit involvement.[23]

HOW TO BIOPSY

Before starting a biopsy it is helpful to know if the nail plate pigment is coming from the proximal or distal matrix. The proximal matrix generates pigment on top of the nail plate, and the distal matrix generates pigment on the bottom or ventral portion of the nail plate. Look at the free edge of the

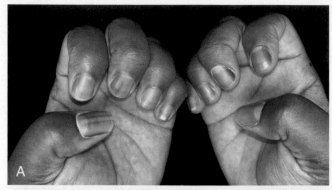

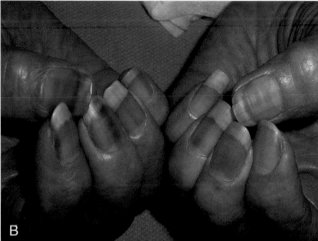

Figure 17.20 (A) Ethnic melanonychia with multiple nails showing hyperpigmented lines in a 34-year-old African American woman. **(B)** Ethnic melanonychia or melanocytic activation in a Hispanic woman. (Copyright Richard P. Usatine, MD.)

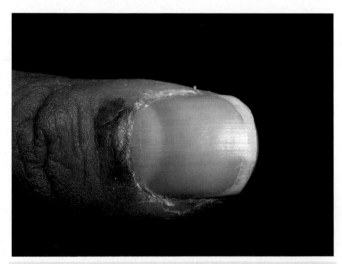

Figure 17.21 SCC *in situ* in a 35-year-old Hispanic woman presenting as pigment on the proximal nail fold. (Copyright Richard P. Usatine, MD.)

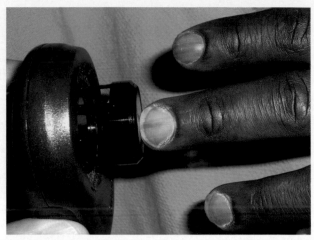

Figure 17.22 Dermoscopy on the edge of the nail plate with longitudinal melanonychia to determine whether the pigment is being produced in the proximal or distal nail matrix. (Copyright Richard P. Usatine, MD.)

PUNCH BIOPSY OF THE NAIL MATRIX (3-MM PUNCH)[8] (FIGURE 17.23)

1. Perform a digital block (lidocaine with epinephrine) first so that the wing block is not painful (Figure 17.4A).
2. Perform a wing block (lidocaine with epinephrine) to obtain good anesthesia and hemostasis (Figure 17.23A).
3. Place a tourniquet on the involved digit (Figure 17.23B).
4. Use a nail elevator to separate the cuticle and proximal nail fold from the nail plate.
5. Use a No. 15 scalpel to cut incisions at the junction of the proximal and lateral nail folds bilaterally (Figure 17.23C, D). The nail elevator can help further separate the proximal nail fold from the nail plate once the cuts have been made.
6. Reflect nail fold back using forceps or skin hooks to see the entire matrix. An alternative method is to place sutures on each side of the nail fold and pull the fold back using the suture to grasp the edges (Figure 17.23E, F).
7. Use a dermatoscope (not touching surface) or good light source to look for the origin of the pigmented band.
8. Biopsy the origin of the pigmented band with a 3- to 4-mm punch through the nail plate and down to the bone (Figure 17.23G–K). There will be fewer nail deformities if the biopsy is in the distal matrix, but if the proximal matrix is the origin of the pigment the biopsy must be at that site.[7]
9. Use the finest forceps available to lift the punch core up, and snip at the deepest base possible (Figure 17.23J, K). One option is to snip with a very fine-tipped scissor without pulling up on the tissue. Whichever method is used, it is crucial to not crush the specimen.[7]
10. The friable matrix tissue may end up in the end of the punch biopsy instrument. If so, use a needle to remove the tissue without damaging it for the pathologist. If this can be performed without forceps, the tissue will have fewer crush artifacts for the pathologist.
11. If needed, use electrocoagulation or a chemical hemostatic agent to stop the punch biopsy from bleeding (Figure 17.23L).

nail with a good source of light and magnification before starting a biopsy. A dermatoscope with clear gel applied directly to the edge of the nail is an excellent method to determine the location of the pigment and the origin of the pigment band (Figure 17.22).

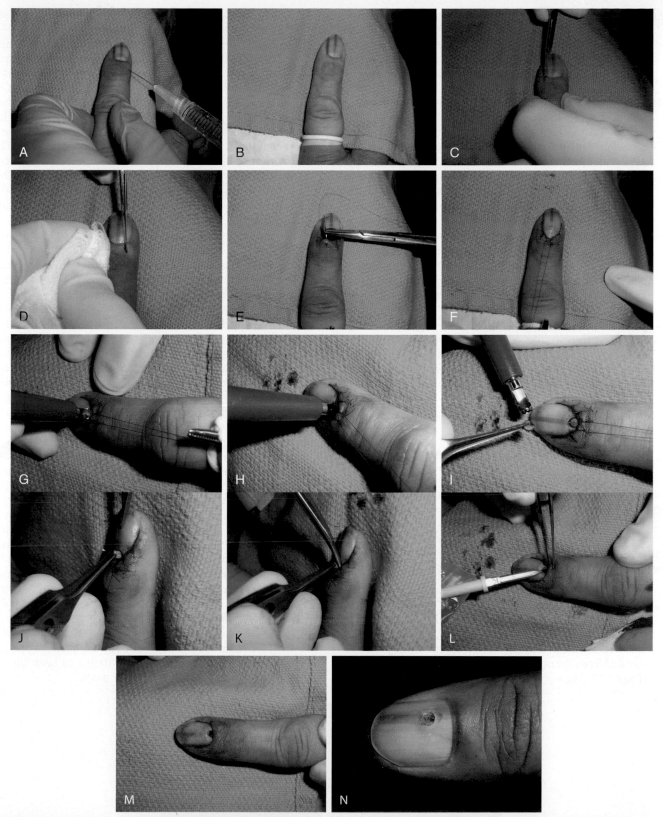

Figure 17.23 Punch biopsy of the nail matrix. **(A)** Wing block being performed after digital block was completed (both with lidocaine and epinephrine). **(B)** Tourniquet applied, and there is blanching of the skin. **(C)** No. 15 scalpel cutting incision at the junction of the proximal and lateral nail folds. **(D)** The second cut is more medial and closer to the pigmented band. **(E)** Suture is being placed to reflect the proximal nail fold back. **(F)** With two sutures placed the proximal nail fold can be more reliably reflected. **(G)** Nail fold reflected back to see the matrix and the 3-mm punch placed over the origin of the pigmented band. **(H)** The punch biopsy is through the nail plate and down to the bone. **(I)** The nail plate is removed and being held in forceps to be sent for pathology along with the tissue from the matrix. **(J)** The punch tissue is being held up with fine forceps. **(K)** Cutting the punch at the base. **(L)** Sharp-tipped electrode for hemostasis. **(M)** The biopsy is complete and the proximal nail fold is now in place. Suturing it is an option, but in this case it was not needed. **(N)** Months later the nail defect is growing out, and the melanonychia is not seen in the new nail. (Copyright Richard P. Usatine, MD.)

12. Send the small circular nail plate specimen along with the matrix tissue for analysis as it may contain cellular remnants, blood, melanocytic pigmentation, or even fungal elements.[24,25] Large cellular remnants of melanocytes in the nail plate can help make the diagnosis of subungual melanoma.[24,25]

13. Return the proximal nail fold to its original location and reapproximate the incision edges. This may be performed with 5-0 nylon or polypropylene (Prolene), Steri-Strips, or the application of a pressure dressing (Figure 17.23M). Suturing these cuts is not always needed.

14. (Optional) Consider injecting Marcaine or Ropivacaine in the wing block area for extended pain relief. Either way, advise the patient on the use of pain medications as needed.

15. Apply petrolatum and a pressure dressing. Typically, there is minimal bleeding with this technique, and often pressure alone will suffice; however, several small pieces of hemostatic gel foam (cut to fit) can be placed in the punch biopsy site for added hemostasis. The gel foam does not need to be removed.

16. If placed, remove sutures in 7 days.

17. Note how the circular defect in the nail plate will grow out (Figure 17.23N). In this case, the diagnosis was benign melanocytic activation (not neoplasia).

18. Figure 17.24 shows a close-up of a 3-mm punch biopsy of melanonychia in which skin hooks were used to reflect the proximal nail fold.

SHAVE BIOPSY OF THE NAIL MATRIX[8]

▶ *See Video 17.4.*

The shave biopsy of the nail matrix provides adequate samples of wider bands (Figure 17.25A) and is less invasive than a deep transversely oriented matrix excision. The reflected proximal nail plate readheres to the nail bed postoperatively and grows out with the nail unit. Even with a wide matrix shave biopsy, there is minimal long-term dystrophy.[8]

1. Perform anesthesia using the same approach as for the punch biopsy of the matrix.

2. Use a No. 15 scalpel to cut incisions at the junction of the proximal and lateral nail folds bilaterally (Figure 17.25B). The nail elevator can help further separate the proximal nail fold from the nail plate once the cuts have been made (Figure 17.25C).

3. Reflect nail fold back using forceps or skin hooks to see the entire matrix (Figure 17.25D).

4. Proximal nail plate evulsion is performed using a nail splitter (English anvil) inserted transversely in one nail sulcus at the level of the proximal third of the nail plate (Figure 17.25E). This is the most challenging part of the procedure, and sometimes it helps to use the scalpel on the nail plate (avoid cutting the skin) to get this process started. It is advanced under the plate transversely until the full width of the nail plate is cut. The proximal plate is then reflected laterally and secured with a hemostat or needle holder (Figure 17.25F). This is like opening the hood of a car (or trap door) as the proximal nail plate is not actually fully removed from its anatomic position.[8]

5. The matrix is examined (Figure 17.25G) to identify the origin of the melanonychia using good light and a dermatoscope (not touching the tissue) if available. Ask a surgical assistant to confirm the origin of the melanonychia, and document that in the chart.

6. A shave biopsy is performed of the origin with 1- to 2-mm margins. This can be performed with a razor blade or scalpel blade. If a No. 15 scalpel blade is used, score the margins first, and then turn the blade horizontally, parallel to the matrix surface, to shave the scored specimen (Figure 17.25H). The specimen should be 1 mm to 1.35 mm (Figure 17.25I) (thickness of a dime) in thickness to provide adequate sampling of the matrix epithelium and a significant portion of dermis.[8]

7. To improve processing and sectioning it may help to place the specimen on a piece of paper or cardboard before placing it into the formalin.[8] A portion of a business card is an easy item to use. This will keep the specimen flat rather than allowing it to roll and curl.

8. Trim the reflected nail plate at its lateral free edge by 2 to 3 mm, and return it to its original position (Figure 17.25J). Trimming the lateral plate will reduce lateral embedding and pain with postoperative edema.[8]

9. The proximal nail fold is returned to its anatomic position and sutured in place using one interrupted suture on each side (Figure 17.25J, K). Use 5-0 nylon or polypropylene (Prolene) suture.

10. Apply petrolatum and a pressure dressing (not too tight).

11. Remove sutures in 7 to 10 days and consider applying adhesive wound closures (Steri-Strips) to keep the integrity of the wound for another week.

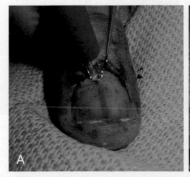
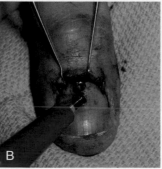

Figure 17.24 **(A)** Proximal nail fold reflected using skin hooks to see where the longitudinal melanonychia begins in the matrix. **(B)** Tissue remains in the punch instrument but is easy to remove since this punch has a window. As this type of punch is no longer available, it is more challenging to get the core out of a solid punch. (Copyright Richard P. Usatine, MD.)

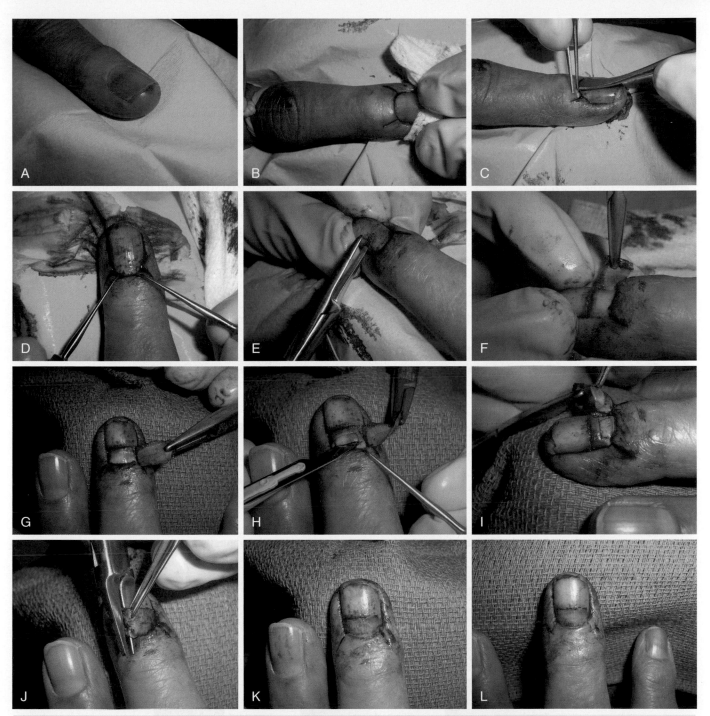

Figure 17.25 **(A)** Longitudinal melanonychia becoming darker and wider. **(B)** No. 15 scalpel is used to cut incisions at the junction of the proximal and lateral nail folds bilaterally. **(C)** Freer elevator can help further separate the proximal nail fold from the nail plate once the cuts have been made. **(D)** Nail fold back reflected using skin hooks to see the entire matrix. **(E)** Proximal nail plate evulsion is performed using a nail splitter (English anvil) inserted transversely in one nail sulcus at the level of the proximal third of the nail plate. **(F)** The proximal plate is then reflected laterally and secured with a hemostat or needle holder. This is like opening a trap door as the proximal nail plate is not actually fully removed from its anatomic position. **(G)** The matrix is examined to identify the origin of the melanonychia. **(H)** A No. 15 scalpel blade was used to score the margins and now is shaving off the scored specimen. **(I)** Specimen visible. **(J)** The reflected nail plate is trimmed at its lateral free edge by 2 to 3 mm before returning it to its original position. Trimming the lateral plate will reduce lateral embedding and pain with postoperative edema. **(K)** The proximal nail fold is returned to its anatomic position. **(L)** It is sutured in place using one interrupted suture on each side. (Copyright Richard P. Usatine, MD.)

FULL-THICKNESS NAIL MATRIX BIOPSY (FIGURE 17.26)

This procedure is performed just as the shave biopsy above except that the tissue is excised using a small elliptical excision. This elliptical defect is closed with 5-0 absorbable sutures and the repair is the same as described for the shave biopsy above.

LATERAL LONGITUDINAL EXCISION[8] (FIGURES 17.27 AND 17.28)

This is a more technically difficult procedure and is used when there is a lateral pigment band on the edge of the nail unit. This is also a good procedure for the treatment of squamous cell carcinoma (SCC) *in situ* of the lateral nail fold.

1. Perform anesthesia using the same approach as for the punch biopsy of the matrix.
2. Soak the finger in chlorhexidine for 10 to 15 minutes to soften the nail plate so that it is easier to pass the suture needle through the plate during the repair.

3. Perform an elliptical excision with narrow margins around the pigmented band. Use a No. 15 scalpel and include the lateral matrix horn. Note that it is probably better to extend the incision more proximally than what was performed in Figures 17.27 and 17.28 to make sure to cut out the full lateral matrix horn. This avoids postoperative spicules and cysts. Extend the incision 3 mm distally into the digital tip. Cut down to the level of bone.
4. Use fine-tipped scissors (curved pointed iris scissor) to remove the tissue to the level of periosteum. The tissue may be stabilized with a skin hook to avoid crush injuries or gently with forceps. Use the scissors with a "tips down" position while cutting out this wedge to ensure that the depth is consistent throughout.
5. Request the pathologist cut the tissue longitudinally and not in the traditional "bread loafed" manner.[8]
6. Excision must remove the entire lateral matrix horn because small matrix remnants can cause postoperative cysts, spicules, and/or pain.[8] A small curette may be used to remove any residual matrix fragments. This

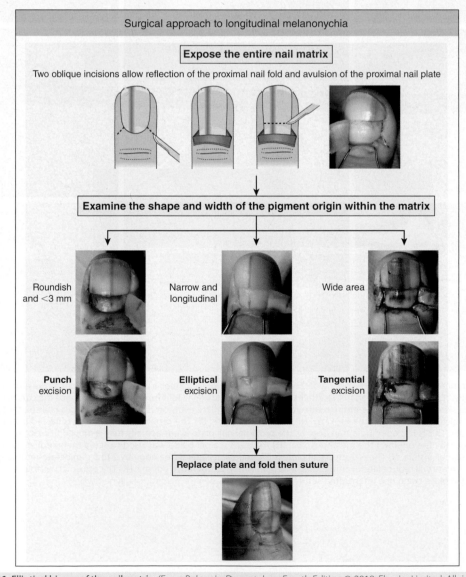

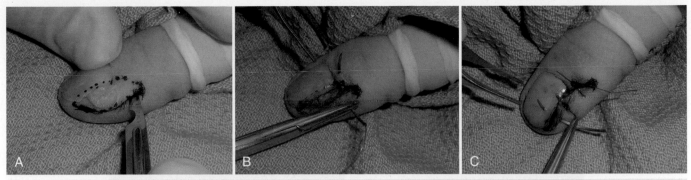

Figure 17.27 Lateral longitudinal excision of a nonpigmented nail fold tumor. **(A)** An ellipse is cut around the tumor including a portion of the nail plate. The ellipse is cut down to the bone. **(B)** Suturing is performed with 4-0 Prolene on a large plastic needle. Note the depth of the incision. **(C)** The needle is passed through the nail starting at the skin and going up through the nail. If this was a biopsy of a pigmented lesion, then it is best to extend the incision more proximally to remove the full lateral matrix horn. (Copyright Richard P. Usatine, MD.)

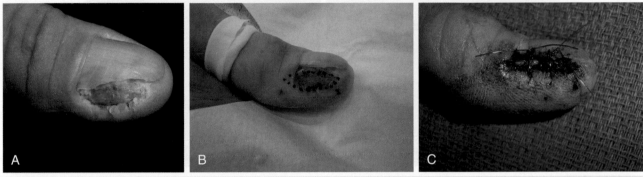

Figure 17.28 **(A)** SCC that was misdiagnosed as a wart for 2 years is about to be biopsied with a lateral longitudinal excision. **(B)** The ellipse is marked, and the tourniquet is in place. **(C)** The final result after suturing with 4-0 Prolene on a large plastic needle. If this surgery was intended to remove the whole tumor, it is best to extend the incision more proximally to make sure to remove the full lateral matrix horn. (Copyright Richard P. Usatine, MD.)

is optional because it may increase the risk of periostitis and postoperative pain while decreasing the risk of spicules or cysts.[8]

7. Repair includes suturing the lateral nail fold to the nail plate with interrupted 4-0 nylon or polypropylene (Prolene). Another option is 5-0 Vicryl on a P3 needle.
8. It is important to run the suture needle from the nail fold into the nail plate (and not the other direction) to avoid creating keratin granulomas in the skin.
9. Apply petrolatum and a pressure dressing (not too tight).
10. Remove sutures in 10 to 14 days.

Notes on Other Lesions

Pincer nails occur when the lateral nail plates dig into the soft tissue of the digits (Figure 17.29). This can eventually lead to pain and discomfort. Partial nail plate excisions bilaterally with destruction of the lateral matrix horn will often give patients relief from this condition (Figures 17.30 and 17.31). In more severe cases, exophytes and dorsal hyperostosis of the distal phalanx may need to be imaged and treated surgically.[26]

Onychogryphosis occurs when a nail plate becomes thickened and curved like a ram's horn (Figure 17.32). While a warm bath or the application of 40% urea cream may make it easier to clip this nail, some patients will want

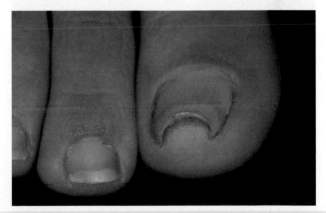

Figure 17.29 Pincer nail. This older man wanted surgery to decrease the pain of this condition. (Copyright Richard P. Usatine, MD.)

to have it removed completely. For this condition the proximal nail evulsion is best, and the nail matrix should be permanently destroyed if the patient does not want the nail to regrow. This may be performed with phenol or electrodestruction.

ONYCHOMATRICOMA

Onychomatricoma is a benign tumor of the nail matrix. It was first described in 1992 and is considered to be a rare

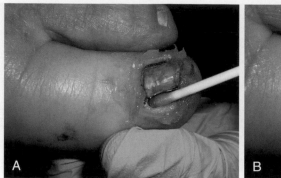
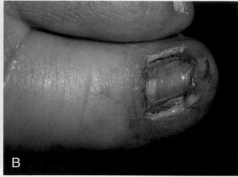

Figure 17.30 (A) Pincer nail that is now undergoing phenol matrixectomy bilaterally with petrolatum to protect surrounding skin. **(B)** Partial nail plate removals on both sides with evidence of bilateral phenol matrixectomy to prevent regrowth (even with petrolatum some normal skin gets affected by the phenol). (Copyright Richard P. Usatine, MD.)

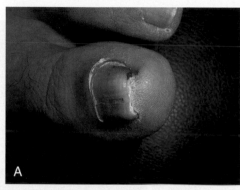
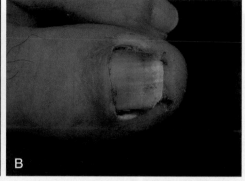

Figure 17.31 (A) Pincer nail. **(B)** Partial nail plate removals on both sides along with matrixectomy to prevent regrowth was performed. (Copyright Richard P. Usatine, MD.)

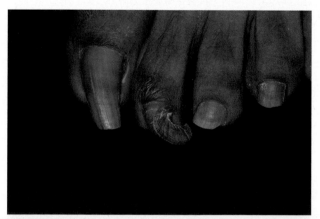

Figure 17.32 Ram's horn nail of second toenail in an older man. This is also known as onychogryphosis. Some patients choose to have a complete nail evulsion with destruction of the matrix to prevent regrowth because this nail is very difficult to cut and can dig into the surrounding toe. (Copyright Richard P. Usatine, MD.)

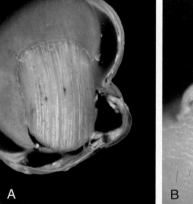
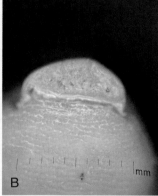

Figure 17.33 (A) Onychomatricoma by dermoscopy showing a discolored thickened nail plate with splinter hemorrhages. **(B)** The honeycomb appearance of the distal edge is easily seen by dermoscopy. (Copyright Richard P. Usatine, MD.)

tumor.[27-29] However, we have seen a number of cases within the last year, and it is helpful to know how to diagnose this tumor.

It is characterized by: (Figure 17.33)

1. Yellowish discoloration and thickening of the nail plate
2. Honeycomb appearance of the distal edge (dermoscopy of the free edge of the nail is a great method for detecting this pattern)

3. Splinter hemorrhages may be present.
4. After removing the nail plate, the matrix tumor has multiple fine filiform projections that extend into the thickened nail plate (causing the honeycomb pattern) (Figure 17.34).

The treatment of onychomatricoma is complete excision of the tumor. This can be done by any clinician competent in nail surgery or can be referred to Mohs surgery.[30,31]

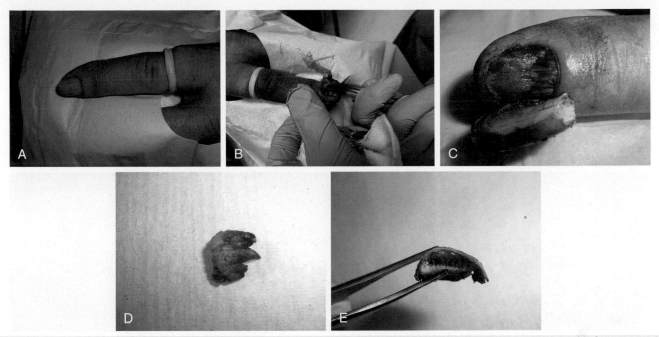

Figure 17.34 Surgical removal of the onychomatricoma in Figure 17.33. **(A)** The digital block is complete, and the tourniquet is applied. **(B)** The thickened nail is removed by clamping it with a hemostat and peeling it off. **(C)** The fine filiform projections of the matrix tumor are readily visible. **(D)** The onychomatricoma after it was excised down to the bone. **(E)** Looking into the proximal end of the thickened nail to see how the filiform projections caused the honeycomb appearance. (Copyright Richard P. Usatine, MD.)

Here is a step-by-step guide to removal of an onychomatricoma: (Figure 17.34)

1. Perform a digital block (lidocaine with epinephrine) first so that the wing block is not painful.
2. Perform a wing block (lidocaine with epinephrine) to obtain good anesthesia and hemostasis.
3. Place a tourniquet on the involved digit.
4. Use a nail elevator to separate the cuticle and proximal nail fold from the nail plate.
5. Clamp a hemostat on the thickened nail plate, and turn it to peel it off.
6. Note the fine filiform projections of the tumor coming from the matrix. Note the hollow nail plate.
7. Cut the corners of the proximal nail fold, and reflect it back to look for the base of the tumor.
8. Cut the onychomatricoma off at its base by cutting down toward the bone. If Mohs surgery is being used, this specimen will be analyzed to make sure the margins are clear. If Mohs surgery is not being performed, gently burn the base of the tumor in the matrix with electrosurgery to avoid recurrence. Be careful to not damage the extensor tendon during this procedure.
9. Suture the proximal nail fold back together.
10. Remove the tourniquet and use electrosurgery if needed for hemostasis.
11. Apply pressure dressing and advise on wound care.
12. Send the tumor and nail plate to pathology in formalin.

Differential diagnosis includes onychopapilloma (Figure 17.35) and SCC (Figure 17.28).

Onychopapilloma (Figure 17.35) is a rare benign tumor of the distal matrix and is the most common cause of localized longitudinal erythronychia. There will be a thin red line running longitudinally from the distal matrix to the end of the nail plate. The tumor may even be seen peeking out at the free edge

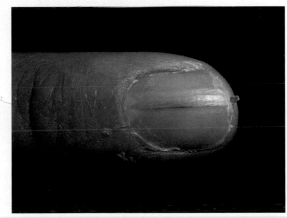

Figure 17.35 Onychopapilloma with erythronychia, subungual keratosis, and abnormal nail matrix in a W shape with the erythronychia coming from the center of the two triangles.

of the nail. The nail matrix makes a W shape with the erythronychia coming from the center of the two triangles.

PERIUNGUAL FIBROMA (FIGURE 17.36)

Periungual fibromas occur around the nails and are seen in tuberous sclerosis. These are benign tumors and do not need to be excised. Figure 17.36 is an example of an elective excision of a periungual fibroma.

SUBUNGUAL HEMATOMA EVACUATION (FIGURE 17.37)

Subungual hematomas form when there is significant trauma to the nail. The pressure of the hematoma can be exquisitely painful, and the patient's pain can be relieved by draining the hematoma through the intact nail. Depending upon the

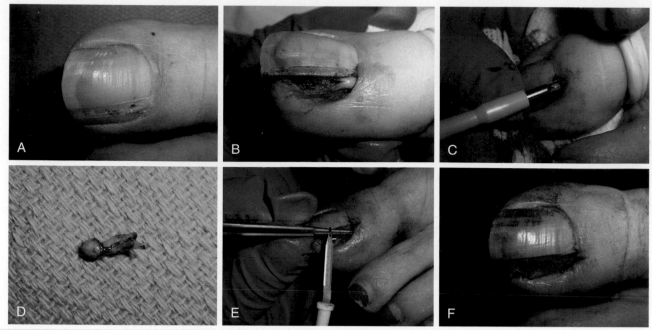

Figure 17.36 (A) Periungual fibroma in a woman with tuberous sclerosis. **(B)** Fibroma visible after partial nail resection. **(C)** Cutting out the fibroma with a punch down to the bone. **(D)** Fibroma. **(E)** Burning the base. **(F)** Completed surgery. (Copyright Richard P. Usatine, MD.)

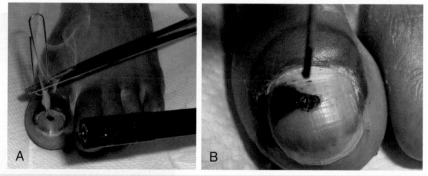

Figure 17.37 Subungual hematoma evacuation. **(A)** A paperclip was held in a hemostat and heated to pierce the patient's nail plate. With minimal pressure the hot point melted through the nail plate. **(B)** The hot paperclip formed a painless hole in the nail plate, and the blood drained out spontaneously. This relieved the pressure and gave the patient immediate pain relief. (Copyright Richard P. Usatine, MD.)

mechanism of trauma and the physical exam, an x-ray of the distal digit may be indicated to investigate for fractures.

Procedure

1. This procedure can be performed without local anesthesia or a tourniquet.
2. There are many ways to pierce the nail plate including a No. 11 scalpel, an 18-gauge needle, a 2-mm punch, a portable hot wire cautery device, or a hot paperclip.
3. The simplest and least expensive method involves heating a paperclip and melting through the nail plate. The paperclip is unbent and can be held in a hemostat. The end of the paperclip is heated with a lighter or other flame (Figure 17.20A).
4. Paperclip is held against the nail, and some pressure is applied until the paperclip pierces the nail plate and blood runs out (Figure 18.20A and B). The patient should only feel pressure and not direct pain.

5. Any remaining blood can be expressed out of the nail opening, to decrease the pain of the hematoma (Figure 17.20C).

Complications of Nail Surgery

The most common complications of nail surgery are infections and scarring, which can cause a permanent nail deformity. In particular, nail matrix biopsy may result in a split nail deformity. Patients should be informed of the risk of permanent nail deformity prior to surgery. Other less common complications include pyogenic granuloma at the surgery site or persistent pain.[32] Another complication is stiffness in the DIP or IP joint. As mentioned above for lateral nail fold excisions, the surgery should remove the entire lateral matrix horn to avoid postoperative cysts, spicules, and/or pain.[8]

Algorithm

The following algorithm is helpful to determine if a pigmented nail needs a biopsy. It is best applied with dermoscopic examination of the nail but can still be useful for those clinicians that don't have the benefit of dermoscopy.

See Algorithm 17.1 that puts this all together based on clinical exam and dermoscopy.

Algorithm 17-1 Nail Lesion

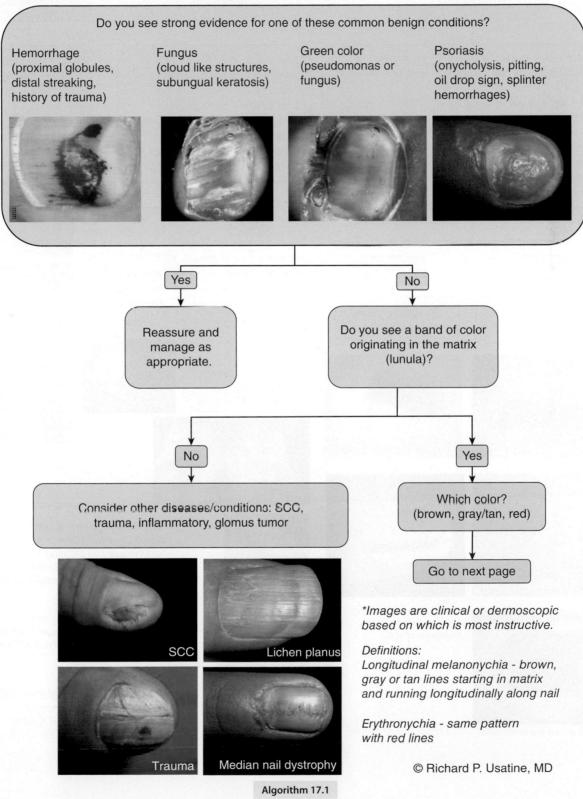

Do you see strong evidence for one of these common benign conditions?

Hemorrhage (proximal globules, distal streaking, history of trauma)

Fungus (cloud like structures, subungual keratosis)

Green color (pseudomonas or fungus)

Psoriasis (onycholysis, pitting, oil drop sign, splinter hemorrhages)

Yes → Reassure and manage as appropriate.

No → Do you see a band of color originating in the matrix (lunula)?

No → Consider other diseases/conditions: SCC, trauma, inflammatory, glomus tumor

Yes → Which color? (brown, gray/tan, red) → Go to next page

SCC   Lichen planus

Trauma   Median nail dystrophy

*Images are clinical or dermoscopic based on which is most instructive.

Definitions:
Longitudinal melanonychia - brown, gray or tan lines starting in matrix and running longitudinally along nail

Erythronychia - same pattern with red lines

© Richard P. Usatine, MD

Algorithm 17.1

Algorithm 17-1 Nail Lesion (continued)

What is the color of the lines originating in the matrix?*

BROWN (melanocytic hyperplasia)

GRAY/TAN (melanocytic activation)

RED lines (erythronychia)

If one of these is positive choose yes to biopsy:

1. Brown pigment band is > 3 mm wide or > 40% nail width
2. It is the only nail involved (in particular, the thumb, index finger, or great toe)
3. Evolving - It is becoming darker or wider (triangular shape)
4. Brown lines are irregular
5. Hutchinson's or micro-Hutchinson's sign
6. It is associated with nail dystrophy, splitting or deformity

Does the pt. have one of these?

1. Multiple affected nails in patient with skin of color
2. Hx of chemotherapy
3. Hx of inflammatory skin disease
4. Trauma history
5. Hyperpigmentation of mucus membranes

Options include:

1. Onychomatricoma
2. Onychopapilloma
3. Darier disease

Yes / **No**

Yes

No

Biopsy matrix for melanoma

Probable nevus and monitor

Consider these:

1. Ethnic (racial) pigmentation
2. Drug related
3. Inflammatory
4. Trauma/friction
5. Laugier-Hunziker syndrome (rare)

Matched to numbers above

Consider dx of lentigo (melanotic macule)

1.

2.

3.

Congenital nevus in child

Hutchinson's sign

Growing nevus in young adult biopsied due to triangular shape

Ethnic (racial)

Ethnic

Chemo induced

All 3 nails above are melanoma

*When the algorithm is difficult to employ due to uncertain color or findings, a noninvasive nail clipping sent to dermatopathology looking for melanocyte remnants could be helpful.

**One exception - wide evolving brown pigment band before age 5 is probably a benign congenital nevus and does not need biopsy

© Richard P. Usatine, MD
Melanoma photos courtesy of
Drs. A. Marghoob and R. Gilson

Algorithm 17.1, cont'd

Nail Plate Dermatopathology

A noninvasive nail clipping sent to dermatopathology looking for melanocyte remnants could be helpful to diagnose nail unit melanoma.[33]

This may be helpful in these settings:

- Dermatopathologist trained in examining nail clippings
- Patients who decline nail matrix biopsy
- Clinician has not been trained to do a matrix biopsy

Tips for submitting a good specimen:[33]

- Patient's nail plate should be allowed to grow long enough to allow for a sample ideally 4 mm in length.
- The nail should be clipped as far back as possible without causing pain or bleeding.
- Submit specimen in formalin.
- For the evaluation of melanonychia, the nail should be clipped in an even fashion, perpendicular to the direction of nail plate growth, and removed in one piece.[33]

Postop Directions for Patients

To prevent some of the pain and throbbing that can occur after any nail surgery, explain to patients to keep their hand or foot elevated once the anesthesia wears off or periodically raise the limb during the day. Oral pain medications may be needed.

If the patient is having trouble with footwear, the diabetic foot shoes with Velcro on top are a good choice while the toe is healing. For toenail surgery, advise the patient to bring an open-toed sandal or comfortable wide shoe for the day of the procedure.

After 24 to 48 hours of keeping the digit dry, the patient should begin soaking the digit in warm, soapy water one to three times a day. Then have them apply clean petrolatum and a clean bandage. This should be continued for 1 or 2 weeks after surgery.

Some amount of pain, redness, and drainage is normal. However, if these signs and symptoms are worsening over time, this may be an infection requiring oral antibiotics.

Coding and Billing Pearls

The following CPT codes are used when billing for nail procedures:

11719 Trimming of nondystrophic nails, any number
11720 Debridement of nail(s) by any method(s); 1 to 5 nails
11721 Debridement of nail(s) by any method(s); 6 or more nails
11730 Removal (avulsion) of one nail plate, partial or complete, simple; single nail
11732 Removal (avulsion) of additional nail plates, partial or complete, simple
11755 Biopsy of nail unit (e.g., plate, bed, matrix, hyponychium, proximal and lateral nail folds)
11750 Removal bed or...Removal of the **entire nail plate or a portion of nail plate** (e.g., ingrown or dystrophic nail) followed by destruction or permanent removal of the associated nail matrix
11760 Repair of nail bed
11765 Wedge excision of skin of nail fold (e.g., for ingrown toenail)
11740 Subungual hematoma drainage

When treating an ingrown toenail the partial removal of the nail plate is coded using CPT 11730. If a partial matrixectomy (chemical or physical) is performed as well, use CPT code of 11750 instead of 11730 (both cannot be used simultaneously). This is not only good medical practice for recurring ingrown toenails but also results in greater compensation.

Debridement of a nail is a procedure that is intended to remove excessive material (e.g., to significantly reduce nail thickness/bulk) or excessive curvature from a clinically and significantly thickened dystrophic or diseased nail. While podiatrists may be more likely to do this procedure, the code is independent and applies to any clinician performing the procedure.

Conclusion

There are many types of nail problems that require surgical intervention. We have covered the most common nail problems in this chapter. With good anesthetic techniques surgery of the nail may be performed in the office setting.

References

1. Haneke E. Nail surgery. *Clin Dermatol.* 2013;31(5):516-525. doi:10.1016/j.clindermatol.2013.06.012.
2. Nielsen LJ, Lumholt P, Hölmich LR. Local anaesthesia with vasoconstrictor is safe to use in areas with end-arteries in fingers, toes, noses and ears. *Ugeskr Laeger.* 2014;176(44):V04140238.
3. Krunic AL, Wang LC, Soltani K, Weitzul S, Taylor RS. Digital anesthesia with epinephrine: an old myth revisited. *J Am Acad Dermatol.* 2004;51(5):755-759.
4. Ilicki J. Safety of epinephrine in digital nerve blocks: a literature review. *J Emerg Med.* 2015;49(5):799-809.
5. Prabhakar H, Rath S, Kalaivani M, Bhanderi N. Adrenaline with lidocaine for digital nerve blocks. *Cochrane Database Syst Rev.* 2015;3:CD010645.
6. Thomson CJ, Lalonde DH, Denkler KA, Feicht AJ. A critical look at the evidence for and against elective epinephrine use in the finger. *Plast Reconstr Surg.* 2007;119:260-266.
7. Lalonde D, Bell M, Benoit P, Sparkes G, Denkler K, Chang P. A multicenter prospective study of 3,110 consecutive cases of elective epinephrine use in the fingers and hand: the Dalhousie Project clinical phase. *J Hand Surg Am.* 2005;30:1061-1067.
8. Jellinek N. Nail matrix biopsy of longitudinal melanonychia: diagnostic algorithm including the matrix shave biopsy. *J Am Acad Dermatol.* 2007;56:803-810.
9. Darouiche RO, Wall Jr MJ, Itani KM. Chlorhexidine-alcohol versus povidone-iodine for surgical-site antisepsis. *N Engl J Med.* 2010;362:18-26.
10. Flatt AE. Tourniquet time in hand surgery. *AMA Arch Surg.* 1972;104:190-192.
11. Chang HC, Lin MH. Comparison of chemical matricectomy with trichloroacetic acid, phenol, or sodium hydroxide for ingrown toenails: a systematic review and network meta-analysis. *Acta Derm Venereol.* 2020;100(4):adv00065. doi:10.2340/00015555-3379.
12. Ramesh S, Shenoi SD, Nayak SUK. Comparative efficacy of 10% sodium hydroxide, 88% phenol, and 90% trichloroacetic acid as chemical cauterants for partial matricectomy in the management of

great toe nail onychocryptosis. *J Cutan Aesthetic Surg.* 2020;13(4): 314-318. doi:10.4103/JCAS.JCAS_183_19.

13. Misiak P, Terlecki A, Rzepkowska-Misiak B, Wcisło S, Brocki M. Comparison of effectiveness of electrocautery and phenol application in partial matricectomy after partial nail extraction in the treatment of ingrown nails. *Pol Przegl Chir.* 2014;86(2):89-93. doi:10.2478/pjs-2014-0016.

14. Zhou Y, Chen W, Liu ZR, Liu J, Huang FR, Wang DG. Modified shave surgery combined with nail window technique for the treatment of longitudinal melanonychia: evaluation of the method on a series of 67 cases. *J Am Acad Dermatol.* 2019;81(3):717-722.

15. Baltz JO, Jellinek NJ. Nail Surgery. *Dermatol Clin.* 2021;39(2): 305-318. doi:10.1016/j.det.2020.12.015.

16. Levit EK, Kagen MH, Scher RK, Grossman M, Altman E. The ABC rule for clinical detection of subungual melanoma. *J Am Acad Dermatol.* 2000;42(2 Pt 1):269-274. doi:10.1016/S0190-9622(00)90137-3.

17. Lee JH, Park JH, Lee JH, Lee DY. Early detection of subungual melanoma *in situ*: proposal of ABCD strategy in clinical practice based on case series. *Ann Dermatol.* 2018;30(1):36-40. doi:10.5021/ad.2018.30.1.36.

18. Tosti A, Piraccini BM, Farias DC. Dealing with melanonychia. *Semin Cutan Med Surg.* 2009;28(1):49-54.

19. Ruben BS. Pigmented lesions of the nail unit: clinical and histopathologic features. *Semin Cutan Med Surg.* 2010;29(3):148-158.

20. Saida T, Ohshima Y. Clinical and histopathologic characteristics of early lesions of subungual malignant melanoma. *Cancer.* 1989; 63(3):556-560.

21. Ronger S, Touzet S, Ligeron C, et al. Dermoscopic examination of nail pigmentation. *Arch Dermatol.* 2002;138(10):1327-1333. doi:10.1001/archderm.138.10.1327.

22. Benati E, Ribero S, Longo C, et al. Clinical and dermoscopic clues to differentiate pigmented nail bands: an International Dermoscopy Society study. *J Eur Acad Dermatol Venereol JEADV.* 2017;31(4): 732-736. doi:10.1111/jdv.13991.

23. Leung AKC, Lam JM, Leong KF, Sergi CM. Melanonychia striata: clarifying behind the Black Curtain. A review on clinical evaluation and management of the 21st century. *Int J Dermatol.* 2019;58(11):1239-1245. doi:10.1111/ijd.14464.

24. Oh SJ, Lee J, Lee JH, et al. Distribution of cellular remnants of melanocytes in the nail plate: clue to the diagnosis of subungual melanoma. *J Cutan Pathol.* 2022;49(4):331-337. doi:10.1111/cup.14150.

25. Rubin AI, Yun SJ, Haneke E. Evaluation of large cellular remnants of melanocytes in the nail plate: an advancement in the correlation of diagnosis and prognosis for nail unit melanocytic lesions. *J Cutan Pathol.* 2022;49(4):418-419. doi:10.1111/cup.14201.

26. Baran R, Haneke E, Richert B. Pincer nails: definition and surgical treatment. *Dermatol Surg.* 2001;27:261-266.

27. Haneke E, Fränken J. Onychomatricoma. *Dermatol Surg Off Publ Am Soc Dermatol Surg Al.* 1995;21(11):984-987. doi:10.1111/j.1524-4725.1995.tb00538.x.

28. Joo HJ, Kim MR, Cho BK, Yoo G, Park HJ. Onychomatricoma: a rare tumor of nail matrix. *Ann Dermatol.* 2016;28(2):237-241. doi:10.5021/ad.2016.28.2.237.

29. Rushing CJ, Ivankiv R, Bullock NM, Rogers DE, Spinner SM. Onychomatricoma: a rare and potentially underreported tumor of the nail matrix. *J Foot Ankle Surg.* 2017;56(5):1095-1098. doi:10.1053/j.jfas.2017.04.008.

30. Lambertini M, Piraccini BM, Fanti PA, Dika E. Mohs micrographic surgery for nail unit tumours: an update and a critical review of the literature. *J Eur Acad Dermatol Venereol.* 2018;32(10):1638-1644. doi:10.1111/jdv.15036.

31. Graves MS, Anderson JK, LeBlanc KGJ, Sheehan DJ. Utilization of Mohs micrographic surgery in a patient with onychomatricoma. *Dermatol Surg.* 2015;41(6):753-755. doi:10.1097/DSS.0000000000000372.

32. Moossavi M, Scher RK. Complications of nail surgery: a review of the literature. *Dermatol Surg.* 2001;27:225-228.

33. Rodriguez O, Elenitsas R, Jiang AJ, Abbott J, Rubin AI. A call for nail clipping histopathology to become an essential component of the routine evaluation of melanonychia: benefitting patients as a triage and surgical planning maneuver. *J Cutan Pathol.* 2023;50(3): 279-283. doi:10.1111/cup.14377.

18 Dermoscopy of Skin Cancer and Benign Neoplasia

RICHARD P. USATINE, MD, and ASHFAQ A. MARGHOOB, MD

SUMMARY

- Algorithms to learn dermoscopy include Triage Amalgamated Dermoscopic Algorithm (TADA), the original two-step algorithm, and the top-down two-step approach.
- The TADA was designed as a method for rapidly learning dermoscopy. TADA is a triage method for differentiating malignant from benign skin lesions.
- The three steps of the TADA algorithm are reviewed in detail, with many figures provided.
- Detailed dermoscopic criteria for skin cancers are described.
- The many variations of benign nevi are reviewed with schematics and dermoscopic figures.
- Ten dermoscopic features of melanomas are listed and described in detail.
- Dermoscopic features of melanoma on the face, palms, and soles are reviewed.

Dermoscopy, by eliminating surface glare, allows clinicians to observe morphologic structures located below the surface of the skin that are otherwise not visible to the naked eye. Many of the dermoscopically observed structures have direct histopathology correlates. In addition, the presence or absence of dermoscopic structures, their association with each other (i.e., certain structures frequently occur together such as milia and comedo openings in a seborrheic keratosis), and their distribution within a lesion allows the clinician to narrow their differential diagnosis, often leading to a specific diagnosis. Multiple metaanalyses have conclusively shown that dermoscopy improves the clinician's diagnostic accuracy.[1,2] Dermatoscopes are relatively inexpensive and easy to use and master. Start with this chapter and consider attending dermoscopy courses, visiting websites and podcasts, and reading books on the subject to extend your learning. *See Video 18.1.*

Advantages of and Evidence for Dermoscopy

Dermoscopy has significantly higher discriminating power than clinical examination for experienced users.[3,4] Improvements in diagnostic accuracy will naturally translate into improved patient management. For example, in one study, the malignant-to-benign biopsy ratio improved in dermoscopy users from 1:18 to 1:4.[5]

Dermoscopy can help in the following ways[6]:

1. Allows the observer to concentrate on a lesion and formulate a logical differential diagnosis
2. Helps differentiate benign from malignant lesions
3. Improves diagnostic accuracy
4. Increases the observer's confidence in his or her clinical diagnosis
5. Confirms naked-eye diagnosis (clinical-dermoscopy correlation)
6. Improves malignant-to-benign biopsy ratio (hence avoiding unnecessary biopsies)
7. Helps isolate suspicious foci within lesions, allowing the clinician to give specific suggestions to the dermatopathologist for tissue processing and step-sectioning
8. Helps more precisely define borders of lesions for improved presurgical margin mapping
9. Helps to reassure patients
10. Helps in the surveillance of patients with many nevi

Equipment

Dermoscopes illuminate the skin via the use of light-emitting diode (LED) lights with or without the use of polarizing filters. Many modern scopes are hybrids, allowing the operator to toggle between polarized and nonpolarized light (Figure 18.1). Most new dermoscopes attach to smartphones for easy dermoscopic photography. Dermoscopic images seen with and without polarization appear different, often providing complementary information.

Algorithms to Learn and Perform Dermoscopy

1. **Triage Amalgamated Dermoscopic Algorithm**
   The Triage Amalgamated Dermoscopic Algorithm (TADA) was designed as a method for rapidly learning dermoscopy.[7] TADA is a triage method for differentiating

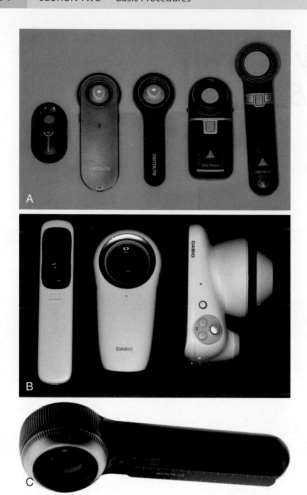

Figure 18.1 An assortment of hybrid dermoscopes. *(Copyright Richard P. Usatine, MD.)*

malignant from benign skin lesions. TADA is organized into three steps as shown in Figure 18.2.

2. **Original two-step algorithm**

   The two-step algorithm is an expanded diagnostic dermoscopic approach for the diagnosis of specific lesions covering a spectrum of skin cancers and benign skin conditions (Figure 18.3). It is a more detailed and complex algorithm that leads to a specific diagnosis.[8,9] It requires separating lesions into melanocytic and nonmelanocytic in step 1. This approach has been criticized because there are a number of nonmelanocytic lesions (dermatofibromas, lentigines, and seborrheic keratoses) that have a network appearance like melanocytic lesions, throwing off the accuracy of step 1.

3. **Top-down two-step approach** (Figure 18.4)

   The *top-down two-step pattern analysis* approach builds upon the previous two-step algorithm and combines it with concepts derived from TADA using a top-down strategy. In this top-down strategy the clinician generates a hypothesis of the most likely clinical diagnosis and performs a targeted search for specific dermoscopic features to confirm or negate the clinical diagnosis in consideration. The hypothesis is based on immediate global pattern recognition within the context of the patient's age, ethnicity, and health status. As a result, the new version of the two-step algorithm eliminates

the former requirement to differentiate melanocytic from nonmelanocytic lesions in *step 1*. Step 1 involves recognizing global patterns associated with common **benign** neoplasms (e.g., nevi, lentigines, seborrheic keratoses [SKs], dermatofibromas, angiomas – an enhancement of TADA step 1). If an unequivocal diagnosis of one of the benign lesions cannot be made with confidence during step 1, then the lesion under consideration will be evaluated in step 2. In *step 2* the observer will determine if the overall pattern of the lesion is **organized or disorganized** (i.e., distribution of colors and structures – same as TADA step 2). Lesions displaying a disorganized pattern (i.e., asymmetric or chaotic) are evaluated in step 2a for known skin cancers, and lesions manifesting in an organized pattern are evaluated in step 2b. Lesions displaying a disorganized pattern have a high likelihood of being malignant, and based on the presence of specific structures these lesions can usually be subclassified as BCC, SCC, or melanoma (step 2a). Lesions that are organized are likely benign; however, organized lesions displaying any of the following should still raise concern for malignancy: starburst pattern, negative network pattern, vessels, ulceration, and blue-black, gray, or white color (Step 2b – same as Step 3 in TADA). With more experience, the expert uses global pattern recognition and if needed will test the presumed diagnosis by looking for specific structures as described in these figures but not necessarily in an algorithmic order. Top-down two-step is essentially an enhanced TADA with the addition of more benign lesions in step 1.

TADA

We will organize this chapter based on TADA due to its inherent simplicity but use some of the enhancements of top-down two-step.

Step 1 – In the first step, commonly encountered and diagnostically unequivocal benign lesions, namely, angiomas, dermatofibromas (DFs), and SKs, are identified. Based on clinical and dermoscopic examination, the patient is reassured, and monitoring is suggested as needed.

Step 2 – The second step of the algorithm requires the observer to judge whether the lesion manifests a disorganized pattern. If the lesion is chaotic/disorganized with asymmetric distribution of colors or structures, then a biopsy or referral is in order.

Step 3 – On rare occasions malignancy can present in an organized and symmetric fashion. Therefore, these organized lesions need to be evaluated further for the presence of other features (structures and colors) for malignancy. The four structures include:

1. Streaks/starburst pattern (found in Spitzoid melanomas)
2. Negative network (found in melanoma)
3. Vessels (found in any skin cancer)
4. Ulceration (found in any skin cancer)

The four colors are blue, black, gray, and white, representing blue-black or gray color (in nodular melanoma and melanoma on sun-damaged skin), shiny-white structures (seen with polarized light in any skin cancer), and white

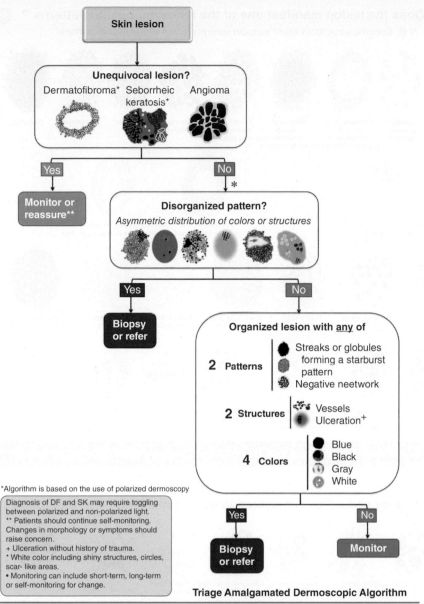

Figure 18.2 The Triage Amalgamated Dermoscopic Algorithm (TADA). (Copyright Ashfaq A. Marghoob, MD.)

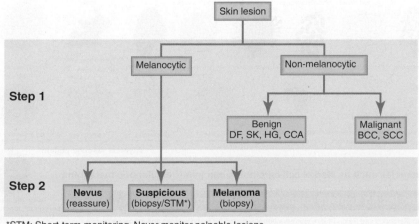

Figure 18.3 The two-step algorithm is a diagnostic dermoscopic approach for the diagnosis of specific lesions covering a spectrum of skin cancers and benign skin conditions. Abbreviations: *CCA*, clear cell acanthoma; *DF*, dermatofibroma; *HG*, hemangioma; *SK*, seborrheic keratosis.

Step 1: Does the lesion manifest one of the following benign patterns ?

N.B: Specific structures must support interpretation of the global pattern!

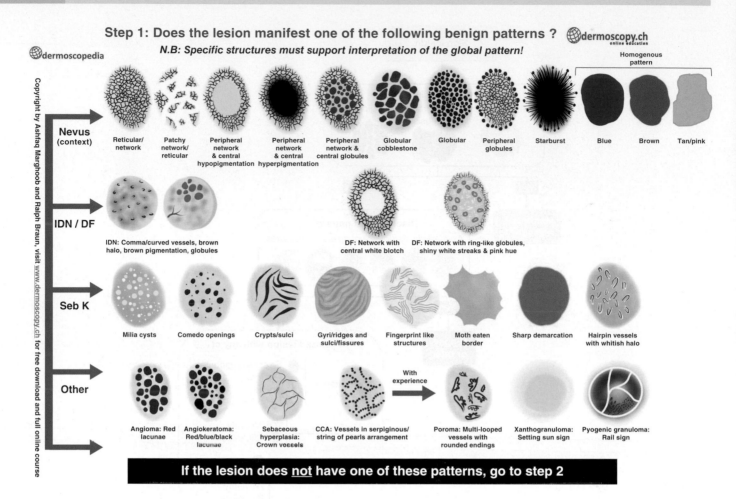

If the lesion does **not** have one of these patterns, go to step 2

Step 2a: Malignancy should be considered in lesions manifesting a "disorganized" pattern

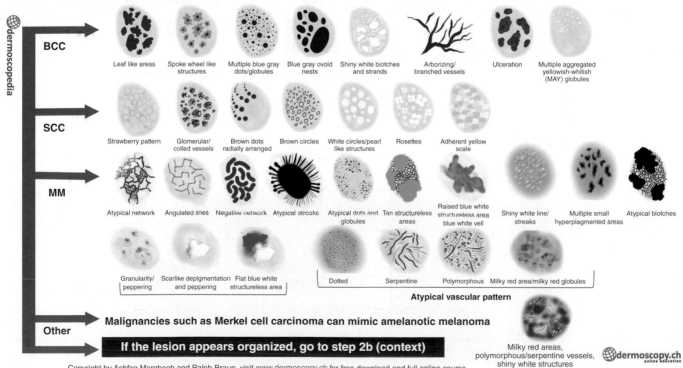

If the lesion appears organized, go to step 2b (context)

Figure 18.4 Top-down two-step approach. (Courtesy of Dermoscopedia.)

Step 2b: Context: If lesion appears organized, the diagnosis of skin cancer should still be considered if it manifests any of the following

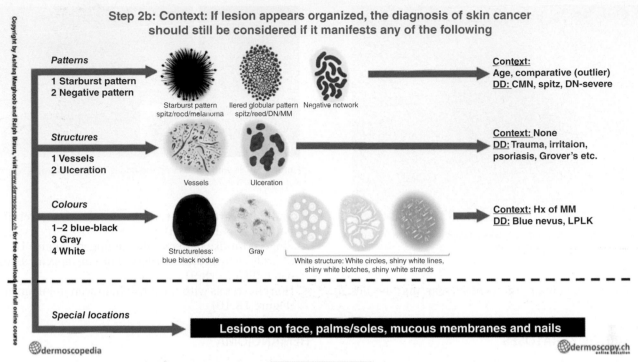

Figure 18.4, cont'd

circles in SCC. Presence of any one of these structures or colors should prompt biopsy or referral for biopsy.

Finally, the lesions that are organized but that lack one of the four structures or colors mentioned above can be safely monitored (most of these are benign nevi). The efficiency of the TADA algorithm was tested in a group of novices, experienced dermatologists, and family physicians. After only one day of training the participants achieved a sensitivity for skin cancer diagnosis (BCC, squamous cell carcinoma, and melanoma) of 93.3% and specificity of 74.1%.[7] There was no difference in the sensitivity between novices and experts, and there was no difference in sensitivity between dermatologists and family physicians.

TADA Step 1 in detail

- Dermatofibroma (DF)
- Seborrheic keratosis (SK)
- Hemangioma

DERMATOFIBROMA

DFs are benign firm tumors that dimple on lateral pressure (Figure 22.12).

Dermoscopic structures visible in DFs are (Figure 18.5):

1. Peripheral fine network
2. Central white or central pink scar
3. Ring-like globules
4. Dotted vessels are seen less often.

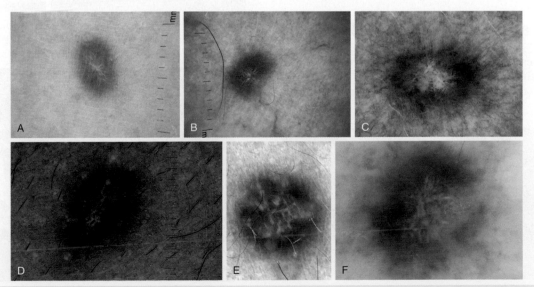

Figure 18.5 Dermatofibromas are benign firm tumors that have peripheral fine network **(A,B)** and a central white scar or central pink scar **(A,B)**. Dermatofibromas with ring-like globules **(C,D,E)**. Dotted vessels visible in central pink white scar **(F)**. (Copyright Richard P. Usatine, MD.)

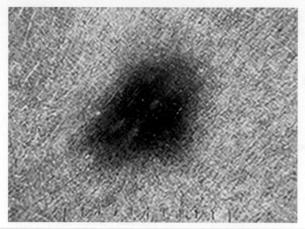

Figure 18.6 Dermatofibromas in Black individuals may lack a central white scar. (Copyright Richard P. Usatine, MD.)

In Black individuals, the central scar may be absent (Figure 18.6).[10]

SEBORRHEIC KERATOSES

SKs are the most common benign tumor in adults. These have some of the following dermoscopic structures.

Milia-like cysts (Figure 18.7a)

■ Round whitish or yellowish structures
■ These represent intraepidermal keratin-filled cysts.
■ Milia-like cysts are shiny with nonpolarized light and dull with polarized light. This leads to a blinking phenomenon seen when switching between polarized and nonpolarized light (blink sign). *See Video 18.2.*

Comedo-Like Openings (Figure 18.7b)

■ Round to elongated brown to black structures corresponding to keratin-filled invaginations of the epidermis

Fissures and Ridges (Figure 18.8)

■ The fissures in seborrheic keratosis are usually filled with keratin and appear darker in color compared to the raised ridge portions of SK. When many fissures

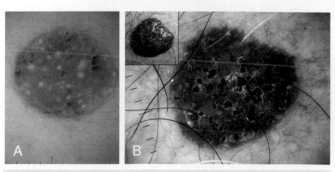

Figure 18.7 SK with **(A)** milia-like cysts and **(B)** comedo-like openings. (Copyright Richard P. Usatine, MD.)

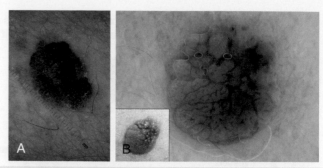

Figure 18.8 SK with **(A)** fissures and ridges, **(B)** cerebriform. (Copyright Richard P. Usatine, MD.)

and ridges are present, they can take on a cerebriform pattern (Figure 18.8b).
■ Fingerprint-like patterns and fat fingers (Figure 18.9)
■ Sharply demarcated borders that can appear as moth eaten (Figure 18.9)
■ Hairpin vessels with a whitish halo seen in inflamed SKs (Figure 18.10)

HEMANGIOMA

Hemangiomas are referring to cherry angiomas and not infantile hemangiomas. These angiomas have red to maroon lacunae with whitish septae (Figure 32.29) (Figure 18.11).

Other Benign Lesions

There are two other common benign lesions that we can add to enhance the specificity of TADA since they both have vessels and step 3 would lead to a biopsy:

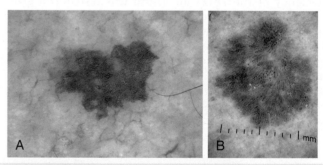

Figure 18.9 **(A)** Flat SKs with fingerprint pattern and moth-eaten borders. **(B)** SK with fat fingers. (Copyright Richard P. Usatine, MD.)

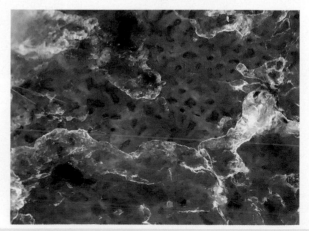

Figure 18.10 Inflamed SK with hairpin vessels surrounded by a whitish halo. (Copyright Richard P. Usatine, MD.)

- Sebaceous hyperplasia (Figure 18.12)
- Intradermal nevi (Figure 18.13)

Sebaceous Hyperplasia

Sebaceous hyperplasia is a common condition in older adults caused by the hyperplasia of sebaceous glands especially on the face. The dermoscopic structures (Figure 18.12) include:

- Crown like vessels
- Popcorn-like structures
- Central opening

Intradermal Nevi

Intradermal nevi are benign and have melanocytes in the dermis. These nevi are pedunculated, and when the dermatoscope is placed upon them they will wobble. This is called the Wobble Sign. *See Video 18.3.*

The dermoscopic structures (Figure 18.13) include:

- Comma vessels, curved vessels
- Small areas of tan, structureless pigmentation
- Globules

TADA Step 2 in detail – Does the lesion have a disorganized pattern?

Dermoscopic asymmetry is not defined by an irregular border but by the distribution of the content within the lesion being assessed. The following malignant lesions are

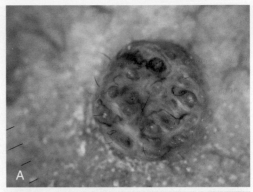
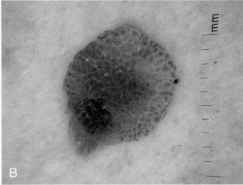

Figure 18.13 Intradermal nevi: **(A)** comma vessels, **(B)** mammilated with comma vessels. (Copyright Richard P. Usatine, MD.)

chaotic/disorganized with asymmetric distribution of colors or structures:

- BCC (Figure 18.14)
- SCC (Figure 18.15)
- Melanoma (Figure 18.16)

TADA Step 3 in detail – Symmetric lesions not called out for biopsy in step 2:

Four structures:

1. Starburst pattern seen in this Spitzoid melanoma (Figure 18.17)
2. Negative network in this melanoma (Figure 18.18)
3. Vessels in BCC, SCC, and melanoma (Figures 18.19, 18.20)
4. Ulcerations found in these skin cancers (Figure 18.21) add 18.19 in paren to say (Figures 18.19 and 18.21)

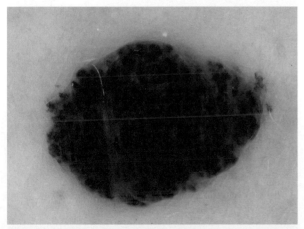

Figure 18.11 Angioma with pink/red lacunae and whitish septae. (Copyright Richard P. Usatine, MD.)

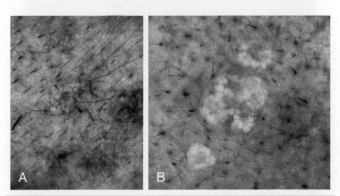

Figure 18.12 Sebaceous hyperplasia. **(A)** Crown vessels and central opening. **(B)** Popcorn-like structures. (Copyright Richard P. Usatine, MD.)

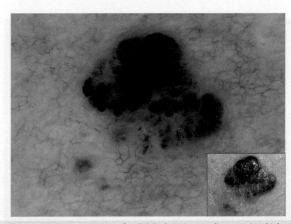

Figure 18.14 Dermoscopy of a BCC showing a disorganized/chaotic pattern. (Copyright Richard P. Usatine, MD.)

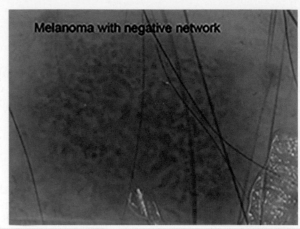

Figure 18.15 Dermoscopy of an SCC showing a disorganized/chaotic pattern. (Copyright Richard P. Usatine, MD.)

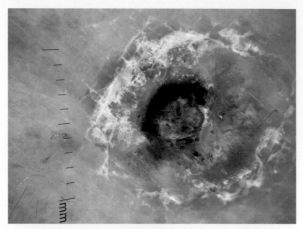

Figure 18.18 Negative network in this melanoma. (Copyright Richard P. Usatine, MD.)

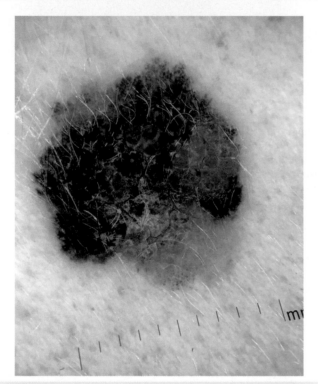

Figure 18.16 Dermoscopy of a melanoma showing a disorganized/chaotic pattern. (Copyright Richard P. Usatine, MD.)

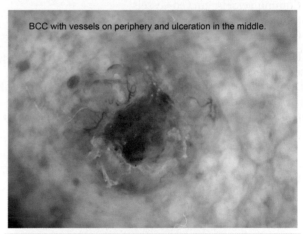

Figure 18.19 Vessels in BCC. (Copyright Richard P. Usatine, MD.)

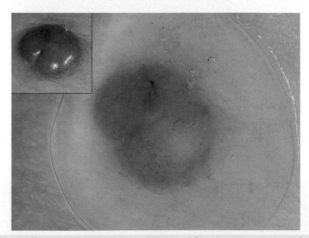

Figure 18.20 Vessels in this amelanotic melanoma. (Copyright Ashfaq A. Marghoob, MD.)

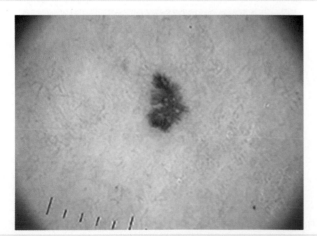

Figure 18.17 Starburst pattern seen in this tiny Spitzoid melanoma. (Reproduced with permission from the International Skin Imaging Collaboration).

Four colors:

1. Blue and black colors in pigmented BCCs and nodular melanomas (Figure 18.22)
2. Gray color seen in these melanomas undergoing regression (Figure 18.23)
3. Shiny white structures in polarized light in this skin cancer (Figure 18.24)
4. White circles in squamous cell carcinomas (Figure 18.25)

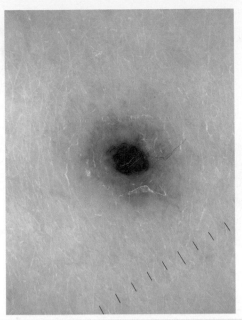

Figure 18.21 Ulceration found in this small BCC on the nose. (Copyright Richard P. Usatine, MD.)

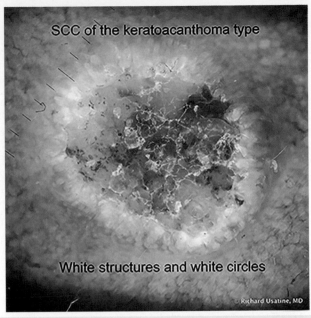

Figure 18.24 Shiny white structures in polarized light in this SCC. (Copyright Richard P. Usatine, MD.)

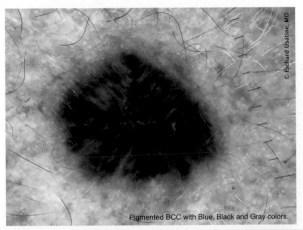

Pigmented BCC with Blue, Black and Gray colors.

Figure 18.22 Blue and black color in this pigmented BCC. (Copyright Richard P. Usatine, MD.)

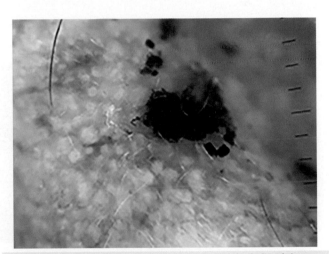

Figure 18.25 White circles in this SCC in situ on the helix of the ear. (Copyright Richard P. Usatine, MD.)

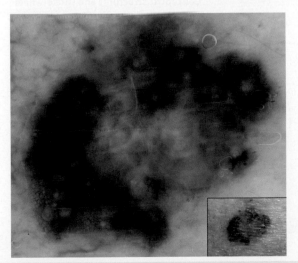

Figure 18.23 Gray color seen in this melanoma undergoing regression. (Copyright Richard P. Usatine, MD.)

Let's look at the structures found in the three most common skin cancers using the detailed descriptions found in any version of the two-step algorithm.

Two-Step Dermoscopy Algorithm for Skin Cancer Criteria

BCCs have at least one of these structures (Figure 18.26 and Table 18.1):

Basal cell carcinoma – The diagnostic criteria for BCC include the lack of a pigment network and the presence of at least one positive feature for BCC.

a. Nonpigmented structures
   - Arborizing vessels
   - Ulceration and small erosions

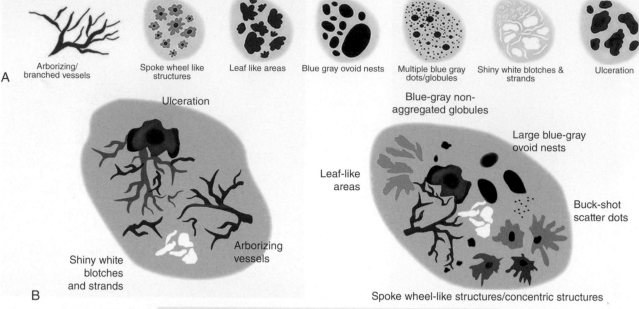

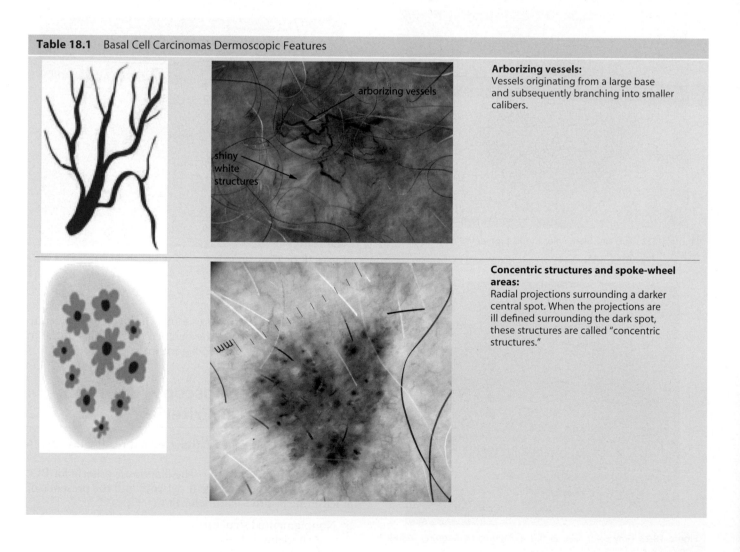

Figure 18.26 Dermoscopic patterns in BCC. (Courtesy of Dermoscopedia.)

Table 18.1   Basal Cell Carcinomas Dermoscopic Features

Arborizing vessels:
Vessels originating from a large base and subsequently branching into smaller calibers.

Concentric structures and spoke-wheel areas:
Radial projections surrounding a darker central spot. When the projections are ill defined surrounding the dark spot, these structures are called "concentric structures."

Table 18.1   Basal Cell Carcinomas Dermoscopic Features—cont'd

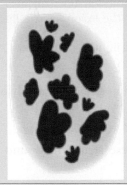

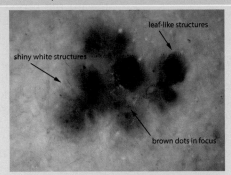

Leaf-like areas:
Brown to blue-gray projections arranged around a common base creating a structure that resembles maple leaves.

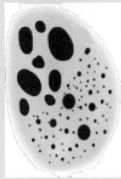

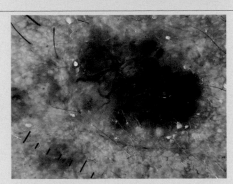

Blue-gray ovoid nests, globules, and dots:
Blue-gray ovoid nests are well-defined, large ovoid areas within a lesion. Blue-gray globules are well-defined, round to oval structures, occupying less space than the ovoid nests yet larger than the blue-gray dots which can appear in a buckshot distribution.

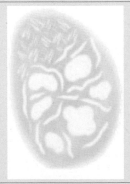

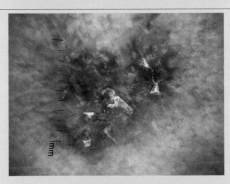

Shiny white structures:
Lines, white, perpendicular, or white structures in the form of circles, oval structures, or large structureless areas that are bright-white, longer and less well-defined lines oriented parallel or distributed haphazardly or forming blotches (shiny white clods). Seen only under polarized dermoscopy.

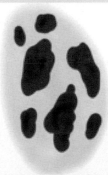

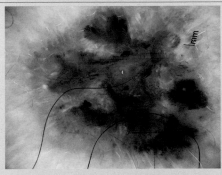

Ulcerations and erosions can appear once or multiple times in a single lesion. They most commonly appear red, covered with black/maroon to orange hue due to a sero sanguinous crust. Multiple, small ulcerations are associated with superficial BCC, while the presence of large ulcerations covering large areas of the lesion is associated with nodular BCC.

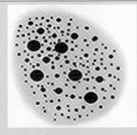

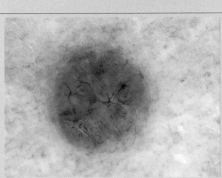

Buckshot (bird-shot) scatter is the presence of clusters of dark fine dots within the BCC.

Schematics courtesy of Dermoscopedia. Photographs copyright Richard P. Usatine, MD.

- Shiny white blotches and strands (seen with polarized dermoscopy)
- Fine, short, superficial telangiectasias

b. Pigmented structures
- Leaf-like areas
- Large blue-gray ovoid nests
- Multiple blue-gray, nonaggregated globules
- Spoke-wheel structures, including concentric globules
- Multiple in-focus, fine brown to gray dots or blue-gray dots in a bird-shot scatter distribution

Criteria for squamous cell carcinoma – The diagnostic criteria for SCC:

- Glomerular or coiled vessels, usually focally distributed toward the periphery of the lesion but can also be diffusely present throughout the lesion or in a linear fashion within the lesion.
- Rosettes (seen with polarized light)
- White circles or keratin pearls
- Yellow scale/rough texture
- Brown dots/globules aligned in straight, radially oriented lines, usually located toward the periphery
- Brown circles

SCCs have at least one of these structures found in Figure 18.27 and Table 18.2:

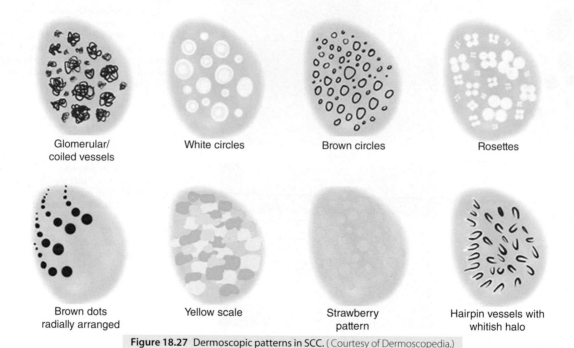

Glomerular/coiled vessels	White circles	Brown circles	Rosettes
Brown dots radially arranged	Yellow scale	Strawberry pattern	Hairpin vessels with whitish halo

Figure 18.27 Dermoscopic patterns in SCC. (Courtesy of Dermoscopedia.)

Table 18.2 Squamous Cell Carcinomas Dermoscopic Features

Glomerular vessels:
They are larger than dotted vessels and can be seen in accumulations; they are typically indicative of SCC.

Table 18.2 Squamous Cell Carcinomas Dermoscopic Features—cont'd

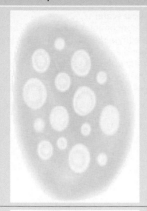 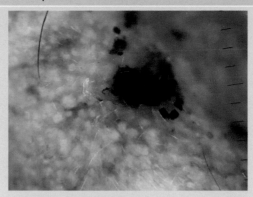

White circles:
White ring-like structures within the hair follicle. The follicle may have a targetoid appearance with central yellowish keratotic plug surrounded by a white halo. This feature is commonly encountered with pigmented AKs.

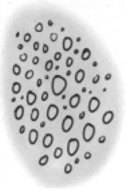 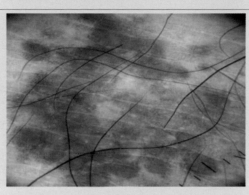

Brown Circles:
These brown circles are usually encountered in pigmented SCC.

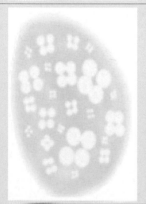 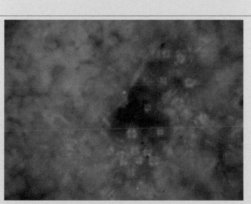

Rosettes:
A white, four-leaf-clover-like formation, apparent only with polarized dermoscopy. It can present at actinic keratoses, BCC, SCC, and actinic damaged skin.

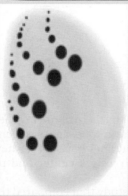 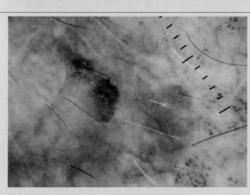

Brown dots:
When arranged as linear radial lines at the periphery of the lesion they can be a strong indicator of pigmented Bowen's disease.

Schematics courtesy of Dermoscopedia. Photographs courtesy of Harold Rabinovitz, MD.

Continued

Table 18.2   Squamous Cell Carcinomas Dermoscopic Features—cont'd

		Yellow scale: The concomitant presence of surface scale (hyperkeratosis) combined with other diagnostic features (i.e., rosettes, white circles, brown dots, brown circles) can lead to the diagnosis of Bowen's disease (SCC in situ).
		Strawberry pattern: Pink-to-red "pseudonetwork" surrounding the hair follicles combined with white-to-yellow scale, and linear vessels surrounding the hair follicles and hair follicle openings filled with yellowish keratotic plugs and/or surrounded by a white halo.
		Hairpin vessels: They have a "U" shape, resembling a hairpin, and they can present with a whitish halo surrounding them. They are typically present in seborrheic keratoses and peripherally in keratoacanthomas (KAs). However, they can also be present in melanocytic lesions and BCCs as well.

Schematics courtesy of Dermoscopedia. Photographs copyright Richard P. Usatine, MD.

MELANOMA/NEVI

Step 2 of the two-step algorithm deals with whether a melanocytic lesion is either a nevus or a melanoma. Step 1 of the top-down two-step involves recognizing benign nevi.

Before we describe the features of melanoma, we will define the patterns of benign melanocytic lesions (nevi).

Nevus Diagnosis Through Pattern Analysis

- Nevi tend to adhere to 1 of 10 recurrent patterns (Figure 18.28).
- These patterns are created by network, dots/globules, and structureless areas that are distributed in an organized and symmetric manner (Table 18.3).

Context for Nevi:

- There are several factors that contribute to different nevi patterns on individuals: skin tone, age, and genetics.
- Patients with darker skin tones have darker nevi in general and more nevi with a dark center and peripheral network (Figure 18.29).
- Tuma et al. performed a study that compared the dermoscopic differences in acquired melanocytic nevi between skin types V/VI and skin types I/II.[11] They concluded that dermoscopy of the acquired melanocytic nevi in skin type V/VI showed a reticular pattern, brown color, and tendency toward central hyperpigmentation, whereas the acquired nevi in skin type I/II showed a

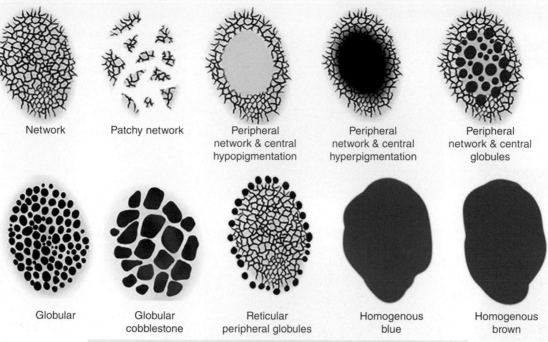

Network   Patchy network   Peripheral network & central hypopigmentation   Peripheral network & central hyperpigmentation   Peripheral network & central globules

Globular   Globular cobblestone   Reticular peripheral globules   Homogenous blue   Homogenous brown

Figure 18.28 Dermoscopic patterns in common nevi. (Courtesy of Dermoscopedia.)

Table 18.3   Benign Nevus Patterns

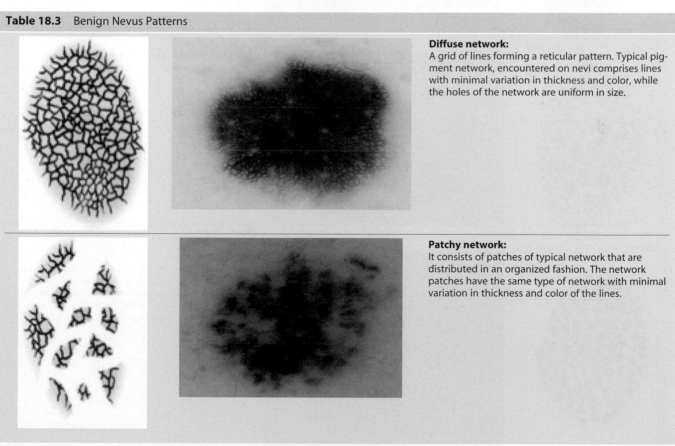

Diffuse network:
A grid of lines forming a reticular pattern. Typical pigment network, encountered on nevi comprises lines with minimal variation in thickness and color, while the holes of the network are uniform in size.

Patchy network:
It consists of patches of typical network that are distributed in an organized fashion. The network patches have the same type of network with minimal variation in thickness and color of the lines.

Continued

Table 18.3   Benign Nevus Patterns—cont'd

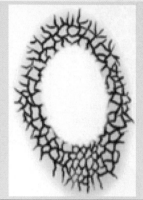
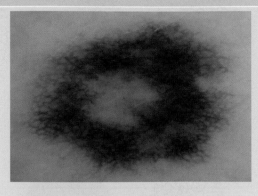

Peripheral network with central hypopigmentation:
Typical network surrounding a hypopigmented central area, which is lighter in color than the network, yet darker than the surrounding skin.

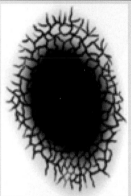
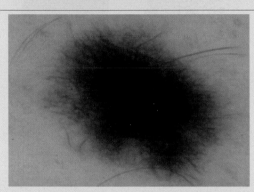

Peripheral network with central hyperpigmentation:
Consists of a typical network surrounding a central hyperpigmented area, called a blotch.

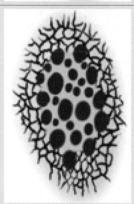
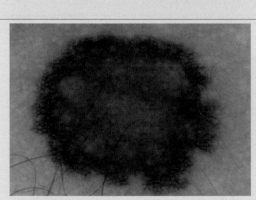

Peripheral network with central globules:
It consists of a typical network surrounding an area of homogeneous brown pigmentation with typical globules.

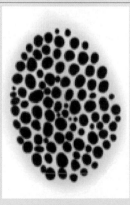
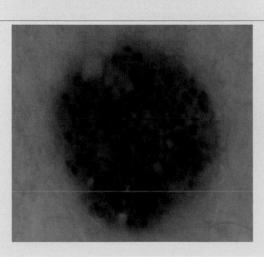

Diffuse globules:
Typical globules are usually black or brown in color, while they can appear blue when the melanocytic nests are located in the dermis. Variation in size and color of the globules makes them atypical and raises suspicion for malignancy.

Table 18.3   Benign Nevus Patterns—cont'd

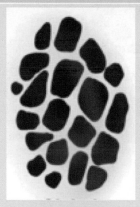
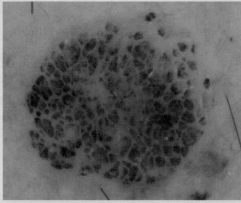

Globular – cobblestone pattern:
It consists of globules that are large in size and angulated, forming a pattern that reminds of that of cobblestones. This pattern is associated with congenital nevi.

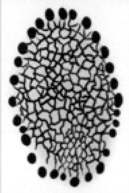
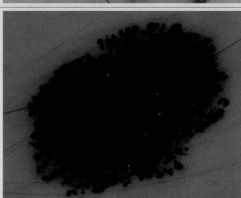

Reticular pattern with peripheral rim of globules:
It consists of a centrally located, typical network, which is surrounded by a rim of regular brown globules. This pattern corresponds with the radial growth phase of some nevi.

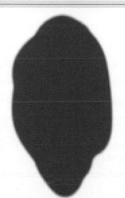
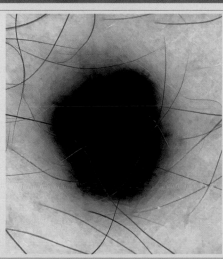

Homogeneous blue:
It consists of a homogeneous blue color (minimal variation of hues), distributed homogeneously across the entire lesion, and is accompanied by a whitish veil.

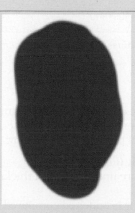
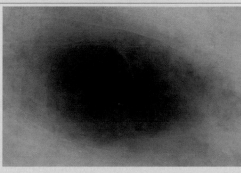

Homogeneous brown:
It consists of a homogeneous brown color encompassing the entity of the lesion without any color variations. Occasionally a few scattered dots or globules or network areas may be discernible within the brown background.

Schematics courtesy of Dermoscopedia. Photographs courtesy of ISIC Archive and Harold Rabinovitz, MD Richard P. Usatine, MD.

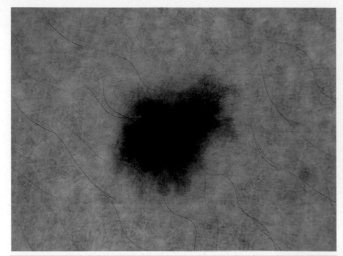

Figure 18.29 Dermoscopy of darker nevus with dark center in patient with darker skin tone. (Copyright Richard P. Usatine, MD.)

light-brown color and a tendency toward structureless pattern and multiple areas of hypopigmentation. Also, nevi in skin type V/VI displayed a higher frequency of gray and black colors.[11]

- A study by Zalaudek et al.[12] showed these trends in nevi with darkening of skin type:
  - Decreasing prevalence of light brown color in nevi
  - Increasing prevalence of dark brown color
  - Decreasing prevalence of central hypopigmentation
  - Increasing prevalence of central hyperpigmentation
- Familiarity with the dermoscopic patterns typically exhibited by nevi provides additional assistance in distinguishing between benign and malignant lesions (Table 18.4).

Melanoma Specific Structures

- Melanoma is a melanocytic lesion that deviates from the 10 benign nevus patterns. That is why it is referred to as the beast in the beauty and the beast sign. A melanoma may also stand out on the skin as an ugly duckling.
- Melanomas almost invariably display some degree of asymmetry of pattern, color, and structure, which is represented by the beast in the beauty and the beast sign. Melanomas most often will display at least one of these local features (Figure 18.30):

1. *Atypical network* and/or angulated lines.
2. *Focal streaks*, that is, pseudopods and radial streaming.
3. *Focal negative pigment network*
4. *Shiny white line* (only seen with polarized dermoscopy)
5. *Atypical dots* are located at the periphery and associated with an atypical network or no network at all. *Atypical globules* consist of globules of different shapes, sizes, and colors distributed in an asymmetric fashion. When reddish in color these are highly suggestive of melanoma.
6. *Off-centered blotch*, a hyperpigmented area that is off-center or multiple hyperpigmented areas
7. *Peripheral brown structureless areas*
8. *Focal blue-white veil over raised areas*
9. *Regressions structures – blue-white veil* and/or *peppering in flat lesions*, that is, regression structures

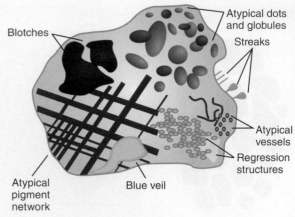

Melanoma specific structures	Odds ratios
Atypical network	1.1–9
Streaks (pseudopods and radial streaming)	1.6–5.8
Negative pigment network	1.8
Shiny white lines (crystalline stryctures)	9.7
Atypical dots and/or globules	2.9–4.8
Off-centered blotch	4.1–4.9
Peripheral tan structureless areas	2.8–2.9
Blue-white veil overlying raised areas	2.5–13
Regression structures • Blue-white veil overlying macular areas, scar-like areas and/or peppering	3.1–18.3
Atypical vascular structures • Dotted vessels, serpentine vessels, polymorphous vessel, milky-red areas, red globules, corkscrew vessels	1.5–7.4
Polygonal structures (zig-zag lines)	

Figure 18.30 Melanoma-specific structures with odds ratios. (Courtesy of Dermoscopedia.)

10. *Vascular structures*, that is, dotted, globular, irregularly linear, serpentine, polymorphous, milky-red, etc., are best seen with noncontact polarized dermoscopy.

1. **Atypical pigment network** (Figure 18.31)
   - The lines of the network are not uniform in thickness and color.
   - The lines are darker and/or broadened compared to a typical network.
   - The "holes" are heterogeneous in size.

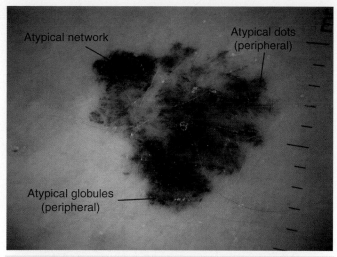

Figure 18.31 Atypical network in a melanoma. (Copyright Richard P. Usatine, MD.)

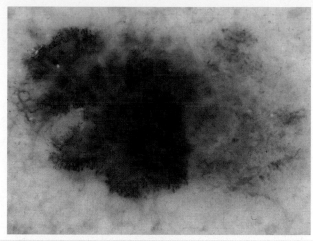

Figure 18.33 Streaks in the form of pseudopods in a melanoma. (Copyright Ashfaq A. Marghoob, MD.)

- The lines end abruptly and are distributed in an asymmetric manner.
- Angulated lines are worrisome.

2. **Streaks and pseudopods** (Figure 18.32)
   - Pseudopods are linear finger-like projections that radiate toward normal skin.
   - They are located at the periphery of the lesion.
   - They have small knobs at their tips that can make them look like tennis rackets.

The term *radial streaming* refers to radial, parallel, linear extensions that resemble pseudopods but do not have a knob at the ends. They are located at the periphery.

Streaks is a term that encompasses both pseudopods and radial streaming. They are seen in the radial growth phase of superficial spreading melanoma and Reed's nevi (Figure 18.33).

3. **A negative network** is a feature associated with Spitz nevi and melanoma (Figures 18.34). It consists of dark, elongated, and curved globular structures surrounded by relative hypopigmentation. This results in the impression

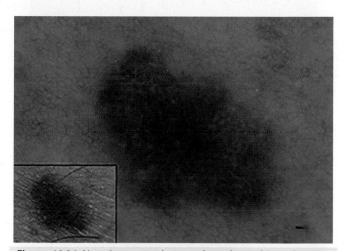

Figure 18.34 Negative network seen throughout this melanoma. (Copyright Ashfaq A. Marghoob, MD.)

that serpiginous hypopigmented lines are present with holes that are darker in color.

4. **Shiny white lines**
   - Seen only with polarized light dermoscopy
   - Consists of linear white lines/streaks that are oriented parallel or orthogonal to each other
   - The shiny white lines (Figure 18.35) represent altered dermal collagen.

5. **Atypical dots and globules**
   Figure 18.36 shows atypical dots and globules aggregated in this melanoma.

6. **Off-centered blotch (black lamella)**
   - A blotch has a large concentration of melanin pigment located in the stratum corneum (aka lamella) or extends throughout the epidermis and/or dermis.
   - The amount of melanin visually obscures the ability to see any underlying structures.
   - A typical blotch in a benign nevus is often centrally located, while an off-center blotch or the presence of multiple blotches may be seen in a melanoma (Figure 18.37).

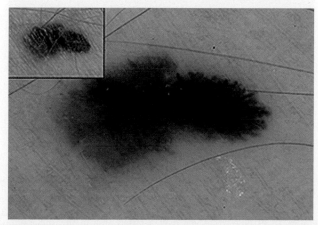

Figure 18.32 Streaks in a melanoma. (Copyright Ashfaq A. Marghoob, MD.)

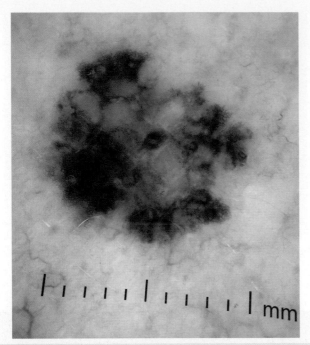

Figure 18.35 Shiny white lines that are orthogonal in this melanoma. (Copyright Richard P. Usatine, MD.)

Figure 18.36 Atypical dots and globules in this melanoma. (Copyright Ashfaq A. Marghoob, MD.)

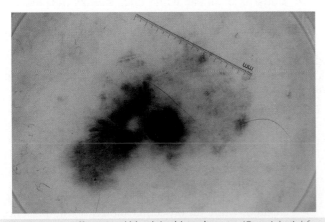

Figure 18.37 Off-centered blotch in this melanoma. (Copyright Ashfaq A. Marghoob, MD.)

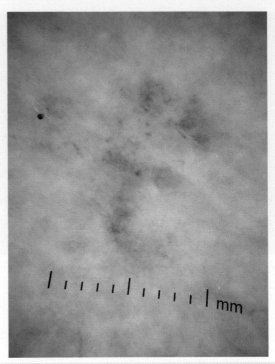

Figure 18.38 Peripheral tan structureless areas in this melanoma. (Copyright Richard P. Usatine, MD.)

7. **Peripheral tan structureless areas** (Figure 18.38)
   - Areas devoid of any discernible structures
   - The color is relatively hypopigmented compared to the surrounding nevus, but it is not white, and it does not manifest any regression structures such as peppering.
   - Results from decreased pigment, attenuated rete ridges, or lack of contrast
8. **Blue-white veil, raised**
   - Area of focal irregular, indistinct, confluent, blue pigmentation (Figure 18.39)
   - Focal overlying white ground-glass haze
   - Aggregation of heavily pigmented cells/melanin in the dermis (blue color) in combination with compact orthokeratosis (white color)

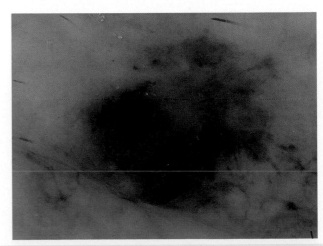

Figure 18.39 Blue-white veil over a raised area in this melanoma. (Copyright Ashfaq A. Marghoob, MD.)

9. Regression structures – peppering

- "Peppering," also known as granularity, is loose melanin in the dermis or melanin in melanophages (Figure 18.40)
- Area of white scar-like depigmentation
- Focal speckled multiple blue-gray granules (blue-white veil over flat area)
- Fibrosis, loss of pigmentation, epidermal thinning, effacement of the rete ridges, and melanin granules free in the dermis or in melanophages scattered in the papillary dermis.

10. Atypical vessels (dotted, serpentine, polymorphous) (Figure 18.41)

Figure 18.42 is a schematic from Dermoscopedia that is helpful for detecting melanoma. These drawings are paired with actual melanoma dermoscopy images in Table 18.5 to enhance your pattern recognition.

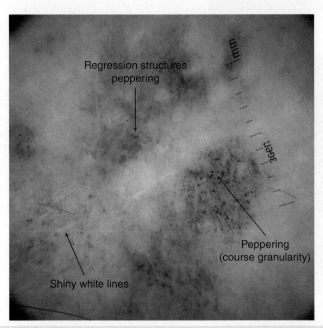

Figure 18.40 Regression structures with peppering in this melanoma in sun-damaged skin. (Copyright Richard P. Usatine, MD.)

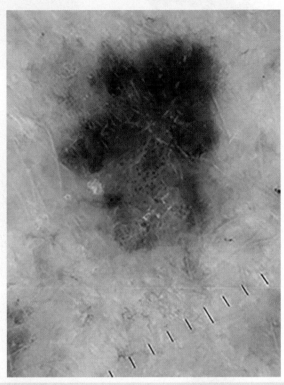

Figure 18.41 Atypical vessels that are polymorphous in this melanoma. (Copyright Richard P. Usatine, MD.)

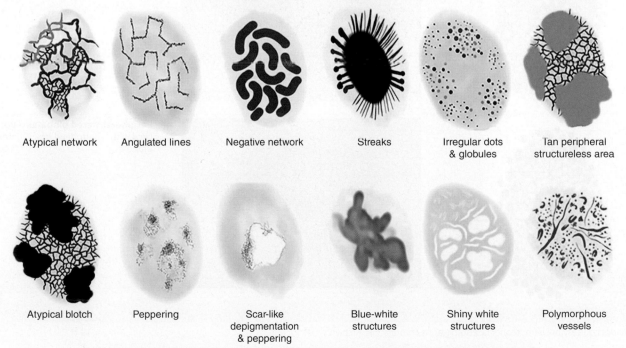

Atypical network   Angulated lines   Negative network   Streaks   Irregular dots & globules   Tan peripheral structureless area

Atypical blotch   Peppering   Scar-like depigmentation & peppering   Blue-white structures   Shiny white structures   Polymorphous vessels

Figure 18.42 Schematic of melanoma structures from Dermoscopedia. (Courtesy of Dermoscopedia.)

Table 18.4   Nevi Requiring Special Attention

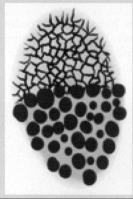

Two-component or kissing nevi:
Nevi that present with two distinct, separate patterns, usually network with globular pattern.

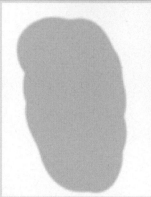
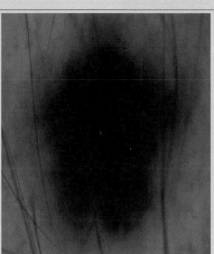

Structureless tan/pink nevi:
Nevi with pink or tan color that present without specific dermoscopic features.

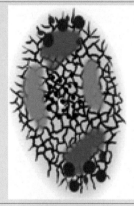
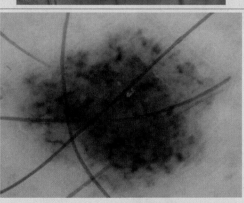

Multicomponent nevi:
Nevi with multiple components that are symmetrically distributed along the lesion.

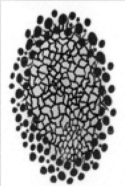
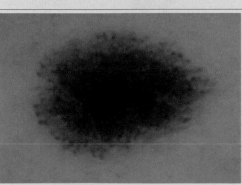

Peripheral/tiered globules nevi:
Nevi with a peripheral rim of tiered globules.

Schematics courtesy of Dermoscopedia. Photographs courtesy ISIC Archive.

Table 18.4   Nevi Requiring Special Attention—cont'd

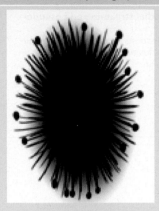

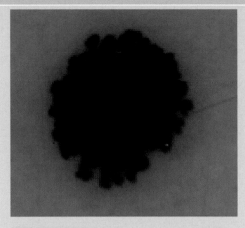

Starburst pattern:
Consists of homogeneous blue-gray or black-brown pigmentation centrally and peripheral structures that give the impression of an exploding star.

Table 18.5   Dermoscopic Features of Melanoma

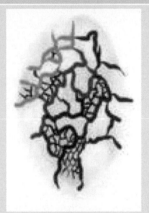

Atypical/irregular pigment network:
Network lines varying in size, color, thickness, and distribution.

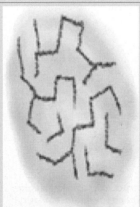

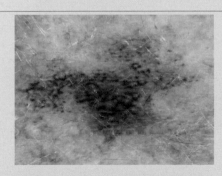

Angulated lines:
Linear brown/gray lines that intersect at acute angles forming a zigzag pattern or polygons, such as rhomboids.

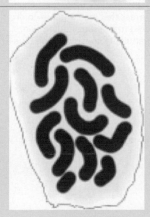

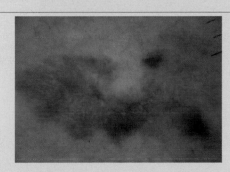

Negative network:
Hypopigmented lines connecting between pigmented structures in a serpiginous fashion.

Schematics courtesy of Dermoscopedia. Photographs courtesy ISIC Archive.

Continued

Table 18.5   Dermoscopic Features of Melanoma—cont'd

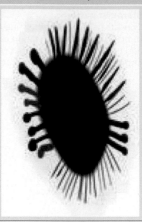

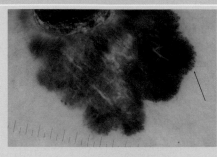

Streaks (radial streaming and pseudo-pods):
Linear projections emerging from the periphery of a lesion and extending into surrounding skin.

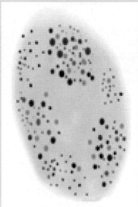

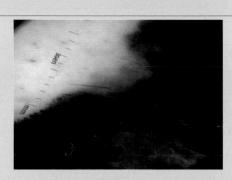

Atypical/Irregular globules:
Globules varying in color, size, and/or shape.

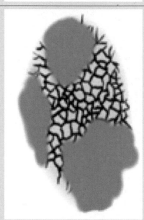

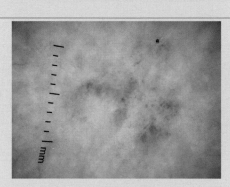

Tan peripheral structureless areas:
Tan or brown structureless areas are abnormal when they cover more than 10% of the lesion and are located on the periphery of the lesion.

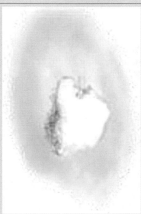

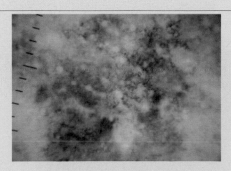

Regression structures (scar-like depigmentation and peppering/granularity):
Scar-like depigmentation appears as white, structureless areas that are lighter in color when compared to the surrounding skin. Peppering/granularity consists of fine blue-gray dots.

Table 18.5   Dermoscopic Features of Melanoma—cont'd

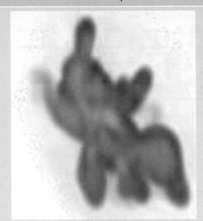 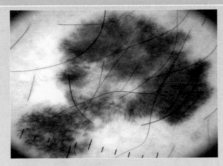

Blue-whitish veil:
Is a whitish ground-glass haze located over a blue, raised area of a lesion.

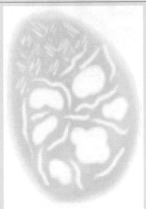 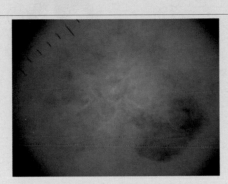

Shiny white lines/streaks:
Usually melanomas appear with shiny white lines, but shiny white blotches and strands can also be present.

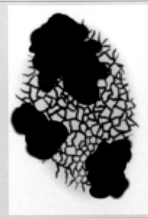 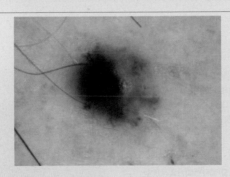

Atypical blotch:
Multiple botches obscuring visualization of underlying structures, or one off-center blotch.

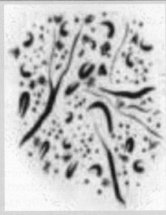 

Polymorphous vessels:
Refers to the combination of two or more vessel morphologies (dotted, coiled, linear irregular and looped vessels).

Schematics courtesy of Dermoscopedia. Photographs courtesy of ISIC Archive, Harold Rabinovitz, MD. and Richard P. Usatine, MD

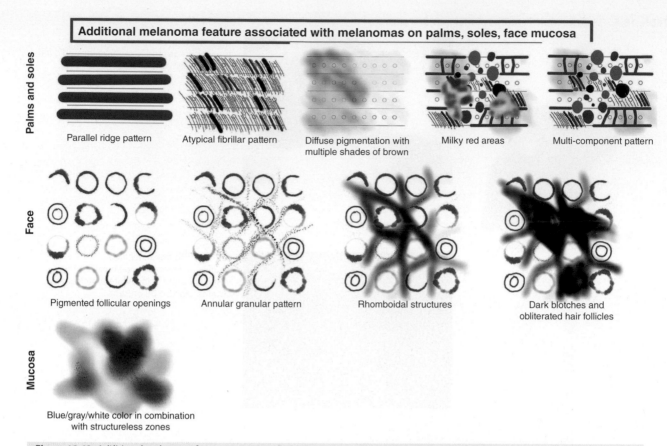

Figure 18.43 Additional melanoma features associated with melanomas on palms, soles, face, and mucosa. (Courtesy of Dermoscopedia.)

Special areas – the original two-step algorithm did not deal with lesions that are on the face or palms and soles. Here are the important basics for these areas that are covered as step 3 in the top-down two-step (Figure 18.43).

Face

The rete ridges that are instrumental in producing network patterns in the nevi on the face are not prominent on the face. Adnexal structures, hair follicles, and sweat glands are more prominent on the face and these produce the pseudonetwork seen in pigmented lesions on the face (Figure 18.44). Lentigo maligna (synonymous with lentigo maligna melanoma in situ) should be recognized on the face before it becomes invasive.

Schiffner et al. described the progression model for lentigo maligna that is detailed in Figure 18.45.[12] Figure 18.46 shows lentigo maligna with rhomboidal structures. Circle in circle pattern is another dermoscopic pattern seen in lentigo maligna melanoma (Figure 18.47).

Three important dermoscopic features are:

1. Asymmetric pigmented follicular openings often with a gray color
2. Angulated lines that create a zigzag pattern and can coalesce to create polygonal shapes, with the most common being a rhomboid (aka, rhomboidal structures)
3. Periadnexal slate-gray dots/granules[12]

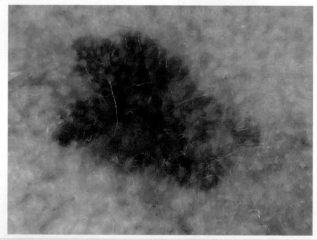

Figure 18.44 Pseudonetwork is the net-like pattern made by lightly colored adnexal openings within pigmented lesions on the face. This is a solar lentigo with a typical moth-eaten border showing the adnexal openings within the pigmented lentigo. (Copyright Richard P. Usatine, MD.)

Acral Areas Palms and Soles

https://dermoscopedia.org/Acrolentiginous_Melanoma

To understand how to differentiate melanoma from other pigmented lesions on the palms or soles, it is important to understand the anatomy of the acral skin. The dermatoglyphics on acral skin consist of ridges and furrows with eccrine

PROGRESSION MODEL FOR LENTIGO MALIGNA

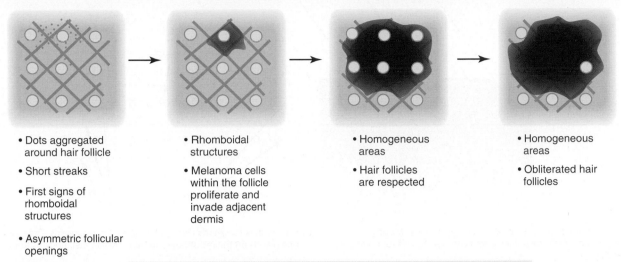

- Dots aggregated around hair follicle
- Short streaks
- First signs of rhomboidal structures
- Asymmetric follicular openings

- Rhomboidal structures
- Melanoma cells within the follicle proliferate and invade adjacent dermis

- Homogeneous areas
- Hair follicles are respected

- Homogeneous areas
- Obliterated hair follicles

Figure 18.45 Progression model for lentigo maligna. (Copyright Richard P. Usatine, MD.)

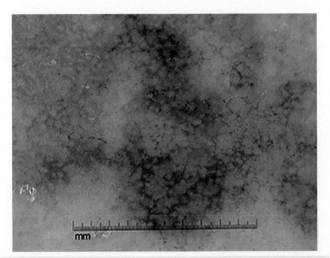

Figure 18.46 Lentigo maligna melanoma on the face with rhomboidal structures. (Copyright Ashfaq A. Marghoob, MD.)

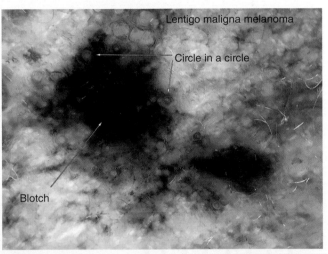

Figure 18.47 Lentigo maligna melanoma on the face with circle in circle pattern. (Copyright Richard P. Usatine, MD.)

sweat glands that are found on the ridges (Figure 18.48). The ridges are wider than the furrows.

Nevi on volar skin have three common patterns: (Table 18.6)

Acral melanomas on volar skin (palms and soles) have five common patterns: (Table 18.7)

It is also important not to confuse subcorneal hemorrhagic lesions on the palms or soles with melanoma since they can also display a parallel ridge pattern (PRP). Frequently the history alone will help to distinguish pigmentation caused by trauma from a malignant lesion. These subcorneal hemorrhages can appear yellow-red to red-black in color and may have globules at the periphery. The heel and bottom of the big toe are common locations for subcorneal hemorrhages seen with sports or ill-fitting shoes. Figure 18.49 is an example of a benign subcorneal hemorrhage.

Many melanomas on the palms and soles have a PRP somewhere within the lesion. Figure 18.50 shows two acrolentiginous melanomas with PRPs on volar surfaces.

The eccrine sweat gland openings are visible in the middle of the ridges, making it easy to distinguish the ridges from the furrows. This pattern is rarely seen in acral nevi.

PRP in Persons of Color

People with darker skin tones tend to have more hyperpigmentation on their palms and soles.[13] This pigmentation has been given many names including ethnic melanosis, racial melanosis, benign volar ethnic melanosis, ethnic pigmented macules, and mottled hyperpigmentation. It is the equivalent of the multiple dark nails that are often seen in persons of color. In the Coleman study the rate of this mottled hyperpigmentation was as high as 52% in individuals of African descent with dark brown skin. We and others have observed that many of the persons with benign volar ethnic melanosis have a PRP despite not having melanoma (Figure 18.51).

ANATOMY

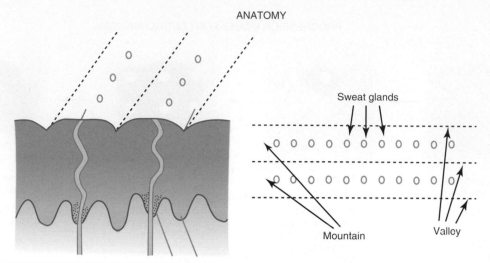

Figure 18.48 Acral skin consists of mountains and valleys (ridges and furrows) with eccrine sweat glands that are found on the mountains. The mountains are wider than the valleys. Melanoma cells tend to be found around the eccrine glands on the mountains, and the normal melanocytes tend to be in the valleys.

Table 18.6   Benign Nevus Patterns on Volar Skin (Palms and Soles)

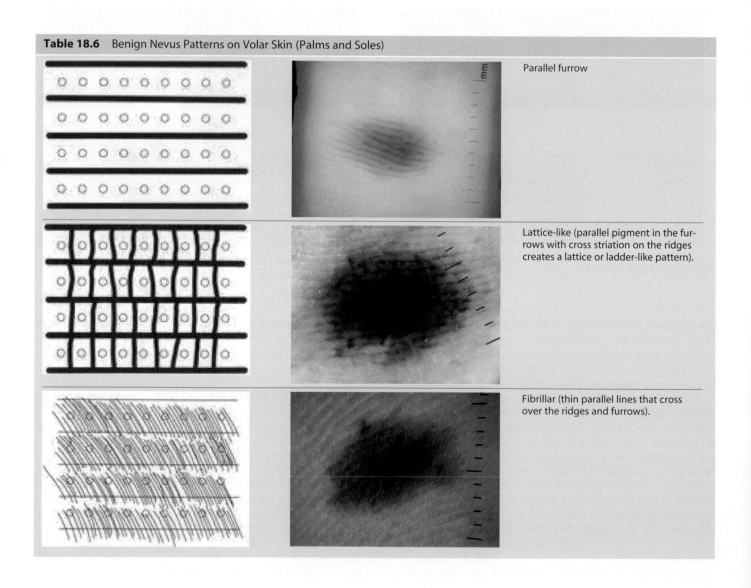

Parallel furrow

Lattice-like (parallel pigment in the furrows with cross striation on the ridges creates a lattice or ladder-like pattern).

Fibrillar (thin parallel lines that cross over the ridges and furrows).

Table 18.7   Acral Melanomas on Volar Skin (Palms and Soles)

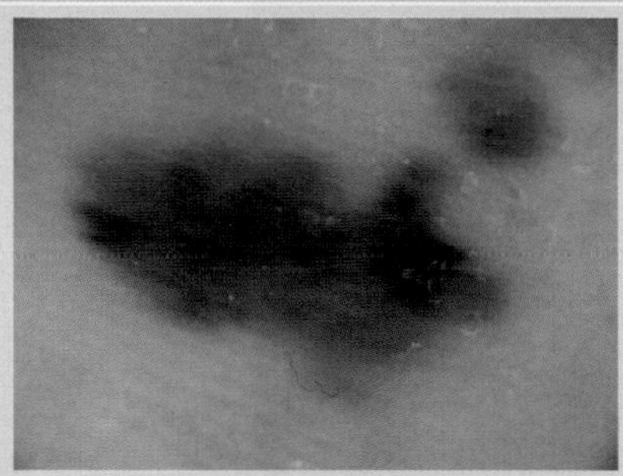

Parallel ridge pattern

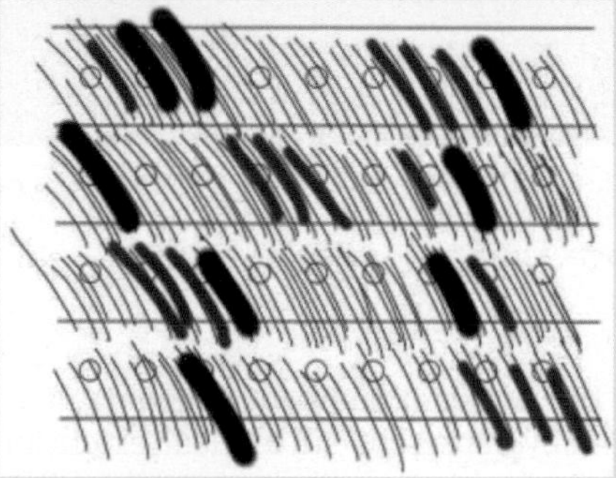

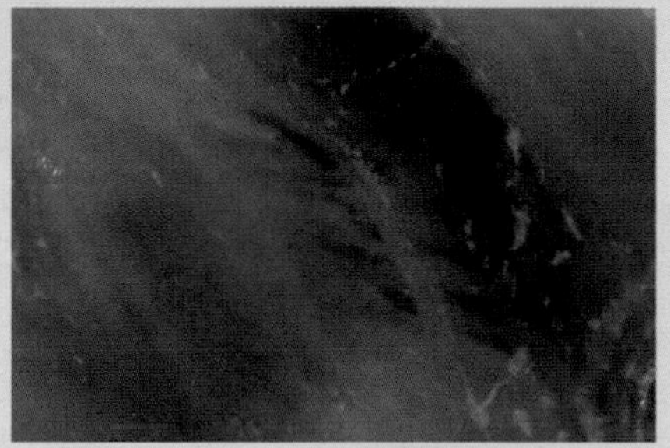

Atypical fibrillar pattern

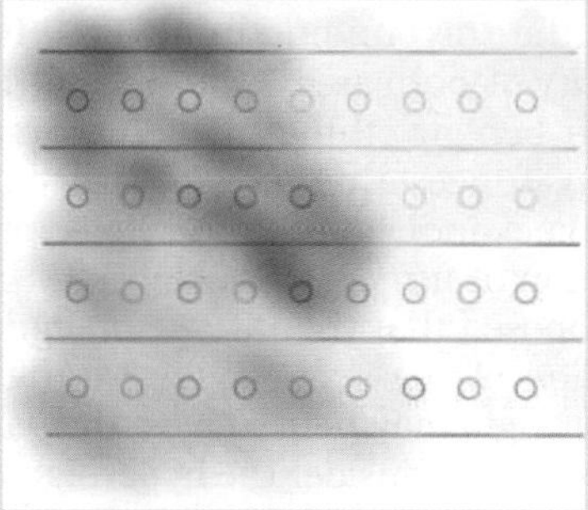

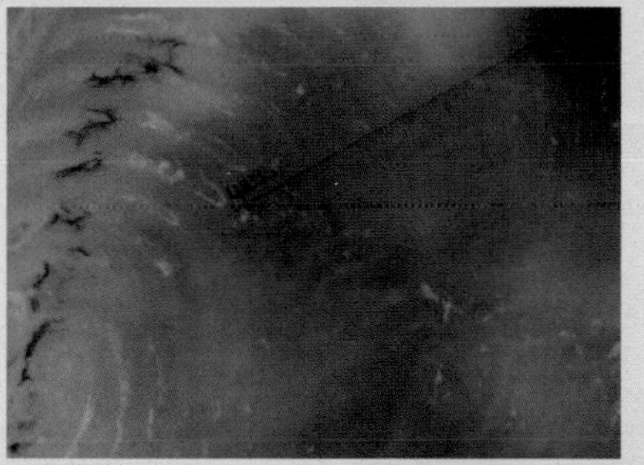

Diffuse pigmentation with multiple shades of brown

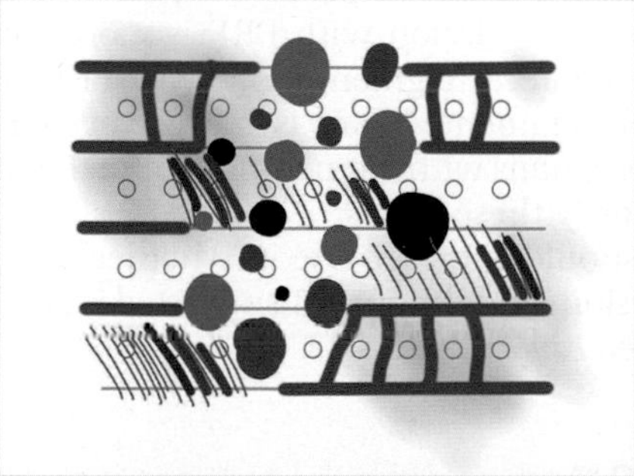

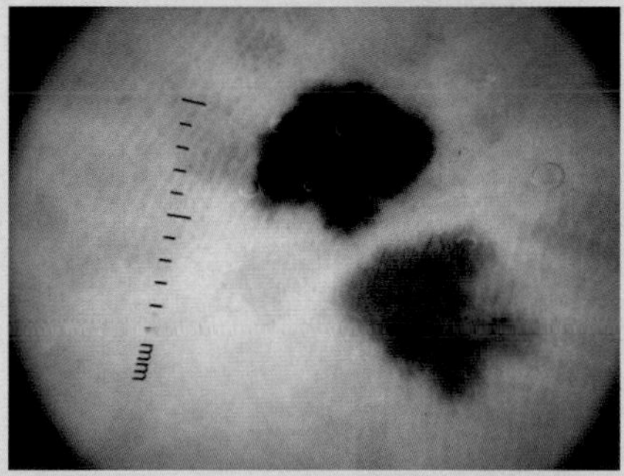

Multicomponent pattern – pigment in large blotches of different colors

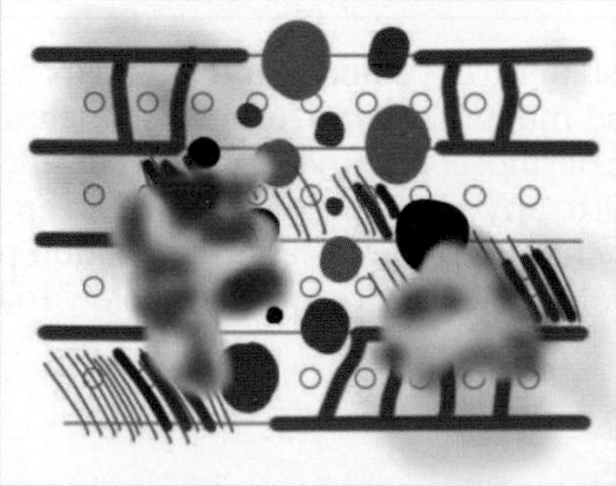

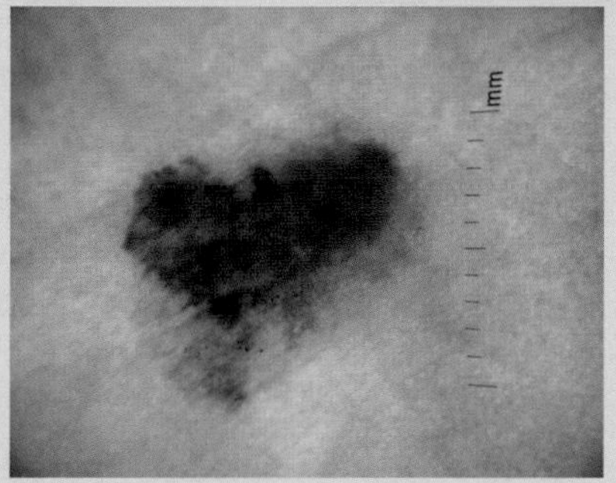

Milky red areas with a multi-component pattern

Schematics courtesy of Dermoscopedia. Photographs copyright Richard P. Usatine, MD. and Ashfaq Marghoob, MD

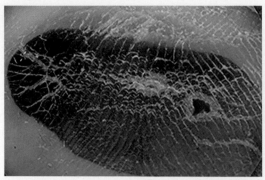

Figure 18.49 Benign subcorneal hemorrhage can resemble a melanoma. The subcorneal blood is sequestered on the ridges creating a pattern that mimics melanoma. (Copyright Ashfaq A. Marghoob, MD.)

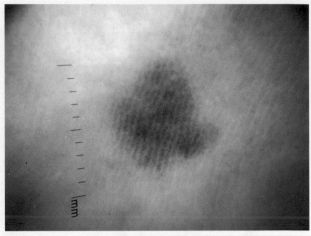

Figure 18.51 This parallel ridge pattern is on the sole of a person of sub-Saharan African descent. This is an example of ethnic melanosis and not melanoma. (Copyright Richard P. Usatine, MD.)

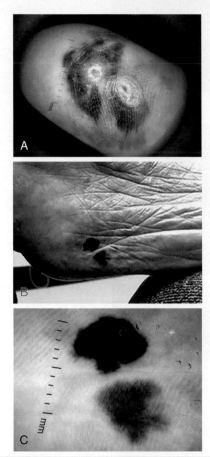

Figure 18.50 (A) Dermoscopy of melanoma of the finger in a Hispanic woman with parallel ridge pattern. (B) Melanoma in situ on the foot of a Hispanic man with multiple colors. (C) Dermoscopy of the melanoma in figure B showing parallel ridge pattern. (A. Courtesy of Leah Shama, DO. B and C. Copyright Richard P. Usatine, MD.)

The PRP has been found to have high sensitivity and specificity for early acrolentiginous melanoma in Caucasian and Asian populations, but it has not been validated in individuals of other races/ethnicities.[14] In a single-institution retrospective study of features of skin cancer in Black individuals, the majority of the plantar melanoma cases demonstrated the PRP.[15] However, these individuals also had the PRP in surrounding uninvolved background skin. The limitation of this finding is that the clinically uninvolved skin

displaying the PRP was not biopsied. Therefore, it is possible that this PRP may represent subclinical extension of the melanomas, though this is unlikely since the PRP was diffusely present in the surrounding uninvolved background skin in the majority of our cases. Additionally, the PRP has been described in benign ethnic pigmented macules.[16,17] These observations suggest that the PRP may lack discriminatory power in Black individuals and when employed may lead to an escalation of unnecessary biopsies.[18,19]

It has been proposed that the PRP in malignant lesions exhibits obliteration of the acrosyringia so that preservation of the acrosyringia may help suggest the pattern is not melanoma.[20] Also, if we consider the hyperpigmentation of nails in benign ethnic melanosis as a model for palms and soles, a solitary volar lesion with PRP is more worrisome than multiple bilateral pigmentation with PRP, just as a solitary heavily pigmented nail is more worrisome than multiple bilateral nails with pigmentation. Further research is needed to clarify these issues.

Finally we should consider size in whether or not to biopsy a volar lesion, and the cut-off suggested is above 7 mm in diameter (see Algorithm 18.1).

Conclusion

Learning the structures, colors, and patterns associated with benign and malignant skin lesions is a necessary prerequisite before dermoscopy can be used in bedside decision making. As with any skill, there exists a steep learning curve, and this chapter serves as an introduction to dermoscopic analysis. Use the list of resources below to continue your learning.

Resources

- Dermoscopedia https://dermoscopedia.org/
- Free dermoscopy app – Dermoscopy: Two Step Algorithm. Available on iTunes and www.usatinemedia.com. Authors: Marghoob AA, Usatine RP, Jaimes N. Released in 2014.

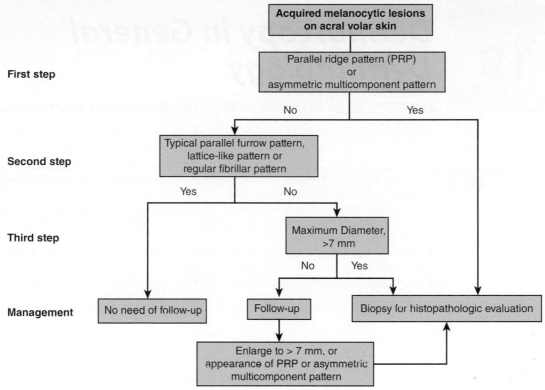

Algorithm 18.1 Adapted from Saida T, Koga H, Uhara H. Key points in dermoscopic differentiation between early acral melanoma and acral nevus. *J Dermatol.* 2011;38(1):25–34.

■ International Dermoscopy Society, http://www.dermoscopy-ids.org/
Multiday dermoscopy courses:
  ■ American Dermoscopy Meeting is a 3-day course held yearly in the summer in a national park
  ■ Mayo Clinic Annual Practical Course in Dermoscopy and Update on Malignant Melanoma – 3 days yearly in early December

Reference

1. Dinnes J, Deeks JJ, Chuchu N, et al. Dermoscopy, with and without visual inspection, for diagnosing melanoma in adults. *Cochrane Database Syst Rev.* 2018;12(12):CD011902. doi:10.1002/14651858.CD011902.pub2.
2. Harkemanne E, Baeck M, Tromme I. Training general practitioners in melanoma diagnosis: a scoping review of the literature. *BMJ Open.* 2021;11(3):e043926. doi:10.1136/bmjopen-2020-043926.
3. Bafounta ML, Beauchet A, Aegerter P, Saiag P. Is dermoscopy (epiluminescence microscopy) useful for the diagnosis of melanoma? Results of a meta-analysis using techniques adapted to the evaluation of diagnostic tests. *Arch Dermatol.* 2001;137:1343-1350.
4. Vestergaard ME, Macaskill P, Holt PE, Menzies SW. Dermoscopy compared with naked-eye examination for the diagnosis of primary melanoma: a meta-analysis of studies performed in a clinical setting. *Br J Dermatol.* 2008;159:669-676.
5. Carli P, De Giorgi V, Crocetti E. Improvement of malignant/benign ratio in excised melanocytic lesions in the "dermoscopy era": a retrospective study 1997–2001. *Br J Dermatol.* 2004;150:687-692.
6. Venuto-Andrade C, Marghoob AA. Ten reasons why dermoscopy is beneficial for the evaluation of skin lesions. *Exp Rev Dermatol.* 2006;1:369-374.
7. Rogers T, Marino ML, Dusza SW, et al. A clinical aid for detecting skin cancer: the Triage Amalgamated Dermoscopic Algorithm (TADA). *J Am Board Fam Med.* 2016;29(6):694-701. doi:10.3122/jabfm.2016.06.160079.
8. Chen LL, Dusza SW, Jaimes N, Marghoob AA. Performance of the first step of the 2-Step Dermoscopy Algorithm. *JAMA Dermatol.* 2015;151:715-721.
9. Marghoob AA, Braun R. Proposal for a revised 2-Step Algorithm for the classification of lesions of the skin using dermoscopy. *Arch Dermatol.* 2010;146:426-428.
10. Giddens T, Seiverling E, Marghoob A, Usatine R. Absence of central white patch in dermatofibromas presenting in darker skin. *JAAD Case Rep.* 2022;21:63-65. doi:10.1016/j.jdcr.2021.12.023.
11. Tuma B, Yamada S, Atallah ÁN, Araujo FM, Hirata SH. Dermoscopy of black skin: a cross-sectional study of clinical and dermoscopic features of melanocytic lesions in individuals with type V/VI skin compared to those with type I/II skin. *J Am Acad Dermatol.* 2015;73(1):114-119. doi:10.1016/j.jaad.2015.03.043.
12. Zalaudek I, Argenziano G, Mordente I, et al. Nevus type in dermoscopy is related to skin type in white persons. *Arch Dermatol.* 2007;143(3):351-356. doi:10.1001/archderm.143.3.351.
13. Coleman WP, Gately LE, Krementz AB, Reed RJ, Krementz ET. Nevi, lentigines, and melanomas in blacks. *Arch Dermatol.* 1980;116(5):548-551.
14. Phan A, Dalle S, Touzet S, Ronger-Savlé S, Balme B, Thomas L. Dermoscopic features of acral lentiginous melanoma in a large series of 110 cases in a white population. *Br J Dermatol.* 2010;162(4):765-771. doi:10.1111/j.1365-2133.2009.09594.x.
15. Manci RN, Dauscher M, Marchetti MA, et al. Features of skin cancer in black individuals: a single-institution retrospective cohort study. *Dermatol Pract Concept.* 2022;12(2):e2022075. doi:10.5826/dpc.1202a75.
16. Phan A, Dalle S, Marcilly MC, Bergues JP, Thomas L. Benign dermoscopic parallel ridge pattern variants. *Arch Dermatol.* 2011;147(5):634. doi:10.1001/archdermatol.2011.47.
17. Saida T, Miyazaki A, Oguchi S. Significance of dermoscopic patterns in detecting malignant melanoma on acral volar skin: results of a multicenter study in Japan. *Arch Dermatol.* 2004;140(10):1233-1238. doi:10.1001/archderm.140.10.1233.
18. Ishihara Y, Saida T, Miyazaki A. Early acral melanoma in situ: correlation between the parallel ridge pattern on dermoscopy and microscopic features. *Am J Dermatopathol.* 2006;28(1):21-27. doi:10.1097/01.dad.0000187931.05030.a0.
19. Tanioka M. Benign acral lesions showing parallel ridge pattern on dermoscopy. *J Dermatol.* 2011;38(1):41-44. doi:10.1111/j.1346-8138.2010.01128.x.
20. Fracaroli TS, Lavorato FG, Maceira JP, Barcaui C. Parallel ridge pattern on dermoscopy: observation in non-melanoma cases. *An Bras Dermatol.* 2013;88(4):646-648. doi:10.1590/abd1806-4841.20132058.

Dermoscopy in General Dermatology

ENZO ERRICHETTI, MD, MARIA BAKIRTZI, and AIMILIOS LALLAS

SUMMARY
- Dermoscopy is also helpful in assisting the diagnosis of nonneoplastic diseases, including inflammatory and infectious dermatoses.
- The inflammatory diseases covered in this chapter include psoriasis, dermatitis, lichen planus, pityriasis rosea, porokeratosis, prurigo nodularis, rosacea, discoid lupus erythematosus, and capillaritis.
- The infectious diseases covered in this chapter include common warts, flat warts, genital warts, molluscum contagiosum, scabies, and tinea corporis.
- Dermoscopic parameters useful in general dermatology include vessels, scales, and follicular findings.

Introduction

Dermoscopy is classically used for the assessment of pigmented and nonpigmented skin tumors, yet it has been shown to be helpful even in assisting the diagnosis of nonneoplastic diseases, including inflammatory and infectious dermatoses.[1-3] Whereas a well-established and structured dermoscopic approach for the analysis of tumors is available, criteria and terminology used for nonneoplastic dermatoses are often metaphoric and inhomogeneous, with consequent lack of a systematic analytic approach.[4] For this reason, a set of five dermoscopic parameters (with a total of 31 subitems) has been proposed by a consensus document of the *International Dermoscopy Society* as a basic guide to use in general dermatology:

1. Vessels (including morphology and distribution)
2. Scales (including color and distribution)
3. Follicular findings
4. "Other structures" (structures other than vessels/scales; including color and morphology) and
5. "Specific clues" (features that, when present, are strongly suggestive of only one diagnosis due to a strict dermoscopic-pathological correlation)[4]

Since vessels and scales are often the main characterizing dermoscopic features of inflammatory and infectious diseases, it is classically advised to use noncontact polarized dermatoscopes as they preserve such findings.[3] However, an interface fluid is sometimes needed to highlight structures covered by overlying scales.[3] Importantly, dermoscopic examination of nonneoplastic dermatoses should be considered the second step of a "2-step procedure," always preceded by the establishment of a differential diagnosis on clinical ground, since such diseases often feature only poorly specific dermoscopic findings that, however, may be useful if interpreted in the context of a specific differential diagnosis.[3] In this chapter, common inflammatory and infectious dermatoses that may significantly benefit from dermoscopic assessment are addressed.

Inflammatory Diseases

PSORIASIS

Psoriasis is probably the dermatosis that benefits most from dermoscopic examination.[1-3] Dermoscopy shows a constant pattern consisting of:

- Dotted vessels distributed in a uniform way
- Diffuse white scales (Figures 19.1, 19.2)[1-3]

Anatomical localization may affect the dermoscopic appearance of psoriasis:

- Humid areas (e.g., genitalia or folds) – vessel pattern predominant (Figure 19.1)
- Scalp/palmoplantar areas – scaling pattern predominant (Figure 19.2)[1-3,5]

Dermoscopic pattern may not vary by clinical variant (plaque, inverse, guttate, erythrodermic, etc.),[1-3,6,7] apart from pustular subtype in which yellow globules (representing pustules) are also seen.[1-3] Sometimes, psoriatic plaques may also feature purpuric (hemorrhagic) dots/areas, especially in scratched lesions (Figure 19.3).[1-3]

DERMATITIS

The term dermatitis (or eczema) encompasses a group of conditions including atopic dermatitis, allergic contact dermatitis, stasis dermatitis, and seborrheic dermatitis. From a dermoscopic point of view, these conditions are usually typified by the presence of:

- Dotted vessels arranged in clusters or in a nonspecific (random) pattern

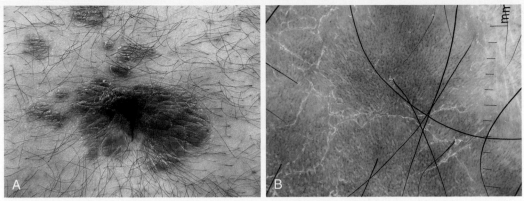

Figure 19.1 Classic vascular pattern of psoriasis, consisting of uniform (regularly distributed) dotted vessels on a pink background. **(A)** Clinical; **(B)** dermoscopic. (Copyright Richard P. Usatine, MD.)

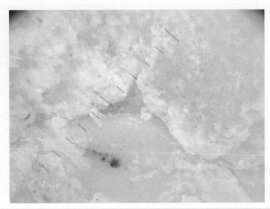

Figure 19.2 Psoriasis of palmoplantar areas usually shows only diffuse white scaling.

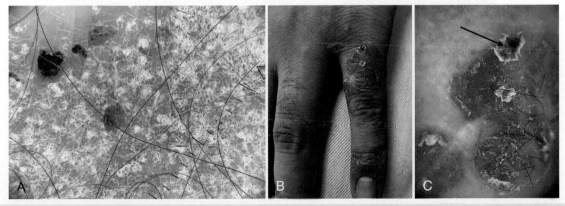

Figure 19.3 **(A)** Dermoscopy of a scratched psoriatic lesion reveals diffuse white scales and purpuric (hemorrhagic) dots/areas. **(B)** Excoriated psoriasis. **(C)** Dermoscopy showing hemorrhagic dots (arrow) and dotted vessels.

- Yellow scales/serocrusts (Figure 19.4)[1-3]
- Vesicles in palmoplantar areas (Figure 19.5)[5]

Vesicles are usually not seen in other areas as they break easily, though they are observed on palmoplantar areas as the thicker epidermis makes them more resistant to rupture.

Importantly, disease stage may affect the dermoscopic pattern of dermatitis as, while in subacute phases both vessels and scales/crusts are usually found, acute lesions mainly display scales/crusts.[1-3] On the other hand, chronic lichenified lesions are commonly characterized by uniform dotted vessels over a white background (differently from psoriasis in which the background is reddish), follicular plugs, and purple (hemorrhagic) dots/areas resulting from scratching (Figure 19.6).[1-3] Fabric fibers stuck to crusts may also be observed in all dermatitis phases.[1-3] Notably, some clinical variants of dermatitis may show some dermoscopic peculiarities:

- Seborrheic dermatitis – linear vessels or linear vessels with branches
- Stasis dermatitis – globular vessels
- Asteatotic eczema – white scales with a double free edge ("rail-like" appearance)[1-3]

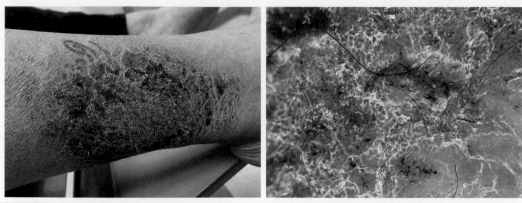

Figure 19.4 Dermatitis mainly displays clustered dotted vessels and yellow scales/crusts on dermoscopy. (Copyright Richard P. Usatine, MD.)

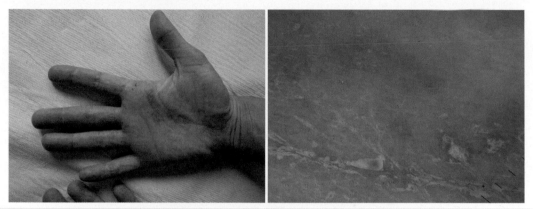

Figure 19.5 Orange globules corresponding to spongiotic vesicles are seen on dermoscopy in chronic hand eczema.

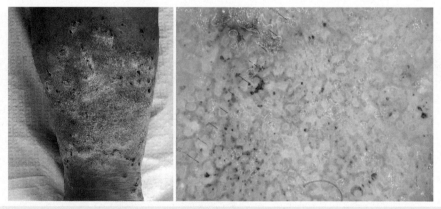

Figure 19.6 Dermoscopic examination of chronic lichenified eczema shows uniform dotted vessels, follicular plugs, and purpuric spots.

LICHEN PLANUS

Lichen planus is one of the most recognizable dermatoses on dermoscopy thanks to the presence of Wickham striae, which appear as white crossing lines forming a network (Figure 19.7). Wickham striae also may also appear to be annular, starlike, dotted, or polygonal.[1-3] This dermoscopic clue is usually observed in active lesions, along with peripheral dotted/linear vessels, whereas in healing phases it may be absent with brown dots (peppering) gradually appearing (Figure 19.8).[1-3] The main dermoscopic clue of hypertrophic lichen planus is the presence of follicular plugs as Wickham striae are usually covered by white hyperkeratosis.[1-3]

PITYRIASIS ROSEA

Diagnosis of pityriasis rosea is straightforward if there is a herald patch, collarette scale, and a Christmas tree–like distribution. Dermoscopy may help visualize the peripheral collarette scale with the inner free edge through better lighting and magnification (Figure 19.9).[1-3] This collarette sign may also be seen in other papulosquamous conditions (e.g., psoriasis and tinea corporis), but in pityriasis rosea vessels are usually limited or absent (mainly with a dotted or linear shape).[1-3] Indeed, in both psoriasis and tinea corporis it is possible to see dotted vessels, with a uniform and (Figure 19.10) nonspecific (random) arrangement,

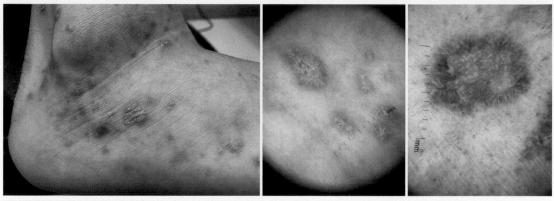

Figure 19.7 Lichen planus with dermoscopic hallmark of Wickham striae, consisting of white crossing lines forming a network. (Copyright Richard P. Usatine, MD.)

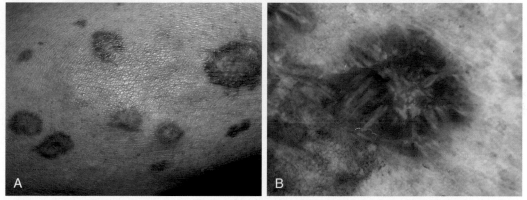

Figure 19.8 **(A)** Clinical lesions of lichen planus on the legs. **(B)** The brown dots (peppering) in the bottom left corner of the dermoscopic image indicate that the lesions are healing. The white lines in the center are those of Wickham's striae. (Copyright Richard P. Usatine, MD.)

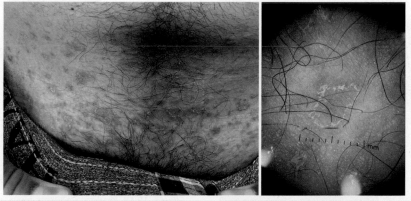

Figure 19.9 Dermoscopy of pityriasis rosea reveals peripheral white scaling with an inner free edge and no vessels. (Copyright Richard P. Usatine, MD.)

respectively.[1-3] Additionally, peripheral scaling of tinea corporis typically shows an outer or mixed (inner and outer) free edge.[1-3]

POROKERATOSIS

All the clinical variants of porokeratosis share the same dermoscopic clue, which is the presence of a white/grey peripheral keratotic tract typified by a double free edge (Figure 19.11).[1-3,6] This double free edge resembles the Great Wall of China seen from above. This structure corresponds to the histological hallmark of this condition,

namely the cornoid lamella.[1-3,6] Sometimes, in nonactive lesions this dermoscopic finding may be absent, and diagnosis becomes more difficult. Besides peripheral keratotic tract, porokeratosis may also display other nonspecific features in the center of the lesions, including vessels, white structureless areas, pigmented structures, and scaling.[1-3,6]

PRURIGO NODULARIS

Dermoscopy may provide significant help in the diagnosis of prurigo nodularis by revealing the so-called "white starburst" pattern, consisting of peripheral white lines over a

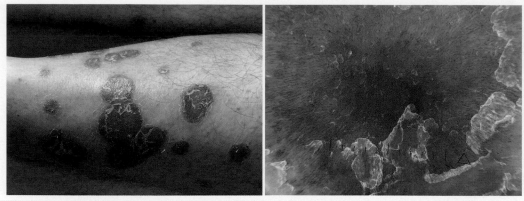

Figure 19.10 Peripheral white scaling may also be seen in psoriasis, yet in this condition uniform dotted vessels are also evident.

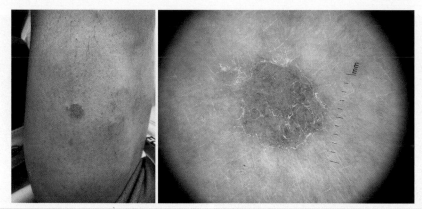

Figure 19.11 Porokeratosis revealing peripheral keratotic rim with a double free edge on dermoscopy. (Copyright Richard P. Usatine, MD.)

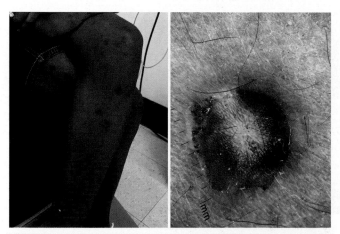

Figure 19.12 Dermoscopic examination of prurigo nodularis shows peripheral white striae ("white starburst" pattern) and central erosion along with linear/linear-curved vessels. (Copyright Richard P. Usatine, MD.)

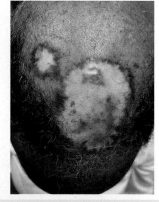

Figure 19.13 Prurigo nodularis may also display follicular plugs surrounded by dotted vessels having a white halo when the scratching is gentler but long-standing.

brown/red background (Figure 19.12).[1-3,7] The center of the lesions may display either erosion or hyperkeratosis/scaling.[1-3,7] Additionally, dermoscopic examination may also reveal another peculiar pattern typified by follicular plugs and perifollicular dotted vessels having a white halo (Figure 19.13).[1-3,7] This pattern is shared with lichen simplex chronicus and is more common when the scratching is more gentle but long-lasting.[1-3,7] Purpuric dots/areas are also commonly encountered in prurigo nodularis lesions.[1-3,7]

ROSACEA

The dermoscopic hallmark of rosacea is represented by the presence of linear vessels arranged in a reticular (netlike) pattern (Figure 19.14).[1-3] They are also commonly known as vascular polygons and correspond to the dilation of subpapillary vascular plexus.[1-3] This finding is very evident in erythemato-telangiectatic rosacea, but it may also be seen in other clinical variants, although it is more subtle.[1-3]

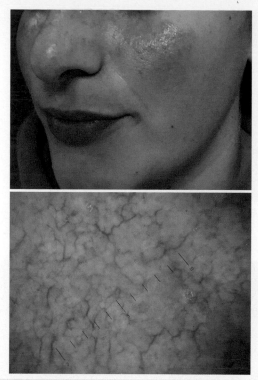

Figure 19.14 Linear vessels arranged in a reticular pattern (vascular polygons) are seen in erythemato-telangiectatic rosacea on dermoscopy.

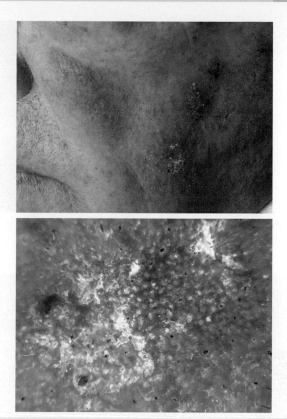

Figure 19.15 Dermoscopy of discoid lupus erythematosus (active lesion): follicular plugs and white scales.

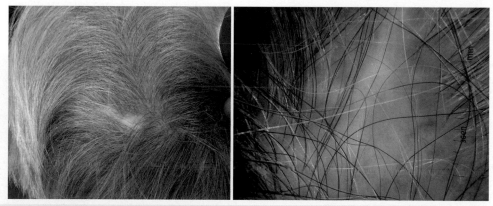

Figure 19.16 Dermoscopy of discoid lupus erythematosus (long-standing healing lesion): white scales, linear-curved and linear branching vessels, and bright white fibrotic areas.

Dermoscopic findings in other clinical variants of rosacea include:

- Papulopustular rosacea – yellow globules (representing pustules)
- Glandular rosacea – polyglobular yellow areas/white areas (due to sebaceous hyperplasia and dermal fibrosis)
- Granulomatous rosacea – orange globules (resulting from the presence of dermal granulomas).[1-3]

DISCOID LUPUS ERYTHEMATOSUS

Dermoscopic features of discoid lupus erythematosus significantly vary according to the disease stage. Indeed, acute/mature lesions are typically characterized by follicular plugs over a red background (Figure 19.15), with or without linear-curved vessels, though the so-called "inverse strawberry" pattern (red follicular dots with perifollicular halos) may also be seen less commonly.[1-3] Scaling, bright white structureless areas and telangiectatic vessels (linear-curved/linear with branches) are the main findings of long-standing/scarring lesions (Figure 19.16).[1-3]

CAPILLARITIS (PIGMENTED PURPURIC DERMATOSES)

The term "capillaritis" encompasses a clinically heterogeneous group of dermatoses typified by erythrocyte extravasation in the dermis with consequent hemosiderin deposition, mainly

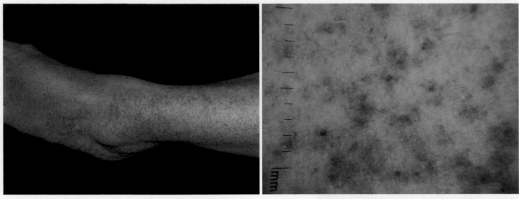

Figure 19.17 Purpuric dots over a rusty background in the dermoscopic hallmark of capillaritis (pigmented purpuric dermatoses). (Copyright Richard P. Usatine, MD.)

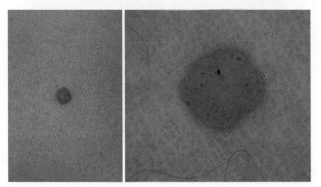

Figure 19.18 A common wart with a mosaic pattern characterized by multiple white roundish areas centered by a dotted or short hairpin vessel.

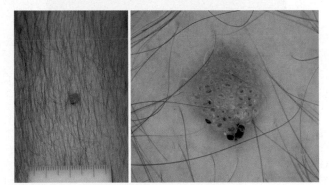

Figure 19.19 A common wart with a papillomatous surface, dermoscopically showing elongated white structures centered by hairpin vessels.

including Schamberg's disease (macular type), eczematid-like purpura of Doucas and Kapetanakis, Majocchi's disease (annular type), lichen aureus, and Gougerot-Blum diseases (lichenoid type).[1-3] All of them are dermoscopically characterized by the presence of small purpuric dots (Figure 19.17), with or without a coppery background, which is particularly pronounced in lichen aureus.[1-3] Additionally, Majocchi disease and eczematid-like purpura of Doucas and Kapetanakis may also show faint telangiectatic vessels (due to dermal vessels dilation) and white/yellow scales (due to hyperkeratosis/spongiosis), respectively.[1-3]

Infectious Skin Diseases

COMMON WARTS

Common warts are a frequent infectious disease caused by human papillomaviruses (most commonly HPV types 1, 2, 4, 27, and 57). They clinically manifest as hyperkeratotic roughened papules or nodules on skin and mucosa, with a characteristic papillomatous surface. Transmission occurs mainly via direct skin-to-skin contact but is also possible via indirect contamination through surfaces. Although considered a self-limiting and self-healing disease, they often persist until being treated.[8]

Dermoscopically, common warts display a mosaic pattern, composed of numerous irregularly shaped whitish areas, typically associated with red or black dots located in the

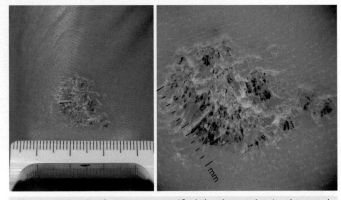

Figure 19.20 A plantar wart typified by hemorrhagic dots and interruption of normal skin dermatoglyphics.

center of each whitish area (Figure 19.18).[9-11] Linear, hairpin, and coiled vessels can also be observed (Figure 19.19). In more exophytic lesions, multiple fingerlike projections contain elongated and dilated vessels.[9-11] In plantar warts, hemorrhagic red to black dots are prominent, and dermatoglyphics are typically interrupted (Figure 19.20).[12-14]

FLAT WARTS

Flat warts are mainly caused by the HPV genotypes 3,10, 28 and 49. They usually develop in children and adolescents,

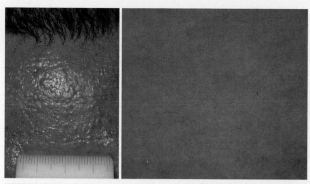

Figure 19.21 Flat warts displaying numerous tiny dotted vessels.

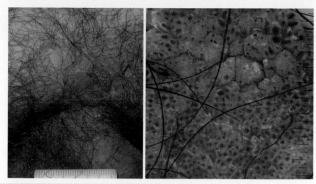

Figure 19.22 Genital warts exhibiting a mosaic pattern of white round structures centered by large dotted vessels.

mainly transmitted via skin-to-skin contact, and can be self-limited.

They manifest as multiple, light brown– or skin-colored, flat-topped, smooth papules, typically on the face.

Dermoscopy of flat warts reveals regularly distributed tiny red dots on a light brown to yellow background (Figure 19.21).[11] The diameter of the red dots is smaller as compared to common warts, because of the mild underlying papillomatosis.[8]

GENITAL WARTS

Genital warts, also known as condyloma acuminata, are a sexually transmitted disease caused by human papillomaviruses. The most common HPV genotypes causing genital warts are 6 and 11, which are considered to possess low oncogenic potential. High-risk HPV genotypes are less frequently found and, among them, types 16 and 18 epidemiologically predominate in most countries.[15] Genital warts usually develop in young adults with sexual activity and without gender predilection. Although nonsexual transmission cannot be excluded with certainty, detection of genital or perianal warts in children should raise suspicion of child abuse and warrant further investigation. Clinically, genital warts manifest as exophytic skin-colored, red, pink, soft gray, or brown papules of variable size. They have the tendency to multiply and become confluent.[15]

The dermatoscopic findings in genital warts are similar to those seen in common warts and usually better visualized because of the minimal hyperkeratosis. Flat sessile lesions display a mosaic pattern consisting of white roundish areas centered by dilated dotted or glomerular vessels, while in more exophytic pedunculated lesions the white areas are more elongated and appear as projections filled with elongated and dilated vessels (Figure 19.22). Pigmented lesions, which are usually flat, typically display numerous brown dots or small globules in addition to the vessels.[16-18]

MOLLUSCUM CONTAGIOSUM

Molluscum contagiosum is a viral cutaneous infection caused by a poxvirus of the Molluscipoxvirus genus, common in children and young adults. Lesions may be spread through close physical contact, autoinoculation, and fomites and are generally self-limiting. Typically, molluscum contagiosum manifests with asymptomatic, smooth, skin-colored,

umbilicated papules. Most lesions are small with a diameter of up to 5 mm, although larger lesions might occasionally develop.[19,20]

Dermoscopy significantly enhances the recognition of molluscum contagiosum. The dermatoscopic hallmark of the disease is yellow-white-yellow structures that project brighter under polarized light. There might be either one large white-yellow central roundish area or multiple smaller ones of variable shapes, including roundish (globular), polylobular, or rosettelike (Figures 19.23 to 19.25). These white-yellow structures are often surrounded by linear vessels that rarely cross the center of the lesion.[21-23]

SCABIES

Scabies is a common parasitic infection caused by *Sarcoptes scabiei*. The mite is easily transmittable by close physical contact and less frequently via fomites.[24,25]

The eruption of scabies consists of macules, papules, vesicles, and mainly excoriations and crusts resulting from an intense itch, that typically worsens at night. The maculopapular and papulovesicular skin changes are mostly an expression of an allergic reaction of the organism to the mite infection. The lesions usually involve the wrists, interdigital spaces, axillae, nipples, and genitalia, although they can be found anywhere on the skin. Multiple members of the family or the close environment are often affected. The diagnosis of scabies is often

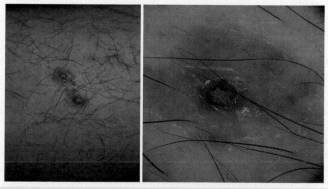

Figure 19.23 Molluscum contagiosum with a single central white-yellow amorphous structure surrounded by vessels.

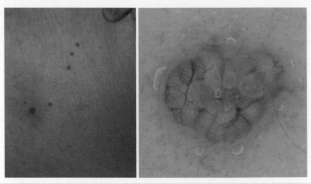

Figure 19.24 Molluscum contagiosum with polylobular central white-yellow structures (molluscum bodies) surrounded by prominent linear vessels that do not cross the midline (described as crown vessels).

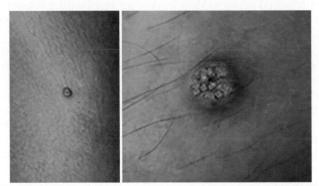

Figure 19.25 Molluscum contagiosum with rosettelike white-yellow structures.

straightforward based on the clinical manifestations but may be challenging at times, so dermoscopy is great to rule scabies in with positive findings or suggest another diagnosis when no signs of mites or burrows are seen with dermoscopy.

Dermoscopy enables the in vivo detection of the mite itself as well as the burrow and is the most efficient method to confirm the diagnosis of scabies. Dermoscopy reveals the pigmented anterior part of the mite as a small dark brown triangle. This triangle is caused by the four anterior legs and the mouth parts of the mite (Figure 19.26). The burrow is seen as a whitish curved line originating from the basis of the brown triangle, resulting in an appearance suggesting a delta-winged jet with contrail (Figure 19.27).[26] Additional dermatoscopic criteria are yellow crusts, resulting from the eczematous reaction and scratching, purpuric dots, resulting from traumatic extravasation of erythrocytes and white/yellow scales (Figure 19.28). The diagnostic accuracy of dermoscopy is at least equal to traditional ex vivo microscopic examination while requiring less time, equipment, and cost.[27-29]

Tips for finding the mites on dermoscopy:

- Look for burrows with the naked eye (often found around the wrist for easy access with the dermatoscope).
- Attach the dermatoscope to a camera or phone camera.
- Use the highest magnification possible to visualize the mite and burrow. Sometimes the video setting will allow for greater magnification.
- Snap photos and blow them up on the screen for further magnification.

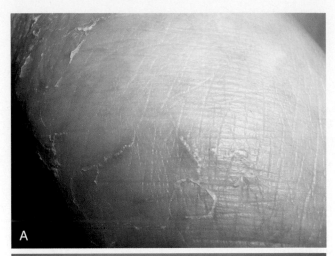

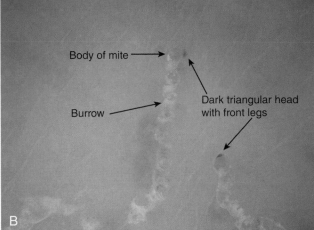

Body of mite

Burrow

Dark triangular head with front legs

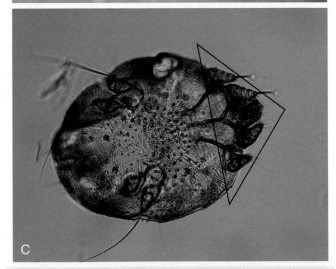

Figure 19.26 Scabies **(A)** clinical **(B)** dermoscopy showing the dark triangular head with front legs on the body of the mite in front of the burrow. **(C)** Microscopic image of the mite showing how the dark front legs and mouth create the dark triangle seen on dermoscopy. (Copyright Richard P. Usatine, MD.)

TINEA CORPORIS

Tinea corporis is a superficial infection of the skin of trunk and extremities caused by dermatophytes belonging to one of the three genera, namely, *Trichophyton*, *Microsporum*, and *Epidermophyton*. Clinically it is characterized by one or

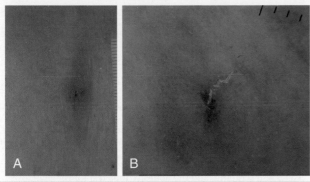

Figure 19.27 Scabies **(A)** clinical **(B)** dermoscopy. The typical jet with contrail of scabies: small brown triangle with a long curved white line.

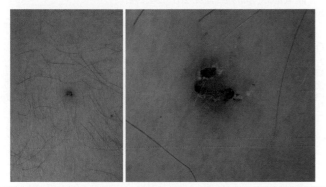

Figure 19.28 In addition to the mite and the furrow, this case of scabies dermoscopy reveals yellow crusts and purpura, reflecting the eczematous reaction and the excoriations.

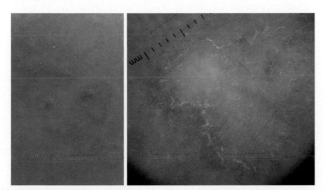

Figure 19.29 Tinea corporis reveals white scales distributed at the periphery of the lesion, with an intact outer edge and a moth-eaten inner edge.

more circular, sharply demarcated, slightly scaly, border-emphasized lesions, which tend to extend centrifugally with central healing.[30]

Dermoscopy of tinea corporis usually reveals white scales distributed at the periphery of the lesion, with an intact outer edge and a moth-eaten inner edge (Figure 19.29). This peculiar inward-to-outward desquamation pattern reflects the centrifugal expansion of the fungus. Dotted or short linear vessels might be present but not as a predominant finding.[31] Dermoscopy might also reveal broken hairs in the center of the lesion, as well as yellow crusts/scales that reflect the eczematous reaction, which is frequent in *Microsporum* infections (Figure 19.30).

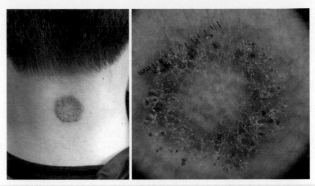

Figure 19.30 Tinea corporis caused by *Microsporum* species, displaying broken hairs in the central part and yellow crusts at the periphery resulting from the eczematous reaction.

Conclusion

Dermoscopy can be used to diagnose many skin problems in general dermatology as evidenced by this introduction. There are whole books devoted to dermoscopy in general dermatology, including books that deal with the spectrum of skin color and how this impacts dermoscopic findings in general dermatology.[32,33]

One area that we have not addressed at all is the use of dermoscopy for diagnosing alopecia and other hair disorders. If these additional areas are of interest there are many articles and books addressing the full range of dermoscopy applications.

References

1. Errichetti E, Stinco G. Dermoscopy in general dermatology: a practical overview. *Dermatol Ther (Heidelb)*. 2016;6(4):471-507.
2. Errichetti E, Stinco G. The practical usefulness of dermoscopy in general dermatology. *G Ital Dermatol Venereol*. 2015;150(5):533-546.
3. Errichetti E. Dermoscopy of inflammatory dermatoses (inflammoscopy): an up-to-date overview. *Dermatol Pract Concept*. 2019;9(3): 169-180.
4. Errichetti E, Zalaudek I, Kittler H, et al. Standardization of dermoscopic terminology and basic dermoscopic parameters to evaluate in general dermatology (non-neoplastic dermatoses): an expert consensus on behalf of the International Dermoscopy Society. *Br J Dermatol*. 2020;182(2):454-467.
5. Errichetti E, Stinco G. Dermoscopy in differential diagnosis of palmar psoriasis and chronic hand eczema. *J Dermatol*. 2016;43(4):423-425.
6. Zaar O, Polesie S, Navarrete-Dechent C, et al. Dermoscopy of porokeratosis: results from a multicentre study of the International Dermoscopy Society. *J Eur Acad Dermatol Venereol*. 2021;35(10): 2091-2096.
7. Errichetti E, Piccirillo A, Stinco G. Dermoscopy of prurigo nodularis. *J Dermatol*. 2015;42(6):632-634.
8. Cardoso JC, Calonje E. Cutaneous manifestations of human papillomaviruses: a review. *Acta Dermatovenerol Alp Pannonica Adriat*. 2011; 20:145-154.
9. Zalaudek I, Giacomel J, Cabo H, et al. Entodermoscopy: a new tool for diagnosing skin infections and infestations. *Dermatology*. 2008; 216:14-23.
10. Haliasos EC, Kerner M, Jaimes-Lopez N, et al. Dermoscopy for the pediatric dermatologist part I: dermoscopy of pediatric infectious and inflammatory skin lesions and hair disorders. *Pediatr Dermatol*. 2013;30:163-171.
11. Lacarrubba F, Verzì AE, Dinotta F, et al. Dermatoscopy in inflammatory and infectious skin disorders. *G Ital Dermatol Venereol*. 2015; 150:521-531.
12. Lee DY, Park JH, Lee JH, et al. The use of dermoscopy for the diagnosis of plantar wart. *J Eur Acad Dermatol Venereol*. 2009;23:726-727.

13. Bae JM, Kang H, Kim HO, Park YM. Differential diagnosis of plantar wart from corn, callus and healed wart with the aid of dermoscopy. *Br J Dermatol.* 2009;160:220-222.

14. Quast DR, Nauck MA, Bechara FG, Meier JJ. A case series of verrucae vulgares mimicking hyperkeratosis in individuals with diabetic foot ulcers. *Diabet Med.* 2017;34:1165-1168.

15. Steben M, Garland SM. Genital warts. *Best Pract Res Clin Obstet Gynaecol.* 2014;28:1063-1073.

16. Micali G, Lacarrubba F. Augmented diagnostic capability using videodermatoscopy on selected infectious and non-infectious penile growths. *Int J Dermatol.* 2011;50:1501-1505.

17. Lacarrubba F, Dinotta F, Nasca MR, Micali G. Enhanced diagnosis of genital warts with videodermatoscopy: histopatologic correlation. *G Ital Dermatol Venereol.* 2012;147:215-216.

18. Paštar Z, Lipozenčić J. Significance of dermatoscopy in genital dermatoses. *Clin Dermatol.* 2014;32:315-318.

19. Brown J, Janniger CK, Schwartz RA, Silverberg NB. Childhood molluscum contagiosum. *Int J Dermatol.* 2006;45:93-99.

20. Alam MS, Shrirao N. Giant molluscum contagiosum presenting as lid neoplasm in an immunocompetent child. *Dermatol Online J.* 2016;22:13030.

21. Morales A, Puig S, Malvehy J, Zaballos P. Dermoscopy of molluscum contagiosum. *Arch Dermatol.* 2005;141:1644.

22. Zaballos P, Ara M, Puig S, Malvehy J. Dermoscopy of molluscum contagiosum: a useful tool for clinical diagnosis in adulthood. *J Eur Acad Dermatol Venereol.* 2006;20:482-483.

23. Ku SH, Cho EB, Park EJ, et al. Dermoscopic features of molluscum contagiosum based on white structures and their correlation with histopathological findings. *Clin Exp Dermatol.* 2015;40: 208-210.

24. Stone SP, Goldfarb JN, Bacelieri RE. Scabies, other mites and pediculosis. In: Wolff K, Goldsmith LA, Katz SI, Gilchrest BA, Paller AS, Leffell DJ, eds. *Fitzpatrick's Dermatology in General Medicine.* 7th ed. McGraw-Hill; 2008:2029-2036.

25. Hicks MI, Elston DM. Scabies. *Dermatol Ther.* 2009;22(4):279-292.

26. Argenziano G, Fabbrocini G, Delfino M. Epiluminescence microscopy. A new approach to in vivo detection of *Sarcoptes scabiei. Arch Dermatol.* 1997;133:751-753.

27. Dupuy A, Dehen L, Bourrat E, et al. Accuracy of standard dermoscopy for diagnosing scabies. *J Am Acad Dermatol.* 2007;56: 53-62.

28. Walter B, Heukelbach J, Fengler G, et al. Comparison of dermoscopy, skin scraping, and the adhesive tape test for the diagnosis of scabies in a resource-poor setting. *Arch Dermatol.* 2011;147: 468-473.

29. Park JH, Kim CW, Kim SS. The diagnostic accuracy of dermoscopy for scabies. *Ann Dermatol.* 2012;24:194.

30. James W, Berger T, Elston D. Diseases Resulting from Fungi and Yeast. In: *Andrews Diseases of the Skin.* 10th ed. *Philadelphia: Elsevier;* 2006:15:311-312.

31. Lekkas D, Ioannides D, Lazaridou E, et al. Dermatoscopy of tinea corporis. *J Eur Acad Dermatol Venereol.* 2020;34:e278-e280.

32. Lallas A, Errichetti Enzo, Ioannidis D. *Dermoscopy in General Dermatology.* CRC Press, Taylor & Francis Group; 2019.

33. Errichetti E, Lallas A, eds. *Dermoscopy in General Dermatology for Skin of Color.* 1st ed. CRC Press; 2022.

SECTION THREE

Advanced Procedures

SECTION OUTLINE

20 Biopsies and Excisions in Challenging Locations

21 Flaps

22 Ultrasound in Dermatology

20 Biopsies and Excisions in Challenging Locations

RICHARD P. USATINE, MD

SUMMARY

■ There are several challenging locations for performing biopsies and excisions related to controlling bleeding, risks of causing vital organ damage, and concerns for cosmetic outcomes.

■ This chapter provides tips for surgery in the following locations: scalp, periocular, nose, ears, lips, oral, genitalia, and soles of the feet.

■ It is safe to use epinephrine in all locations for skin surgery, and it is especially helpful in the challenging locations we address in this chapter.

There are several challenging locations for performing biopsies and excisions. Some of the challenges include difficulties controlling bleeding, risk of causing vital organ damage, and concerns for cosmetic outcomes. In this chapter we will provide tips for surgery in the following locations:

■ Scalp
■ Periocular
■ Nose
■ Ears
■ Lips
■ Oral
■ Genitalia
■ Soles of the feet

It is safe to use epinephrine in all locations for skin surgery, and it is especially helpful in the challenging locations we address in this chapter.[1-4] It is especially important to wait at least 10 minutes after injecting the lidocaine and epinephrine so that the epinephrine has time to work. This is especially true for the scalp and lips, which are very vascular.

Scalp

CHALLENGES TO OVERCOME

■ Very vascular site, so one may cut into an artery and have a pumping vessel
■ Even without cutting into an artery, the scalp is very vascular, and hemostasis can be challenging.
■ Hair can get in the way of cutting and sewing.
■ It is difficult to dress the resultant wound when hair is present.

PEARLS TO APPROACH THE SCALP

■ Give the epinephrine time to work after injecting lidocaine with epinephrine – at least 10 minutes.

■ While shave biopsies can remove hair, reassure the patient that usually these are not deep enough to remove the follicles and cause alopecia.
■ When a shave is sufficient for a biopsy, it is less likely to cause the bleeding problems that occur with a punch biopsy.

For punch biopsies and excisions:

■ In a punch biopsy for alopecia, always include affected hair follicles in the specimen.
■ Do the punch to the depth of the upper subcutaneous fat and avoid going deeper to avoid larger vessels that can bleed profusely.
■ Make sure the punch specimen separates easily from the surrounding skin and lift up the plug to cut the specimen off in the subcutaneous fat.
■ Use suture of a color different from the patient's hair color (e.g., blue Prolene if hair is black or black nylon if hair is blond).
■ Keep the tail of suture long enough when doing instrument ties to not get tangled in the hair.
■ If a vessel is pumping vigorously, it might help to put pressure on the unsevered portion of the vessel under the uncut scalp as it approaches the bleeding site. Injecting another 3 mL of lidocaine with epinephrine can help stop or slow the bleeding enough to use electrocoagulation or a suture. See the Steps to Take With Nonstop Bleeding in Surgery (Chapter 4, *Hemostasis*).
■ Pressure dressings can be applied using self-adhering bandages (e.g., Coban) that are wrapped around the head to keep underlying gauze in place.
■ Absorbable gelatin foam sponges such as Surgifoam and Gelfoam can be placed into the hole of a punch biopsy that is not sutured (Figure 4.12). This can be very helpful when performing a punch biopsy on the scalp.[5]

INSTRUMENT TAMPONADE FOR THE SCALP

- Instrument tamponade is a method described by Whalen et al. for hemostasis during a punch biopsy of the scalp.[6] An assistant uses the circular handle of an instrument to surround the punch biopsy site and apply pressure 360 degrees around the site (Figure 4.15).[6] This compresses the surrounding vessels, allowing the surgeon to remove the punch tissue with better visualization and then obtain hemostasis with a suture or absorbable gelatin sponge.[6]

PEARLS SPECIFIC TO PERFORMING TWO PUNCH BIOPSIES ON THE SCALP
(See Video 20.1)

Two punch biopsies are often done for the diagnosis of alopecia. This gives the dermatopathologist a chance to see the hair follicle cut vertically and horizontally.

- When doing two punch biopsies, close the first one before starting the second one because two simultaneously bleeding sites can be harder to deal with than one at a time.
- Use a 4-mm punch because it provides a good specimen size for the pathologist and will allow for a cotton-tipped applicator (CTA) to be inserted into the punch space to prevent bleeding before putting in a hemostatic stitch (Figure 20.1).
- An alternative approach involves using one 6- to 8-mm punch and then bisecting the specimen once it has been removed with a scalpel running in the direction of the hair follicles.
- Place both punches or one bisected punch in a single formalin container so that it can be cut horizontally and vertically for analysis.

PEARLS SPECIFIC TO AN ELLIPTICAL EXCISION
(See Video 20.2)

- Have at least two hemostats ready to clamp bleeding vessels.
- Be prepared to tie off any bleeding vessels with a figure-of-eight using absorbable suture (4-0 Vicryl on a 16-mm reverse cutting needle is a good choice).
- Cut the ellipse down to the loose alveolar tissue (Figure 20.2), which is white below the yellow fat (see Chapter 11, *Elliptical Excision*). To find this level the scalpel will cut close to the bone as this level is just right above the periosteum. This avascular tissue is like white tissue paper with no blood vessels and is easily spread apart with blunt dissection. Cutting the ellipse off at this level will stop the bleeding from the base of the ellipse. This is also the correct level for undermining.
- The worst bleeding problems are often in the walls of the ellipse above this level. The bleeding from the walls will often need to be stopped before the white glistening alveolar tissue can be seen. It is not unusual to need to stop the ellipse wall bleeding while cutting the ellipse so that the white base can be seen. When undermining at this avascular level, there should be no additional bleeding.
- When hair is in the way, it is better not to shave the hair as shaving increases the risk of infection. Other methods to try to keep hair away from the surgical site include using hair clips and petroleum jelly. Snipping the hairs with a scissor can help keep them out of the way without increasing the risk of postoperative infections (Figure 20.3).
- Try to do all closures with a single external layer as deep sutures may compromise the integrity of the hair follicles and lead to unintended hair loss.

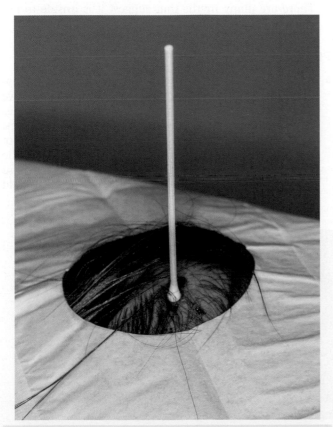

Figure 20.1 After the first of two 4-mm punch biopsies on the scalp is performed a cotton-tipped applicator is used for temporary hemostasis. (Copyright Richard P. Usatine, MD.)

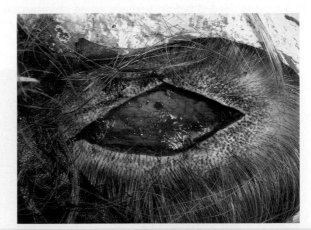

Figure 20.2 Loose alveolar tissue visible during the elliptical excision of a BCC on the scalp. Note that it is somewhat shiny and white. It is below the galea aponeurotica and above the periosteum and can look and feel like tissue paper. This is the most avascular layer of the scalp and the best layer for undermining. Cutting down to this layer will diminish bleeding during scalp surgery. (Copyright Richard P. Usatine, MD.)

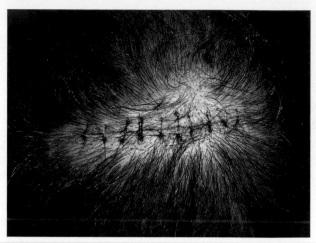

Figure 20.3 Note how some of the hairs around the scalp incision were snipped (not shaved) to make it easier to suture the defect after a nevus sebaceous was excised. (Copyright Richard P. Usatine, MD.)

Periocular

CHALLENGES TO OVERCOME

- Concerns with cutting the globe and the eyelid margins
- Concerns about getting aluminum chloride and chlorhexidine into the eye or having a spark from electrosurgery contact the globe

PEARLS

- Plan biopsies and excisions to be as far from the globe as possible.
- It is safe to prep the eyelids with an alcohol wipe prior to injecting anesthesia.
- Use the orbital rim as a protection when injecting local anesthesia and cutting with the scalpel. This is accomplished by moving the skin so that it is as much over the orbital rim as possible during the invasive portions of the procedure (Figure 20.4A).
- If a prep is needed before surgery, avoid chlorhexidine and use Betadine. Chlorhexidine can cause damage to the cornea, and Betadine is considered safe and has been used by ophthalmology for years in eye surgeries.
- If aluminum chloride is to be used, then make sure that the CTA has been dried thoroughly after it was dipped into the aluminum chloride. This can be done by sitting the CTA on top of gauze. Then use extreme care so that there is no aluminum chloride running into the eye.
- If electrosurgery is to be used, keep the wattage as low as possible to avoid sparking that could affect the eye and as above shift the skin away from overlying the globe.
- If a lesion suspicious for cancer is touching the eyelid margin (Figure 20.4B), do the shave biopsy of the tissue furthest from the eyelid margin, leaving the eyelid margin undisturbed.
- When surgery around the eye is beyond your level of skill, do not hesitate to refer to a Mohs surgeon, oculoplastic surgeon, or ophthalmologist.

Nose

CHALLENGES TO OVERCOME

- The nose is the most prominent cosmetic portion of the face, so scars and deformities can be very disturbing to patients.
- The nose has many convex surfaces that show indentations and scars more than flat surfaces. Shave biopsies on convex surfaces of the nose such as the nasal ala are likely to leave a visible divot when the lesion is flat.
- There are many myths that suggest it is unsafe to use epinephrine on the nose.

PEARLS

- Always use lidocaine with epinephrine when doing biopsies and surgery on the nose. Multiple studies have shown it to be safe[7] (see Chapter 3, *Anesthesia*). Surgeries of the nose will often demonstrate profuse bleeding even with epinephrine (Figure 20.5). Don't think about not using it. Use a needle attached with a Luer lock to the syringe, as injecting into the thick tissue of the nose requires significant pressure and the needle could

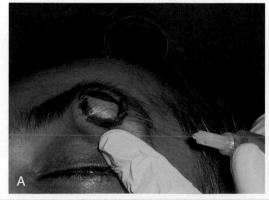
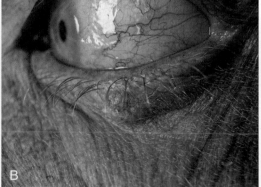

Figure 20.4 (A) The orbital rim is used as a protection when injecting local anesthesia and cutting with the scalpel. This is accomplished by moving the skin so that it is over the orbital rim as much as possible during the invasive portions of the procedure. **(B)** A BCC close to the edge of the eyelid. Do the shave biopsy of the tissue starting furthest from the eyelid margin and leave the eyelid margin undisturbed. (Copyright Richard P. Usatine, MD.)

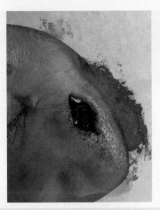

Figure 20.5 The nose is very vascular, and even when epinephrine is used there is plenty of bleeding during surgery as noted in this elliptical excision. It is best to use lidocaine with epinephrine when anesthetizing a lesion for biopsy or excision on the nose. (Copyright Richard P. Usatine, MD.)

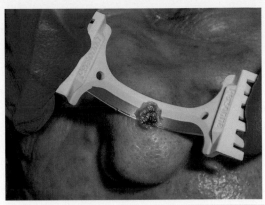

Figure 20.7 A shave biopsy is performed of a pigmented BCC with a DermaBlade on the nose after lidocaine with epinephrine anesthesia was injected. (Copyright Richard P. Usatine, MD.)

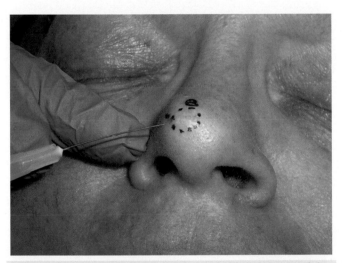

Figure 20.6 Lidocaine and epinephrine injected into the tip of the nose prior to a shave biopsy of a suspected BCC. Note there is blanching due to the hydrostatic pressure, and eventually the epinephrine will help to control bleeding when the shave biopsy is performed. (Copyright Richard P. Usatine, MD.)

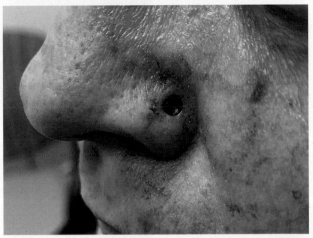

Figure 20.8 A punch biopsy was performed of a suspicious lesion on the nares. It was packed with Surgifoam to avoid possible distortion of the anatomy that might occur with a suture. The punch was chosen because the lesion was small and a shave biopsy would likely leave a divot that would be visible if the lesion turned out to be benign and no further surgery was needed. (Copyright Richard P. Usatine, MD.)

- After confirmation of malignancy, excisions on the nose should most likely be referred to a Mohs surgeon (see Chapter 27).

Ears

CHALLENGES TO OVERCOME

- Concerns over cutting the cartilage (Figure 20.9) and causing deformities of the ear
- Doing procedures on the pinna when the tumor is difficult to reach
- Removing large keloids that are on the pinna but not the earlobe
- Doing surgery on chondrodermatitis nodularis

PEARLS

- It is best to avoid cutting into cartilage when biopsying the ear. On the helical rim a shave biopsy with a razor (DermaBlade) usually works well (Figure 20.10).

otherwise pop off the syringe. Use eye protection when injecting since medication can sometimes spray out of the normal pores of the nose. The nasal tissue should blanch with injection initially from the hydrostatic pressure and then from the epinephrine (Figure 20.6).

- A raised lesion on the nose can often be biopsied with a shave technique keeping flat with the skin and avoiding a divot (Figure 20.7). A No. 15 blade scalpel instead of a flexible razor blade is one option to keep the biopsy flat.
- Flat lesions on the concave surfaces of the nose may be best biopsied with a punch biopsy or small ellipse that can be closed with sutures. Small punch biopsies such as 3 to 4 mm can be closed with minimal distortion to the nose. Sometimes a 3-mm punch may be chosen for cosmetic purposes even though the tissue given to the pathologist is smaller. Another option is to use a hemostatic gel (Figure 20.8) to stop the bleeding rather than a suture (*video 20-7*).

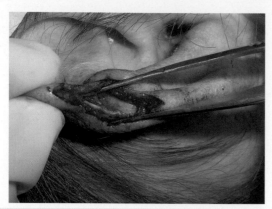

Figure 20.9 An elliptical excision of the lesion on the helix shows the underlying cartilage. (Copyright Richard P. Usatine, MD.)

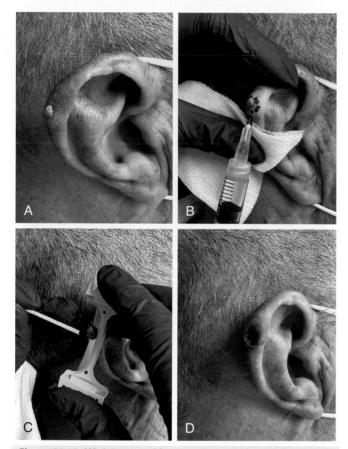

Figure 20.10 (A) A 72-year-old man presents with a tender growth (cutaneous horn) on the right helical rim. **(B)** Local anesthesia with lidocaine and epinephrine. **(C)** Shave biopsy with a DermaBlade. **(D)** Note that the biopsy did not need to cut into the cartilage. The result was an SCC. (Copyright Richard P. Usatine, MD.)

- The inside of the conchal bowl or other portions of the ear that are not easily reachable with a razor blade are best biopsied with a No. 15 scalpel on a handle (Figure 20.11). When that proves to be too difficult, a 2- to 4-mm curette can obtain tissue in tight areas (Figure 20.12). One alternative is to refer directly to ENT or a Mohs surgeon.
- Excisions of keloids on the ear vary by location. Many of the earlobes can be just shaved off, and the base burned

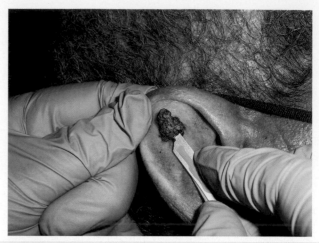

Figure 20.11 A shave biopsy is being performed with a No. 15 blade scalpel on the ear in the location where it may be challenging to use a razor blade. (Copyright Richard P. Usatine, MD.)

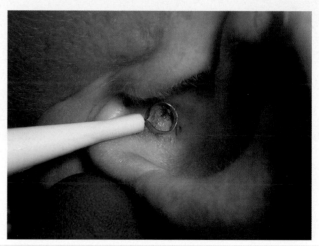

Figure 20.12 This lesion in the ear is not amenable to a biopsy with a razor blade but could be biopsied with a curette or a No. 15 blade. (Copyright Richard P. Usatine, MD.)

with electrocoagulation (see Chapter 23). Larger keloids on the helical rim can be excised, and it is helpful to leave enough normal skin to sew up the defect (Figure 20.13).
- Chondrodermatitis nodularis can be effectively treated with an ellipse (Figure 20.14). See Figure 23.8 for a step-by-step demonstration of the procedure. *See video 20.3.*
- An advanced procedure on the ear is the wedge excision. *See video 20.4.*

Lips

See Video 20.5 for the excision of a mucocele.

CHALLENGES TO OVERCOME

- The lips can be very vascular and bleed excessively with biopsies and excisions.
- It is important to line up the vermillion border after excising a lesion on the outer lip.

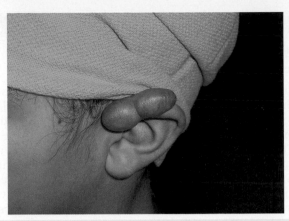

Figure 20.13 The removal of this keloid on the helix is challenging, and sufficient skin must be preserved on either side of the keloid to allow the defect to be closed for primary intention healing. (Copyright Richard P. Usatine, MD.)

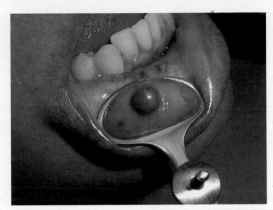

Figure 20.15 A chalazion clamp has been applied to the lip for excision of this fibroma in a manner to avoid excessive bleeding. Once the chalazion clamp has been applied effectively, it is easy to stabilize the lip for surgery. (Copyright Richard P. Usatine, MD.)

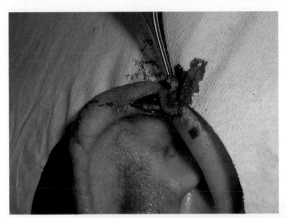

Figure 20.14 Chondrodermatitis nodularis is being removed on the helix, and the cartilage is exposed. Lidocaine and epinephrine was used for local anesthesia. (Copyright Richard P. Usatine, MD.)

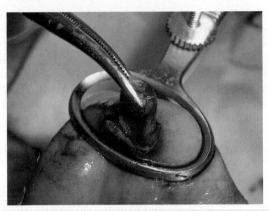

Figure 20.16 A chalazion clamp applied to the lower lip allows for the removal of a mucocele with minimal bleeding. (Copyright Richard P. Usatine, MD.)

Oral

CHALLENGES TO OVERCOME

- The tongue is very vascular, and some lesions can be hard to reach.
- Lesions on the inside cheek can also be hard to reach.
- Most healthcare providers, aside from oral surgeons, have had little to no training in doing biopsies inside the mouth.

PEARLS

Oral Biopsies

- Use epinephrine with lidocaine for local anesthesia and wait at least 10 minutes.
- Hemostasis can be obtained using topical aluminum chloride and/or electrocoagulation.
- Aluminum chloride is safe to use in the mouth and is considered a preferred method for hemostasis in dental surgery.[10]
- The clinician or an assistant can grasp the tongue with a dry gauze to stabilize it or pull on it to facilitate biopsies, excisions, or suturing.
- Advise the patient not to eat or chew until the anesthetic has worn off.

PEARLS

- Use lidocaine with be careful not to use too much volume because the lip becomes swollen easily and the swelling will persist for days.
- Give the epinephrine at least 10 minutes to work.
- A chalazion clamp can be extremely helpful due to its tourniquet effect and it allows the surgeon or assistant to stabilize the area being cut during an excision (Figure 20.15).[8,9]
- The ones used for dermatologic purposes are larger than the ones used by ophthalmologists to remove a chalazion from the eyelids.
- Chalazion clamps come in different sizes and shapes, so it is helpful to have at least two sizes available in the office. The size we use most often is 12×21 mm, but other sizes and shapes can be useful (Figure 20.16).
- The chalazion clamp can be used to stabilize the lip while giving anesthesia and then kept on during the surgery for hemostasis and stabilization.
- Soft absorbable sutures such as Vicryl are more comfortable for use on the lip. Silk is another option.

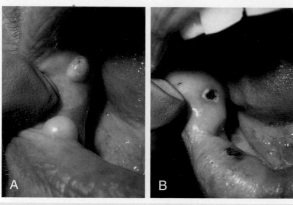

Figure 20.17 (A) Two fibromas are visible on the lower lip. **(B)** After local anesthesia with lidocaine and epinephrine, the fibromas were shaved off, and the base treated with electrocoagulation. (Copyright Richard P. Usatine, MD.)

- A razor blade or No. 15 scalpel works well for these oral benign fibromas (Figure 20.17). Electrosurgery was used for hemostasis.
- The biopsy of flat lesions on the cheek (e.g., oral leukoplakia) are usually performed with a punch instrument (Figure 20.18a). While the cheek appears such that you might go through from the inside to the outside this should not occur. The punch biopsy does not need to be driven all the way to the hilt to get adequate tissue and therefore will not go through the muscle and the skin on the other side. Hemostasis can be obtained with aluminum chloride and/or electrocoagulation.
- In this biopsy of a lesion suspicious for SCC, a chalazion clamp was used to stabilize the area and help with hemostasis during the procedure (Figure 20.18B and C). Another hemostasis option is to use a hemostatic gelatin sponge (Figure 20.18D).

Lesions on the inside of the cheek

- Suturing the buccal mucosa may be challenging unless the biopsy is close to the oral opening. Soft braided suture (Vicryl or silk) is less irritating in the mouth than monofilament suture.
- The tongue can be biopsied after sufficient lidocaine and epinephrine are injected. Make sure to hold the tongue with a 4 × 4 gauze so it does not move away as a reflex during the injection. Shave or punch techniques work well and should be chosen based on the appearance of the lesion (Figure 20.19).
- Fortunately, the oral mucosa and tongue reepithelialize very quickly.

Genitalia

PENIS

Challenges to overcome

- Fear of damaging the penis and causing erectile dysfunction
- Fear that the anesthesia will hurt more here than in other locations

Pearls

- Biopsies of the penis can be performed with a shave biopsy (Figure 20.20).

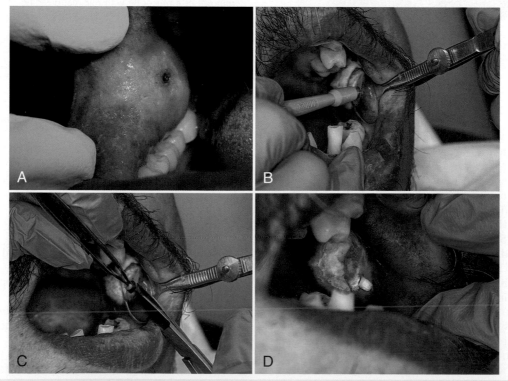

Figure 20.18 Biopsies of the buccal mucosa. **(A)** A punch biopsy was performed on the inner cheek for leukoplakia. Hemostasis was obtained with electrocoagulation, and the punch was left open to heal. **(B)** A chalazion clamp applied around the biopsy site of this suspicious lesion allowed the punch biopsy to be performed with no bleeding. **(C)** Note how the specimen is removed with the benefit of good stabilization from the chalazion clamp and a field that is not obscured by bleeding. **(D)** Hemostatic gelatin sponge was inserted before the chalazion clamp was removed and there was no bleeding after removal of the clamp.

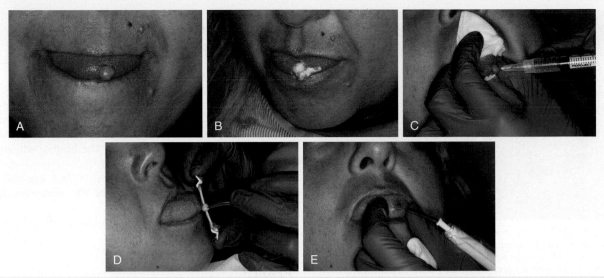

Figure 20.19 (A) New growth on the tongue. **(B)** Topical lidocaine/prilocaine cream applied for initial anesthesia. **(C)** Injecting 1% lidocaine with epinephrine for improved anesthesia and to prevent bleeding. **(D)** Shave biopsy with a DermaBlade. **(E)** Hemostasis with electrosurgery. (Copyright Richard P. Usatine, MD.)

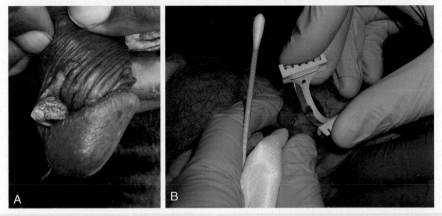

Figure 20.20 (A) This suspicious lesion on the penis was biopsied after local anesthesia was obtained with lidocaine and epinephrine. The shave biopsy was easily performed, and hemostasis was obtained with aluminum chloride and electrocoagulation. This patient with HIV turned out to have an invasive SCC. **(B)** Shave biopsy of a penis with nonhealing ulcers on the glans penis. (Copyright Richard P. Usatine, MD.)

- While this may appear frightening to the patient and surgeon at first, local anesthesia with lidocaine and epinephrine will allow for a painless and simple shave biopsy.
- Generally, a shave biopsy is preferred to a punch biopsy to avoid a deep biopsy that would cut into the corpus cavernosum, the urethra, or large superficial blood vessels.
- Common reasons for biopsy include diagnosing SCC, lichen planus, psoriasis, and lichen sclerosus (Figure 20.21). A DermaBlade or bendable razor works well.
- Large excisions on the penis are best referred to a urologist or Mohs surgeon.

VULVA AND INTROITUS

Challenges to overcome

- Patient and clinician fear over the sensitive and private area involved

Pearls

- Biopsies in this area can be performed as a shave or punch after anesthesia with lidocaine and epinephrine.
- For a punch biopsy, we usually place a suture for hemostasis and to speed healing but second intention healing works well in this location too (Figure 20.22).

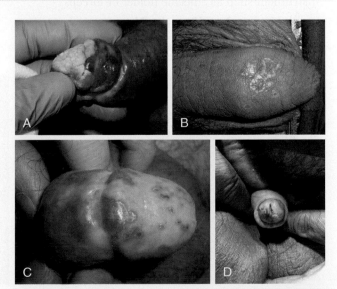

Figure 20.21 Various penile lesions that were biopsied with shave biopsies. **(A)** Leukoplakia and erythroplasia that was diagnosed as SCC after a shave biopsy. **(B)** The patient presented with these annular lesions on the penis and no other skin lesions. Lichen planus was suspected and confirmed with a shave biopsy. **(C)** Psoriasis of the penis proven by shave biopsy. **(D)** Lichen sclerosus proven by shave biopsy. (Copyright Richard P. Usatine, MD.)

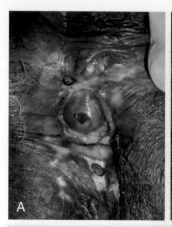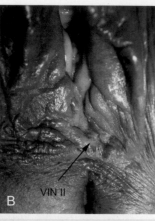

Figure 20.22 **(A)** This patient with a prolapsed uterus also had leukoplakia of the atrophic vulva suspicious for cancer. Two punch biopsies were performed of the most suspicious areas, and both were found to have vulvar intraepithelial neoplasia (VIN2). Hemostasis of these 4-mm punch biopsies was obtained with aluminum chloride and then allowed to heal by second intention. **(B)** A small painful ulcer turned out to be vulvar intraepithelial neoplasia II on punch biopsy. A 3-mm punch biopsy was performed on the edge of the ulcer. (Copyright Richard P. Usatine, MD.)

- Bleeding and hematoma formation can occur due to the vascular nature of the vulva. Have suture available on a needle large enough to encompass the biopsy site and underneath the defect, in case a hemostatic stitch is required.
- The tissue here may be very mobile, and usual methods of tissue stabilization during a shave biopsy may be less effective. Pinching the skin after anesthesia is still the simplest method to keep the skin from moving back and forth during the cutting. Other methods involve placing a skin hook or suture in the skin to be cut and pulling up on it to stabilize the skin. Pull up on the skin for biopsy with the skin hook or suture and cut the piece for pathology. A substitute skin hook can be created by carefully bending the needle used for anesthesia with a surgical instrument such as a needle holder or forceps.

Sole of the Foot

(See Videos 20.6 and 20.7)

CHALLENGES TO OVERCOME

- Biopsies in this area are problematic because the patient will most likely need to walk on the site afterward.
- Shave biopsies are one option, but the stratum corneum is thick, and it is possible that the biopsy will not yield useful tissue.
- Punch biopsies are an alternative but are difficult to close because of the tension of the skin and may not provide enough tissue.
- An elliptical biopsy or excision can be daunting for the inexperienced clinician.

PEARLS

- Use a dermatoscope to avoid the biopsy of benign nevi (see Chapter 18, *Dermoscopy*).
- An incisional biopsy of the fusiform or elliptical shape is ideal for providing sufficient tissue, and the geometry is better for a closure (Figure 20.23).
- Punch biopsies with suture closures are possible despite the fact that the tension on the suture will be greater than in other areas. *See video 20.6.* If the suture tears, the wound will still heal by secondary intention.
- One option is to perform a punch biopsy and leave it open to heal. A hemostatic gel or foam can be placed (Figure 20.24). Otherwise, aluminum chloride or electrosurgery may be used to stop the bleeding.
- It is possible to obtain a deep enough shave for an adequate diagnosis (Figure 20.25). *See video 20.7.* If the pathology of any partial biopsy is not as expected, a full sample will be needed.
- If a referral is difficult to obtain, an attempt to get a deeper shave biopsy or adequate punch may be step one before needing to resort to a referral (Figure 20.26).

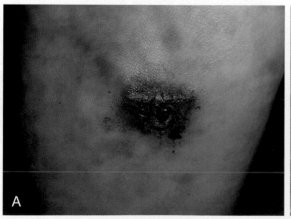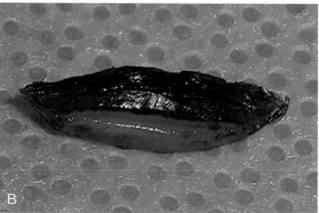

Figure 20.23 **(A)** This suspicious pigmented lesion on the sole of a Black man needed a biopsy. A punch biopsy was performed at a previous visit, and the pathologist reported that there was insufficient tissue for diagnosis. This photograph was taken after an incisional biopsy was performed with a narrow ellipse. **(B)** The tissue before sending to pathology. This sample was adequate. (Copyright Richard P. Usatine, MD.)

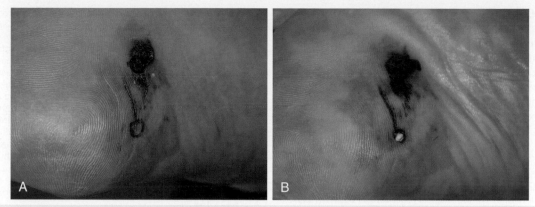

Figure 20.24 (A) Suspected acral lentiginous melanoma on the sole of this Black man. Two punch biopsy sites were marked and performed a with 4-mm punch. **(B)** Hemostatic gelatin foam was placed in the punch biopsy sites for hemostasis. (Copyright Richard P. Usatine, MD.)

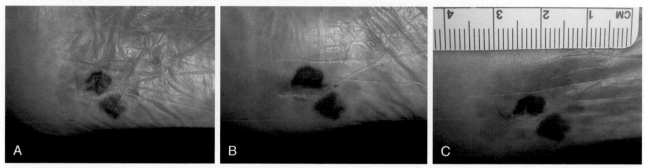

Figure 20.25 (A) This 63-year-old Hispanic man presented with this large multicolored pigmented area on the sole. **(B)** A deep shave biopsy was performed to include the three areas of abnormal pigmentation. **(C)** The biopsy area is healing well. The sample was adequate to diagnose melanoma in situ. (Copyright Richard P. Usatine, MD.)

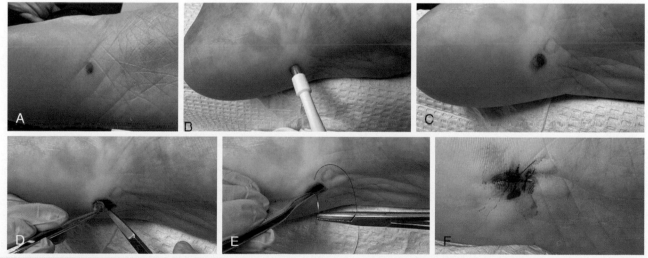

Figure 20.26 Punch biopsy
(A) New and growing pigmented lesion on the sole of the foot
(B) 6.mm punch biopsy performed.
(C) The punch has encircled the whole lesion.
(D) Carefully cutting the base of the punch
(E) Suturing the punch with 4-0 Prolene
(F) Even with multiple interrupted sutures and a figure-of-eight suture the punch biopsy is not completely closed due to the tension. This was adequate for wound healing. The final diagnosis was a benign melanocytic nevus.
(Copyright Richard P. Usatine, MD.)

Conclusion

Performing biopsies and excisions in challenging areas is rewarding as it allows you to do the surgeries that patients need in your office. This can result in earlier diagnoses of skin cancers and earlier reassurance when there is no cancer and help patients that would otherwise need to wait to see another consultant.

References

1. Häfner HM, Röcken M, Breuninger H. Epinephrine-supplemented local anesthetics for ear and nose surgery: clinical use without complications in more than 10,000 surgical procedures. *J Dtsch Dermatol Ges.* 2005;3(3):195-199.
2. Ilicki J. Safety of epinephrine in digital nerve blocks: a literature review. *J Emerg Med.* 2015;49(5):799-809.
3. Krunic AL, Wang LC, Soltani K, Weitzul S, Taylor RS. Digital anesthesia with epinephrine: an old myth revisited. *J Am Acad Dermatol.* 2004;51(5):755-759.
4. Prabhakar H, Rath S, Kalaivani M, Bhanderi N. Adrenaline with lidocaine for digital nerve blocks. *Cochrane Database Syst Rev.* 2015; 3:CD010645.
5. Hansen LM, Wu DJ, Liu D, Aires DJ, Elston DM. Gelatin foam instead of suturing for punch biopsies on the scalp. *J Am Acad Dermatol.* 2021;84(1):e15-e16. doi:10.1016/j.jaad.2020.07.083.
6. Whalen JG, Gehris RP, Kress DW, English JC. Surgical pearl: instrument tamponade for punch biopsy of the scalp. *J Am Acad Dermatol.* 2005;52(2):347-348. doi:10.1016/j.jaad.2004.06.042.
7. Seiverling EV, Ahrns HT, Bacik LC, Usatine R. Biopsies for skin cancer detection: dispelling the myths. *J Fam Pract.* 2018;67(5):270-274.
8. Garcia RL, Davis CM. Chalazion clamp for dermatological surgery. *Arch Dermatol.* 1970;102(6):693. doi:10.1001/archderm.102. 6.693.
9. Jha AK, Ganguly S. Chalazion clamp in dermatology revisited. *Indian J Dermatol Venereol Leprol.* 2015;81(3):280-281. doi:10.4103/0378-6323.154797.
10. Khater AGA, Al-Hamed FS, Safwat EM, Hamouda MMA, Shehata MSA, Scarano A. Efficacy of hemostatic agents in endodontic surgery: a systematic review and network meta-analysis. *J Evid Based Dent Pract.* 2021;21(3):101540. doi:10.1016/j.jebdp.2021. 101540.

21 *Flaps*

RYAN O'QUINN, MD, and RICHARD P. USATINE, MD

SUMMARY	■ Although the surgeon should always first consider primary linear closure of a skin defect, there are many circumstances in which a skin flap may be the ideal choice for reconstruction.
	■ The chapter focuses on random pattern flaps that are divided into advancement, transposition, and rotation flaps.
	■ The following terms are explained to better understand the use of flaps: primary defect, secondary defect, primary motion, secondary motion, flap tip, flap pedicle, key suture, and standing cones.
	■ The advancement flaps include single pedicle flaps, bilateral advancement flaps, T-plasty, L-plasty, and island pedicle flaps.
	■ Rotation flaps include the single rotation flap and the bilateral rotation flap.
	■ Transposition flaps include the rhombic flap and the bilobed flap.
	■ Performing cutaneous flaps is an advanced skill that takes considerable experience to master and should begin under the guidance of a mentor.

Overview

The proper development and implementation of the skin flap is a key skill in reconstruction of cutaneous wounds. Flaps may be employed for reconstructing wounds created by trauma or wounds created by the extirpation of benign or malignant lesions of the skin or subcutaneous tissues. Although the surgeon should always first consider primary linear closure of a skin defect, there are many circumstances in which a skin flap may be the ideal choice for reconstruction.[1,2]

Skin flaps may be chosen instead of a primary linear closure in order to:

- Recruit skin from areas of lower tension to areas of higher tension
- Prevent the retraction of a free margin such as the lip or eyelid
- Avoid distortion of critical normal anatomy such as pulling up the nasal tip
- Maintain a reconstructive maneuver in a single cosmetic subunit
- Realign wound closure lines in a more cosmetically acceptable manner
- Shorten the final closure length

In addition, flaps can also perform very well in situations that would not be ideal for skin grafts; flaps can be employed to fill deeper defects that would lead to poor contours with skin grafting, or to cover anatomical structures that may prevent the use of grafts (bone, cartilage, or tendon).

It is critical to understand the advantages and disadvantages of the different types of flaps rather than apply a "cookbook" approach to flap planning. When selecting the best choice of flap for a particular defect, the relative benefits and risks of each flap should be considered beforehand. A deep understanding of both flap theory and anatomy can lead to the best results.

Terminology

Flaps can be classified by their blood supply into *axial pattern flaps*, which have a larger typically named artery supplying their vascular needs (such as the paramedian forehead flap, which depends on the supratrochlear arteries of the medial lower forehead), and *random pattern flaps*, which rely on the unnamed vasculature of the dermis, subcutaneous fat, and in some cases the superficial musculature of facial structures. Axial pattern flaps are often quite large and often require more than one stage to complete and are typically only performed by the most experienced surgeons. Most skin flaps used to repair facial defects following skin cancer removal are random pattern flaps. Because the blood supply of the skin and soft tissues of the scalp, face, and neck is so rich, the random pattern flaps enjoy very high rates of success. These local random pattern flaps are by far the more commonly employed flaps and will be the focus of this chapter. These flaps are smaller and more manageable and can be successfully performed by specialties outside of plastic surgery.

The random pattern flap is further classified by its movement. The three basic types of movement are (Figure 21.1):

1. Advancement
2. Transposition
3. Rotation

The initial wound that is to be reconstructed is the *primary defect*, and here it refers to the result of the removal of a skin tumor (Figure 21.2). Once a flap has been advanced, transposed, or rotated into position to close the primary defect, the wound that remains behind at the donor site of the flap is the *secondary defect*. The *primary motion* of a flap is the movement that the flap makes when it advances, transposes, or rotates into and closes the primary defect (Figure 21.2). The *secondary motion* is the movement that the tissue adjacent to and surrounding the flap makes when

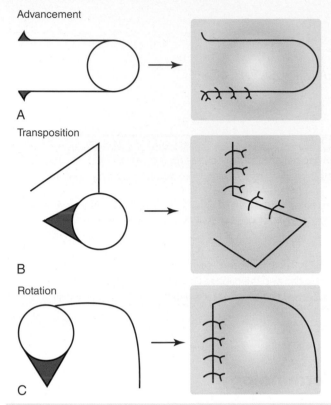

Advancement

A

Transposition

B

Rotation

C

Figure 21.1 The three basic types of random pattern flap movement are **(A)** advancement, **(B)** transposition, and **(C)** rotation. (Courtesy of Ryan O'Quinn, MD.)

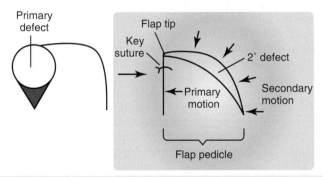

Primary defect

Flap tip

Key suture

2° defect

Primary motion

Secondary motion

Flap pedicle

Figure 21.2 The initial wound to be reconstructed is the primary defect, and the wound that remains behind at the donor site of the flap is the secondary defect. The primary motion of a flap is the movement that the flap makes when it advances, transposes, or rotates into and closes the primary defect. The secondary motion is the movement that the tissue adjacent to and surrounding the flap makes when the final defect is closed. (Courtesy of Ryan O'Quinn, MD.)

the final defect is closed. Both the primary and secondary motion of a flap are important in proper flap design. The very end of the flap that fills the primary defect, farthest from the donor site, is the *flap tip*. The *flap pedicle* is that portion of the flap that connects it to the surrounding skin and is the conduit for the vascular supply of the flap. The *key suture* of a local flap is the location in which the first suture is typically placed to provide the initial correct alignment of

a flap to fill the primary defect and to direct additional placement of sutures to close the secondary defect. *Standing cutaneous cones* (dog-ears) are areas of local tissue redundancy that occur in wound closure but that can be minimized, eliminated, or moved to more cosmetically advantageous locations by the correct choice and meticulous planning of a flap.

Use of Flaps Following Treatment of Malignant Tumors

While it is always important that malignant tumor clearance is achieved, it is even more critical prior to employing flap reconstruction. If a flap is used and later the surgical margins are determined to be positive histologically for persistence of tumor, it may lower the cure rate for a subsequent excision due to the loss of the true surgical margins by the significant movement of tissue that occurs in flap mobilization. In addition, using a flap prematurely may "burn bridges" and prevent further reconstruction using adjacent tissue if a reexcision is necessary. A potentially worse scenario can arise if there is a persistence of tumor that is buried under a flap. Such tumors can grow to great size and depth before they become clinically obvious and may lead to severe morbidity and need for extensive reconstruction at the time of reexcision. Mohs micrographic surgery can achieve cure rates up to 99% in primary tumors and is the gold standard for margin clearance of cutaneous malignancy and should be strongly considered for more aggressive tumors or those in critical anatomic areas. Margin control of skin tumors can also be achieved through standard frozen section pathology, but if this is not available in the primary care setting, wounds can be bandaged following tumor excision with a plan for delayed repair following clearance of the tumor with permanent section pathology.

Contraindications

Although there are no absolute contraindications, factors to consider when planning for the use of a flap include underlying disorders that may lead to increased rates of intraoperative or postoperative complications. These include patients who are highly anticoagulated or with bleeding diatheses who may experience troublesome intraoperative bleeding or postoperative hematoma formation. Patients who smoke excessively experience a higher risk of flap tip necrosis and flap failure and encouraging smoking cessation in the perioperative and postoperative course is helpful to achieve the best healing. The use of flaps must also be carefully weighed in those patients who may have underlying skin conditions that can lead to increased complications. Decreased flexibility and therefore impaired movement of skin can be seen in patients with extensive scarring from burns or other injuries, previous radiotherapy, or an underlying skin disease such as scleroderma. Decreased perfusion of skin leading to flap failure or infection can be seen in conditions such as diabetes mellitus, lung disease, or poor circulation secondary to atherosclerosis, especially in peripheral areas. Finally, the use of a flap may not be possible in patients with extremely thin skin that will not bear the stresses of flap movement, such as elderly patients with extreme photodamage or long-term users of corticosteroids.

Planning the Flap

Careful planning is essential for successful flap reconstruction. Following confirmed tumor clearance of the surgical margins, the primary defect is lightly infiltrated with local anesthetic so that it may be manipulated without patient discomfort. Local anesthetic with epinephrine can be used in flap surgery without fear of compromising the flap. It is important that the surgeon not immediately proceed with an anticipated flap procedure before carefully considering the ramifications of tissue movement for surrounding structures. At this point the defect should be evaluated for surrounding tissue laxity, and any potential reservoirs of loose skin that may be recruited for repair. This may be done by pinching the skin with gloved fingers, but the fingers may be inadequate in more inflexible areas, and a skin hook is a very useful surgical instrument to gauge tissue movement without tissue damage even in large defects of inflexible skin. Careful flap planning will then include not only the evaluation of possible sources of skin for flap creation but also the consideration of nearby anatomical structures that could be distorted by either the primary or secondary movement of the flap. Especially vulnerable areas are the free margins of the eyelids, lips, and nasal tip. The vectors of flap movement should be placed perpendicular to such structures, lest tissue movement distort their anatomy.

Tissue texture and color should be matched whenever possible, as a flap from similar adjacent skin will lead to the best results. A defect on the nose should be filled with similar-appearing skin from the nose instead of skin from a flap on the cheek. Finally, anticipated tissue redundancies from wound closure should be considered, with thought to how these redundancies or dog-ears may be best camouflaged along anatomic borders. The proposed flap should always

be drawn out prior to incision, and this may be done with a surgical marker.

Advancement Flap

CONCEPTUAL

The primary motion of the advancement flap is the sliding of the flap, usually in a single linear vector as it advances into the primary defect. This sliding motion may be unidirectional (single advancement flap) or bidirectional (double advancement flap).[3] Although there are several variations of this type of flap, the two main benefits of the advancement flap are:

1. Redirection of tissue movement – It may be critical to keep the repair within a single cosmetic subunit or to selectively move certain skin into the primary defect. This can be helpful when a defect lies within an eyebrow or the mustache, and the advancing primary motion can restore uninterrupted hair growth (Figure 21.3).
2. Reorientation of tissue redundancy – When closing a skin defect, tissue redundancies (dog-ears) are inevitable. A properly employed advancement flap can redistribute tissue redundancies to more acceptable locations that may be far from the primary defect. This is useful in moving the tissue redundancies away from a certain structure (lips or eyebrow) or aligning them along the boundary of an anatomic subunit (alar crease) to camouflage the scar (Figure 21.4).

It is important to realize that the purpose of the advancement flap is not to increase laxity to close a wound under high tension. Although it may appear that an advancement flap may provide superior tissue movement over a primary linear closure, this is rarely the case. If more mobility is needed, another flap should be considered. In preoperative planning, if a defect cannot be approximated primarily by pinching the skin or mobilizing the skin edges with hooks, an advancement flap will not be the best option because the amount of additional tissue movement that it provides over primary closure is often minimal.

Advancement flap
Redirection of tissue movement

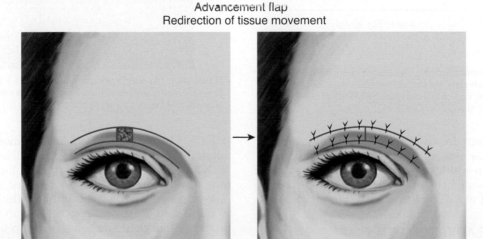

Figure 21.3 Double advancement flap (bidirectional) within an eyebrow to restore uninterrupted hair growth after resecting a tumor within the eyebrow. (Courtesy of Ryan O'Quinn, MD.)

Advancement flap
Reorientation of tissue redundancy

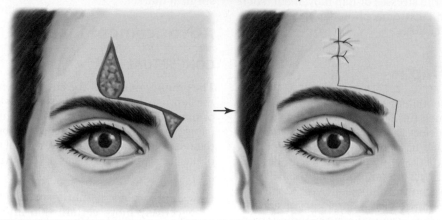

Figure 21.4 Reorientation of tissue redundancy to a more acceptable location away from the primary defect. (Courtesy of Ryan O'Quinn, MD.)

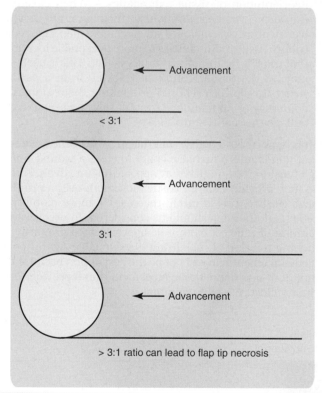

Figure 21.5 Advancement flaps are also limited by their blood supply, so the length-to-width ratio should not exceed 3:1. A long, thin advancement flap in violation of this ratio runs a high risk of distal flap tip necrosis. (Courtesy of Ryan O'Quinn, MD.)

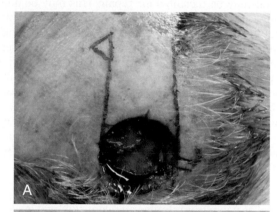

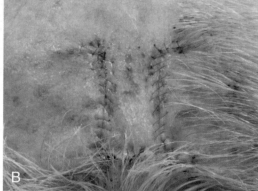

Figure 21.6 (A) Single-pedicle advancement flap (U-plasty) on the forehead may fit in well with horizontal relaxed skin tension lines in this area. **(B)** The flap is sutured in place. (Courtesy of Ryan O'Quinn, MD.)

Advancement flaps are also limited by their blood supply. The pedicle of skin and soft tissue must not be compromised. A length-to-width ratio should ideally not exceed 3:1. A long, thin advancement flap in violation of this ratio runs a high risk of distal flap tip necrosis (Figure 21.5).

SINGLE-PEDICLE ADVANCEMENT FLAP (U-PLASTY)

The classic form of the advancement flap is the single-pedicle advancement flap, also known as the U-plasty

(Figure 21.6). This is an older technique that has been advocated for repairs on the forehead, as it may fit in well with horizontal relaxed skin tension lines in this area. It may also be used on the sideburn or eyebrow to move hair-bearing skin together and hide the scars in the hair. A significant disadvantage to the flap is that it creates numerous surgical lines and, in an area such as the forehead, may provide an inferior surgical result than a primary linear closure. It has been advocated as well for use on the glabella and nasal bridge, but other flaps are nearly always preferable in these areas.

BILATERAL ADVANCEMENT FLAP (H-PLASTY)

The H-plasty flap is similar to the classic single-pedicle advancement flap except that another pedicled advancement flap is created on the opposite side of the defect. The two flaps need not necessarily be symmetrical or parallel but may be curved or slightly shortened on one side as anatomic structures allow. Unfortunately, this flap creates even more incisions than the single-pedicle advancement flap, and therefore its clinical usefulness is limited. This flap could be useful for the closure of a defect in the eyebrow, as the lines could be camouflaged along the brows edges (Figure 21.7). It may also be reserved for situations in which a single pedicle is first employed and judged inadequate to close a defect, at which time a second pedicle is created to provide farther tissue movement. Occasionally when a wound lies between two forehead wrinkles, a bilateral H-plasty flap can be useful to camouflage the closure in these two wrinkles.

T-PLASTY (O-T FLAP)

This bilateral advancement flap has great utility in facial reconstruction. It is best suited for the repair of defects at the edge of a free margin, such as the lip, or at the junction of two cosmetic subunits when it is preferable to keep the repair from crossing the junction, such as when closing a chin defect and preventing the closure from crossing the mental crease. The final suture line, in the T configuration, is a result of a Burow's triangle excision on one side of the defect, which is approximately the length of the defect, and two incisions (each the width of the defect) on the other side to create the bilateral flaps. These incisions need not be completely straight and can be somewhat curved and tailored to the necessary skin tension lines (Figure 21.8). The resulting redundancies along the flap edges can be sewn out by the rule of halves or resolved with small Burow's triangle excisions. The O to T flap can be utilized also for wounds above the eyebrow (to prevent extension of a Burow's triangle into the eyebrow) or wounds on the upper cutaneous lip inferior to the nose (to prevent involvement of the nose in the closure).

L-PLASTY

The L-plasty is a single advancement flap that is employed to redirect tissue redundancy and maintain the repair in a single cosmetic subunit. The tissue redundancy has been distributed along the edge of the advancing flap and thereby avoid cutting into an adjacent cosmetic unit such as the lip (Figure 21.9). The L-plasty can be considered to be simply one-half of an O to T bilateral advancement flap.

Advancement Flap

Step-by-Step Instructions (Figure 21.10)

a) Moderately large wound resulting from the removal of a BCC using the Mohs surgical technique. The location immediately above the eyebrow presents a dilemma. Horizontal linear closure would result in unnatural elevation of the eyebrow margin. Vertical linear closure would extend the Burow's triangle through the brow into the upper eyelid.

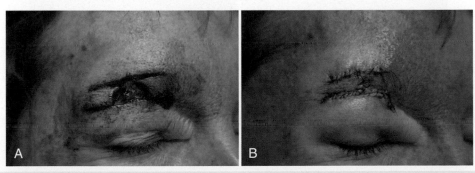

Figure 21.7 Bilateral advancement flap (H-plasty) could be useful for the closure of a defect in the eyebrow, as the lines could be camouflaged along the brows edges. **(A)** The "H" is cut. **(A)** The "H" is sutured in preserving the eyebrow anatomy. (Courtesy of Ryan O'Quinn, MD.)

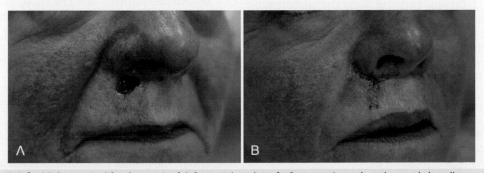

Figure 21.8 T-plasty (O-T flap) is best suited for the repair of defects at the edge of a free margin, such as the nasal ala or lip, or at the junction of two cosmetic subunits. **(A)** The "O" shaped defect. **(B)** The "T" shaped repair. (Courtesy of Ryan O'Quinn, MD.)

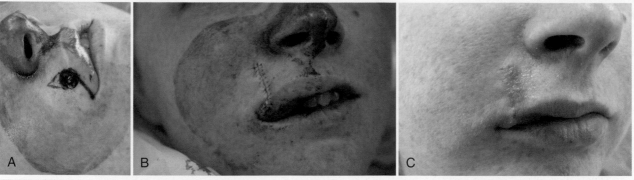

Figure 21.9 L-plasty is a single advancement flap that is employed to redirect tissue redundancy and maintain the repair in a single cosmetic subunit. In this case, the purpose of this flap is to avoid cutting beyond the vermillion border into the lip. **(A)** The defect on the lip margin. **(B)** The "L" shaped repair. **(C)** Repair healing one week after surgery. (Courtesy of Ryan O'Quinn, MD.)

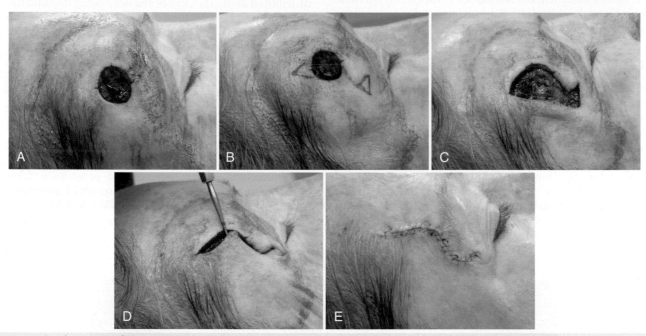

Figure 21.10 Advancement flap:
(A) Circular wound from the removal of a BCC using the Mohs surgical technique.
(B) The Burow's triangle is drawn superiorly, and the inferior edge of the flap is created running along the lateral margin of the brow. A smaller Burow's triangle is drawn to anticipate skin redundancy.
(C) The flap is incised, and both Burow's triangles are removed.
(D) A skin hook is used here to illustrate the location of the buried key suture for this flap.
(E) The final result achieves excellent closure of the primary defect without anatomical distortion. (Courtesy of Ryan O'Quinn, MD.)

b) A laterally based advancement flap is planned. The Burow's triangle is drawn superiorly, and the inferior edge of the flap is created running along the lateral margin of the brow. A smaller Burow's triangle is drawn to anticipate skin redundancy.

c) The flap is incised, and both Burow's triangles are removed. The level of undermining in this area is fairly superficial with the flap containing epidermis, dermis, and several millimeters of subcutaneous fat. This is to avoid injury to the underlying superficial temporal branch of the facial nerve. The depth of most advancement flaps is to the subcutaneous adipose tissue. All surrounding wound edges are undermined. Hemostasis was achieved with electrosurgery.

d) A skin hook is used here to illustrate the location of the buried key suture for this flap. This initial suture advances the tissue into the defect and shows proper alignment of the final closure. At this point, the deep absorbable sutures are placed to secure the flap and hold tension. Once the flap is in place, a running polypropylene suture is placed to nicely approximate epidermal edges.

e) The final result achieves excellent closure of the primary defect without anatomical distortion.

Island Pedicle Flap

CONCEPTUAL

Although the primary movement is advancement of tissue into the defect, the island pedicle flap is so fundamentally different from the previously described advancement flaps

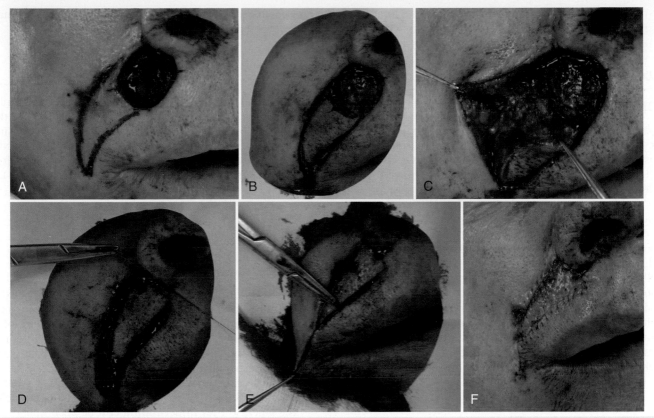

Figure 21.11 Island pedicle flap:
(A) Large defect of the upper cutaneous lip. The lines are drawn such that the flap fits nicely into the nasolabial fold laterally. The curvilinear shape of the flap assures that the secondary defect will be closed horizontally to avoid raising the lip.
(B) Here the flap is incised along planned lines.
(C) All surrounding wound edges are undermined. The pedicle is not undermined.
(D) The key suture is placed in the center of the advancing edge of the island pedicle flap.
(E) The secondary defect is then closed with a buried suture at the inferior tip of the flap. Vector of tension here is horizontal, avoiding pull on the upper lip.
(F) The final result reconstructs the upper cutaneous lip with no anatomic distortion (perioperative swelling will resolve).
(Courtesy of Ryan O'Quinn, MD.)

that it occupies a class of its own. Unlike the other advancement flaps, it does provide significantly increased tissue movement over primary closure. Uniquely, the epidermis and dermis of the island pedicle flap is completely severed from the surrounding skin, and instead the pedicle is an "island" of rich vascular subcutaneous and muscle tissue underneath the flap. Because of the robust blood supply, it is very rare to experience ischemic necrosis of a properly designed and executed island pedicle flap. The flap can avoid the 3:1 rule of advancement flaps and move a thinner flap over a greater distance. It may be an ideal choice in patients with poorly perfused skin or smokers. Another advantage of the flap is that it may limit reconstruction of a large or complex defect to a single cosmetic subunit. This is the case in the area of the lateral upper cutaneous lip, where the flap is the most useful. Island pedicle flaps are also utilized on the nasal bridge and eyebrow.

Island Pedicle Flap

Step-by-Step Instructions (Figure 21.11)

a) Reconstruction of a large defect of the upper cutaneous lip presents a particular challenge. Care must be taken to avoid anatomic distortion of the upper lip and nasal ala. An island pedicle flap is drawn inferiorly and lateral to the angle of the mouth. This will allow the lax skin of the area to be moved upward into the primary defect. The lines are drawn such that the flap fits nicely into the nasolabial fold laterally. The curvilinear shape of the flap assures that the secondary defect will be closed horizontally to avoid raising the lip.

b) Here the flap is incised along planned lines. The depth of incision is to the deep subcutaneous layer. The central deep portion of the flap is left undisturbed to avoid compromising vascular supply. The flap tip and primary defect edges are trimmed so that the advancing edge of the island flap fits nicely.

c) All surrounding wound edges are undermined. Here the richly supplied pedicle is visible. It is not undermined to avoid vascular compromise. Hemostasis is achieved with electrosurgery.

d) The key suture is placed in the center of the advancing edge of the island pedicle flap. As the flap is advanced, it fills the primary defect and creates a smaller secondary defect lateral to the angle of the mouth.

e) The secondary defect is then closed with a buried suture at the inferior tip of the flap. Vector of tension here is horizontal, avoiding pull on the upper lip.

f) After completion of the layered closure, the final result nicely reconstructs the upper cutaneous lip with no anatomic distortion (perioperative swelling will resolve).

Rotation Flap

CONCEPTUAL

The rotation flap consists of tissue rotating in an arc to fill the primary defect. The rotation flap differs from primary closure and the advancement flap in that the tension is directed not in a single, linear vector but rather from several different directions. Once the flap is put into position with the first key suture, the primary defect is filled, leaving a much longer curvilinear secondary defect. Closing this secondary defect results in the redirection of wound tension, as well as the redirection of tissue redundancy. This redistribution of wound tension is the great advantage of a well-chosen rotation flap. It can recruit significant laxity from surrounding tissue and greatly aid in closing defects under significant tension, such as large, tight scalp defects, or it can result in moving the secondary motion of a flap away from a critical anatomic structure, such as when a rotation flap is used to close a wound in the infraorbital region and prevent downward pull on the free margin of the lower eyelid.[4]

Single Rotation Flap

This is the rotation flap in its most basic form. A single flap is rotated into the defect. A single Burow's triangle is excised to remove tissue redundancy created by primary flap movement (Figure 21.12).

Bilateral O-Z Rotation Flap

The bilateral rotation flap is helpful with wounds under high tension. Often, a wound can be approached with a single rotation flap. If it is inadequate to close a very tight wound, another rotation flap can be incised and rotated in to provide more movement for final wound closure. Often, no Burow's triangle needs to be excised (Figure 21.13).

Rotation Flap

(See Video 21.1)
Step-by-Step Instructions (Figure 21.14)

a) The rotation flap works very well in areas of inflexible skin or wounds under considerable tension where a primary closure may be impossible. Here, a single rotation flap is planned, with a Burow's triangle drawn inferiorly.
b) The rotation flap is incised, and the Burow's triangle removed. The depth of undermining should be in the plane of the subcutaneous adipose for most rotation flaps. On the scalp the flap may be incised down below the galea so that undermining can be accomplished in the relatively avascular loose connective tissue. This can create a thick, hearty flap and avoid unnecessary hemorrhage. Of course, the primary defect will need to be the appropriate depth to accommodate the thickness of

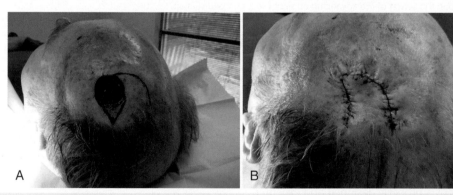

Figure 21.12 (A) A single rotation flap is drawn to repair this scalp defect. A single Burow's triangle is drawn to remove tissue redundancy created by primary flap movement. **(B)** The flap is rotated into the defect and sutured. (Courtesy of Ryan O'Quinn, MD.)

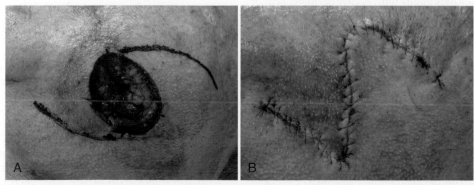

Figure 21.13 (A) Bilateral O-Z rotation flap on the scalp is drawn. **(B)** The flap is sutured and resembles a "Z." (Courtesy of Ryan O'Quinn, MD.)

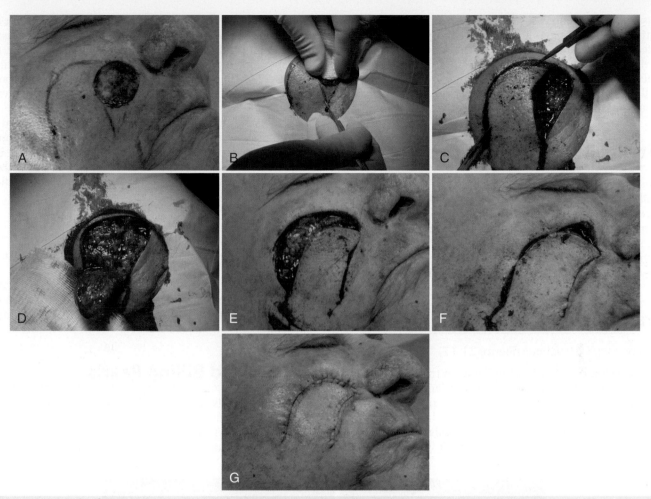

Figure 21.14 Rotation flap
(A) The rotation flap works very well in areas of inflexible skin or wounds under considerable tension where a primary closure may be impossible. Here, a single rotation flap is planned, with a Burow's triangle drawn inferiorly.
(B) The Burow's triangle is incised and removed.
(C) The rotation flap is incised.
(D) The flap and all wound edges are widely undermined and hemostasis achieved with electrosurgery.
(E) The flap is rotated in to fill the primary defect, and the key suture is placed. Note that a long curved secondary defect is created.
(F) The secondary defect is then closed with buried sutures by the "rule of halves." This effectively redistributes the tension from the initial primary defect over a much larger area.
(G) The final result is achieved with running sutures to approximate the epidermis.
(Courtesy of Ryan O'Quinn, MD.)

the flap. All wound edges are widely undermined and hemostasis achieved with electrosurgery.
c) The flap is rotated in to fill the primary defect, and the key suture is placed. Note that a long curved secondary defect is created.
d) The secondary defect is then closed with buried sutures by the "rule of halves." This effectively redistributes the tension from the initial primary defect over a much larger area.

Transposition Flap

CONCEPTUAL

Both the design and tissue movement of the transposition flap is more difficult than with the other random pattern flaps. Like the rotation flap, tissue is harvested from an area of laxity to be used to repair the primary defect, but instead of advancing or rotating into the defect, the flap is transposed over an area (Figure 1B) of normal skin. The great advantage of the transposition flap is its ability to redirect the wound closure tension. A wound inferior to the free margin of the lower eyelid is often at high risk for ectropion. A transposition flap can transpose skin into the defect to close the wound while reorienting the tension parallel to the eyelid margin. Similarly, a wound of the lower nose can often be difficult to close without pulling up on the nasal tip. A transposition flap can be employed to redirect the tension away from the tip while moving more pliable skin from the upper nose to resurface the wound. Proper use of transposition flaps for prevention of distortion of the nasal tip and lower eyelid requires a certain amount of experience and artistry.

Rhombic Transposition Flap

The rhombic flap may be the most commonly used type of transposition flap. Although many variants exist, the classic rhombic flap is easily visualized as a parallelogram, with the flap tip having a 60-degree angle. The primary defect may be cut to fit the flap, or the flap may be trimmed to fit the defect when it is placed. It is useful to redirect wound tension away from the primary defect. This type of flap is often deployed on the upper nose and periorbital areas (Figure 21.15).

Zitelli Bilobed Transposition Flap

This more specialized variant of the transposition flap, while more complex, is included due to its great usefulness in reconstruction of wounds of the sebaceous and inflexible skin of the lower nose. The bilobed flap is excellent for closing small- to intermediate-sized wounds less than 1.5 cm in diameter. The placement of the extra lobe allows greater movement of tissue from the upper nose (Figure 21.16).[5,6]

Transposition Flap

Step-by-Step Instructions (Figure 21.17)

a) The primary defect is a small one on the inflexible sebaceous skin of the distal nose. The rhombic flap taps into the more mobile skin of the proximal nose.
b) The flap is incised, and the laterally placed Burow's triangle is removed. On the mid- to distal nose, the flap will be incised slightly deeper to improve flap perfusion. A small amount of nasalis musculature is included at the bottom of the flap. The rich vasculature of the nasalis will almost always ensure a healthy flap. Of course, the depth of the primary defect will need to equal the thickness of the flap to avoid "trapdoor" formation. All wound edges are undermined, and hemostasis is obtained with electrodesiccation.
c) The key suture is placed initially to close the secondary defect. Transposition flaps always close the widest portion of the distal secondary defect first. This pushes the flap into place. Usually the flap tip is trimmed to fit the primary defect.
d) The remainder of the flap is sutured in a layered fashion.

Learning the Techniques

Performing cutaneous flaps is an advanced skill that takes considerable experience to master. Initial experience can be gained in a workshop using pigs' feet. It is recommended to begin to practice their use on patients with the help of a mentor, such as a dermatologic, Mohs, or plastic surgeon.

Coding and Billing Pearls

The adjacent tissue transfer (flaps) or rearrangement procedures (plasties) are described by the series of codes from 14000-14300. These codes are for the excision of the lesion and/or repair by adjacent tissue transfer or

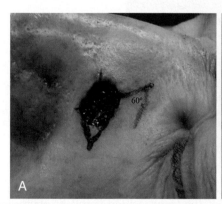
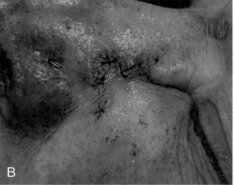

Figure 21.15 Rhombic transposition flap is useful to redirect wound tension away from the primary defect and is often used on the upper nose. **(A)** Flap drawn with 60-degree angle. **(B)** Repaired flap looks like a parallelogram. (Courtesy of Ryan O'Quinn, MD.)

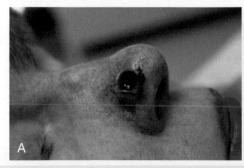
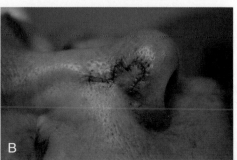

Figure 21.16 The bilobed transposition flap is excellent for closing small- to intermediate-sized wounds less than 1.5 cm in diameter on the lower nose. The placement of the extra lobe allows greater movement of tissue from the upper nose. **(A)** Small lower nose defect after excising a BCC. **(B)** Bilobed transposition flap completed. (Courtesy of Ryan O'Quinn, MD.)

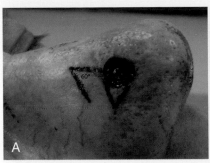 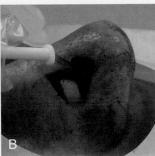 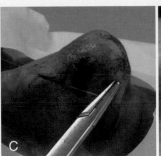 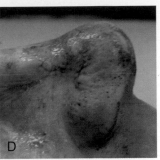

Figure 21.17 Transposition flap:

(A) The primary defect is a small one on the inflexible sebaceous skin of the lower nose. The rhombic flap is drawn to use the more mobile skin of the upper nose.

(B) The flap is incised, and the laterally placed Burow's triangle is removed. All wound edges are undermined, and hemostasis is obtained with electrodesiccation.

(C) The key suture is placed initially to close the secondary defect. This pushes the flap into place. The flap tip is trimmed to fit the primary defect.

(D) The remainder of the flap is sutured in a layered fashion.

(Courtesy of Ryan O'Quinn, MD.)

rearrangement. Routine excision of the lesion, whether it is benign or malignant, is included with codes 14000-14300 and should not be coded or billed separately.

The specific code is determined by the location and the size of the defect. The term "defect" includes the primary defect resulting from the excision and the secondary defect resulting from flap design to perform the reconstruction. The areas of both defects are added together to determine the code (see Box 21.1 for the actual CPT Codes).

Box 21.1 CPT Codes for Adjacent Tissue Transfer (Flaps)

14000 trunk; defect 10 sq cm or less
14001 trunk; defect 10.1 sq cm to 30.0 sq cm
14020 scalp, arms, and/or legs; defect 10 sq cm or less
14021 scalp, arms, and/or legs; defect 10.1 sq cm to 30.0 sq cm
14040 forehead, cheeks, chin, mouth, neck, axillae, genitalia, hands, and/or feet; defect 10 sq cm or less
14041 forehead, cheeks, chin, mouth, neck, axillae, genitalia, hands, and/or feet; defect 10.1 sq cm to 30.0 sq cm
14060 eyelids, nose, ears, and/or lips; defect 10 sq cm or less
14061 eyelids, nose, ears, and/or lips; defect 10.1 sq cm to 30.0 sq cm
14300 more than 30 sq cm, unusual or complicated, any area

References

1. Bowman PH, Fosko SW, Hartstein ME. Periocular reconstruction. *Semin Cutan Med Surg.* 2003;22:263-272.
2. Chen EH, Johnson TM, Ratner D. Introduction to flap movement: reconstruction of five similar nasal defects using different flaps. *Dermatol Surg.* 2005;31:982-985.
3. Krishnan R, Garman M, Nunez-Gussman J, Orengo I. Advancement flaps: a basic theme with many variations. *Dermatol Surg.* 2005;31:986-994.
4. Seline PC, Siegle RJ. Scalp reconstruction. *Dermatol Clin.* 2005;23:13-21, v.
5. Aasi SZ, Leffell DJ. Bilobed transposition flap. *Dermatol Clin.* 2005;23:55-64, vi.
6. Collins SC, Dufresne Jr RG, Jellinek NJ. The bilobed transposition flap for single-staged repair of large surgical defects involving the nasal ala. *Dermatol Surg.* 2008;34:1379-1385.

22 Ultrasound in Dermatology

DAVID SWANSON, MD

SUMMARY

- Ultrasound in dermatology usually involves determining if a subcutaneous mass is an epidermal cyst, lipoma, lymph node, vascular lesion, or malignancy. It is used to determine the size and depth of a mass.
- These ultrasound terms are defined: hyperechoic, isoechoic, hypoechoic, acoustic shadow, acoustic enhancement, and mirror artifact.
- Ultrasound markedly improves diagnostic accuracy for subcutaneous nodules, especially for the differentiation between epidermal inclusion cysts and lipomas.
- Other subcutaneous lesions covered include pilomatrixomas, ganglion cysts, digital mucous cysts, thyroglossal cysts, subcutaneous fat necrosis, and osteomas.

Point-of-care ultrasound (POCUS) is the use of diagnostic and interventional ultrasound by clinicians at the bedside. Almost always, it refers to the use of ultrasound by nonradiologists. POCUS is becoming commonplace in offices and hospital settings, such as emergency rooms. The use of ultrasound has increasingly become a part of medical school and residency curricula, and it is now commonplace for medical students to acquire personal devices in their first year of training.[1] Eugene Braunwald has stated, "Inspection, palpation, percussion, and auscultation have been the 4 pillars of clinical bedside medicine. Time to add a Fifth Pillar to bedside physical examination: Inspection, Palpation, Percussion, Auscultation, and Insonation."[2]

The general adoption of POCUS has in great part been a result of the development of technology that is durable and affordable. At the time of this writing, the cost for high-quality portable instruments has fallen to the range of US$2000 to US$12,000. The instruments commonly fit into a white coat pocket. They have either built-in image screens or, more commonly, they may use iOS- or Android-based devices for displaying images.[3]

For cutaneous applications, the clinical questions are usually very straightforward. Is a subcutaneous mass an epidermal cyst, lipoma, lymph node, vascular lesion, or malignancy? How large is the lesion? What other structures are affected by it? Is there any cellulitis or an abscess present? We will see how all interpretations of POCUS are performed in the context of the clinical history and examination.

Targets of ultrasound are classified descriptively by the intensity of the reflection of the sound waves and the resulting brightness of the structures relative to the surrounding tissue (Figure 22.1).

- *Hyperechoic* structures are more highly reflective and appear brighter than surrounding tissue. They may create a partial *acoustic shadow* beyond them (Figure 22.2) or, as in the case of bone, be acoustically opaque. Hyperechoic structures are most commonly structurally complex or contain calcium found in bones, cysts, or calcinosis cutis.

- *Isoechoic* structures have a similar brightness to surrounding tissues and are distinguished anatomically by the morphologic differences from surrounding tissue.

- *Hypoechoic* are less reflective and appear darker, and anechoic structures are completely black. Dark anechoic structureless areas often contain fluid such as blood, pus, mucus, urine, and lymphatic or synovial fluid. Because hypoechoic and anechoic structures are less reflective, the tissue beyond them often appears brighter than surrounding tissue – *acoustic enhancement* (Figure 22.1).

Ultrasound images are generated by software that assumes that the reflective sound waves travel in a straight line and reflect back once. Occasionally, especially from a hypoechoic structure with a hyperechoic lining, the software will create a *mirror artifact* from two or more reflections occurring before the sound waves return to the transducer (Figures 22.3, 22.16). Although infrequent, mirror artifacts can create confusion unless recognized.

Most examinations are performed with *grayscale*, two-dimensional cross-sections of tissue, but most devices have other image options. *Color Doppler* can identify the presence and direction of flow of blood; red color occurs with motion of fluid toward the probe, and blue with motion away ("red forward, blue back") (Figure 22.4 and 22.5). *Power Doppler* is more sensitive for detecting vascular flow but does not provide directional information. A limitation of Doppler ultrasound is that it depends on the probe position and is invisible if the probe is perpendicular to the direction of flow. This is easily remedied by simply adjusting the probe tilt angle. Most devices have *M-mode* capability, which is an anatomical one-dimensional view displayed over time to document motion. It has little utility in dermatology.

Knobology refers to adjustments available in the device to improve image quality, depending on the target. Fortunately, most POCUS devices have presets for different examinations. This can include presets for nerves, OB/GYN, vascular, cardiac, abdomen, aorta/gallbladder, and musculoskeletal examinations. For cutaneous and subcutaneous

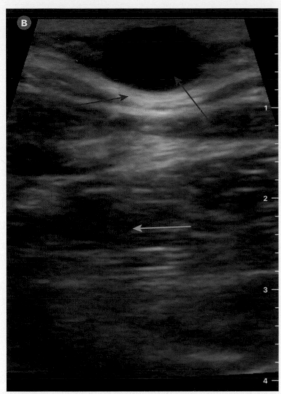

Figure 22.1 Epidermal cyst. Note the relatively bright acoustic enhancement deep to the cyst. Red arrow: hyperechoic fascia with acoustic enhancement. Green arrow: isoechoic muscle. Blue arrow: hypoechoic cyst. (Copyright Richard P. Usatine, MD.)

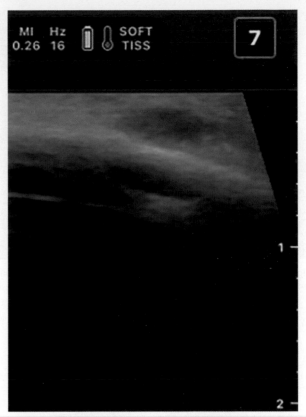

Figure 22.3 Pilar cyst of upper forehead, showing cyst above the calvarium and a mirror artifact below. (Courtesy of David Swanson, MD.)

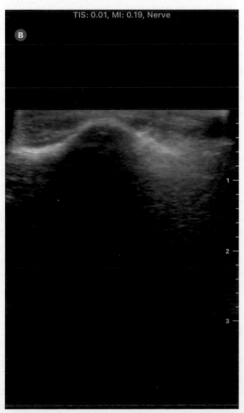

Figure 22.2 Boney exostosis of scalp. Note the dark acoustic shadow that results for the hyperechoic calcified surface. (Copyright Richard P. Usatine, MD.)

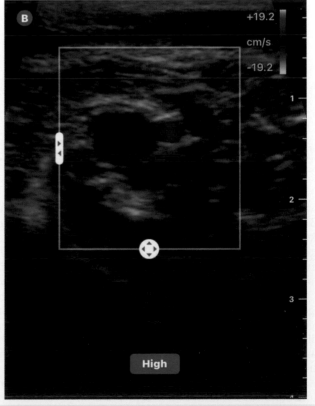

Figure 22.4 Color Doppler image of popliteal artery between two veins. The probe is pointing proximally, resulting in a red Doppler signal from the arterial flow. (Courtesy of David Swanson, MD.)

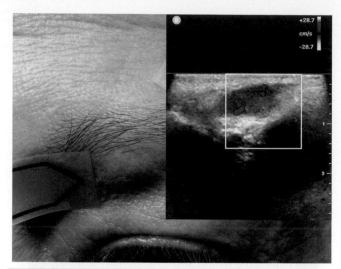

Figure 22.5 Ultrasound of suborbital desmoid tumor showing lesional vascular signals with color doppler. (Courtesy of David Swanson, MD.)

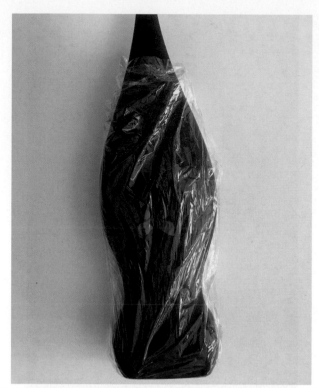

Figure 22.7 Demonstration of the use of common disposable plastic wrap to protect probe. (Courtesy of David Swanson, MD.)

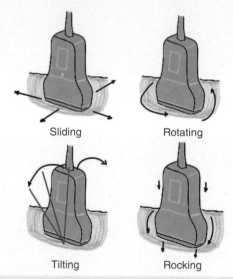

Figure 22.6 Motions when moving ultrasound probe. (Courtesy of David Swanson, MD.)

examinations, we have found the nerve presets most useful (3 cm depth). When greater depth is needed, the musculoskeletal preset is a good option (4 cm depth). All devices have simple adjustments that are simple for gain, depth, and mode. Gain adjustments beyond the presets can enhance resolution and reduce noise but are not often needed.

Ultrasound imaging is performed by placing the probe against the skin using an ultrasound gel to match the acoustic impedance of the tissue. One applies the gel liberally to the probe allowing for full application of the probe and the elimination of air bubbles. It is usually easy to find the target structure with cutaneous examinations.

Structures are always examined in at least two dimensions, and the examination is dependent on probe motions (Figure 22.6). These motions are sliding, rotating, tilting, rocking, and stabbing. The stabbing motions are used to assess compressibility or to look around structures, such as

the costal margin. It is common for novices to combine several motions at the same time, but motions are best made slowly, smoothly, and one motion at a time.

Ultrasound is extremely safe technology. Hygiene is one important consideration, particularly when examining potentially contaminated tissue. For normal examinations, probes can be cleaned with common, high-efficiency and high-intensity bacterial/viral antiseptic cleansers such as Cidex OPA, Trophon2, Virusolve+ EDS, and Virusolve+. The device manufacturer usually provides specific recommendations. For obviously contaminated tissue encountered in cellulitis and hidradenitis, many manufacturers have disposable protective caps that attach to probes or one can obtain standard sheaths available from Civco, ProTek, Medline, Sheathes, and other retailers. A simple, inexpensive alternative hygiene solution is to apply ultrasound gel to the end of the probe, wrap it in a cling-type clear food wrap, and then use the combination as the examining probe (Figure 22.7). After the examination, the wrap can be pulled off and discarded.

Normal Anatomy

The epidermis is usually not seen with standard imaging, except on the palms and soles, where it shows as a superficial hyperechoic band. The dermis (Figure 22.8) is a homogeneous isoechoic band that with age and chronic sun damage may have a superficial hypoechoic band component. The latter is a consequence of structural degradation of the dermis (solar elastosis).

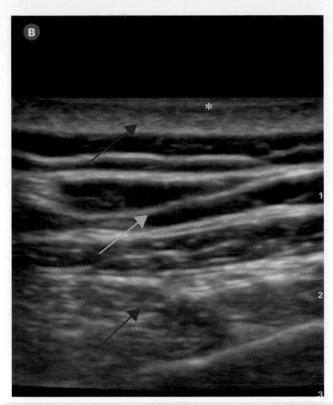

Figure 22.8 Normal skin. Arrows: red, dermis; green, subcutaneous fat; blue, muscle. Asterisk: epidermis, mostly stratum corneum. (Courtesy of David Swanson, MD.)

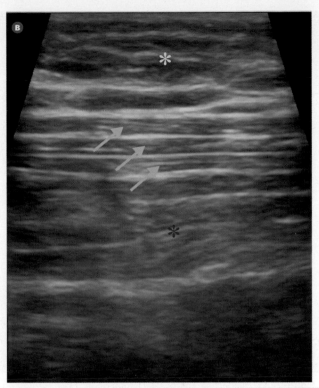

Figure 22.9 Distal thigh, longitudinal view, showing tendons (arrows) overlying muscle (red asterisk) and beneath fat (yellow asterisk). (Courtesy of David Swanson, MD.)

Below the dermis is a layer of subcutaneous fat (Figure 22.8). As expected from observation of fat when performing skin surgery, fat is lobulated on ultrasound. These lobulations are seen as hypoechoic structures separated by hyperechoic fibrous septae. Fascia is a homogeneous hyperechoic band that commonly overlies muscle. Muscle (Figure 22.8) typically appears grouped into compartments, separated by fat. Tendons (Figure 22.9) can be differentiated from muscle by their greater hyperechoic density, narrow linear structure, and tighter parallel-fibrillar pattern. Nerves also show a tight parallel-fibrillar pattern but are differentiated by being hypoechoic and having a hyperechoic sheath (Figure 22.10).

Lymph nodes, especially enlarged reactive nodes, are common findings that may be confused with cysts. Lymph nodes most commonly are oval in shape, but they may be round if inflamed or infiltrated. Normal lymph nodes may be hypoechoic (Figure 22.11) or isoechoic (Figure 22.12) or show a defined hypoechoic cortex at the perimeter, with a hyperechoic hilum or medulla (Figure 22.13). The cortical rim is normally thin, but it thickens in inflammatory nodes (Figure 22.14). Doppler ultrasound may not demonstrate flow or may show low flow in the hilum of the node. Doppler ultrasound may help differentiate reactive nodes from cysts. Cysts never show Doppler signals except by artifact.

Bone and extraosseous calcifications appear as hyperechoic lines and cast strong acoustic shadows.

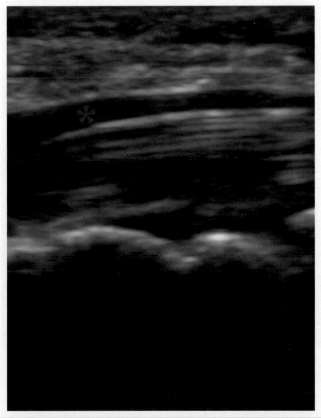

Figure 22.10 Wrist, longitudinal view. Median nerve (asterisk) overlying flexor tendons in carpal tunnel. (Courtesy of David Swanson, MD.)

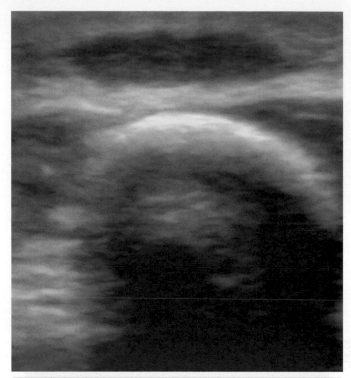

Figure 22.11 Hypoechoic epitrochlear lymph node. (Courtesy of David Swanson, MD.)

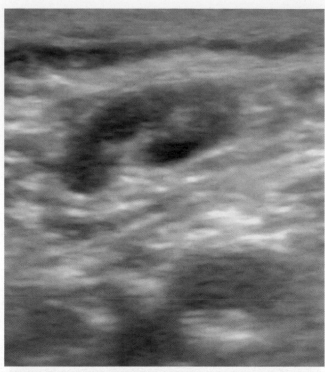

Figure 22.13 Lymph node with hypoechoic cortex and hyperechoic hilum. (Courtesy of David Swanson, MD.)

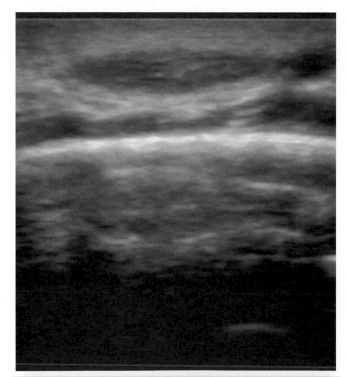

Figure 22.12 Isoechoic epitrochlear lymph node. (Courtesy of David Swanson, MD.)

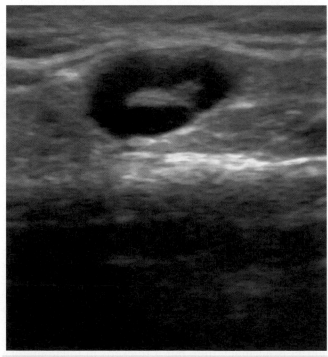

Figure 22.14 Preauricular lymph node in a patient with facial herpes zoster. Note the hilum and thickened reactive cortex. (Courtesy of David Swanson, MD.)

Applications

Ultrasound markedly improves diagnostic accuracy for subcutaneous nodules (Table 22.1), especially for the differentiation between epidermal inclusion cysts and lipomas (Table 22.2).

Epidermal inclusion cysts (EICs) (Figure 22.15) are cutaneous nodules composed of fluid and keratinaceous debris. *See video 22.1.* They are usually hypoechoic and may appear empty (Figure 22.16) but more commonly have particulate echo reflections within them (Figures 22.17, 22.18). EICs adhere to the dermis; a particularly useful finding is when the cyst occupies 50% or more of the dermis (Figure 22.19). In about half of cases, one can identify a communication with the surface, described as the "submarine sign" (Figure 22.20).[4] This is thought to be a visualization of the punctum.[4]

EICs may show mass effect as they displace surrounding structures. They usually show acoustic enhancement deep to the cyst wall, which helps differentiate them from lipomas in similar locations, and accordingly may show a hyperechoic deep wall. They may be simple or complex in structure with lobulation (Figure 22.21). When inflamed, there will be evident cellulitis (Figure 22.32).

Table 22.1 Diagnostic Accuracy of Ultrasound of Subcutaneous Nodules Compared to Palpation

Pathologic Diagnosis	Total Number of Each Tumor	Agreement With Pathologic Diagnosis	
		After Palpation	After Ultrasonography
Lipoma	42	23	37
Epidermal cyst	44	19	29
Ganglion cyst	18	5	7
Others	79	6	12

From Kumano et al. (2009).[5]

Table 22.2 Epidermal Cyst vs Lipoma, Clinical and Ultrasound Features

Clinical	Epidermal Cyst	Lipoma
Visible punctum	Often	No
Malodorous discharge	Often	No
Ultrasound	**Epidermal Cyst**	**Lipoma**
Submarine sign	Often	No
Hyperechoic inferior wall	Yes	No
Echoic enhancement below wall	Yes	No
Lateral demarcation line	Yes	No
Hypoechoic areas internally	Yes	Sometimes
Internal chaotic debris	Yes	No
Hyperechoic striated echoes – horizontal reflections running through them	No	Yes
Doppler shows significant vascularity	No	No

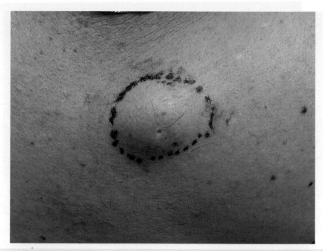

Figure 22.15 Epidermal inclusion cyst. (Copyright Richard P. Usatine, MD.)

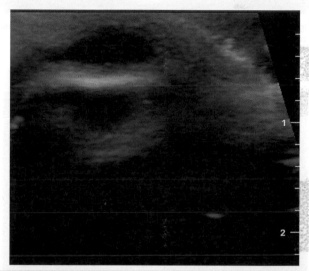

Figure 22.16 Hypoechoic epidermal cyst, also showing mirror artifact. (Courtesy of David Swanson, MD.)

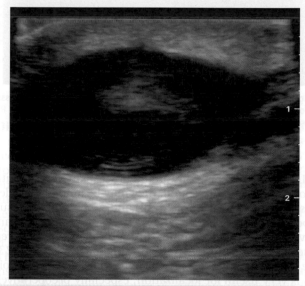

Figure 22.17 Epidermal inclusion cyst with echogenic contents and acoustic enhancement. (Copyright Richard P. Usatine, MD.)

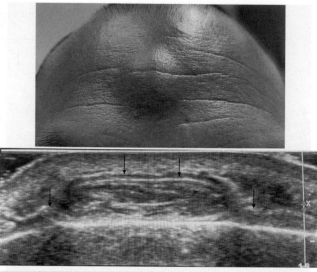

Figure 22.26 Lipoma of forehead lying deep to and displacing the frontalis muscle (arrows). (Note acoustic echo artifact from reflection off calvarium).

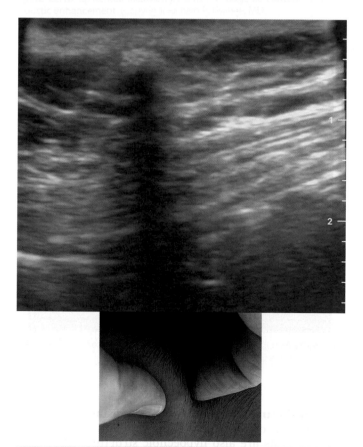

Figure 22.27 Pilomatrixoma at margin of the scalp in a young girl with shadowing seen in the ultrasound from the calcifications present. (Copyright Richard P. Usatine, MD.)

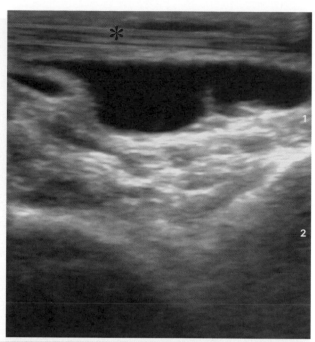

Figure 22.28 Ganglion cyst. Note the extension circumferentially around tendon (asterisk). (Courtesy of David Swanson, MD.)

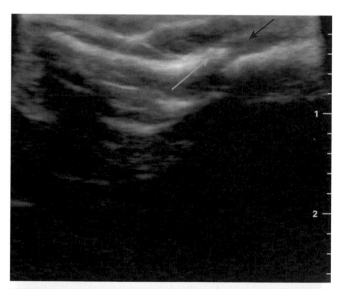

Figure 22.29 Digital mucous cyst, longitudinal view, overlying the DIP joint of a second toe. Note the presence of an osteophyte (green arrow) and the communication with the joint space (red arrow). (Courtesy of David Swanson, MD.)

represent the only functional thyroid tissue in given patients. Likewise, **lateral brachial cleft cysts** can be deep to the platysma, abut or extend between the internal and external carotid artery and internal jugular vein, and potentially extend superiorly to the skull base. Formal ultrasound is preferred in both of these settings along with a referral to ENT.

As noted above, normal subcutaneous fat has distinct hypoechoic lobules divided by discrete isoechoic septa. When **cellulitis** is present, the lobules are less distinct and can be separated by hypoechoic edema, often giving a cobblestone appearance (Figures 22.31 and 22.32). *See video 22.3.* The cellulitis can be infectious, or in the context of venous insufficiency or other disorders; the findings are nonspecific. The principal value of POCUS in cellulitis is to identify the presence of abscess, which will be collections of hypoechoic areas within the cellulitis (Figures 22.33 and 22.34).

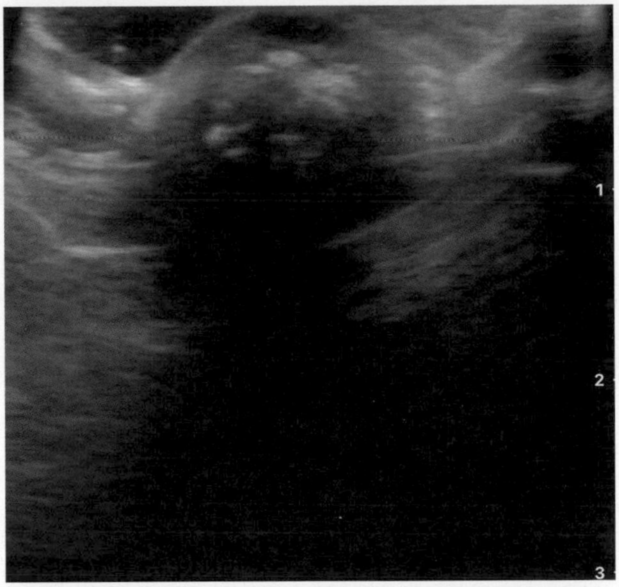

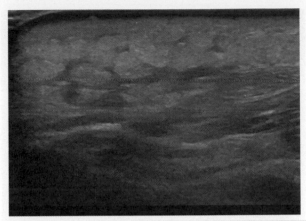

Figure 22.32 Cellulitis of lower extremity, higher resolution, showing edema of fat and cobblestone pattern. (Courtesy of Dr. E.J. Mayeaux, Jr.)

Figure 22.30 Digital mucous cyst, transverse view. (Courtesy of David Swanson, MD.)

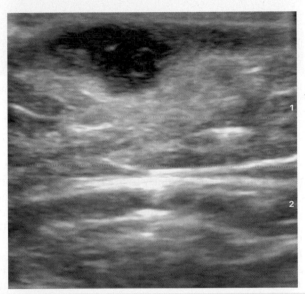

Figure 22.33 Inflamed cyst with rupture, abscess formation, and surrounding cellulitis. (Courtesy of David Swanson, MD.)

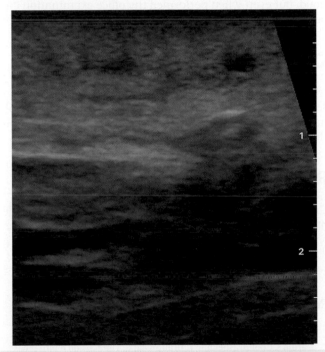

Figure 22.31 Cellulitis of lower extremity, showing edema of fat and cobblestone pattern. (Courtesy of David Swanson, MD.)

Subcutaneous fat necrosis is most commonly from trauma; the injury may have been minor and forgotten by the patient. It presents as a palpable subcutaneous nodule, sometimes tender, usually slightly firmer than a lipoma. Ultrasound findings resemble a lipoma, except that there are usually discrete hypoechoic features within the lesions (Figure 22.35).

Osteomas are firm subcutaneous nodules most frequently encountered on the forehead and scalp. These are fixed, and firmer than cysts, lymph nodes, and lipomas, but

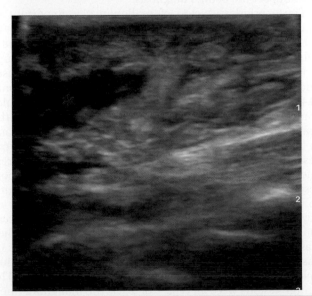

Figure 22.34 Cellulitis with abscess formation (asterisk). (Courtesy of David Swanson, MD.)

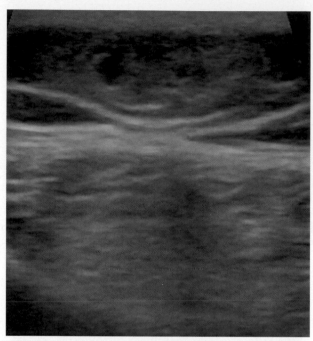

Figure 22.35 Subcutaneous fat necrosis above bone, showing hypoechoic pockets within lipoma-like nodule. (Courtesy of David Swanson, MD.)

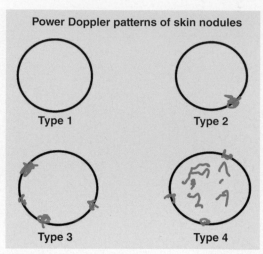

Power Doppler patterns of skin nodules

Type 1

Type 2

Type 3

Type 4

Figure 22.36 Power Doppler image classification for benign and malignant lesions (from Giovagnorio et al.). (Courtesy of David Swanson, MD.)

can fool a clinician particularly in areas of poor skin mobility, such as the forehead. The skin can be moved over them, causing them to appear movable. However, on ultrasound they show a characteristic protuberance of the calvarium with acoustic shadowing (Figure 22.2).

Benign vs malignant subcutaneous masses. A common application of ultrasound is differentiation of benign from malignant subcutaneous nodules. Usually, ultrasound allows a positive diagnostic identification of benign lesions, such as a lipoma. There are specific features that additionally support the benign diagnosis.

The a priori suspicion of malignancy is important in interpretation, but high-resolution ultrasound (10 to 20 MHz) with color Doppler is a powerful tool to evaluate subcutaneous nodules. Giovagnorio reported the findings in 68 nodules, of which 23 were malignant (21 metastases and 2 lymphomas). The primary cancers were melanoma (44%), breast (28%), and lung (28%). No benign nodules showed vascularity on color Doppler examination. Of the malignant lesions, all showed signs of vascularity in one or more peripheral poles and 11 of 21 showed internal vessels.[6] Metastases had a polycyclic shape, but the presence of sharp borders, circular or oval shape, or hypoechoic resolution did not distinguish benign from malignant.[6] In another study, the same author showed that color or power Doppler differentiated 71 nodules, of which 32 were malignant, with a 90% sensitivity and 100% specificity.[7] They classified lesion vascularity based on absence of flow (type 1), based on the presence of flow in a single pole (type 2) or multiple poles (type 3), or internally (type 4) (Figure 22.36). The benign lesions were all type 1 or 2. Of the malignant ones, three were type 1 and the remainder type 3 or 4. Office assessment usually will be followed by formal examination depending on the clinical context and preprobability likelihood, but even when performed the office examination can be very comforting to patients.

Conclusion

Ultrasound can greatly enhance dermatological diagnoses. The emergence of high-quality, affordable instruments has created the opportunity to easily adopt ultrasound into the diagnosis of skin and subcutaneous lesions.

Resources

Great site to explore the various ultrasound options available: https://www.pocus.org/pocus-devices-and-manufacturers/

References

1. Available at: https://medicine.temple.edu/news/temple-medicine-students-butterfly-ultrasounds. Accessed December 19, 2021.
2. Narula J, Chandrashekhar Y, Braunwald E. Time to add a fifth pillar to bedside physical examination: inspection, palpation, percussion, auscultation, and insonation. *JAMA Cardiol.* 2018;3(4):346-350. doi:10.1001/jamacardio.2018.0001.
3. Available at: https://www.pocus.org/pocus-devices-and-manufacturers/. Accessed February 2, 2022.
4. Lee DH, Yoon CS, Lim BJ, et al. Ultrasound feature-based diagnostic model focusing on the "submarine sign" for epidermal cysts among superficial soft tissue lesions. *Korean J Radiol.* 2019;20(10):1409-1421. doi:10.3348/kjr.2019.0241.
5. Kuwano Y, Ishizaki K, Watanabe R, Nanko H. Efficacy of diagnostic ultrasonography of lipomas, epidermal cysts, and ganglions. *Arch Dermatol.* 2009;145(7):761-764. doi:10.1001/archdermatol.2009.61.
6. Giovagnorio F, Valentini C, Paonessa A. High-resolution and color Doppler sonography in the evaluation of skin metastases. *J Ultrasound Med.* 2003;22(10):1017-1025. doi:10.7863/jum.2003.22.10.1017.
7. Giovagnorio F, Andreoli C, De Cicco ML. Color Doppler sonography of focal lesions of the skin and subcutaneous tissue. *J Ultrasound Med.* 1999;18(2):89-93. doi:10.7863/jum.1999.18.2.89.

Putting It All Together

SECTION OUTLINE

23 Procedures to Treat Benign Conditions

24 Diagnosis and Treatment of Malignant and Premalignant Lesions

25 Wound Care

26 Complications: Postprocedural Adverse Effects and Their Prevention

27 When to Refer/Mohs Surgery

28 Coding Common Skin Procedures

23 Procedures to Treat Benign Conditions

DANIEL STULBERG, MD, HAMID QAZI, MD, ROBERT FAWCETT, MD, and
RICHARD P. USATINE, MD

SUMMARY

- Multiple benign skin conditions may be treated in the primary care office with the right surgical supplies and techniques.
- Cryosurgery using a liquid nitrogen gun is a fast and efficient treatment for seborrheic keratoses, lentigos, and keloids.
- Cryo Tweezers chilled in liquid nitrogen are excellent for treating acrochordons, filiform warts, genital papillomas, and other small, raised lesions with minimal pain.
- Electrodesiccation is an inexpensive destructive treatment for many lesions and particularly well suited for vascular lesions like hemangiomas and for small lesions including sebaceous gland hyperplasia.
- Two cycles of electrodesiccation with curettage are useful for pyogenic granulomas and an option for seborrheic keratoses.
- Dermatofibromas require full-thickness excision for complete removal.
- There are multiple treatment options for common and plantar warts if over-the-counter salicylic acid products are not effective.
- Laser and intense pulsed light are effective destructive treatments for many benign lesions, though availability is limited in the primary care office due to the cost.

Many skin tumors and growths are benign and can be diagnosed based on their clinical appearance and history. These lesions can arise from the epidermis, the dermis, or the subcutaneous tissues. This chapter provides a detailed discussion of the most common benign skin lesions and their treatment options. Chapter 14, *Cysts and Lipomas*, covers epidermal cysts, lipomas, digital mucous cysts, and hidrocystomas, so these will not be covered here.

Acne Surgery

Acne surgery is the name given to the removal of open comedones (blackheads) with a comedone extractor in the clinician's office. It can also be performed on actinic comedones or senile comedones. It is often performed for cosmetic reasons but can also decrease pain around a comedone that is under pressure. Large inflammatory nodules and cysts are best treated with intralesional steroids rather than acne surgery (see Chapter 15, *Intralesional Injections*).

After informed consent, the comedones are cleaned with alcohol. No anesthesia is needed. The comedone is nicked with a No. 11 blade, a sterile needle, or the sharp end of a comedone extractor. Sebum, cells, and other debris are expressed out using pressure from a comedone extractor (Figure 23.1A–C). If a comedone extractor is not available, a small diameter dermal curette (1 to 3 mm) can also be

used, but make sure you apply the blunt side to the patient's skin and not the sharp edge. One can bend a small paperclip to produce a homemade device. Clean the paperclip with an alcohol wipe before using it. Bill using acne surgery CPT code = 10040.

Acrochordons

- Also known as skin tags, fibroepithelial polyps when large, papillomas

DIAGNOSIS

- Flesh-colored, raised lesions, often pedunculated
- Common on the neck, axillae, inguinal regions, and under the breasts
- More common in persons with obesity, diabetes, impaired glucose tolerance, or pregnancy (second and third trimester)
- Some people develop hundreds of skin tags in conjunction with acanthosis nigricans (Figure 23.2).

TREATMENT

Treatment is done for cosmetic reasons or if the skin tags are getting caught in or irritated by clothing or jewelry.

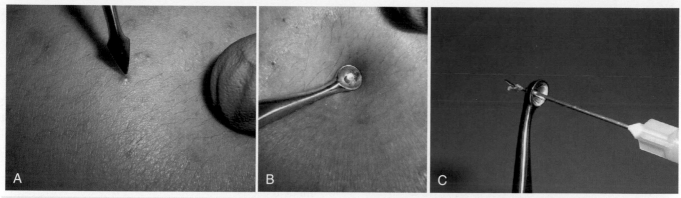

Figure 23.1 Acne surgery: **(A)** Pierce the comedone with the sharp side of the comedone extractor (a No. 11 scalpel blade works even better). **(B)** Press the comedone extractor against the skin until the pilosebaceous material comes out. **(C)** The comedone extractor can be used multiple times after cleaning between uses with a 21-gauge needle and then sterilized. (Copyright Richard P. Usatine, MD.)

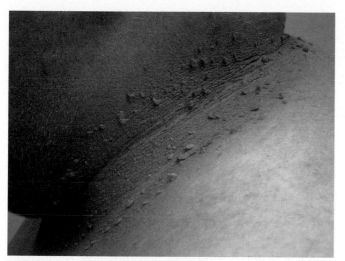

Figure 23.2 Multiple skin tags (acrochordons) on the neck of a man with acanthosis nigricans. (Copyright Richard P. Usatine, MD.)

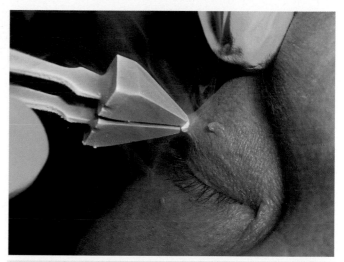

Figure 23.3 Cryosurgery using the Cryo Tweezer on a skin tag located on the eyelid. Grasp the acrochordon and pull the eyelid away from the globe. (Copyright Richard P. Usatine, MD.)

Cryo Tweezers (See Also Chapter 17, Cryosurgery, for More Details)

Freeze with Cryo Tweezer down to normal tissue (Figure 23.3).

- Tags will necrose and fall off over 1 to 2 weeks.
- Works better for smaller pedunculated skin tags. Only a small percentage will fail to necrose.
- This is a clean procedure; no bleeding or anesthetic needed – the patient feels a mild pinch.
- Great for skin tags on eyelids or around the eyes (Figure 23.3)

Snip With Iris Scissors (Figure 23.4)

- Simple and quick with immediate results
- Use lidocaine with epinephrine if skin tags have a wide base.
- Minimal bleeding for small lesions
- Direct pressure, aluminum chloride for hemostasis if needed. Electrocoagulation without anesthesia can be tolerated if needed but is not pleasant.
- *See videos 23.1 and 23.2 (9.9 and 9.10).*

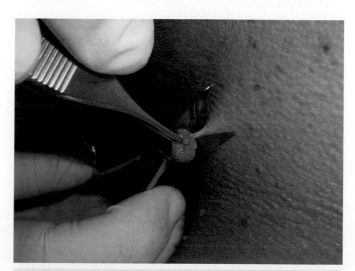

Figure 23.4 Snip excision of a pedunculated acrochordon. (Copyright Richard P. Usatine, MD.)

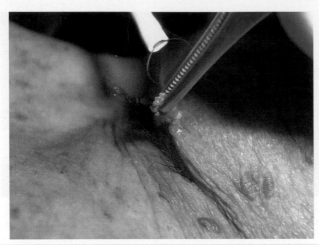

Figure 23.5 Removing a skin tag from the eyelid using an electrosurgical loop. This requires local anesthetic and is no longer preferred now that the Cryo Tweezer is available. (Copyright Richard P. Usatine, MD.)

Electrosurgery

- Electrodesiccate to destroy the skin tag with settings between 2.1 and 2.5 without anesthesia.
- Radio-frequency (RF) loop to cut through base of the lesion is an option only after local anesthesia.
- Even for the Hyfrecator, use local anesthetic unless the skin tags are very small. Patients report that this hurts more without anesthesia than snipping or freezing.
- Also good for skin tags on eyelids or around the eyes because the electrosurgery minimizes bleeding and avoids the use of caustic hemostatic chemicals near the eye (Figure 23.5)

SPECIAL CONSIDERATIONS/BILLING

- Cosmetic procedures are not covered by insurance unless interfering with the visual axis. Rarely insurance will cover removal when irritated by clothing or jewelry.
- Treated lesions can recur, and more commonly new ones will form.
- No need to send for pathology unless diagnosis is uncertain.
- Code 11200 once for the first 1 to 15 lesions destroyed by any method.
- Code 11201 for each additional 10 lesions beyond 15.

Angiomas/Angiokeratomas/ Angiofibromas

DIAGNOSIS

Cherry Angiomas[1]

- Red papules that appear with aging
- Dermoscopy shows red, pink, or purple lacunae with white septae (see Figure 18.11).
- Found most commonly on the trunk
- Benign and can be treated if they are bleeding or for cosmetic reasons. As mentioned above, usually not covered by insurance

- Shave biopsy/excision if diagnosis is not certain or a malignancy, such as angiosarcoma is suspected.

See Video 23.3.

Angiokeratomas

- Red to dark red or purple papules that appear with aging
- Dermoscopy shows red and black lacunae with white veil/septae.
- Found most commonly on the scrotum or vulva
- Benign and can be treated if they are bleeding or for cosmetic reasons
- Shave biopsy/excision if solitary and not genital as these may mimic melanomas

Angiofibromas

- Skin-colored to pink papules found around the nose (Figure 23.6)
- Referred to as adenoma sebaceum when found in clusters around the nose in patients with tuberous sclerosis
- Shave biopsy/excision if diagnosis is not certain or a malignancy is suspected

Multiple facial angiofibromas are now being treated safely and effectively with topical sirolimus (rapamycin).[2]

TREATMENT

The following treatments are used for angiomas, angiokeratomas, or angiofibromas.

Electrodesiccation for Small Lesions

Low-power setting 2 to 3 W on Hyfrecator (or similar instrument) without anesthesia. Start at 2 and only increase power if needed.

- Consider using lidocaine and epinephrine for larger angiomas and angiokeratomas in the genital area or by patient preference (Figure 23.7).

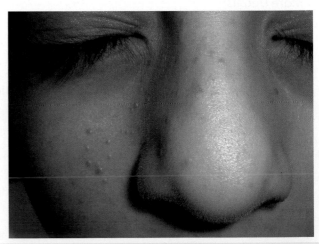

Figure 23.6 Multiple angiofibromas on the face of a young child. Topical sirolimus is now the treatment of choice for multiple angiofibromas associated with tuberous sclerosis. (Copyright Richard P. Usatine, MD.)

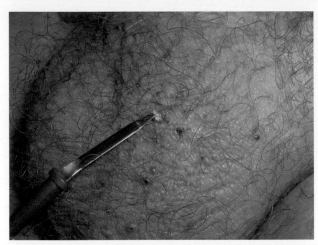

Figure 23.7 Multiple angiokeratomas on the scrotum. The patient requested removal, so after obtaining consent, lidocaine with epinephrine was injected for local anesthesia. The Hyfrecator was used to electrocoagulate the angiokeratomas. (Copyright Richard P. Usatine, MD.)

Shave Excision With Electrodesiccation of the Base for Larger Lesions

- Anesthetize with lidocaine and epinephrine, and send specimen for histology if diagnosis is in doubt.

Cryosurgery With Compressive Probe

- Cryosurgery works best if the vascular lesion is compressed with a probe during the freeze time. A compressive probe can be attached to the liquid nitrogen spray gun, or the nitrous oxide and carbon dioxide powered guns with their solid metal tips can also be used to compress the lesion for better effect. A narrow-diameter liquid nitrogen spray or nitrous oxide spray may also be used. See Chapter 13, *Cryosurgery*, for details.

Lasers

- Lasers and intense pulsed light (IPL) devices used for treatment of red vascular ectasias are effective for angiomas.[3]

Chondrodermatitis Nodularis Helicis

DIAGNOSIS

- Skin-colored or erythematous firm nodule of the helix of the ear (Figure 23.8A)
- Frequent shallow central scale or crust
- Usually very tender to palpation or when trying to sleep on the affected ear
- More common in men, and prevalence increases with age over 40. Less commonly, the nodule may be on the antihelix.
- SCC is in the differential diagnosis, so consider a shave biopsy if the diagnosis is uncertain.

TREATMENT

See Video 23.4.

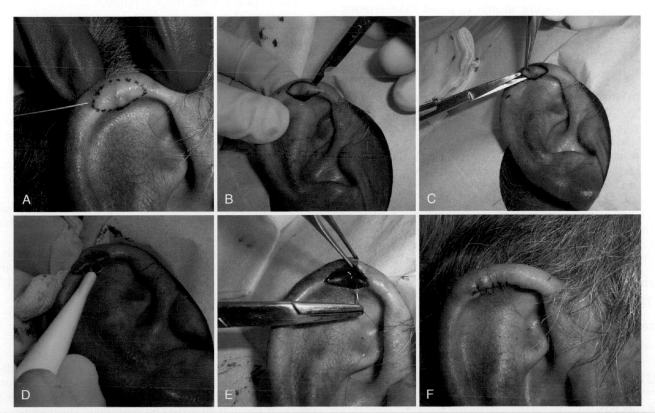

Figure 23.8 (A) 1% Lidocaine with epinephrine was injected into the helical rim to excise chondrodermatitis nodularis helicis. **(B)** A 15c blade was used to cut the ellipse. **(C)** A sharp iris scissor was used to cut off the bottom of the ellipse. **(D)** A curette was used to curette away the affected cartilage. **(E)** 5-0 Polypropylene was used to close the defect. **(F)** Three interrupted sutures produced an excellent closure. (Copyright Richard P. Usatine, MD.)

Topical or Pillow Use[4]

- Pressure-relieving padding or pillows with a cut-out are available commercially. Routine use may alleviate the symptoms and lead to resolution of the lesion.
- High-potency steroid with occlusion
- Nitroglycerine 2% paste applied twice daily
- Photodynamic therapy
- Diltiazem topical cream

Injection

- Use this treatment method only if you are certain of the diagnosis clinically or by previous biopsy.
- Triamcinolone acetonide 10 to 40 mg/mL injected into the lesion can reduce the size and tenderness.
- Injections may be repeated at 2- to 4-week intervals, but the overall success rate is low.

Elliptical Excision

See Video 23.4.

- Elliptical excision around the lesion has a high success rate (Figure 23.8A–F).
- Draw the ellipse around the nodule and follow ear anatomy.
- Anesthetize with 1% lidocaine and epinephrine (epinephrine is not contraindicated and helps to produce a field not obscured by blood).
- Lightly curette the underlying diseased cartilage with a 3-mm curette or snip it off with a sharp scissor.
- Close the defect with a few simple interrupted sutures using 5-0 monofilament nonabsorbable suture such as polypropylene on a small plastic needle (13 to 16 mm). Use a reverse cutting needle to avoid inadvertently cutting the normal skin on the ear when placing the sutures.
- Bill for excision of benign growth on the ear based on size.

Electrodesiccation and Curettage

- Do a shave biopsy for diagnosis (if not already done).
- Scrape off abnormal tissue with 3-mm curette.
- Use electrodesiccation to destroy any remaining abnormal tissue.
- Repeat another cycle of curettage and electrodesiccation if needed for any remaining abnormal tissue.
- Cover with petrolatum, and let heal by secondary intention.
- The remaining scar may be less cosmetically appealing than the sutured closure done with the ellipse.
- Can only bill for destruction of a benign growth (same charge as cryosurgery of benign lesion)

Cryosurgery

- This method can be attempted, but it is not very effective.

Laser

- Ablate with CO_2 laser and leave open to granulate in.

Cutaneous Horn

DIAGNOSIS

- Thickened keratin that grows from the skin like an animal's horn (Figure 23.9).

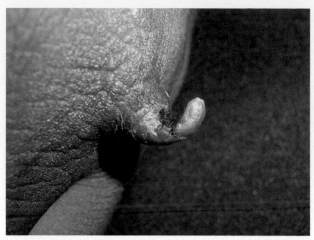

Figure 23.9 A cutaneous horn turned out to be a wart when it was biopsied and sent to pathology. (Copyright Richard P. Usatine, MD.)

TREATMENT

- Shave off the horn including tissue at the base using a blade (razor or scalpel). Use electrocautery or aluminum chloride for hemostasis. Always send for pathology because the underlying lesion may be a squamous cell carcinoma, hypertrophic actinic keratosis, wart, or other diagnoses.
- The thick keratin itself is difficult to cut and nondiagnostic unless the biopsy includes the tissue below the horn itself.
- Cryosurgery of the base may be performed as a second step if the original shave showed the base to be a wart, SK, or AK and some tissue is remaining.
- Ablative CO_2 and neodymium-doped yttrium aluminum garnet lasers may be preferred for aesthetics.[5]

Dermatofibromas

DIAGNOSIS

- Firm nodular thickening of the dermis that may have a hyperpigmented halo (Figure 23.10). It can be hypopigmented, hyperpigmented, or pink.
- Most commonly found on the legs, particularly in women (Figure 23.11A, B). It is not unusual to see them on the arms or trunk.
- Displays retraction sign (i.e., Fitzpatrick's sign). Lesion seems to retract or dimple downward when pinching around it (Figure 23.12).
- Dermatofibromas have a specific dermoscopic pattern of a central scar or starburst pattern with peripheral hyperpigmentation that helps with the diagnosis (Figure 23.13 and see Chapter 18, *Dermoscopy*).
- Dermatofibromas are most often diagnosed clinically.

TREATMENT

Discuss with the patient that a dermatofibroma is not dangerous and can be left alone. The scar from treatment may be more unsightly and more uncomfortable than the original DF. If the patient insists on treatment, the options consist of the following:

- Punch excision if smaller than 6 mm

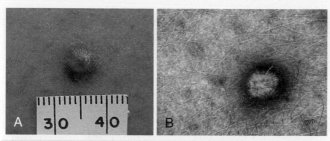

Figure 23.10 **(A)** Dermatofibroma with a hyperpigmented halo and a white and pink scar at the center. **(B)** Dermatofibroma in patient with skin of color with brown tones instead of pink or red. (Copyright Daniel L. Stulberg, MD.)

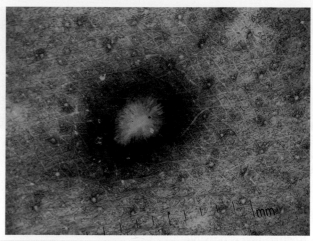

Figure 23.13 Dermoscopy of dermatofibroma with central starburst scar pattern and peripheral pigmentation in a patient with dark skin. (Copyright Daniel L. Stulberg, MD.)

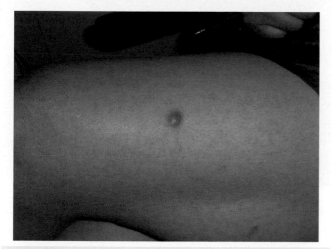

Figure 23.11 Large dermatofibroma on the leg that was not dermatofibrosarcoma protuberans. (Copyright Richard P. Usatine, MD.)

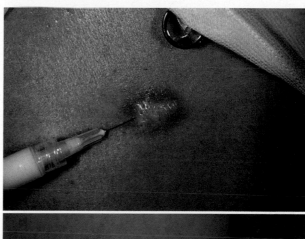

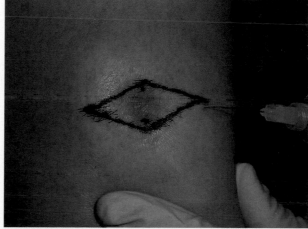

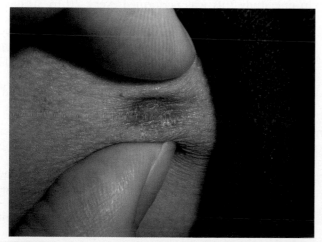

Figure 23.12 Positive pinch test showing how the dermatofibroma dimples down when pinched from the sides. (Copyright Richard P. Usatine, MD.)

Figure 23.14 Elliptical excision of a dermatofibroma on the arm. (Copyright Richard P. Usatine, MD.)

- Elliptical excision (full thickness down to subcutaneous [SQ] fat) for larger lesions (Figure 23.14)
- Always send tissue to confirm diagnosis and rule out dermatofibrosarcoma protuberans (DFSP) (see Chapter 24, *Diagnosis and Treatment of Malignant and Premalignant Lesions*).
- A shave biopsy can be combined with cryosurgery, but this is not proven to be effective.

- Cryosurgery is less effective than surgery but can shrink the lesion if that is what the patient desires. Using liquid nitrogen (spray or probe), freeze to a 2-mm freeze margin for a 15-second freeze time. Allow to thaw completely, and consider a second freeze for another 15 seconds. Regrowth is not uncommon with this method. A closed probe may allow a deeper freeze (Figure 23.15A, B).

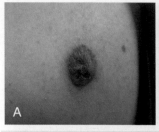
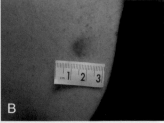

Figure 23.15 (A) Dermatofibroma blistering 2 days after treatment with cryosurgery. **(B)** Dermatofibroma with reduced pigmentation 1 year after cryosurgery. (Copyright Daniel L. Stulberg, MD.)

SPECIAL CONSIDERATIONS/BILLING

- Recurrence is possible.
- Send for pathology if excised.
- Bill for the excision of a benign lesion based on the size of the excision.
- If cryosurgery is used, bill for the destruction of a benign lesion.

Keloids and Hypertrophic Scars

DIAGNOSIS

- Thickened, dense proliferation at site of trauma may be pink, red, or brown.
- May itch or be irritated
- Keloids extend beyond the margin of scar site in contrast to hypertrophic scar (Figure 23.16).
- More common in people with darker skin tones
- More common on ear, midchest, and back

TREATMENT

Cryosurgery

See Video 13.7.

- Use a 10-second freeze with 1-mm freeze margin, thaw, and then repeat or inject with steroid. Schedule monthly

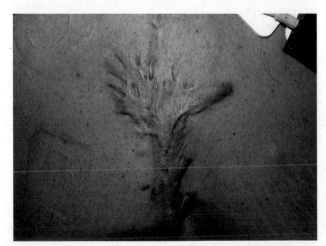

Figure 23.16 Keloid with thickened abnormal tissue beyond the original skin trauma. (Copyright Daniel L. Stulberg, MD.)

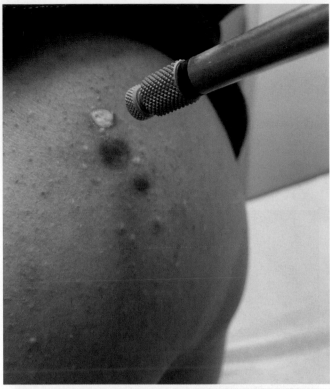

Figure 23.17 Third cryosurgery of keloids with thinning and lightening of pigmentation. (Copyright Daniel L. Stulberg, MD.)

visits for retreatment until symptoms, thickening, and appearance have improved to the patient's satisfaction. In one study this was performed every 20 to 30 days until flattening with a 73% success rate (Figure 23.17).[2]

- As an adjunct before intralesional injection, some recommend waiting 10 to 15 minutes after cryosurgery to allow softening of keloids (Figure 23.18A, B). We could find no data to support waiting.
- Cryosurgery and intralesional steroids can be combined.
- May cause hypopigmentation in addition to pain

Injection

See Video 13.7.

- Inject triamcinolone acetate 10 to 40 mg/mL infiltrated with a 27-gauge needle into keloids until tissue blanches (Figure 23.18B).
- Use needle with Luer lock since this requires significant pressure injecting into the dense keloid tissue.
- Start at 10 mg/mL and titrate up to 40 mg/mL as needed if no effect and no atrophy.
- Repeat every 2 to 4 weeks until nearly flat.
- May cause telangiectasias and atrophy

Excision of Keloid

See Video 23.5.

- Results in a high rate of recurrence, so this method should not be used as sole therapy
- After excision, inject with triamcinolone 10 to 40 mg/mL into wound margins at time of surgery and every 2 to 4 weeks for 6 months. *Or* one reinjection at 4 weeks only.

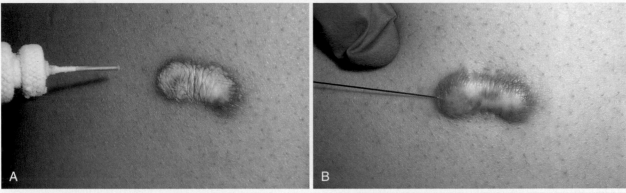

Figure 23.18 (A) Using cryosurgery on a keloid to soften it prior to injection with steroids. **(B)** Injecting an acne keloid with triamcinolone using a 27-gauge needle. (Copyright Richard P. Usatine, MD.)

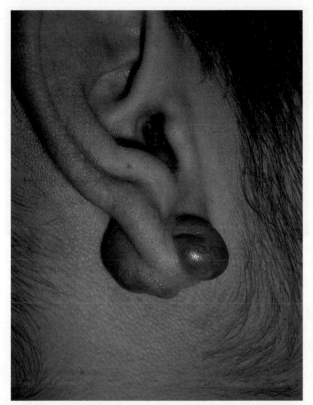

Figure 23.19 Keloids formed on both sides of the earlobe secondary to ear piercing. (Copyright Richard P. Usatine, MD.)

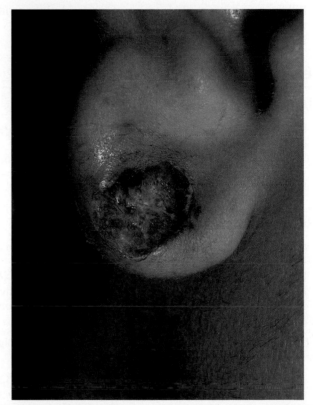

Figure 23.20 The front side of an earlobe after the keloid was excised. The base was electrocoagulated, and steroid suspension was injected at the base. (Copyright Richard P. Usatine, MD.)

- Earlobe keloids (Figure 23.19) can be shaved off, injected with triamcinolone, and allowed to heal by secondary intent (Figure 23.20). If possible, have the patient return in 1 month for a second triamcinolone injection to prevent regrowth.
- Large keloids on the ear can be excised and sutured (Figure 23.21A, B).
- After a keloid excision in any location (Figure 23.18), consider injections with triamcinolone to prevent keloids from recurring.

Lasers

- Ablative devices, including erbium and CO_2 lasers, and nonablative devices, including pulsed dye (585- and 595-nm) and fractional (1550-nm) devices, can reduce the thickness and texture of scars.[6]
- Nonablative lasers and IPL devices for treatment of red vascular ectasias can reduce the erythema associated with scars.

Other Treatments

- Use topical silicone sheeting or other occlusive dressings for up to 1 year.

SPECIAL CONSIDERATIONS/BILLING

- Recurrence and future lesions are common.

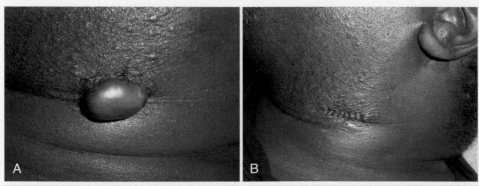

Figure 23.21 **(A)** Keloid on the neck. **(B)** Keloid excised, and defect closed with 6-0 Prolene. The incision site was injected with triamcinolone to prevent recurrence. (Copyright Richard P. Usatine, MD.)

- Bill for cryosurgery (destruction of benign lesion) or intralesional injections based on treatment.
- If excised, bill for the excision of a benign lesion.

Lentigines (Solar)

DIAGNOSIS

- Benign pigmented macules in sun-exposed areas (Figure 23.22).
- Single or multiple, starting in adulthood and increase with age and sun exposure.
- Do not regress with sun avoidance.

TREATMENT

- Sunscreen and sun avoidance may decrease occurrence.
- Use makeup to cover lentigines.
- Depigmentation with cryosurgery with short superficial freezing. Warn patients that this is not an exact science and that there is a risk of hypopigmentation or occasionally postinflammatory hyperpigmentation.

Lasers and IPL devices used for treatment of benign pigmented lesions are also effective for solar lentigines.[7,8]

- In general, devices with shorter wavelengths (e.g., 532- and 755-nm lasers and IPLs with lower cutoff filters) and Q-switched lasers are most effective for lentigines, where melanin is located superficially in the skin.
- Lentigines typically darken immediately after treatment and spontaneously exfoliate over a few weeks.
- One to three treatment sessions are typically needed.
- Topical retinoids may lighten lesions.
- Tretinoin nightly. (Retin-A multiple strengths available; use lower strengths for sensitive or dry skin.)
- Adapalene 0.1% to 0.3% gel (Differin) nightly
- Light chemical peels

SPECIAL CONSIDERATIONS/BILLING

- Treatment for lentigines is cosmetic, so insurance likely will not cover.
- Consider lentigo maligna and lentigo maligna melanoma in the differential diagnosis. Use dermoscopy to help with this differential diagnosis and if still uncertain, perform a shave biopsy.

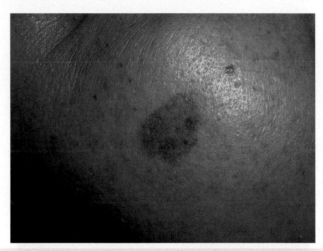

Figure 23.22 Large solar lentigo on the face of a 54-year-old Hispanic woman. (Copyright Richard P. Usatine, MD.)

Milia

DIAGNOSIS

- Superficial 1- to 3-mm white keratinized cysts (Figure 23.23).
- Common in the normal newborn but usually regresses spontaneously.
- May occur later in children and adults where they are more persistent.
- Most common on the face and genital region.

TREATMENT

See Video 23.6.

- Nick top of lesion with a No. 11 blade, sterile needle, or the sharp end of a comedone extractor (Figure 23.23B).
- Express white keratin contents by pressure with comedone extractor or paperclip (Figure 23.23C, D).[9]
- This is performed without anesthesia to avoid obscuring the milia and because the small cut should be less painful than the anesthetic.
- If this does not work the first time, make a slightly larger incision. Some comedone extractors work better than others depending on the size and location of the milia. It

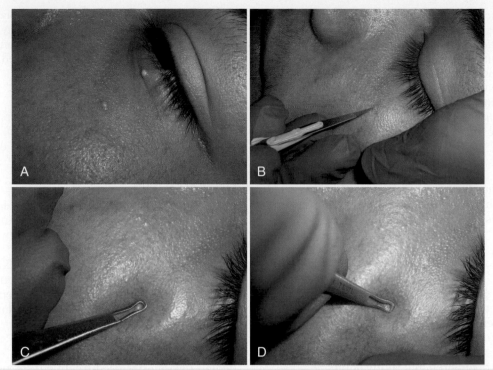

Figure 23.23 (A) Milia on the lower eyelid. **(B)** Milia incised with a No. 11 blade. **(C)** Milia within comedone extractor. **(D)** Milia removed. (Copyright Richard P. Usatine, MD.)

is therefore good to have a few types of comedone extractors in the office.

SPECIAL CONSIDERATIONS/PATHOLOGY/ BILLING

- Bill using the CPT code for acne surgery = 10040.

Molluscum Contagiosum

DIAGNOSIS

- Clustered, flesh-colored epidermal papules; dome shaped often with central umbilication
- Molluscum contagiosum virus infection is seen commonly in children.
- In adults it can be a sexually transmitted infection.

TREATMENT

Treatments induce an inflammatory response, which helps the immune system fight off the virus and includes the following[10]:

- Spontaneous resolution may take months to years.
- Cryosurgery to a 1-mm freeze margin, approximately 5- to 10-second freeze, thaw, and repeat (Figure 23.24)
- Curette the papules off with a skin curette (or scrape with an 18-gauge needle).
  - Pretreat with topical anesthetic in children (lidocaine/prilocaine cream or others).
  - Any bleeding may be stopped with aluminum chloride.
- Cantharidin (blister beetle extract) topically applied in office once. This method does not hurt when initially

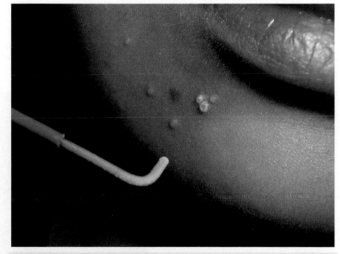

Figure 23.24 Molluscum contagiosum receiving cryosurgery with a bent tip spray. (Copyright Richard P. Usatine, MD.)

applied, so it is easier to use for children who are afraid of liquid nitrogen. Apply with the wooden end of a cotton-tipped applicator (CTA). If applied carefully it can be well tolerated and effective.

- Trichloroacetic acid 20% to 30% applied in office once
- Tretinoin (Retin-A) nightly (off-label)
- Imiquimod 5% (Aldara) was previously recommended but is now off-label, as the FDA has deemed it equivalent to placebo.
- Electrodesiccation lightly performed; no need to destroy entire lesion. The risk of scarring is probably greatest with electrodesiccation.

Results from the Cochrane database suggest:

No single intervention has been shown to be convincingly effective in the treatment of molluscum contagiosum. They found moderate-quality evidence that topical 5% imiquimod was no more effective than vehicle in terms of clinical cure but led to more application site reactions. They concluded that the natural resolution of molluscum contagiosum remains a strong method for dealing with the condition.[11]

BILLING

- 17110 used once for treatment of 1 to 14 lesions.
- 17111 used once for treatment of 15 or more lesions, and these codes are mutually exclusive.

Mucocele

DIAGNOSIS

- Bluish to clear or mucosal-colored fluid collection, not a true cyst with epithelial lining
- Most common on inner lower lip (Figure 23.25A)
- Mucin collection due to disruption of minor salivary duct
- Most common in children and young adults
- Often due to biting inner lip

TREATMENT

Cryosurgery

- This is an especially good technique for children old enough to permit this procedure.[12,13]

- Freeze the closed probe, and then apply to the mucocele with pressure. A second treatment may be needed.
- Alternatively, aspirate the mucin contents, and then freeze using CTAs or cryoprobe pressed against the base of the mucocele.

Shave Excision

- If the mucocele protrudes above the lip, a shave excision may be performed (Figure 23.25B). Then the base may be destroyed with cryosurgery or electrosurgery (Figure 23.25C).

Elliptical Excision

- This is best performed using a chalazion clamp on the lower lip to minimize bleeding and to control the site during surgery (see Chapter 20 for more details). *See video 20.5.*
- Suture with absorbable suture or silk. Consider using buried absorbable sutures so that the ends of the sutures do not irritate the patient.[14] If a deep excision is performed be careful not to cut a labial artery. If so, ligate the artery on both ends.[12]

Nevi

Benign nevi do not need treatment for medical purposes. However, patients may ask for their "moles" to be removed, and this would be a cosmetic procedure.

Pigmented lesions that are suspicious for melanoma need to be biopsied for a definitive diagnosis. Dermoscopy is the best way to distinguish between nevi and melanoma and to help determine when a nevus might require a biopsy. (See Chapter 18, *Dermoscopy of Skin Cancer.*)

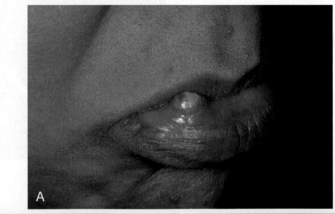

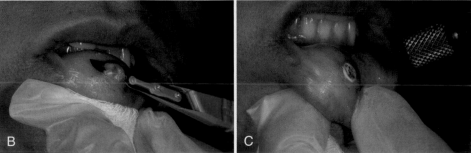

Figure 23.25 (A) Mucocele on the inner lip. **(B)** Mucocele shaved off with scalpel. **(C)** Mucocele being frozen with liquid nitrogen spray. (Copyright Richard P. Usatine, MD.)

ACQUIRED NEVI

The three most common acquired nevi are junctional, compound, and intradermal nevi. Some nevi evolve over time from junctional to compound to intradermal nevi.

Junctional Nevi

- Flat, pigmented brown to black with nevus cells at the dermal epidermal junction

Compound Nevi

- Have nevus cells in the epidermis and dermis
- Slightly raised and pigmented brown to black
- Slightly irregular surface

Intradermal Nevi

- Raised, flesh-colored; pink or brown to black
- Often cerebriform/variegated surface especially on scalp. The nevus cells are in the dermis.

Dysplastic Nevi (Atypical Moles)

- Have atypical features similar to an early melanoma clinically and dermoscopically.
- These are not precancerous lesions and only need to be biopsied when melanoma is suspected. If biopsied, and the result is mild-moderate atypia, then it may help to ensure that the lesion was fully excised clinically. If there is severe atypia, most clinicians treat this similarly to melanoma in situ with reexcision using 3- to 5-mm margins.

There are many other types of nevi including epidermal nevi, speckled nevi, nevus sebaceous, Becker's nevi, halo nevi, Spitz nevi, nevus depigmentosus, and nevus anemicus. The most important issue is to make a clear diagnosis when melanoma is suspected. Dermoscopy is the key to a good clinical diagnosis before initiating a biopsy (see Chapter 18, *Dermoscopy of Skin Cancer*). Also, see Chapter 24 for further information on biopsy/excision techniques for lesions suspicious for melanoma.

TREATMENT

Remember, benign nevi do not need treatment for medical purposes. Do not perform cryosurgery or electrodesiccation on nevi in general as you may be treating a melanoma inadvertently. Also, if a nevus that was benign grows back after cryosurgery, a biopsy may show histology suggestive of a melanoma (pseudomelanoma). Whether excising a suspicious nevus or a benign-appearing one, it is best to send the tissue to pathology for diagnosis.

Shave

See Videos 23.7–23.10.

- Intradermal nevi may be shaved flat with the surrounding surface to provide good cosmesis and adequate tissue for diagnosis (Figure 23.26). These may have features suggestive of a BCC such as telangiectasias, so a shave biopsy is a good technique to differentiate between these diagnoses.
- Scalp nevi that appear benign can be removed with a shave excision.
- Nevi may recur partially, but if the pathology is normal, it need not be removed again unless the patient wants it done for cosmetic reasons.
- Shave biopsy/excision may be performed with electrosurgery using an RF loop electrode (Figure 23.27).

See Video 23.11.

- Dysplastic nevi may be removed with a deep shave excision (also called *saucerization*). Shave deep enough to remove all pigmentation using a 1- to 2-mm circumferential margin. It helps to mark around the pigmented lesion before cutting (Figure 23.28A–D).

Punch Excision

- If the nevus is less than 6 mm, it is small enough to be biopsied completely with a punch. For example, a 4-mm nevus can be removed with a 1-mm margin using a 6-mm punch excision (Figure 23.29). If greater than 6 mm, a deep shave excision or an elliptical excision is preferred.
- A full-thickness excision is good for pathology and diagnostic depth (as is a deep shave that completely removes the lesion without requiring suturing).

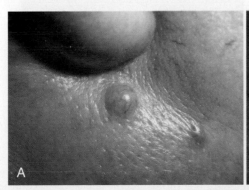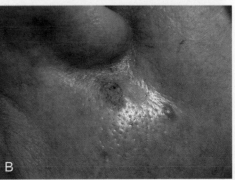

Figure 23.26 (A) Benign intradermal nevus that looks like a BCC because of its pearly nature and telangiectasias. **(B)** Intradermal nevus after a simple shave excision. (Copyright Richard P. Usatine, MD.)

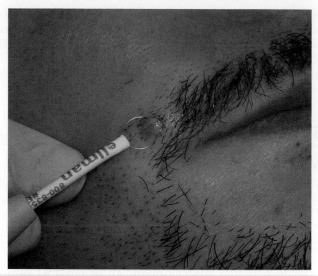

Figure 23.27 Excising an intradermal nevus with a radio-frequency loop. (Copyright Richard P. Usatine, MD.)

■ Junctional nevi are flat and if not suspicious for melanoma, these are best left alone. If a patient insists on removal for cosmetic purposes, a punch biopsy will give a good cosmetic result if the nevus is less than 6 mm.

Elliptical Excision

■ Use for lesions greater than 6 mm when a full-thickness excision is preferred.

■ Nevi with hair will do better cosmetically with a full-thickness excision because most shave biopsies will not be deep enough to remove the hair follicles.
■ A full-thickness excision is good for pathology and diagnostic depth if it turns out to be a melanoma.
■ Usually heals well with linear scar
■ Takes more time than other techniques

Dysplastic Nevus (Atypical Mole)

■ Possible dysplastic nevi suspicious for melanoma may be biopsied using a deep shave, a punch, or an elliptical excision based on size.
■ Figure 23.28A–D above shows how a dysplastic nevus can be fully removed with a deep shave biopsy, confirming that there is no remaining pigmentation at the deep margin.
■ If the pathology shows severe dysplasia and the margins were not clear, it is best to reexcise the area with 5-mm margins.

Studies show that 30% of melanomas appear to arise from preexisting nevi. The annual risk of an individual nevus transforming into a melanoma is estimated to be only 1 in 200,000.[15] The annual risk for an individual dysplastic nevus (DN) is extremely low as well, but estimates are higher: 1 in 10,000 may transform into a melanoma in 1 year.[16]

The only statistically significant association found with nevus recurrence was with the superficial shave technique being significantly associated with recurrence.[17]

Goodson et al.'s results[17] are consistent with those of Kmetz et al.,[18] who found that no melanomas developed during a 5-year period after biopsy of 55 atypical nevi

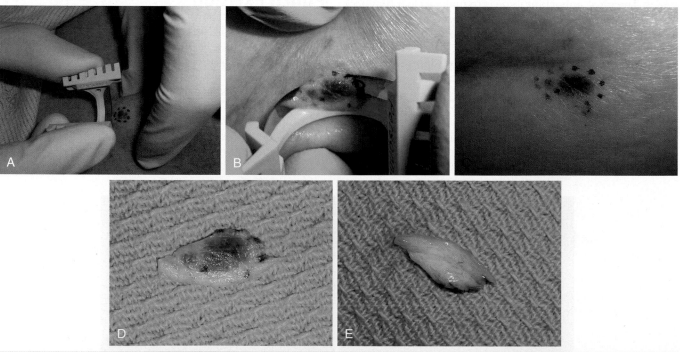

Figure 23.28 (A) Physician has pinched the skin for stabilization before cutting this possible dysplastic nevus off with a shave biopsy to pathology. **(B)** Completing the deep shave excision, aka saucerization. Note the outlines with a 1-mm margin. **(C)** The resultant defect with no residual pigmentation. **(D)** The removed specimen before placing in formalin. **(E)** Confirming no residual pigmentation on the underside of the removed specimen, which turned out to be a dysplastic nevus with clear margins. (Copyright Richard P. Usatine, MD.)

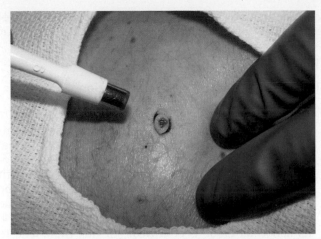

Figure 23.29 Punch biopsy done of a pigmented lesion. Note the elongated ellipse achieved on purpose by pulling the skin away from the biopsy site perpendicular to the skin lines. (Copyright Daniel L. Stulberg, MD.)

(26 lesions with at least 1 positive margin and 29 with clear margins) that were not reexcised.[16] Both studies suggest that lesions that demonstrate only mild or moderate dysplasia may not need to be reexcised given their low likelihood of recurrence and can be followed clinically for evidence of recurrence or development of any concerning features.[15,16] As above, DN demonstrating severe dysplasia should be reexcised with 3- to 5-mm margins given the risk of early or evolving melanoma.

Congenital Nevi

Congenital nevi are frequently large and very rarely can transform into melanoma (larger congenital nevi have a higher risk of malignant transformation). The clinical diagnosis of congenital nevus is made based on history because they have been present since birth or occurred within the first year after birth (tardive congenital nevus). Biopsy is indicated if a congenital nevus changes in color, there is a new growth within the nevus, or bleeding without trauma occurs within the nevus. The most recent approach recommends following these lesions as with any other nevus and removing them for any observed changes or concerns.

Neurofibromas

DIAGNOSIS

- Neurofibromas are soft fleshy papules that can feel like pushing tissue through a buttonhole when compressed downward.
- Persons without neurofibromatosis can have a few isolated neurofibromas.
- Neurofibromatosis type 1 (NF1) is associated with multiple neurofibromas.

Diagnosis of NF1 is made if an individual has two or more of the seven National Institutes of Health criteria present:

1. Multiple café au lait macules (6 or more)
2. Axillary or inguinal freckling
3. Multiple neurofibromas
4. Characteristic skeletal disorders
5. Family history of NF1
6. Iris hamartomas (Lisch nodules)
7. Optic gliomas

TREATMENT

- Individual lesions can be removed if desired by the patient.
- A narrow elliptical incision around a neurofibroma is an effective method for removal.
- An alternative approach involves a shave across the base with razor, scalpel, or electrosurgical cutting electrode (Figure 23.30A).
- Often the underlying tissue will elevate above the skin surface (pouch out).
- Remove the remaining tissue from the surrounding skin using a scalpel or scissors while using a forceps to stabilize the abnormal tissue (Figure 23.30B).
- If the defect is small and flat, allow it to heal by secondary intention. Otherwise suture the defect with a single-layer closure. Use deep sutures only if there is tension.
- Convert to an ellipse if there are standing cones (dogears) (see Chapter 11, *The Elliptical Excision*).

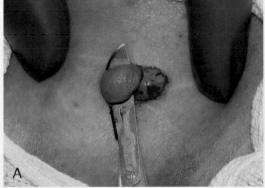
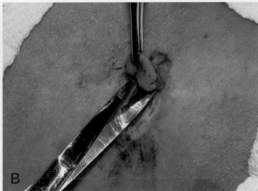

Figure 23.30 (A) Shave excision of a neurofibroma revealed an outpouching of soft tissue. **(B)** The remainder of the neurofibroma was excised with a sharp iris scissor. (Copyright Daniel L. Stulberg, MD.)

Pilomatricoma

DIAGNOSIS

- Dermal or subcutaneous nodule containing calcium (also known as calcifying epithelioma of Malherbe) (Figure 23.31)
- Often presents in childhood on the neck or upper extremities
- Firm to palpation

TREATMENT

- Elliptical excision is the treatment of choice (Figure 23.31A, B).

Pyogenic Granuloma (Lobular Capillary Hemangioma)

DIAGNOSIS

- Glistening, friable, easily bleeding vascular tissue often with a narrowed base (Figure 23.32A).
- Initial rapid growth and failure to heal
- Often at site of trauma or irritation
- Common on extremities, especially fingers
- May occur as an umbilical granuloma of the newborn or on gums of pregnant woman

In a randomized controlled trial that compared cryotherapy with liquid nitrogen versus curettage and electrodesiccation of patients with PG, the curettage and electrodesiccation had the advantage of requiring fewer treatment sessions to achieve resolution and had better cosmetic results.[19] Treatment of the PGs resulted in complete resolution of all lesions after one to three sessions (mean 1.42) in the cryosurgery group and after one to two sessions (mean 1.03) in the curettage group ($P < 0.001$). Twenty-three patients (57.5%) in the cryotherapy group and 25 patients (69%) in the curettage group had no scar or pigmentation abnormality. From this study and personal experience, we conclude that curettage and electrodesiccation is the preferred treatment option over cryosurgery.

TREATMENT

Shave, Curettage, and Electrodesiccation

See Video 14.5.

- Use lidocaine with epinephrine, and wait at least 10 minutes for the epinephrine to work. Shave off the abnormal tissue, and send this for pathology (the differential diagnosis includes amelanotic melanoma). This can be done with a razor blade, scalpel, or electrosurgical loop. Curette the base and use electrodesiccation to stop the bleeding. The curettage and desiccation may need to be repeated until all abnormal tissue is destroyed.[20] If not, these tend to recur. Two cycles are routine; see Figure 23.32B–E demonstrating the procedure.

Elliptical Excision

- PGs on the lips or face may not be adequately treated using the above method, and the scarring may be unacceptable. Another option is to elliptically excise the PG. Figure 23.33A and B show how the PG on the lip is excised with the ellipse running vertically for the best cosmetic result.

Cryosurgery

- Children may be afraid of needles and may not allow one to anesthetize the skin to cut off their PG. In Figure 17.26 of Chapter 17, *Cryosurgery*, a young child has a PG on the face and allowed the physician to use a Cryo Tweezer to treat her. While it is best to obtain tissue for pathology in most cases, it is safe to treat a benign-appearing PG in a child with cryotherapy.

Silver Nitrate

- Silver nitrate may be used to treat umbilical granulomas. Be careful, however, because excessive application of silver nitrate can burn and/or tattoo the surrounding skin of an infant.[21]

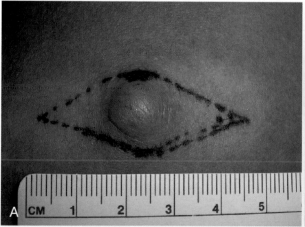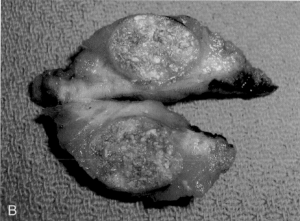

Figure 23.31 (A) Pilomatricoma on the left arm of a 17-year-old girl. The nodule is tender, and she requests it to be resected. **(B)** After elliptical excision, the pilomatricoma was analyzed by cutting the specimen in half. Note the white calcium granules within the tissue. (Copyright Richard P. Usatine, MD.)

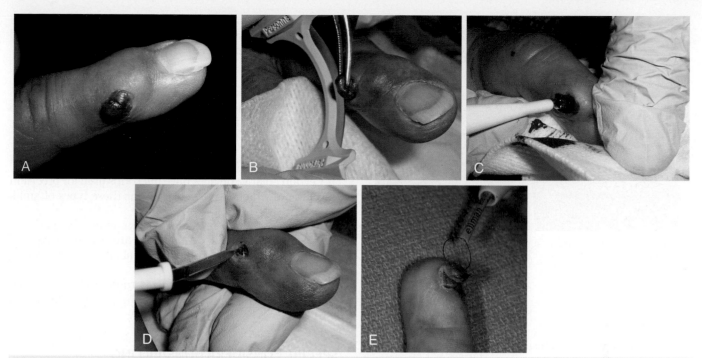

Figure 23.32 **(A)** Pyogenic granuloma on a finger. **(B)** Shave excision of the pyogenic granuloma using a DermaBlade. **(C)** The base was then curetted. **(D)** Electrodesiccation of the base. Often a second cycle of curettage and electrodesiccation is needed. **(E)** Using an Ellman Surgitron to remove a different pyogenic granuloma. (Copyright Richard P. Usatine, MD.)

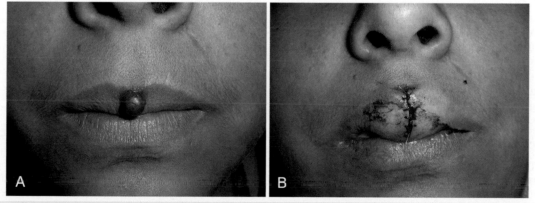

Figure 23.33 **(A)** Suspected pyogenic granuloma on the lip. **(B)** Pyogenic granuloma excised elliptically with direction of the ellipse being perpendicular to the vermilion border. The swelling is secondary to the anesthesia, and the cosmetic result looked great the following week. (Copyright Richard P. Usatine, MD.)

SPECIAL CONSIDERATIONS/BILLING

- Differential diagnosis includes amelanotic melanoma, so send tissue for pathology.
- Bill for a skin neoplasm (ICD-10 D48.5) because the diagnosis is not completely certain until the pathologist reviews the slides, or hold the billing until pathology is complete, and then code as indicated. Use CPT codes 11400-11446 for full-thickness excision based on location and size, or 17000 for destruction of benign lesion as indicated.
- Recurrence is common, so aggressive removal is prudent.

Sebaceous Hyperplasia

DIAGNOSIS

Flesh-colored to slightly pale papular clusters of enlarged sebaceous glands (Figure 23.34).

- Usually, multiple lesions on forehead and face help to differentiate them from BCC.
- Often doughnut shaped around central gland opening.
- Telangiectasias run radially without crossing the midline (called crown vessels) (Figure 23.35A)

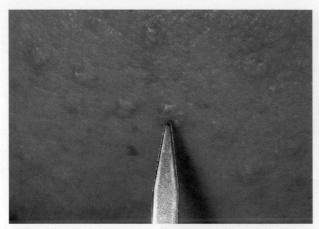

Figure 23.34 Blunt electrode about to electrodesiccate sebaceous hyperplasia. (Copyright Richard P. Usatine, MD.)

TREATMENT

Electrodesiccation

- This is done without anesthesia using low settings as for cherry angiomas and telangiectasias (Hyfrecator 2 to 3 joules). Start at 2.1 and only increase power if needed. *See video 23.12.*
- Lightly electrodesiccate the rim of sebum-laden tissue around the central pore. Using the blunt electrode can be easier than using the sharp-tipped electrode (Figure 23.34).
- Results can be seen immediately (Figure 23.35C).
- Many lesions (especially larger lesions) may need re-treatment after 1 to 2 months.
- Consider local anesthesia if lesions are large or multiple or if patients request it. Topical EMLA may be sufficient. If injecting lidocaine, use a surgical marker before administering the anesthesia because the sebaceous hyperplasia may be hard to see afterward.

Shave Excision

- If the diagnosis is not clear and a BCC is in the differential diagnosis, a shave biopsy is a good method medically and cosmetically. Do not forget to mark the lesion with a surgical marker before administering the anesthesia.
- For sebaceous hyperplasia that has not cleared with electrosurgery, shave excisions can provide long-lasting

results. The most common complication of this method is to leave a divot at the site of removal, so care is needed not to shave too deeply.

Cryotherapy

- Not as effective as electrosurgery but it is another option
- Light freezing with liquid nitrogen of the lesions can help slough them off in about a week.[22]

Lasers

- Ablative lasers (e.g., 2940 nm and CO_2) can be used.[23,24] Certain ablative devices have microtips used for precision ablation, which is very effective for these types of small lesions.[25]
- Nonablative 1450-nm diode lasers can also be used.[26]
- A series of four to six treatments are usually necessary with nonablative lasers, whereas ablative lasers require only one or two treatments.
- Photodynamic therapy utilizes topical photosensitizing medication activated by light (lasers, LEDs, and IPL devices).[27]

SPECIAL CONSIDERATIONS/BILLING

- Often appears similar to BCC; if any question, perform the shave and send to pathology. Code these as skin neoplasms ICD-10 48.5.
- May leave depressed area/scar that over time will usually partially fill in but may not
- Initial diagnostic E&M (evaluation and management) service and shave biopsy if needed to rule out BCC should be covered.
- Electrosurgery or laser for cosmesis is usually not covered by insurance.

Seborrheic Keratoses and Dermatosis Papulosa Nigra

DIAGNOSIS

- Benign stuck-on tumors with tan, brown, or black colors.
- Dermatosis papulosa nigra (DPN) is a collection of seborrheic keratoses (SKs) found on the cheeks and face – most commonly on the face in skin of color and bilaterally distributed (Figure 17.22 in Chapter 17, *Cryosurgery*).[28]

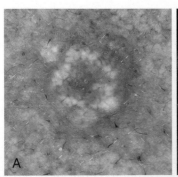
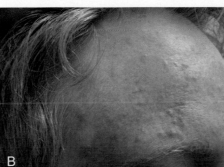
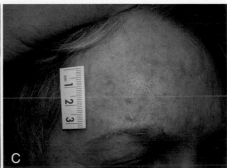

Figure 23.35 **(A)** Dermoscopy of sebaceous hyperplasia showing crown vessels popcorn-like structures. *(Copyright Richard P. Usatine, MD.)* **(B)** Sebaceous hyperplasia prior to electrosurgical treatment. **(C)** Clearance of sebaceous hyperplasia after treatment. (B Copyright Daniel L. Stulberg, MD.)

- Verrucous or smooth surface, often with keratin pearls (horn cysts, comedo-like openings, and milia cysts) and crevices seen on magnification and dermoscopy (see Chapter 18, *Dermoscopy*).
- Sharply demarcated, stuck-on appearance
- Superficial layers peel away easily, leaving capillary bleeding at base.
- Sudden appearance of multiple seborrheic keratosis lesions (sign of Leser-Trelat) may require workup for a possible malignancy, likely GI or pulmonary cancers.[29]

TREATMENT

- No treatment necessary if classic appearance and asymptomatic

Cryosurgery of SK (Figure 23.36)

See Videos 23.13 and 23.14.

- No anesthesia required
- Use an approximate 10-second freeze to a 1- to 2-mm freeze margin to avoid leaving a rim or remaining SK, thaw, and then consider a second freeze at the same visit.
- May be erythematous for weeks
- Can cause hypo- or hyperpigmentation (especially hypopigmentation in persons of darker color)
- This method is quick and clean with initial erythema in the office, necrosis of the lesion (sometimes with vesicle formation), and sloughing in 1 to 2 weeks.

Alternative treatment methods that require local anesthesia include the following:

- Shave biopsy/excision with blade and aluminum chloride or electrosurgery for hemostasis (Figure 23.37). This allows tissue to be sent for pathology if diagnosis is uncertain. Even if an SK is most likely, send for pathology to avoid missing a melanoma.
- Shave excision with electrosurgical loop.
- Curettage followed by electrodesiccation or aluminum chloride for hemostasis (Figure 23.38). It may help to

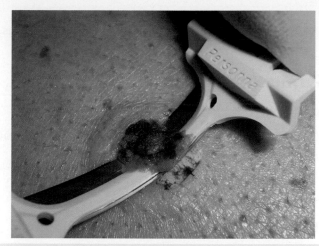

Figure 23.37 Shave biopsy/excision of a suspicious-looking pigmented lesion that turned out to be a seborrheic keratosis. (Copyright Richard P. Usatine, MD.)

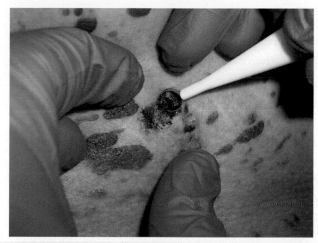

Figure 23.38 Curettage of a seborrheic keratosis in a patient where the diagnosis was certain. No tissue was sent for pathology. (Copyright Richard P. Usatine, MD.)

apply the electrodesiccation first because that will make the curettage step easier.

Electrodesiccation With Local Anesthesia

- Desiccate the raised tissue.
- Wipe off destroyed tissue with moistened gauze.
- Repeat as needed until lesion is removed and flat skin remains.

Electrodesiccation Without Local Anesthesia for DPN

- This is less likely to cause hypopigmentation and can be done with a Hyfrecator using settings of 2.1 to 2.5 W as needed and tolerated by the patient.
- *See video 23.15.*

SPECIAL CONSIDERATIONS/BILLING

- Consider malignant melanoma in differential diagnosis if atypical appearance.
- Be careful when freezing SKs or DPN on the face of a darkly pigmented person –hypopigmentation can be permanent.

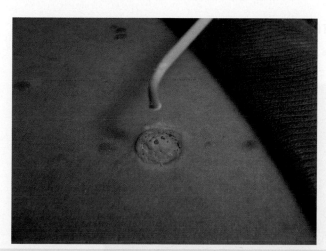

Figure 23.36 Cryosurgery of a seborrheic keratosis using an open spray approach with a bent tip. The comedo-like openings can be seen. (Copyright Richard P. Usatine, MD.)

- 17110 used once for treatment of 1 to 14 lesions.
- 17111 used once for treatment of 15 or more lesions. These codes are mutually exclusive.

Syringomas

DIAGNOSIS

- Benign periorbital adnexal tumors commonly seen on both lateral lower eyelids
- Diagnosis is clinical based on appearance (Figure 23.39A).
- Only of cosmetic concern and not a sign of any underlying illness.

TREATMENT

Treatment may be reassurance in many patients. If the patient insists on treatment, electrosurgery or laser treatments are most effective.

Electrodesiccation

- Apply a topical anesthetic such as EMLA. Wait for it to take effect.
- Use a Hyfrecator or other electrosurgical device using 2 to 3 W (Figure 23.39B). Use the ball electrode with the Surgitron.
- Deliver short bursts with standard electrodes or an epilation needle.[30]

Cryosurgery

Cryosurgery with tight control, as with the bent tip in Figure 23.39A, or a needle tip, due to proximity to the eyes may be used.

Laser

- Ablative lasers (e.g., 2940 nm and CO_2) can be used.[30]

Telangiectasias and Spider Angiomas

DIAGNOSIS

- Telangiectasias are frequently found on the nose as patients age. Persons with rosacea may have many telangiectasias on the nose and face.

TREATMENT

Telangiectasias may be treated for cosmetic reasons using electrosurgery or laser treatments.

- Electrodesiccation is performed without anesthesia using a Hyfrecator or other electrosurgical device set at 2 to 3 W (Figure 23.40). *See video 14.1.*
- Short bursts of energy are delivered with a sharp-tipped electrode or epilation needle. Enough electricity should be delivered to see the vessel blanch but avoid leaving a burn on the skin. Epilation needles are inserted into the vessel to avoid skin scarring and provide electrodesiccation to the blood vessel.
- Telangiectasias on the legs do not respond well to electrosurgery and are best treated by sclerotherapy or vascular surgery.

Spider angiomas (Figure 23.41) are often larger than telangiectasias and have a central feeding vessel. These are seen more commonly in patients with liver disease. Apply the electrosurgical sharp-tipped electrode to the central feeding vessel using 2 to 3 W and a quick pulse of electrical energy. Then the spider-like peripheral vessels can be treated the same way.

Cryosurgery is not very effective for telangiectasias and spider angiomas, and we do not recommend it.

Lasers (e.g., 532, 595, and 980 nm) and IPL devices used for treatment of red vascular ectasias are effective for facial telangiectasias.[31]

Trichoepithelioma

DIAGNOSIS

- Papular lesions most commonly of the head and upper trunk
- May be single or multiple and may occur in childhood (Figure 23.42)
- Shave biopsy to confirm suspected diagnosis because a single trichoepithelioma may resemble a BCC
- Desmoplastic trichoepitheliomas are more aggressive and should be removed with clear margins. Consider Mohs surgery if this is on the face.[32]

TREATMENT

- Shave excision may be adequate.

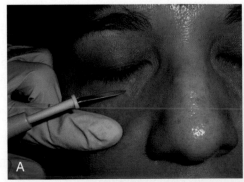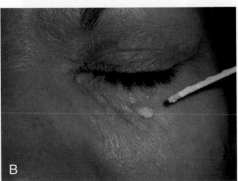

Figure 23.39 **(A)** Syringomas being treated with electrosurgery after topical lidocaine/prilocaine anesthetic. **(B)** Cryosurgery of syringomas. (Copyright Richard P. Usatine, MD.)

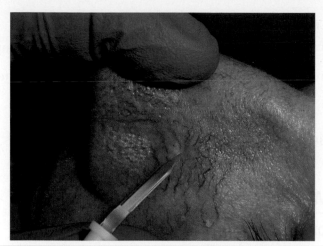

Figure 23.40 Electrosurgery of telangiectasias on the nose using the sharp tip electrode on the Hyfrecator without anesthesia. (Copyright Richard P. Usatine, MD.)

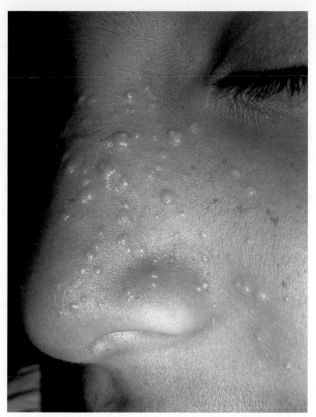

Figure 23.42 Multiple trichoepitheliomas are seen around the nose of a 9-year-old girl. Treatment was initiated with cryosurgery and topical tretinoin. (Copyright Richard P. Usatine, MD.)

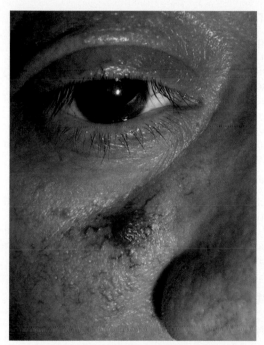

Figure 23.41 Spider angioma on the face. (Copyright Richard P. Usatine, MD.)

- Punch or elliptical excision is an alternative.
- For multiple trichoepitheliomas on the face in children, the treatment choices include cryosurgery along with topical medications (Figure 23.42). Although no clinical trials have been done that could help guide treatment, topical imiquimod and topical tretinoin have been used alone or in combination for treatment.[33]

Warts, Common

DIAGNOSIS

- Benign human papillomavirus (HPV) infection
- Most common on extremities
- Range from flat to dome shaped, smooth, or rough surface

TREATMENT

Topical Salicylic Acid

- These preparations are up to 75% effective and per the Cochrane Database are the first choice treatment.[34]
- Topical liquid 17% (Compound W, Duofilm, and others) or wax-based applicator (Wart Stick) applied nightly after soaking the wart in water and debriding loose skin
- Topical 40% salicylic acid plasters applied before bed
- May take weeks to months, and advise patients to use it for at least 3 to 4 months before being considered a treatment failure.

Cryosurgery

- Use a liquid nitrogen spray to a 1- to 2-mm freeze margin, allow to thaw, and then a repeat freeze. The second freeze usually takes less time to achieve the same effect due to the chilling of the tissues. A pulsatile spray can be used in order to get a deep enough freeze without too much superficial spread.
- One study showed that a 10-second sustained freeze to reach a 1- to 2-mm freeze margin was more effective than a shorter freeze.[35] This was an RCT, and the 10-second sustained freeze led to more pain and blistering.
- Even a short freeze can be divided into multiple freeze-thaw cycles if the patient can't tolerate one longer freeze.
- Use longer total freeze time if warts are thick, large, or resistant to previous cryosurgery.

- Cryo Tweezers can be used for pedunculated warts (especially around the face and eyes); *see video 13.9.*
- Pain, erythema, possible blistering, and skin sloughing are expected.
- A prolonged freeze can cause hematoma or temporary local nerve damage on occasion.
- Hypopigmentation is especially problematic in skin of color.
- Scarring is possible, but not common.
- Schedule additional visits for cryosurgery every 3 to 4 weeks with more frequent treatments being more effective in our experience.

In-Office Topicals

- Cantharidin may be used as for molluscum.
- Trichloroacetic acid 20% to 30% applied weekly after paring the wart down
- Topical sensitizers can be used. They require inducing immune system sensitization and resultant local reaction before treatment. The dinitrochlorobenzene sensitizer has cure rates from 38% to 80%.[37]

Curettage and Desiccation

- In resistant warts, may curette or dissect out the wart and electrodesiccate the base
- Leaves large initial defect
- Scarring is the norm.
- Electrodesiccation can aerosolize viral particles, so use a smoke evacuator and wear a mask.

Immunotherapy

- *Candida* antigen is a useful method to treat recalcitrant warts
- Intralesional *Candida* antigen with 0.1 to 0.2 mL of undiluted antigen injected into the largest 1 to 2 warts; may repeat monthly until resolution
- A recent RCT found it to be more effective than cryosurgery. There was complete clearance of warts in 63.3% of the *Candida* antigen group, 50% of the bivalent HPV vaccine group, 20% in the cryotherapy group, and 0% of the control group (Nassar).[36]
- A detailed description of how to inject *Candida* antigen is given in Chapter 15, *Intralesional Injections.*[37]

Special Considerations/Billing

- Biopsy if persistent or atypical appearance to rule out malignancy, especially if patient is immunocompromised because SCC can mimic warts.
- 17110 used once for treatment of 1 to 14 lesions.
- 17111 used once for treatment of 15 or more lesions. These codes are mutually exclusive.

Warts, Filiform

DIAGNOSIS

- Finger-like projection of warty tissue
- Common on face

TREATMENT

- Cryosurgery with Cryo Tweezers down to normal skin; thaw and repeat
- Due to small base can snip or shave and electrodesiccate the base
- Electrodesiccation can aerosolize viral particles.

BILLING

- As above for common warts.

Warts, Flat

DIAGNOSIS

- Slightly raised multiple flat flesh-colored lesions, 2 to 4 mm.
- Common on face, extremities of children, and legs (if shaving legs).

TREATMENT

- Imiquimod (Aldara).
- Tretinoin (Retin-A) nightly.
- Topical 5-fluorouracil (Efudex) nightly in refractory cases in adults.
- Intralesional *Candida* antigen with 0.1 to 0.2 mL of undiluted antigen injected into the largest 1 to 2 warts. May repeat monthly until resolution.
- Cryosurgery to a 1-mm freeze margin; approximately 5- to 10-second freeze.

See video 13.5.

- Electrosurgery with light fulguration (use topical anesthetic first)
- Light curettement with a disposable sharp curette is one option and can be performed either without anesthesia or after topical anesthetics have been applied.

Warts, Plantar

DIAGNOSIS

- Warts on the sole of the foot (plantar surface) (palmar are on the palm of the hand)
- Pain with walking or pressure
- Thickened, slightly raised
- To differentiate from calluses, warts disrupt the normal dermatoglyphic pattern and have visible thrombosed capillaries causing small black dots (Figure 23.43).

TREATMENT

- Cryosurgery with a 2-3-mm freeze margin; approximately 5- to 10-second freeze. Note that the Cochrane Database indicates that a more aggressive freeze has better success rates than a less aggressive freeze, but there is variation in how that is delineated.[37] A 3-mm freeze margin, thaw and repeat freeze is more likely to be effective, but there is discomfort during the cryosurgery and can cause pain with walking the next day.
- Consider adequate trial of topical therapy, which is 3 to 4 months of daily application following soaking in water, before more aggressive treatment.

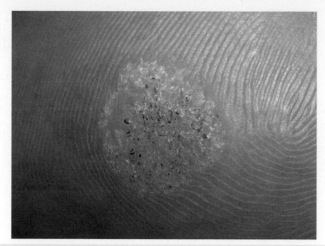

Figure 23.43 Plantar wart on the sole of the foot disrupting skin lines and showing black dots caused by thrombosed capillaries. (Copyright Richard P. Usatine, MD.)

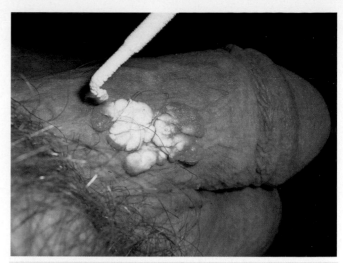

Figure 23.44 Cryosurgery of condyloma acuminata on the penis. (Copyright Richard P. Usatine, MD.)

SPECIAL CONSIDERATIONS/BILLING

- As above for common warts.
- Resistant and recurrent warts may respond to laser treatment.

Warts, Venereal (Condyloma Acuminata)

DIAGNOSIS

- Fleshy, polypoid, or verrucous flesh-colored raised lesions of the genital region and perirectal areas caused by HPV.

TREATMENT

Imiquimod 5% (Aldara)

- Topically QHS three times per week; wash off after 6 to 10 hours
- Use up to 16 weeks.

Podofilox 0.5% Solution or Gel (Condylox)

- Apply topically BID for 3 days to lesions; repeat weekly for 1 to 4 weeks.
- Gel for perianal lesions

Intralesional Candida Antigen

- Intralesional *Candida* antigen with 0.1 to 0.2 mL of undiluted antigen injected into the largest 1 to 2 warts. May repeat monthly until resolution.

Cryosurgery

- Use a 1- to 2-mm freeze margin and a freeze-thaw-freeze cycle (Figure 23.44).

Excision

- Large lesions can be anesthetized and excised with dissecting scissors or a scalpel with suture repair of any large defect.
- Condyloma can be excised using electrosurgery and a loop electrode as demonstrated with other types of lesions (Figures 23.5 and 23.32). Make sure to use a smoke evacuator to reduce risk of clinician infection with aerosolized viral particles.
- Scarring is possible.

Electrodesiccation or Laser

- Electrodesiccation or laser treatment can also aerosolize viral particles; use a vacuum filter.
- Use local anesthetic, general if large areas.
- Results are immediate.
- Scarring is possible.

SPECIAL CONSIDERATIONS/PATHOLOGY/BILLING*

- Viral infection is not cleared by removal of the condyloma. Recurrence is always possible.
- Caution to not miss cervical, penile, anal, and vulvar cancer, which is often caused by HPV
- Caution to not miss syphilitic condyloma lata
- Use site specific codes to bill for destruction of condyloma. See Table 28.2 in Chapter 28, *Coding and Billing for Dermatologic Procedures.*

Xanthelasma

DIAGNOSIS

- Superficial lipid deposits around the eyes and eyelids (Figure 23.45)
- Pale, raised, rubbery
- Fifty percent of patients have hyperlipidemia, so evaluate lipid levels and treat as appropriate.

TREATMENT

- Elliptical excision by a clinician skilled at eyelid surgery
- Cryosurgery or electrosurgical destruction may be attempted, but do not expect great results.
- Ablative lasers, including erbium and CO_2, and pulsed dye lasers (585 and 595 nm)[38]

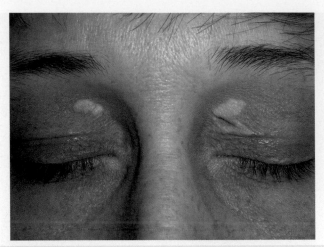

Figure 23.45 Xanthelasma in a woman with cholesterol over 300. (Copyright Richard P. Usatine, MD.)

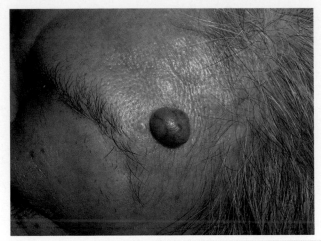

Figure 23.47 Spiradenoma on the forehead. (Copyright Richard P. Usatine, MD.)

Less Common Benign Adnexal Tumors

- Eccrine poroma (Figure 23.46).
- Spiradenoma (Figure 23.47).

These will most likely be diagnosed when an unusual growth is removed, and the pathology report comes back with one of these descriptions. Their photos are included in this chapter as an introduction to their existence. In most cases the definitive treatment involves complete excision with clear margins.

Conclusion

Benign skin tumors will be seen daily in any clinical practice involving the skin. It is important to realize that many, once diagnosed, do not require treatment or intervention. If a patient desires to have the lesion removed, there are usually multiple techniques to achieve removal with reasonable cosmetic results. Clinicians should consider their array of instruments, equipment, and their own skills and practice flow to choose the appropriate technique for the individual situation. If the diagnosis is uncertain or malignancy is high in the differential diagnosis, do not hesitate to remove the lesion and send for pathology. When in doubt cut it out.

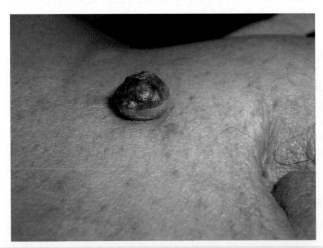

Figure 23.46 Eccrine poroma on the abdomen. (Copyright Richard P. Usatine, MD.)

References

1. Qadeer HA, Singal A, Patel BC. Cherry hemangioma. In: *StatPearls [Internet]*. 2021. Available at: https://www.ncbi.nlm.nih.gov/books/NBK563207/#article-19379.s12.
2. Cortell Fuster C, Martínez Gómez MA, Cercós Lleti AC, Climente Martí M. Topical rapamycin in the treatment of facial angiofibromas in tuberous sclerosis: a systematic review based on evidence. *J Dermatolog Treat*. 2022;33(4):1804-1810. doi:10.1080/09546634.2021.1905768.
3. Goldberg DJ, Marcus J. The use of the frequency-doubled Q-switched Nd:YAG laser in the treatment of small cutaneous vascular lesions. *Dermatol Surg*. 1996;22:841-844.
4. Gupta G, Hohman MH, Kwan E. Chondrodermatitis nodularis helicis. In: *StatPearls [Internet]*. 2021. Available at: https://www.ncbi.nlm.nih.gov/books/NBK482507/#article-32734.s2.
5. Thiers BH, Strat N, Snyder AN, Zito PM. Cutaneous horn. In: *StatPearls [Internet]*. 2023. Available at: https://www.ncbi.nlm.nih.gov/books/NBK563280/#article-22999.s2.
6. Katz TM, Glaich AS, Goldberg LH, Friedman PM. 595-nm long pulsed dye laser and 1450-nm diode laser in combination with intralesional triamcinolone/5-fluorouracil for hypertrophic scarring following a phenol peel. *J Am Acad Dermatol*. 2010;62:1045-1049.
7. Ross EV, Smirnov M, Pankratov M. Intense pulsed light and laser treatment of facial telangiectasias and dyspigmentation: some theoretical and practical comparisons. *Dermatol Surg*. 2005;31:1188-1198.
8. Small R. Aesthetic procedures in office practice. *Am Fam Physician*. 2009;80:1231-1237.
9. Gallardo Avila PP, Mendez MD. Milia. In: *StatPearls [Internet]*. 2021. Available at: https://www.ncbi.nlm.nih.gov/books/NBK560481/.
10. Badri T, Gandhi G. Molluscum contagiosum. 2021. Available at: https://www.ncbi.nlm.nih.gov/books/NBK441898/#article-25233.s2.
11. van der Wouden JC, van der Sande R, Kruithof EJ, Sollie A, van Suijlekom-Smit LW, Koning S. Interventions for cutaneous molluscum contagiosum. *Cochrane Database Syst Rev*. 2017;5(5):CD004767. doi:10.1002/14651858.CD004767.pub4.
12. Marcushamer M, King DL, Ruano NS. Cryosurgery in the management of mucoceles in children. *Pediatr Dent*. 1997;19:292-293.

13. Essaket S, Hakkou F, Chbicheb S. Mucocèle de la muqueuse buccale [Mucocele of the oral mucous membrane]. *Pan Afr Med J.* 2020;35: 140. doi:10.11604/pamj.2020.35.140.21079.

14. Tran TA, Parlette HL III. Surgical pearl: removal of a large labial mucocele. *J Am Acad Dermatol.* 1999;40:760-762.

15. Tsao H, Bevona C, Goggins W, Quinn T. The transformation rate of moles (melanocytic nevi) into cutaneous melanoma: a population-based estimate. *Arch Dermatol.* 2003;139:282-288.

16. Naeyaert JM, Brochez L. Clinical practice. Dysplastic nevi. *N Engl J Med.* 2003;349:2233-2240.

17. Goodson AG, Florell SR, Boucher KM, Grossman D. Low rates of clinical recurrence after biopsy of benign to moderately dysplastic melanocytic nevi. *J Am Acad Dermatol.* 2010;62:591-596.

18. Kmetz EC, Sanders H, Fisher G, et al. The role of observation in the management of atypical nevi. *South Med J.* 2009;102:45-48.

19. Ghodsi SZ, Raziei M, Taheri A, et al. Comparison of cryotherapy and curettage for the treatment of pyogenic granuloma: a randomized trial. *Br J Dermatol.* 2006;154:671-675.

20. Sarwal P, Lapumnuaypol K. Pyogenic granuloma. In: *StatPearls [Internet].* 2021. Available at: https://www.ncbi.nlm.nih.gov/books/ NBK556077/#_NBK556077_pubdet.

21. Daniels J, Craig F, Wajed R, Meates M. Umbilical granulomas: a randomised controlled trial. *Arch Dis Child Fetal Neonatal Ed.* 2003; 88:F257.

22. Farci F, Rapini RP. Sebaceous hyperplasia. In: *StatPearls [Internet].* 2021. Available at: https://www.ncbi.nlm.nih.gov/books/ NBK562148/#_NBK562148_pubdet_.

23. Krupashankar DS. Standard guidelines of care: CO_2 laser for removal of benign skin lesions and resurfacing. *Indian J Dermatol Venereol Leprol.* 2008;74(suppl):S61-S67.

24. Riedel F, Bergler W, Baker Schreyer A, et al. Controlled cosmetic dermal ablation in the facial region with the erbium: YAG laser. *HNO.* 1999;47:101-106.

25. Khatri KA. Treatment of cutaneous lesions using a novel 2.94 erbium laser with micron tips. Presented at American Society for Laser Medicine and Surgery; 2009; National Harbor, MD.

26. No D, McClaren M, Chotzen V, Kilmer SL. Sebaceous hyperplasia treated with a 1450-nm diode laser. *Dermatol Surg.* 2004;30: 382-384.

27. Richey D, Hopson B. Treatment of sebaceous hyperplasia with photodynamic therapy. *Cosm Dermatol.* 2004;17:525-529.

28. Xiao A, Muse ME, Ettefagh L. Dermatosis papulosa nigra. In: *StatPearls [Internet].* 2021. Available at: https://www.ncbi.nlm.nih.gov/books/NBK534205/#_NBK534205_pubdet_.

29. Greco MJ, Bhutta BS. Seborrheic keratosis. In: *StatPearls [Internet].* 2021. Available at: https://www.ncbi.nlm.nih.gov/books/NBK5 45285/#_NBK545285_pubdet_.

30. Karam P, Benedetto AV. Syringomas: new approach to an old technique. *Int J Dermatol.* 1996;35:219-220.

31. Goldman MP, Bennett RG. Treatment of telangiectasia: a review. *J Am Acad Dermatol.* 1987;17:167-182.

32. Mamelak AJ, Goldberg LH, Katz TM, et al. Desmoplastic trichoepithelioma. *J Am Acad Dermatol.* 2010;62:102-106.

33. Urquhart JL, Weston WL. Treatment of multiple trichoepitheliomas with topical imiquimod and tretinoin. *Pediatr Dermatol.* 2005;22:67-70.

34. Kwok CS, Gibbs S, Bennett C, Holland R, Abbott R. Topical treatments for cutaneous warts. *Cochrane Database Syst Rev.* 2012; 9:CD001781. doi:10.1002/14651858.CD001781.pub3.

35. Connolly M, Bazmi K, O'Connell M, Lyons JF, Bourke JF. Cryotherapy of viral warts: a sustained 10-s freeze is more effective than the traditional method. *Br J Dermatol.* 2001;145(4):554-557. doi:10.1046/j.1365-2133.2001.04449.x.

36. Nassar A, Alakad R, Essam R, Bakr NM, Nofal A. Comparative efficacy of intralesional *Candida* antigen, intralesional bivalent human papilloma virus vaccine, and cryotherapy in the treatment of common warts. *J Am Acad Dermatol.* 2022;87(2):419-421. doi:10.1016/j.jaad.2021.08.040.

37. Phillips RC, Ruhl TS, Pfenninger JL, Garber MR. Treatment of warts with *Candida* antigen injection. *Arch Dermatol.* 2000;136:1274-1275.

38. Karsai S, Czarnecka A, Raulin C. Treatment of xanthelasma palpebrarum using a pulsed dye laser: a prospective clinical trial in 38 cases. *Dermatol Surg.* 2010;36:610-617.

24 Diagnosis and Treatment of Malignant and Premalignant Lesions

RICHARD P. USATINE, MD, and DANIEL L. STULBERG, MD

SUMMARY

- The goal of this chapter is to look at procedures and treatments organized by diagnosis so that one can compare the various treatment options available to an individual patient.
- The diagnoses covered in detail include actinic keratosis, squamous cell carcinoma *in situ*, keratoacanthoma, squamous cell carcinoma, basal cell carcinoma, melanoma, cutaneous T-cell lymphoma, dermatofibrosarcoma protuberans, and Merkel cell carcinoma.
- Treatments reviewed include surgical excisions, Mohs surgery, cryosurgery, electrodessication and curettage, curettage alone, photodynamic therapy, ultraviolet light, radiotherapy, and topical treatments.
- Small lesions that are not near important structures, have distinct margins, and are not high-grade cancers can usually be managed by clinicians with good basic skills in their office.
- For high-risk locations and lesions, the best results of complete lesion removal are typically obtained by Mohs micrographic surgery or surgical oncology.

Skin cancer is the most common cancer in the United States; fortunately, however, it is not one of the most common causes of death. Skin cancers can be divided into melanoma and nonmelanoma skin cancers (NMSC). In light skin tones the most common skin cancers are basal cell carcinomas (BCC) and squamous cell carcinomas (SCC) in that order. In persons with the darkest skin tones, skin, cancers are much less common, but when they do occur, SCC is more common, than BCC.[1] Also, SCC occurs more frequently on non-sun-exposed sites in Black individuals.[1,2] Melanomas are usually the least common of the top three skin cancers regardless of skin color. Ultraviolet radiation (UVR) plays a larger role in melanoma in lighter skin tones. Acral melanomas, which account for a higher percentage of melanomas in persons with darker skin tones, are often unrelated to UVR exposure. Some of the rare skin cancers include Merkel cell carcinoma, dermatofibrosarcoma protuberans, and cutaneous T-cell lymphoma. These account for less than 1% of skin cancers.

In Figure 24.1, the relative burden of the top three skin cancers from 2005 to 2019 can be visualized.[3] The incidence of BCC exceeds SCC and melanoma, but the mortality rates are highest for melanoma followed by SCC. The mortality rate for BCC during this time was zero.

Nonmelanoma skin cancer typically refers to BCC and SCC. Cutaneous metastases (of nonskin cancers), human papilloma virus–related cancers, tumors arising from dermal fibroblasts, neuroendocrine cells, and cutaneous lymphomas also occur. Both BCC and SCC have an increased incidence in people with fair skin, with increased sun exposure, and with aging. Patients with xeroderma pigmentosum have a very high rate of skin cancers due to sun exposure and UVB damage because they are unable to correct errors in their sun-damaged skin, leading to multiple skin cancers. SCCs are also more frequent in skin that is exposed to carcinogens or affected by chronic wounds or burns. BCCs very rarely metastasize, but can cause severe complications from local invasion if left untreated. High risk SCCs can metastasize and lead to death.[3]

For melanoma, risk factors include family history, large congenital nevi, the familial atypical mole and melanoma syndrome (FAMMS; previously dysplastic nevus syndrome) (Figure 24.2) and sun exposure, particularly blistering burns in fair-skinned individuals. After initial biopsy, Breslow's classification by depth of invasion is used to guide re-excision margins and the need for sentinel lymph node biopsy and to predict general survival rates.

The treatment of most skin cancers begins with a biopsy (see Chapter 8, *Choosing the Biopsy Type*). In most cases this will be shave or saucerization biopsy. Having a histologic diagnosis can prevent a large unnecessary excision if the pathology turns out to be benign and can help guide the treatment of choice if malignancy is confirmed. The choice of treatment can be guided by the subtype of the skin cancer and how aggressive it is found to be on histology. Precancers can often be diagnosed clinically and dermoscopically so may not need a biopsy prior to treatment.

Mohs Surgery Appropriate Use Criteria (AUC) App (see Figure 27.13)

Many of the skin cancers in this chapter will be candidates for Mohs surgery (see Chapter 27) depending upon the location of the cancer and how aggressive it is.

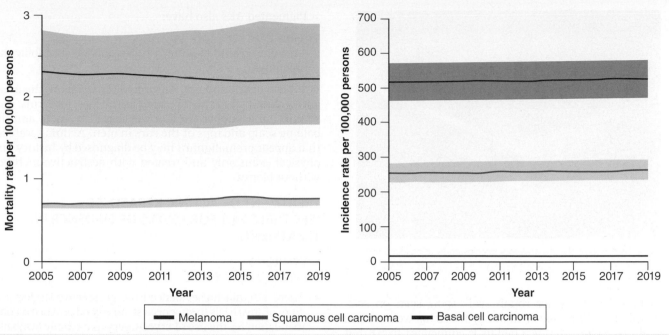

Figure 24.1 Changes in age-standardized mortality and incidence rates of skin cancers in the United States from 2005 to 2019. Shaded area represents the 95% uncertainty interval. Basal cell carcinoma had a mortality rate of zero from 1990 to 2019. Courtesy of Aggarwal P, Knabel P, Fleischer AB Jr. United States burden of melanoma and non-melanoma skin cancer from 1990 to 2019. J Am Acad Dermatol. 2021 Aug;85(2):388-395. doi: 10.1016/j.jaad.2021.03.109. Epub 2021 Apr 20. PMID: 33852922.

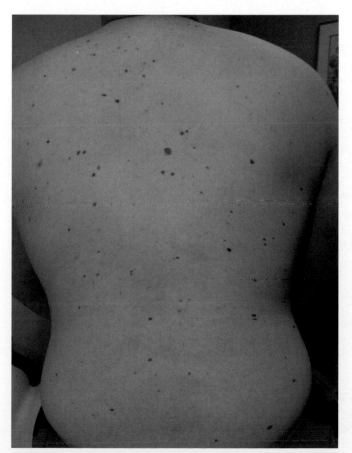

Figure 24.2 Young man with familial atypical mole and melanoma syndrome (FAMMS; previously called dysplastic nevus syndrome). (Copyright Daniel L. Stulberg, MD.)

The Mohs surgery appropriate use criteria (AUC) app is an incredible free resource we highly recommend for making decisions about the need for Mohs referral.

This interactive app provides detailed guidance on appropriate use in real time, as you visit with the patient.

Highlights of the app include:

- Decision support on the appropriateness of Mohs surgery for 270 unique scenarios
- Guided interactive navigation through tumor and patient characteristics
- Color-coded body maps for high-, medium-, and low-risk areas
- Supplemental clinical algorithms
- Quick reference guide that can be shared with referring physicians and patients

Actinic Keratoses

Actinic keratoses (AK) and actinic cheilitis (on lips) are all caused by cumulative sun exposure and have the potential to become invasive squamous cell carcinomas. The rate of malignant transformation has been variably estimated but is probably no greater than 6% per AK over a 10-year period.[4] On a spectrum of malignant transformation, Bowen's disease is squamous cell carcinoma *in situ* before the squamous cell carcinoma becomes invasive. In one large prospective trial, the risk of progression of AK to primary SCC (invasive or *in situ*) was 0.6% at 1 year and 2.6% at 4 years.[5] Approximately 65% of all primary SCCs and 36% of all primary BCCs diagnosed in the study group arose in lesions that had been previously diagnosed clinically as AKs.[5]

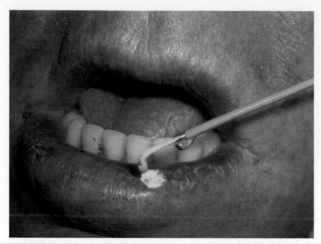

Figure 24.3 Actinic cheilitis undergoing cryosurgery. (Copyright Richard P. Usatine, MD.)

Actinic keratoses are rough scaly spots seen on sun-exposed areas that may be found by touch, as well as close visual inspection. Actinic cheilitis is equivalent to AK but found on the lips (Figure 24.3).

Dermoscopic features of AK include:

1. Rosette sign
2. Surface scale
3. Strawberry pattern.[6]

Pigmented AKs also have:

1. Gray dots
2. Annular-granular pattern (gray dots around follicular openings)[6]

Typical distribution of AKs and SCC *in situ* are the areas with greatest sun exposure such as the face, forearms, dorsum of hands, upper chest, lower legs of women, and the balding scalp and tops of the ears in men. Actinic keratoses that appear premalignant may be diagnosed by history and physical exam only and treated with destructive methods without biopsy.

TREATMENT OF ACTINIC KERATOSES (SEE TABLE 24.1 FOR LEVELS OF EVIDENCE IN TREATMENT)

Cryosurgery -

See Videos 24.1 and 24.2

- There is significant evidence from prospective studies and comparative trials to support a strong, good practice recommendation for the use of cryosurgery as a readily available, rapid, and effective lesion-directed treatment for AKs.[7]
- Primary treatment for isolated AKs
- Cryosurgery with liquid nitrogen with up to a 1-mm freeze margin
- Treating AKs with liquid nitrogen using a 1-mm halo freeze demonstrated complete response of 39% for freeze

Table 24.1 Recommendations for the Management of Actinic Keratoses (AK)[7]

Recommendation (supporting evidence)	Strength	Quality of Evidence
UV PROTECTION		
For patients with AK, we recommend the use of UV protection. *Remark: UV protection may include sun avoidance, sun-protective clothing, and broad-spectrum sunscreen.*	Strong	Good practice statement
TOPICAL AGENTS		
For patients with AKs, we recommend field treatment with 5-fluorouracil.	Strong	Moderate
For patients with AKs, we recommend field treatment with imiquimod.	Strong	Moderate
For patients with AKs, we conditionally recommend the use of diclofenac.	Conditional	Low
CRYOSURGERY		
For patients with AKs, we recommend the use of cryosurgery.	Strong	Good practice statement
For patients with AKs, we conditionally recommend treatment with cryosurgery over CO_2 laser ablation.	Conditional	Moderate
PDT - Aminolevulinic acid (ALA)		
For patients with AKs, we conditionally recommend ALA red light-PDT.	Conditional	Low
For patients with AKs, we conditionally recommend I- to 4-hour 5-ALA incubation time to enhance complete clearance with red light-PDT.	Conditional	Low
For patients with AKs, we conditionally recommend ALA-daylight-PDT as less painful than, but equally effective as, ALA and light-PDT.	Conditional	Moderate
For patients with AKs, we conditionally recommend treatment with ALA red light PDT over trichloroacetic acid peel.	Conditional	Moderate
For patients with AKs, we conditionally recommend ALA blue light-PDT.	Conditional	Moderate
For patients with AKs, we conditionally recommend against pretreatment with alpha hydroxy acid solution prior to ALA blue light-PDT.	Conditional	Very low
For patients with AKs, we conditionally recommend treatment with ALA red light- PDT over cryosurgery alone.	Conditional	Low
COMBINATION THERAPY		
For patients with AKs, we conditionally recommend the combined use of 5-FU and cryosurgery over cryosurgery alone.	Conditional	Moderate

Table 24.1   Recommendations for the Management of Actinic Keratoses (AK)—cont'd

Recommendation (supporting evidence)	Strength	Quality of Evidence
For patients with AKs, we conditionally recommend the combined use of 5-FU and cryosurgery over cryosurgery alone.	Conditional	Low
For patients with AKs, we conditionally recommend against the use of diclofenac in addition to cryosurgery compared to cryosurgery alone.	Conditional	Low
For patients with AKs, we conditionally recommend against the use of topical adapalene in addition to cryosurgery compared to cryosurgery alone.	Conditional	Low
For patients with AKs, we conditionally recommend against the addition of imiquimod following ALA blue light-PDT.	Conditional	Low
For patients with AKs, we conditionally recommend against the addition of imiquimod following ALA blue light-PDT.	Conditional	Moderate

times of less than 5 seconds, 69% for freeze times greater than 5 seconds, and 83% for freeze times greater than 20 seconds.[8]

- Considerably more hypopigmentation is caused by 20 seconds of freeze time, so base the freeze time on the size, location, and thickness of the AK along with the patient's skin color. Risks of visible hypopigmentation increase with darker skin tones.
- Excellent for a small number of lesions
- Adjunct before and after topical therapies

Curettage (Single Cycle for AK)

- Not in current AAD guidelines
- Use local anesthetic by injecting lidocaine with epinephrine.
- Useful for thicker lesions
- Adjunct before or after topical therapies
- One option is to use curettage alone.[9]

Photodynamic Therapy

- Requires special equipment not covered in this textbook but is a standard of care therapy endorsed by the AAD guidelines.[7] There is sufficient good evidence to support its use for AK.[7]

Topical Medications

Topical medications are useful for a large area or large number of lesions in a region. Treatment with topical medications is useful for field cancerization when there are many AKs clustered in one area, such as the scalp, face, or forearms. Cryosurgery should often be combined with topical therapy for the best long-term outcomes.[7]

Fluorouracil

- Topical fluorouracil is the topical treatment with the greatest level of evidence.[7]
- 5% cream (Efudex), 1% cream (Fluoroplex), 0.5% microspore cream (Carac). The generic 5% fluorouracil cream is most affordable, and there is no evidence that one type of fluorouracil cream is better than another.
- 5-FU is applied twice daily for 2 to 4 weeks. Usually 3-4 weeks are needed for the arms and the back of the hands. Patients should stop if the skin becomes ulcerated, extremely painful, or infected. An alternative regimen for the face (or any other area as desired) is to

apply the cream twice daily for 1 week, then wait 1 month to allow for healing, and then apply twice daily for another 2-3 weeks.

- Causes marked inflammation and patients should be advised of this at the time the prescription is being considered (Figure 24.4). It is not recommended to give topical steroids routinely with topical fluorouracil as it may decrease effectiveness. Topical steroids may be considered if the reaction is greater than expected and the patient is very symptomatic.
- Consider treating remaining lesions with cryosurgery or curettage after full healing has occurred.

Imiquimod 5% (Aldara)

- Should be avoided in immunosuppressed individuals
- To be applied 3 to 4 times per week before bed up to 16 weeks
  FDA approved for area up to 5 × 5 cm
- Causes considerable skin inflammation with symptoms similar to 5-FU
  Can cause influenza-like side effects[7]
- Probably not as effective as 5-FU

Diclofenac Gel 3% (Solaraze)

- Not as effective as 5-FU, and we don't recommend it as first line
- Apply twice daily for 90 days.
- Long treatment period and more expensive than 5-FU

SCC in situ (Bowen's disease)

Bowen's disease (BD) appears similar to actinic keratosis but tends to be larger in size and thicker with a well-demarcated border (Figure 24.5). Bowen's disease requires a biopsy for diagnosis because it is difficult to distinguish it from invasive SCC and hypertrophic AK clinically in many cases. Bowen's disease and suspected invasive SCC should be biopsied prior to treatment even if the treatment is performed at the time of biopsy. A shave biopsy or saucerization should usually produce enough tissue and depth for histopathology.

Dermoscopic features of Bowen's disease include:

1. Surface scale
2. Peripheral brown/gray dots arranged linearly (pigmented BD)
3. Glomerular (coiled)/dotted blood vessels[6]

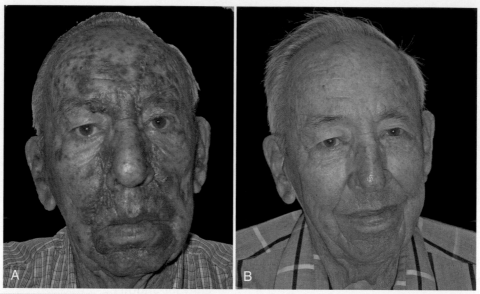

Figure 24.4 **(A)** Erythema and scaling secondary to 5-FU use to treat multiple actinic keratoses on the face. **(B)** The skin is much improved after the erythema resolves. (Copyright Richard P. Usatine, MD.)

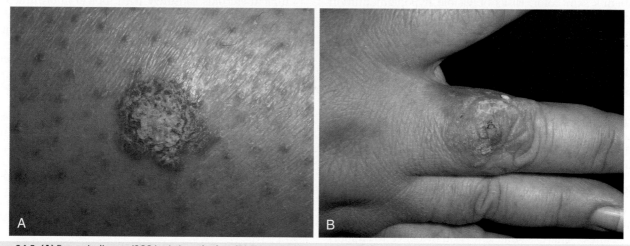

Figure 24.5 **(A)** Bowen's disease (SCC *in situ*) on the leg. **(B)** Bowen's disease on the finger secondary to human papilloma virus. Evidence for HPV was seen in the biopsy specimen performed with a shave. (Copyright Richard P. Usatine, MD.)

TREATMENT OF BOWEN'S DISEASE (BD) (SCC *IN SITU*)

- The risk of progression to invasive cancer is about 3%. This risk is greater in genital BD and particularly in perianal BD. A high risk of recurrence, including late recurrence, is a particular feature of perianal BD, and prolonged follow-up is recommended for this variant.
- There is reasonable evidence to support use of 5-fluorouracil (5-FU).[10] It is more practical than surgery for large lesions, especially at potentially poor healing sites, and has been used for "control" rather than cure in some patients with multiple lesions.
- Topical imiquimod is also used for BD.[11]
- One prospective study suggests that curettage and electrodesiccation treatment is superior to cryotherapy in treating BD, especially for lesions on the lower leg.[12] Curettage with electrodessication was associated with a

significantly shorter healing time, less pain, fewer complications, and a lower recurrence rate when compared with cryotherapy.[12]

See video 24.3 for ED&C

- Cryosurgery has good evidence, of efficacy, but discomfort and time to healing are inferior to photodynamic therapy (PDT) or curettage. With discretion, SCC *in situ* can be treated by cryotherapy with liquid nitrogen spray by a 20-30-second freeze for 1-2 cycles (see Chapter 13, *Cryosurgery*).
- Photodynamic therapy has been shown to be equivalent to cryosurgery and 5-FU, either in efficacy and/or in healing.[10] PDT may be of particular benefit for lesions that are large, on the lower leg, or at otherwise difficult sites, but it is costly.
- Excision should be an effective treatment with low recurrence rates, but the evidence base is limited and for the most part does not allow comment on specific sites of

Table 24.2 Summary of the Main Treatment Options for SCC *in situ*[13]

Summary of the main treatment options for squamous cell carcinoma (SCC) *in situ*. The suggested scoring of the treatments listed takes into account the evidence for benefit, ease of application or time required for the procedure, wound healing, cosmetic result, and current availability/costs of the method or facilities required. Evidence for interventions based on single studies or anecdotal cases is not included.

Lesion Characteristics (small, < 2 cm)	Topical 5-FU	Topical Imiquimod[b]	Cryotherapy	Curettage	Excision	PDT	Radiotherapy	Laser
Small, single/few, good healing[a]	3	3	2	1	3	3	5	4
Large, single, good healing[a]	3	3	3	4	5	2	4	—
Multiple, good healing[a]	2	3	2	3	5	3	4	4
Small, single/few, poor healing site[a]	2	2	3	2	2	2	5	—
Large, single, poor healing site[a]	3	2	5	4	5	1	6	—
Facial	3	3	4	2	4	3	4	—
Digital	3	3	4	5	2	3	3	3
Nail bed	—	4	—	—	2[c]	3	4	4
Penile	3	3	4	5	4[c]	3	3	3
Lesions in immunocompromised patients	5	4	3	3	4	3	—	—

FU, fluorouracil; PDT, photodynamic therapy; 1, probably treatment of choice; 2, generally good choice; 3, generally fair choice; 4, reasonable but not usually required; 5, generally poor choice; 6, probably should not be used; —, insufficient evidence available. [a]Refers to the clinician's perceived potential for good or poor healing at the affected site. [b]Does not have a product license for SCC *in situ*. [c]Consider micrographic surgery for tissue sparing or if poorly defined or recurrent.

lesions. Lower leg excision may be limited by lack of skin mobility. Although elliptical excision with clear margins is an effective and acceptable treatment for Bowen's disease, it is too aggressive for actinic keratoses.

- Mohs surgery is a good option for BD at sites such as the digits or penis where it is important to limit removal of unaffected skin. However, topical and other methods are not contraindicated in these areas. These options should be presented to the patient so that shared decision making can occur.
- Mohs surgery is useful for poorly defined or recurrent head and neck BD.
- See Table 24.2 for a summary of all recommended treatments for Bowen's disease based on location and other characteristics.

SPECIAL CONSIDERATIONS/BILLING

- AK and actinic cheilitis treatment are coded as premalignant.
- 17000 for first lesion treated
- 17003 repeated for each lesion 2–14
- 17004 stand-alone code if more than 15 lesions treated
- Treatment of Bowen's disease is coded the same as invasive SCC (see below).

Squamous Cell Carcinoma

DIAGNOSES

- Erythematous plaque with scale and/or ulceration, frequently found on the face, ears, and lower lip (Figure 24.6). May occur in any sun-exposed area or on mucous membranes of the mouth and anus
- Transplant patients on chronic immunosuppression are at high risk to develop SCC (Figure 24.7).
- May be at the base of actinic horns or thick actinic keratoses

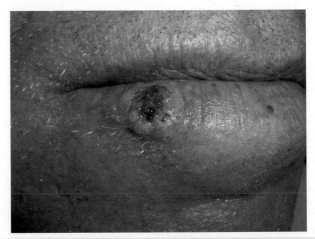

Figure 24.6 Squamous cell carcinoma of the lower lip related to sun exposure. (Copyright Richard P. Usatine, MD.)

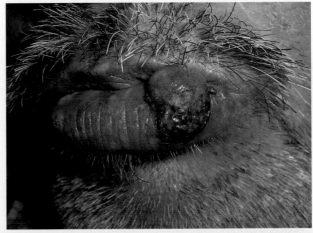

Figure 24.7 Large quickly growing SCC on the lip of a patient on immunosuppression after a renal transplant. (Copyright Richard P. Usatine, MD.)

- May occur in areas of chronic irritation or burns
- A shave or punch biopsy is useful for diagnosis.

Dermoscopic features include (see Chapter 18):

1. Yellow keratin mass/scale crust
2. White circles ("keratin pearls")
3. Rosette sign
4. Glomerular (coiled) blood vessels
5. Hairpin vessels, usually with whitish halo
6. Ulceration/blood spots/hemorrhage[6]

TREATMENT (TABLES 24.3 AND 24.4)

See Videos 24.4 and 24.5
Recurrence rates of SCC and SCCIS following nonsurgical treatments:

- Electrodessication with curettage (2.0%; 95% CI, 1.1-3.0)
- Cryotherapy with curettage (1.6%; 95% CI, 0.4-2.8)
- Photodynamic therapy (29.0%; 95% CI, 25.0-33.0)
- 5-Fluorouracil (26.6%; 95% CI, 16.9-36.4)
- Imiquimod (16.1%; 95% CI, 10.3-21.8)[15]

Table 24.3   Recommendations for the Surgical Treatment of cSCC[14]

A treatment plan that considers recurrence rate, preservation of function, patient expectations, and potential adverse effects is recommended.

C&E may be considered for low-risk, primary cSCC in nonterminal hair—bearing locations.

For low-risk primary cSCC, standard excision with a 4- to 6-mm margin to a depth of the mid-subcutaneous adipose tissue with histologic margin assessment is recommended.

Standard excision may be considered for select high-risk tumors. However, strong caution is advised when selecting a treatment modality for high-risk tumors without a complete margin assessment.

MMS is recommended for high-risk cSCC.

C&E, Curettage and electrodessication; cSCC, cutaneous squamous cell carcinoma; MMS, Mohs micrographic surgery.
Keep in mind that there is only B and C level evidence for these recommendations.

Table 24.4   Recommendations for the Nonsurgical Therapy of cSCC[14]

If surgical therapy is not feasible or preferred radiation therapy (e.g., superficial radiation therapy, brachytherapy external electron beam therapy, and other traditional radiotherapy forms) can be considered when tumors are low risk, with the understanding that the cure rate may be lower.
Cryosurgery may be considered for low-risk cSCC when more effective therapies are contraindicated or impractical.
Topical therapies (imiquimod or 5-FU) and PDT are not recommended for the treatment of cSCC on the basis of available data.
There is insufficient evidence available to make a recommendation on the use of laser therapies or electronic surface brachytherapy in the treatment of cSCC.

cSCC, Cutaneous squamous cell carcinoma; 5-FU, 5-fluorouracil; PDT, photodynamic therapy.

In another meta analysis, the authors found no RCTs investigating surgical modalities for SCC, which are the first-line treatment. This lack of evidence is reflected in the most recent American Academy of Dermatology (AAD) guidelines on SCC.[14,16] For invasive SCC, no treatment recommendation was made with an A grade (consistent good-quality patient-oriented evidence).[14,16] Additional comparative studies are needed to inform treatment decisions for patients with SCC.[16] Good practice entails presenting the pros and cons of the treatment options to patients and engaging in shared decision making.

- Electrodesiccation and curettage (for 2-3 cycles just as in BCC) may be used for Bowen's disease and for early small SCC (see Chapter 14, *Electrosurgery*).
- 5-FU combined with epinephrine injected weekly has shown success in small trials.[11] This is not a mainstay of therapy.
- On the trunk or extremities, SCC can be excised with an elliptical excision.
- Removal margins for elliptical excision:
    - 4 mm if clinically feasible with SCC less than 2 cm in diameter
    - 6 mm if high-grade lesions or with SCC greater than 2 cm in diameter
- SCC on the ears and lips have higher rates of metastasis, and referral for Mohs surgery is often recommended.

SPECIAL CONSIDERATIONS

- Use the Mohs surgery appropriate use criteria (AUC) app described at the beginning of the chapter to help make decisions about referral for Mohs surgery.
- Consider referral for Mohs surgery if lesions affect sensitive structures including the eyelids, nose, and ear.
- Consider referral for Mohs if aggressive SCC, SCC greater than 2 cm, or if recurrent lesion.
- After one or more SCCs, many patients are at higher risk of additional and future BCC and SCC, so reexamination for additional lesions is required at least annually.[17]
- Transplant patients are at high risk of developing SCCs, so an annual full skin exam is recommended.

Keratoacanthoma

Most pathologists and skin experts consider KA to be one type of SCC. The controversy revolves around the fact that it was considered a precancer for years, in part, because some KAs will spontaneously resolve.

DIAGNOSIS

- Rapidly enlarging, often erythematous dome-shaped lesion (Figure 24.8)
- A central keratin plug is the classic distinguishing feature.
- Frequently on the hands or face
- Considered a type of squamous cell cancer
- Use a shave biopsy for pathology.

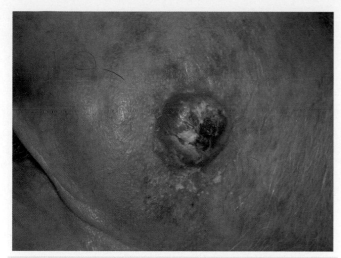

Figure 24.8 Keratoacanthoma-type SCC growing rapidly over the temple region of the face. The central keratin core is a distinct feature of a keratoacanthoma. (Copyright Richard P. Usatine, MD.)

Table 24.5	Stratification of Low- Versus High-Risk cSCC[14]	
Parameters	**Low Risk**	**High Risk**
Clinical Location*/size[†]	Area L <20 mm Area M[‡] 20 mm	Area L ≥20 mm Area M ≥10 mm Area H[§]
Borders	Well defined	Poorly defined
Primary vs recurrent	Primary	Recurrent
Immunosuppression	No	Yes
Site of prior radiation therapy or chronic inflammatory process	No	Yes
Rapidly growing tumor	No	Yes
Neurologic symptoms	No	Yes
Pathologic		
Degree of differentiation	Well to moderately differentiated	Poorly differentiated
High-risk histologic subtype[‖]	No	Yes
Depth (thickness or Clark level)[¶]	<2 mm, or I, II, III	≥2mm or IV, V
Perineural, lymphatic, or vascular involvement	No	Yes

cSCC, Cutaneous squamous cell carcinoma.
*Area L consists of trunk and extremities (excluding hands, feet, nail units, pretibia, and ankles); area M consists of cheeks, forehead, scalp, neck, and pretibia; and area H consists of central face, eyelids, eyebrows, periorbital skin, nose, lips, chin, mandible, preauricular and postauricular skin/sulci, temple, ear, genitalia, hands, and feet.
[†]Greatest tumor diameter, including peripheral rim of erythema.
[‡]Location independent of size may constitute high risk.
[§]Area H constitutes high-risk on the basis of location, independent of size.
[‖]Adenoid (acantholytic), adenosquamous (showing mucin production), desmoplastic, or metaplastic (carcinosarcomatous) subtypes.
[¶]A modified Breslow measurement should exclude parakeratosis or scale/crust and should be made from base of the ulcer if present. If clinical evaluation of incisional biopsy suggests that microstaging is inadequate, consider narrow-margin excisional biopsy.

- An unknown percentage may spontaneously regress over 2 to 12 months, but it is safer to remove it than wait.

  Dermoscopic features include:

1. Central keratin mass
2. Hairpin (looped) or serpentine (linear-irregular) blood vessels, usually at the periphery, with white-yellow halo

REMOVAL

- Electrodesiccation and curettage (see pages 177–178)
- Excision by ellipse with 3- to 5-mm margins
- Inject 5-FU, methotrexate, or interferon.
- Radiation therapy if unable to treat by measures above

Decisions about how to treat any cutaneous SCC should take into account the features that make it low risk or high risk. See Table 24.5.

Basal Cell Carcinoma

DIAGNOSES BY CLINICAL FEATURES

- Frequent on the face, neck, arms, back, upper chest, and any sun-exposed skin
- Nodular is the most common form (Figure 24.9):
  - Raised, waxy, translucent, or pearly border
  - Central erosion, telangiectasias, and bleeding are common.
  - Usually flesh colored or pale, but may be pigmented, confusing it with melanoma
- Superficial BCC (Figure 24.10)
  - Flat or slightly raised, often red to brown
  - Look for a thready border that may be pearly.
  - More often on the trunk and arms than face
- Morpheaform, sclerosing, infiltrating (Figure 24.11)
  - Usually has nondiscrete margins
  - More aggressive growth
  - Higher recurrence rate

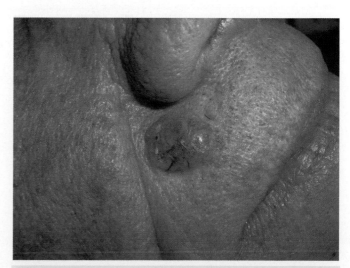

Figure 24.9 Typical nodular BCC on the face of a 53-year-old man. Note the pearly borders and telangiectasias. (Copyright Richard P. Usatine, MD.)

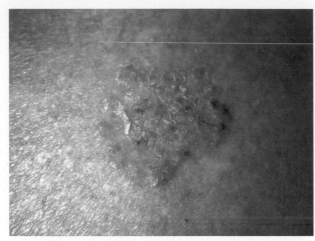

Figure 24.10 Superficial BCC on the back with erythema, scale, and a thready border. (Copyright Richard P. Usatine, MD.)

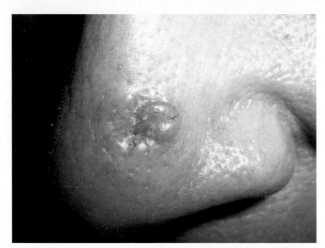

Figure 24.11 Infiltrating BCC on the nose of a 58-year-old White woman. She was referred for Mohs surgery. (Copyright Richard P. Usatine, MD.)

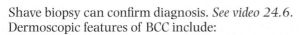

Shave biopsy can confirm diagnosis. *See video 24.6.* Dermoscopic features of BCC include:

1 Leaflike structures
2 Blue-gray ovoid nests
3 Multiple blue-gray dots and globules (buckshot scatter)
4 Spoke wheel-like structures/concentric structures
5 Ulceration/erosion
6 White shiny blotches and strands
7 Arborizing blood vessels
8 Short fine telangiectasias (superficial BCC)[6]

https://academy.dermoscopedia.org/Basal_cell_carcinoma

TREATMENT OPTIONS FOR BCC

Recurrence rates give a general idea about the effectiveness of the treatment options without being specific to any one BCC. However, it is always important to consider whether one is dealing with a low-risk or high-risk BCC (Table 24.6). The treatment plan should always consider recurrence

Table 24.6 Stratification of Low- Versus High-Risk BCC[18]

Parameters	Low Risk	High Risk
Clinical		
Location*/size†	Area L <20 mm Area M‡ <10 mm	Area L ≥20 mm Area M ≥10 mm Area H§
Borders	Well defined	Poorly defined
Primary vs recurrent	Primary	Recurrent
Immunosuppression	No	Yes
Site of prior radiation therapy	No	Yes
PATHOLOGIC		
Growth pattern	Nodular superficial‖	Aggressive¶
Perineural involvement	No	Yes

BCC, Basal cell carcinoma.
*Area L consists of trunk and extremities (excluding hands, feet, nail units, pretibia, and ankles); area M consists of cheeks, forehead, scalp neck, and pretibia; and area H consists of central face, eyelids, eyebrows, periorbital skin, nose, lips , chin, mandible, preauricular and postauricular skin/sulci, temple, ear, genitalia, hands, and feet.
†Greatest tumor diameter.
‡Location independent of size may constitute high risk.
§Area H constitutes a high-risk area on the basis of location, independent of size.
‖Other low-risk growth patterns include keratotic, infundibulocystic, and fibroepithelioma of Pinkus.
¶Having morpheaform, basosquamous (metatypical), sclerosing, mixed infiltrative, or micronodular features in any portion of the tumor.

Table 24.7 Recommendations for the Surgical Treatment of BCC[18]

A treatment plan that considers recurrence rate, preservation of function, patient expectations, and potential adverse effects is recommended.
C&E may be considered for low-risk tumors in non—terminal hair—bearing locations.
For low-risk primary BCC, surgical excision with 4-mm clinical margins and histologic margin assessment is recommended.
Standard excision may be considered for select high-risk tumors. However, strong caution is advised when selecting a treatment modality without complete margin assessment for high-risk tumors.
Mohs micrographic surgery is recommended for high-risk BCC.

BCC, Basal cell carcinoma; C&E, curettage and electrodessication.

rate, preservation of function, potential adverse effects, and patient expectations and preferences (Table 24.7).

The recurrence rates reported in a meta-analysis in 2018 follow.[19]

Estimated recurrence rates were similar for:

- Excision (3.8% [95% CI, 1.5% to 9.5%])
- Mohs surgery (3.8% [CI, 0.7% to 18.2%])
- Curettage and electrodesiccation (6.9% [CI, 0.9% to 36.6%])
- External-beam radiation (3.5% [CI, 0.7% to 16.8%])
Recurrence rates were higher for:
- Cryotherapy (22.3% [CI, 10.2% to 42.0%])
- Curettage and cryotherapy (19.9% [CI, 4.6% to 56.1%])
- 5-Fluorouracil (18.8% [CI, 10.1% to 32.5%])
- Imiquimod (14.1% [CI, 5.4% to 32.4%]).

- Photodynamic therapy using methyl-aminolevulinic acid (18.8% [CI, 10.1% to 32.5%]) or aminolevulinic acid (16.6% [CI, 7.5% to 32.8%])

An earlier evidence-based review of recurrence rates after cryosurgery for BCC found rates to be less than 10%.[20]

Recommendations for the surgical treatment of BCC are found in Table 24.7 and for nonsurgical therapy in Table 24.8. Level of evidence and SOR for nonsurgical treatment of BCC is found in Table 24.9.

Elliptical Excision (Fusiform)

See Video 24.7

- Remove with 3-mm surgical margin if discrete border and clinically feasible, 4 to 5 mm if indiscrete border[21] (Figure 24.12).
- If the borders of the BCC are not clear, consider using a curette to define the borders, and then redraw the ellipse as needed (Figure 24.13).
- Heals with linear scars, which can be hidden in skin lines
- Provides immediate closure

Table 24.8 Recommendations for the Nonsurgical Therapy of BCC[18]

Cryosurgery may be considered for low-risk BCC when more effective therapies are contraindicated or impractical.

If surgical therapy is not feasible or preferred, topical therapy (e.g., imiquimod or 5-FU), MAL- or ALA-PDT, and radiation therapy (e.g., superficial radiation therapy, brachytherapy, external electron beam, and other traditional radiotherapy forms for BCC) can be considered when tumors are low risk, with the understanding that the cure rate may be lower.

Adjustment of topical therapy dosing regimen on the basis of side effect tolerance is recommended.

There is insufficient evidence to recommend the routine use of laser or electronic surface brachytherapy in the treatment of BCC.

ALA, Aminolevulinic acid; BCC, basal cell carcinoma; 5-FU, 5-fluorouracil; MAL, methylaminolevulinate; PDT, photodynamic therapy.

Table 24.9 Level of Evidence and Strength of Recommendations for the Nonsurgical Treatment of BCC as Alternatives to Surgical Therapy

Recommendation	Strength of Recommendation	Level of Evidence	References*
Cryosurgery	A	I	36,41,46, 60-63
Topical therapy			
▪ Imiquimod	A	I	39,64-77
▪ 5-FU	A	I, II	46,64,74-76, 78,79
PDT			
▪ ALA	A	I, II	38,47,61,74, 76,77,80-85
▪ MAL	A	I, II	35,37,60,64, 74,76,77,83, 86,87

*Reference numbers refer to references in source article:
Kim JYS, Kozlow JH, Mittal B, Moyer J, Olencki T, Rodgers P. Guidelines of care for the management of basal cell carcinoma. J Am Acad Dermatol. 2018;78(3):540-559.
Aminolevulinic acid; BCC, basal cell carcinoma; 5-FU, 5-fluorouracil; MAL, methylaminolevulinate; PDT, photodynamic therapy

- Provides tissue for pathology and assurance of removal
- If you find evidence of the BCC at the base or edges (Figure 24.14) of the removed specimen, take another piece of skin or fascia at a deeper and/or wider level, and put it in a second formalin container with a stitch used to mark its orientation in the body.

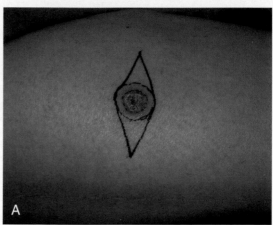
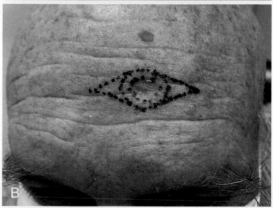

Figure 24.12 4-mm margins marked around these previously biopsied BCCs before drawing a 3:1 ellipse. **(A)** BCC on the thigh. **(B)** BCC on the forehead. (Copyright Richard P. Usatine, MD.)

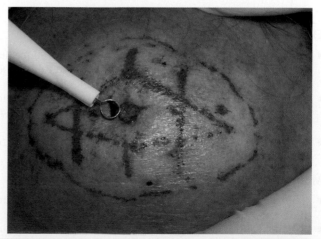

Figure 24.13 After marking the margins and anesthetizing the area, a curette is being used to determine the full margins of the BCC more accurately. An adjusted ellipse can then be drawn to avoid incomplete excision. (Copyright Richard P. Usatine, MD.)

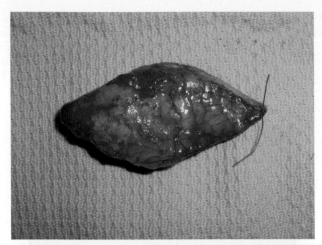

Figure 24.14 Basal cell carcinoma palpable and barely visible (whiter than the yellow fat) at the base of this elliptical excision. A second layer should be removed more deeply before closing up the surgical defect. (Copyright Richard P. Usatine, MD.)

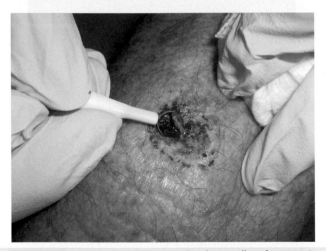

Figure 24.15 A curette is scooping out the abnormally soft cancer tissue from this basal cell carcinoma on the arm as the first step of an electrodesiccation and curettage. (Copyright Richard P. Usatine, MD.)

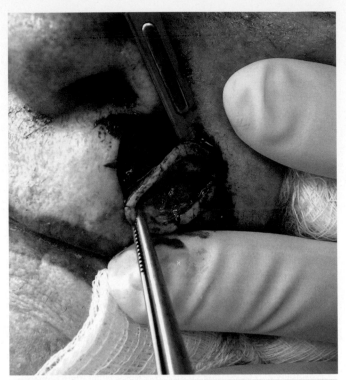

Figure 24.16 Mohs surgery being performed on a basal cell carcinoma of the upper lip region. First the tumor was debulked, and now a thin sliver of tissue is being removed 360 degrees around the original tumor to look for adequate margin control. (Courtesy of Ryan O'Quinn, MD.)

Electrodesiccation and Curettage

- BCC tissue is softer than the surrounding normal tissue, so a skin curette can remove the BCC without taking too much normal tissue around it (Figure 24.15).
- Firmly curette in all directions, then electrodesiccate and repeat to a total of 2-3 cycles at one visit (see Chapter 14, *Electrosurgery*, pages 177–178).
- Useful for smaller lesions (preferably <2 cm) or where closure of a full-thickness excision would be difficult

Mohs Micrographic Surgery (Figure 24.16)

- The most effective in achieving cure with clean margins—99%
- Specialized skin surgeon examines pathology for margin control at time of excision.
- Further resection as needed at time of surgery until margins are clear
- Can minimize impact on adjacent structures

- Useful for uncertain borders or aggressive forms of BCC (i.e., sclerosing or morpheaform)
- Consider for H-zone on face (see Figure 27.12), especially for recurrent BCC.[22]
- Consider referral for Mohs surgery if lesions affect sensitive structures including the eyelids, nose, and the ear.
- Consider referral for Mohs if aggressive lesion or if recurrent lesion.
- Basosquamous carcinoma is an aggressive subtype of basal cell cancer that has metastatic potential and high recurrence rates that should be managed by Mohs surgery.

Topical Immunotherapy

- Imiquimod locally boosts immune response and is approved for immunocompetent patients.
- FDA approved for superficial BCC (not for other subtypes) lesions up to 2 cm in diameter; not approved for use on the face, hands, or feet

Cryosurgery (cryotherapy)

- An option for smaller nonaggressive BCCs using liquid nitrogen spray for a 30-second freeze (thaw and refreeze 30 seconds unless it is a superficial BCC on the trunk in which a single freeze may be adequate) (Figure 24.17) (see Chapter 15).

Radiation Therapy

- Usually reserved for those not able to tolerate other treatments

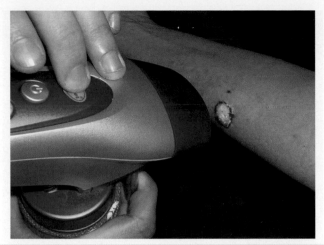

Figure 24.17 Cryosurgery being performed on a superficial BCC of the arm. A 5-mm margin of freeze is the goal with two freezes each of 30-seconds duration. (Copyright Richard P. Usatine, MD.)

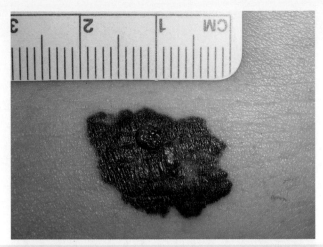

Figure 24.18 Superficial spreading melanoma with all features of the ABCDE. This was on the abdomen of a 41-year-old Hispanic woman. Breslow depth 0.85 mm. (Copyright Richard P. Usatine, MD.)

Photodynamic Therapy (PDT)

- PDT has a number of limitations in the treatment of BCC.

Special Consideration

- High risk of additional and future BCC and SCC, so frequent reexamination for additional lesions is required at least annually.[17]

Melanoma

DIAGNOSIS

- The **ABCDE** guidelines for diagnosing melanoma (Figure 24.18) are a good start but alone may miss 50% of melanomas. Dermoscopy is the most important method to increase sensitivity and specificity of diagnosing melanoma (see Chapter 18).
    - **A = Asymmetry.** Most melanomas are asymmetrical: a line through the middle will not create matching halves.
    - **B = Border.** The borders of melanomas are often uneven and may have scalloped or notched edges.
    - **C = variation in Color.** Melanomas are often varied shades of brown, tan, or black. As melanomas progress, they may appear red, white, and blue.
    - **D = Diameter** greater than or equal to 6 mm. Melanomas tend to grow larger than most nevi. (*Note:* Congenital nevi are often large.)
    - **E = Evolving or Elevated.** Any enlarging nevus is suspect for melanoma even though benign nevi may also grow. Melanoma is often elevated, at least in part, so that it is palpable.

Dermoscopic features include:

1. Atypical pigment network
2. Blue structures (blue-white veil, blue-gray structures)
3. White shiny lines (crystalline structures)
4. Negative network
5. Irregular dots/globules
6. Irregular streaks (radial streaming, pseudopods)

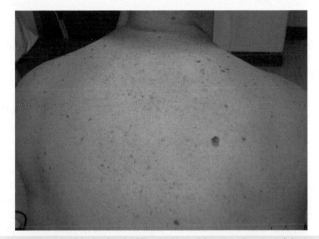

Figure 24.19 The "ugly duckling" sign with one pigmented lesion standing out on the upper right side of the back. This was indeed a malignant melanoma caught early by careful observation. (Copyright Richard P. Usatine, MD.)

7. Regression structures (white scarlike area and/or peppering)
8. Peripheral brown structureless area
9. Angulated lines (extrafacial)
10. Atypical vascular pattern, polymorphous vessels (2+ types of blood vessels, e.g., linear irregular and dotted vessels)
11. Atypical blotch[6]

For photographic examples of each feature see:
https://academy.dermoscopedia.org/Melanoma_(overview_of_features)

Clinical Appearance

- The "ugly duckling" rule: If a mole looks different from the patient's other moles, there is a higher likelihood that it is malignant (Figure 24.19).
- May be friable, ulcerating, nonhealing, or bleeding.

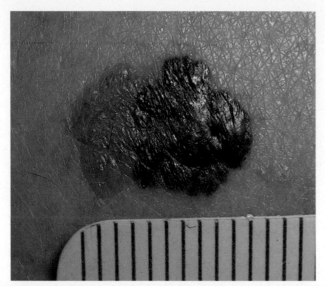

Figure 24.20 Superficial spreading melanoma in its radial growth phase on the back of the patient above (0.35 mm in depth). (Copyright Richard P. Usatine, MD.)

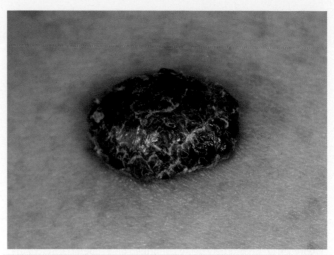

Figure 24.21 Nodular melanoma on the shoulder of a young woman. Breslow depth 8.5 mm. (Copyright Richard P. Usatine, MD.)

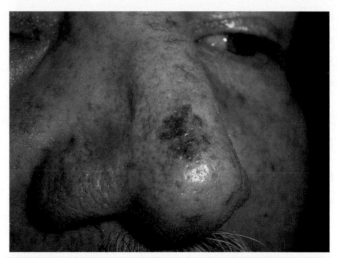

Figure 24.22 Lentigo maligna melanoma in situ on the nose of a 68-year-old Hispanic man. (Copyright Richard P. Usatine, MD.)

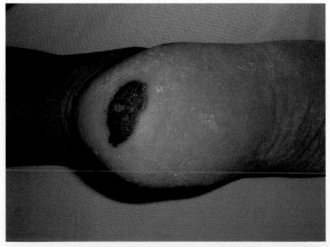

Figure 24.23 Acral lentiginous melanoma on the heel of a young Black woman. (Copyright Richard P. Usatine, MD.)

The four major categories of cutaneous melanomas are as follows:

1. *Superficial spreading melanoma* is the most common type of melanoma, accounting for about 70% of melanomas in the United States.[23] This melanoma has a radial growth pattern before dermal invasion occurs (Figure 24.20). The first sign is the appearance of a flat macule or slightly raised discolored plaque that has irregular borders and is somewhat geometrical in form. The color varies with areas of tan, brown, black, red, blue, or white. These lesions can arise in an older nevus. The melanoma can be seen almost anywhere on the body, but is most likely to occur on the trunk in men, the legs in women, and the upper back in both. Most melanomas found in the young are of the superficial spreading type.

2. *Nodular melanoma* occurs in approximately 15% of melanoma cases.[23,24] The color is most often black, but occasionally is blue, gray, white, brown, tan, red, or nonpigmented (Figure 24.21). It is often ulcerated and bleeding at the time of diagnosis. The nodule in Figure 24.21 is multicolored. Although it is often evolving and elevated, it may lack the ABCD criteria.

3. *Lentigo maligna melanoma* (LMM) is found most often in the elderly and arises on the chronically sun-damaged skin of the face. The term *lentigo maligna* is used for the melanoma precursor in the setting of atypical melanocytic hyperplasia alone, and the term *melanoma in situ, LM type,* is used to represent the true *in situ* melanoma. LM is the precursor to LMM and not a nevus (Figure 24.22). Globally, LM/LMM is estimated to account for 4% to 15% of all melanomas, and 10% to 26% of all head and neck melanomas.[25]

4. *Acral lentiginous melanoma* (ALM) is the least common subtype of melanoma among non-Hispanic Whites and accounts for 2% to 3% of melanomas overall in the US.[23] ALM is the most common subtype of cutaneous melanoma among people of color.[26] It occurs on the soles or palms or in the nail unit (Figure 24.23). ALM has 5- and

10-year melanoma-specific survival rates of 80.3% and 67.5%, respectively, which is less than those for all cutaneous malignant melanomas overall (91.3% and 87.5%, respectively; $p < 0.001$).[23] ALM disproportionately affects people of color, who tend to present with thicker tumors and advanced disease stages, factors associated with lower survival rates.[27] Subungual melanoma may manifest as diffuse nail discoloration or a longitudinal pigmented band within the nail plate. When subungual pigment spreads to the proximal or lateral nail fold, it is referred to as Hutchinson's sign and is highly suggestive of acral lentiginous melanoma (Figure 24.24).

Less common variations of melanomas include the following:

- *Amelanotic melanoma* (<5% of melanomas) is nonpigmented and appears pink or flesh colored, often mimicking BCC or SCC or a ruptured hair follicle. It may be a nodular melanoma subtype or melanoma metastasis to the skin, because of the inability of these poorly differentiated cancer cells to synthesize melanin pigment (Figure 24.25).

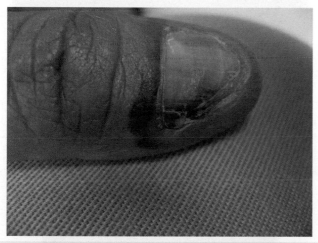

Figure 24.24 Subungual melanoma that has spread to the proximal nail fold producing a positive Hutchinson sign. (Courtesy of Ryan O'Quinn, MD.)

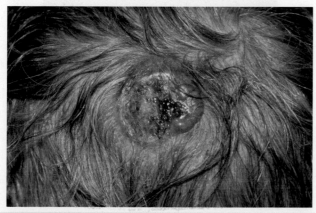

Figure 24.25 Amelanotic melanoma arising on the scalp. (Copyright Richard P. Usatine, MD.)

- Other rare melanoma variants include (1) desmoplastic/neurotropic melanoma, (2) mucosal (lentiginous) melanoma, (3) malignant blue nevus, and (4) melanoma arising in a giant congenital nevus. There is a newer WHO complex way to categorize melanoma into nine subtypes that also takes into account the role of cumulative sun damage.[28]

Diagnosis starts with history (change) and physical exam (ABCDE).

- Use dermoscopy if available (see Chapter 18, *Dermoscopy*).
- Biopsy per recommendations in Chapter 8, *Choosing the Biopsy Type*.
- It is better to give the pathologist the whole lesion or a large representative portion of the lesion rather than a few small punch biopsies.
- A broad deep shave is often better than a single punch biopsy unless the punch biopsy will remove the whole lesion. *See videos 24.8 and 9.11.*

TREATMENT

Definitive treatment is based on Breslow depth and other factors.

- If there is any doubt about the best treatment for any melanoma, consult a dermatologist with expertise in melanoma treatment. Melanoma treatment is more complicated now that we have excellent systemic treatments along with surgical therapy.
- Recommended surgical margins are based on tumor thickness and summarized in Table 24.10.
- If depth greater than 1.0 cm, refer to surgical oncologist for excision and simultaneous sentinel node biopsy (SNLB). For depths between 0.8 mm and 1.0 cm, factors such as ulceration are considered when it comes to referrals for SNLB. The NCCN guidelines discuss the rationale of how to approach a patient who may need SNLB.[30]
- If SLNB is not needed and the melanoma is on the trunk or extremities, the definitive surgical treatment with margins up to 1.0 cm can potentially be performed in the office by any provider skilled in a large elliptical excisions with 2-layer closures. If it is melanoma *in situ*, then a 5-mm margin is the standard. The excision should be marked before giving anesthesia (Figure 24.26), and

Table 24.10 Surgical Margin Recommendations for Primary Cutaneous Melanoma[29]

Tumor Thickness (Breslow)	Surgical Margin (cm)*
In situ	0.5- 1[†]
≤1.0 mm	1
>1.0–2.0 mm	1
>2.0 mm	2

*Recommended surgical excision margins are clinically measured from the edge of the lesion or prior biopsy at the time of surgery; they are not histologic margins as measured by the pathologist. Margins may be modified for functional considerations or anatomic location.
[†]Margins larger than 0.5 cm may be necessary for melanoma *in situ*, lentigo maligna type.

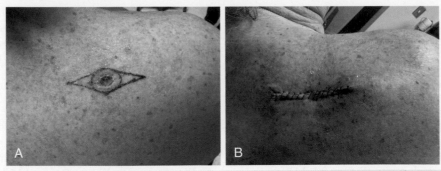

Figure 24.26 (A) Melanoma *in situ* on the back about to be excised with 5-mm margins. Note how the margins and Burow's triangles are drawn to guide the anesthesia and cutting with the scalpel. The ellipse has a 3:1 ratio to avoid creating standing cones. **(B)** Incision closed with 2 layers – deep 4-0 Vicryl and running 4-0 Prolene. Some bulging on the lateral corners is normal and should flatten over time. (Copyright Richard P. Usatine, MD.)

the depth of the ellipse should be to fascia (which should be preserved).[30]

- Always send the excision for dermatopathology because sometimes the final depth will be larger than seen with an incomplete biopsy.
- Of course, if the melanoma is large or the clinician lacks the skillset to do this excision, referral can be to dermatology, Mohs surgery, plastics, or surgical oncology.
- When dealing with facial, acral, or anogenital melanomas, Mohs surgery may be preferable to allow reduced margins and conservation of tissue.[31]
- Staging of the melanoma is accomplished using the TNM system.
- Oncology referral is based on staging (including if sentinel node positive or depth >4 mm). Of course, any metastatic melanoma should be referred immediately to oncology.
- Close clinical follow-up starting with quarterly and tapering to annual complete skin examinations – is recommended to be done by a clinician with experience detecting and treating melanoma. Total body photography may be indicated for certain high-risk melanoma patients.
- Teach the patient to perform self-skin exams (with or without partner help).

Cutaneous T-Cell Lymphomas (Including Mycosis Fungoides)

DIAGNOSIS

- Mycosis fungoides is the most frequent of the cutaneous T-cell lymphomas.
- Erythematous scaling plaques and patches are seen in early localized forms (Figure 24.27).
- Plaques and patches may be hyperpigmented or hypopigmented (Figure 24.28).
- Can progress to diffuse erythema (erythroderma) in later disseminated stage Sézary – syndrome
- May present as refractory or recurrent eczema
- Most often starts on the trunk, but there are variations that start on the face or elsewhere. Folliculotropic MF is one type that is often on the face (Figure 24.29).
- Itching and photosensitivity are common.
- May develop into a tumor stage (see nasal lesion in Figure 24.30).

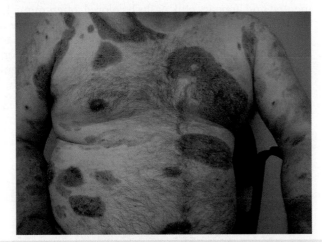

Figure 24.27 Plaque-type mycosis fungoides on the extremities and trunk. Biopsy a few years before this was read as atopic dermatitis only. Lack of response to medications and the suspicious appearance led to a new biopsy and the correct diagnosis. (Courtesy of Deborah Henderson, MD.)

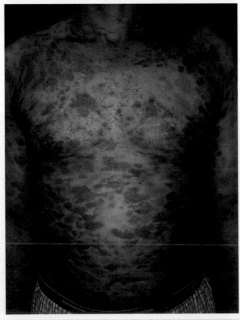

Figure 24.28 Cutaneous T-cell lymphoma causing large hyperpigmented patches and plaques. (Copyright Richard P. Usatine, MD.)

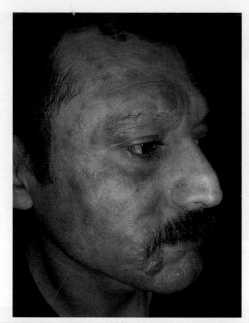

Figure 24.29 Folliculotropic mycosis fungoides on the face with loss of some eyebrow hair and pink plaques. (Copyright Richard P. Usatine, MD.)

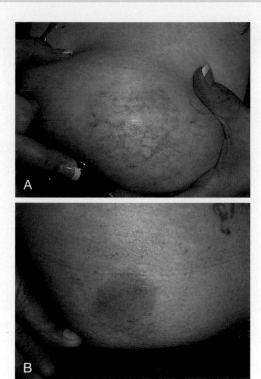

Figure 24.31 Two cases of patch stage localized mycosis fungoides being treated successfully with clobetasol cream. **(A)** On the breast of a 60-year-old woman. **(B)** On the abdomen. (Copyright Richard P. Usatine, MD.)

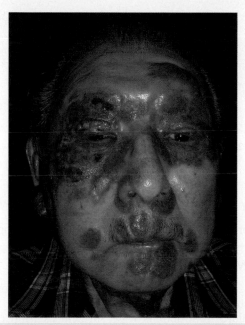

Figure 24.30 Widespread advanced tumor stage mycosis fungoides on the face but also present from the trunk to the feet. (Copyright Richard P. Usatine, MD.)

BIOPSY

- Perform a broad saucerization biopsy of involved skin. This is generally better than a punch biopsy as more tissue is better than less. Consider doing two sites to maximize the opportunity to make the diagnosis.
- Alert the pathologist that this is on your differential diagnosis so that special stains can be done.
- The first biopsy may not show the disease, so consider repeating the skin biopsies if the clinical suspicion remains high.

- Flow cytometry can be done on peripheral blood to look for abnormal lymphocytes.
- Palpate for lymph nodes, and consider referring for a lymph node biopsy if the skin biopsies and flow cytometry are not definitive.
- CT of the abdomen and pelvis can be used to look for enlarged lymph nodes and/or splenomegaly.
- Consult specialists if needed – this can be a hard diagnosis to make.

TREATMENT AND PROGNOSIS

- Early stages are treated locally with topical steroids, nitrogen mustards, psoralen, and UVA, UVB with excellent prognosis for remission and preventing progression of disease.
- For the earliest stages, ultra-high potency topical steroids such as clobetasol are the main-stay of therapy (Figure 24.31).
- More advanced disease carries a poor prognosis and is treated with a combination of topical medications as above, radiation therapy, and systemic immune system modulators and chemotherapy.

Dermatofibrosarcoma Protuberans

DIAGNOSIS

- Flesh-colored gradually enlarging nodule from one to several or more centimeters in diameter. It may be shiny with a look of multiple deep nodules (Figure 24.32).

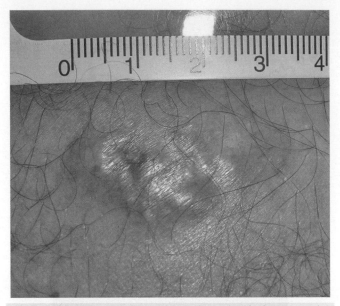

Figure 24.32 Dermatofibrosarcoma protuberans on the leg. (Copyright Richard P. Usatine, MD.)

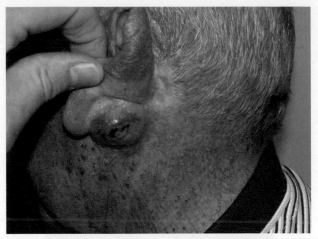

Figure 24.33 Merkel cell carcinoma on the ear. (Courtesy of Frank Miller, MD.)

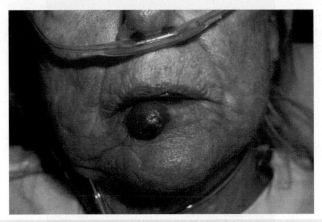

Figure 24.34 Merkel cell carcinoma on the lip. (Courtesy of Jeff Meffert, MD.)

- It is of different origin than a dermatofibroma and is not a dermatofibroma becoming malignant.
- May be erythematous or occasionally pigmented
- Site distribution is typically 45% head and neck and 55% trunk and extremities.[32]

BIOPSY

- Use a 4-cm punch biopsy or larger incisional biopsy to provide adequate tissue for diagnosis.

TREATMENT AND PROGNOSIS

- The tumor can invade into adjacent deep structures, becoming locally invasive and highly recurrent.
- Mohs surgery is the preferred treatment to decrease the recurrence rate.
- Wide local excision with 2–4 cm margins is the alternative with lower cure rates.
- One study using pooled data from the literature reported a recurrence rate of 1.3% with Mohs surgery and 20.7% with wide local excision.[33]
- Frequent clinical follow-up is indicated for more than 5 years because 25% of recurrences occur after 5 years.[32]

Merkel Cell Carcinoma

DIAGNOSES

- Blue red nodular lesion most commonly of the head and neck (Figures 24.33 and 24.34)
- Mostly older patients and/or immunosuppressed persons
- Rapidly growing
- Usually in sun-exposed areas (Figure 24.34)
- Merkel cell polyomavirus is associated with about 80% of Merkel cell carcinomas.[34]

BIOPSY

- Perform a shave, 4-mm punch, or excisional biopsy.

TREATMENT AND PROGNOSIS

- Surgery, radiation, chemotherapy, and immunotherapy are current options.
- Standard treatment is wide surgical excision (2-3 cm margins) followed by adjuvant radiotherapy.
- An alternative treatment option for advanced MCCs, especially those in anatomically challenging locations, is radiotherapy.[35]
- Chest x-ray to check for lung cancer as primary site with cutaneous metastasis.
- Refer for multidisciplinary management that includes surgical oncology, radiation oncology, and oncology.

Coding and Billing Pearls

- Bill for malignant lesion removals after pathology is determined because malignancies have different codes and higher reimbursements.

- When calculating the size of the excised lesion, it is important to include the necessary margins. Therefore if you are excising a 1-cm basal cell carcinoma with 4-mm margins, you would bill for an excision at 1.8 cm. Do not forget to make these measurements so that you get paid for what you do.

Conclusion

There are a number of choices among the methods of removal of malignant lesions. Small lesions that are not near important structures, have distinct margins and are not high-grade cancers can usually be managed by clinicians with good basic skills in their office. For high-risk locations and lesions, the best results of complete lesion removal are typically obtained by Mohs micrographic surgery or surgical oncology. This chapter has provided a general guideline for malignant lesion management, but as always providers must use their best clinical judgment and adjust the specific treatment based on their individual patient's needs. Also, guidelines evolve and change so it is best to consult the literature and expert clinicians when in doubt.

Resources

Selected Guidelines

Kim JYS, Kozlow JH, Mittal B, Moyer J, Olencki T, Rodgers P. Guidelines of care for the management of basal cell carcinoma. *J Am Acad Dermatol.* 2018;78(3):540-559. doi:10.1016/j.jaad.2017.10.006.

Kim JYS, Kozlow JH, Mittal B, Moyer J, Olenecki T, Rodgers P. Guidelines of care for the management of cutaneous squamous cell carcinoma. *J Am Acad Dermatol.* 2018;78(3):560-578. doi:10.1016/j.jaad.2017.10.007.

Swetter SM, Tsao H, Bichakjian CK, et al. Guidelines of care for the management of primary cutaneous melanoma. *J Am Acad Dermatol.* 2019;80(1):208-250. doi:10.1016/j.jaad.2018.08.055.

Swetter SM, Thompson JA, Albertini MR, et al. NCCN Guidelines® Insights: melanoma: cutaneous, version 2.2021. *J Natl Compr Cancer Netw JNCCN.* 2021;19(4):364-376. doi:10.6004/jnccn.2021.0018.

Dermoscopic resources can be found in Chapter 18.

References

1. Gloster HMJ, Neal K. Skin cancer in skin of color. *J Am Acad Dermatol.* 2006;55(5):741-760; quiz 761-764. doi:10.1016/j.jaad.2005.08.063.
2. Singh B, Bhaya M, Shaha A, Har-El G, Lucente FE. Presentation, course, and outcome of head and neck skin cancer in African Americans: a case-control study. *Laryngoscope.* 1998;108(8 Pt 1):1159-1163. doi:10.1097/00005537-199808000-00011.
3. Aggarwal P, Knabel P, Fleischer AB. United States burden of melanoma and non-melanoma skin cancer from 1990 to 2019. *J Am Acad Dermatol.* 2021;85(2):388-395. doi:10.1016/j.jaad.2021.03.109.
4. Anwar J, Wrone DA, Kimyai-Asadi A, Alam M. The development of actinic keratosis into invasive squamous cell carcinoma: evidence and evolving classification schemes. *Clin Dermatol.* 2004;22:189-196.
5. Criscione VD, Weinstock MA, Naylor MF. Actinic keratoses: natural history and risk of malignant transformation in the Veterans Affairs Topical Tretinoin Chemoprevention Trial. *Cancer.* 2009;115:2523-2530.
6. Fried LJ, Tan A, Berry EG, et al. Dermoscopy proficiency expectations for US dermatology resident physicians: results of a modified Delphi survey of pigmented lesion experts. *JAMA Dermatol.* 2021;157(2):189-197. doi:10.1001/jamadermatol.2020.5213.
7. Eisen DB, Asgari MM, Bennett DD, et al. Guidelines of care for the management of actinic keratosis: executive summary. *J Am Acad Dermatol.* 2021;85(4):945-955. doi:10.1016/j.jaad.2021.05.056.
8. Thai KE, Fergin P, Freeman M, et al. A prospective study of the use of cryosurgery for the treatment of actinic keratoses. *Int J Dermatol.* 2004;43(9):687-692. doi:10.1111/j.1365-4632.2004.02056.x.
9. Peris K, Calzavara-Pinton PG, Neri L, et al. Italian expert consensus for the management of actinic keratosis in immunocompetent patients. *J Eur Acad Dermatol Venereol.* 2016;30(7):1077-1084. doi:10.1111/jdv.13648.
10. Cox NH, Eedy DJ, Morton CA. Guidelines for management of Bowen's disease: 2006 update. *Br J Dermatol.* 2007;156:11-21.
11. Ridky TW. Nonmelanoma skin cancer. *J Am Acad Dermatol.* 2007;57:484-501.
12. Ahmed I, Berth-Jones J, Charles-Holmes S, O'Callaghan CJ, Ilchyshyn A. Comparison of cryotherapy with curettage in the treatment of Bowen's disease: a prospective study. *Br J Dermatol.* 2000;143(4):759-766. doi:10.1046/j.1365-2133.2000.03772.x.
13. Stewart JR, Lang ME, Brewer JD. Efficacy of nonexcisional treatment modalities for superficially invasive and in situ squamous cell carcinoma: a systematic review and meta-analysis. *J Am Acad Dermatol.* 2022;87:131-137. doi:10.1016/j.jaad.2021.07.067.
14. Kim JYS, Kozlow JH, Mittal B, Moyer J, Olenecki T, Rodgers P. Guidelines of care for the management of cutaneous squamous cell carcinoma. *J Am Acad Dermatol.* 2018;78(3):560-578. doi:10.1016/j.jaad.2017.10.007.
15. Drucker AM, Adam GP, Rofeberg V, et al. Treatments for primary squamous cell carcinoma and squamous cell carcinoma in situ of the skin: a systematic review and network meta-analysis: summary of an Agency for Healthcare Research and Quality Comparative Effectiveness Review. *J Am Acad Dermatol.* 2020;82(2):479-482. doi:10.1016/j.jaad.2019.06.030.
16. Marcil I, Stern RS. Risk of developing a subsequent nonmelanoma skin cancer in patients with a history of nonmelanoma skin cancer: a critical review of the literature and meta-analysis. *Arch Dermatol.* 2000;136:1524-1530.
17. Drucker AM, Adam GP, Rofeberg V, et al. Treatments of primary basal cell carcinoma of the skin: a systematic review and network meta-analysis. *Ann Intern Med.* 2018;169(7):456-466. doi:10.7326/M18-0678.
18. Kokoszka A, Scheinfeld N. Evidence-based review of the use of cryosurgery in treatment of basal cell carcinoma. *Dermatol Surg.* 2003;29(6):566-571.
19. Ricotti C, Bouzari N, Agadi A, Cockerell CJ. Malignant skin neoplasms. *Med Clin North Am.* 2009;93:1241-1264.
20. Mosterd K, Krekels GA, Nieman FH. Surgical excision versus Mohs' micrographic surgery for primary and recurrent basal-cell carcinoma of the face: a prospective randomised controlled trial with 5-years' follow-up. *Lancet Oncol.* 2008;9:1149-1156.
21. Bradford PT, Goldstein AM, McMaster ML, Tucker MA. Acral lentiginous melanoma: incidence and survival patterns in the United States, 1986–2005. *Arch Dermatol.* 2009;145:427-424.
22. Kalkhoran S, Milne O, Zalaudek I. Historical, clinical, and dermoscopic characteristics of thin nodular melanoma. *Arch Dermatol.* 2010;146:311-318.
23. Swetter SM, Boldrick JC, Jung SY. Increasing incidence of lentigo maligna melanoma subtypes: northern California and national trends 1990–2000. *J Invest Dermatol.* 2005;125:685-691.
24. Huang K, Fan J, Misra S. Acral lentiginous melanoma: incidence and survival in the United States, 2006–2015, an analysis of the SEER Registry. *J Surg Res.* 2020;251:329-339. doi:10.1016/j.jss.2020.02.010.
25. Yan BY, Barilla S, Strunk A, Garg A. Survival differences in acral lentiginous melanoma according to socioeconomic status and race. *J Am Acad Dermatol.* 2022;86(2):379-386. doi:10.1016/j.jaad.2021.07.049.
26. Elder DE, Bastian BC, Cree IA, Massi D, Scolyer RA. The 2018 World Health Organization Classification of cutaneous, mucosal, and uveal melanoma: detailed analysis of 9 distinct subtypes defined by their evolutionary pathway. *Arch Pathol Lab Med.* 2020;144(4):500-522. doi:10.5858/arpa.2019-0561-RA.
27. Swetter SM, Thompson JA, Albertini MR, et al. NCCN Guidelines® Insights: melanoma: cutaneous, version 2.2021. *J Natl Compr Cancer Netw.* 2021;19(4):364-376. doi:10.6004/jnccn.2021.0018.
28. Garbe C, Peris K, Hauschild A. Diagnosis and treatment of melanoma: European consensus-based interdisciplinary guideline. *Eur J Cancer.* 2010;46:270-283.

stimulate fibroblast proliferation and angiogenesis. As more cells migrate and proliferate, an increased amount of blood is needed to adequately deliver gas and perform metabolite exchange.[1] Keratinocytes proliferate and migrate from the intact epidermis around the wound as well as from remaining structures in the wound base, including the epidermis from hair follicles, which are deeper structures and may be partially intact. This is characterized as horizontal healing. The rate of reepithelialization is directly related to moistness of the wound; open, dry wounds reepithelialize significantly more slowly than occluded moist wounds.[2] One week after injury, myofibroblasts initiate contraction by pulling the wound edges closer together. Hair follicles are spared unless the wound is full thickness. Vertical healing involves collagen synthesis, tissue regeneration of epidermis and dermis, and tissue scarring in muscle and subcutaneous tissue.

REMODELING

This phase lasts from 3 weeks to 2 years. Contraction continues, and an organized form of collagen gradually replaces the immature collagen. Wounds created by destructive techniques such as cryosurgery heal more slowly than those caused by a scalpel. Wound tensile strength increases over weeks to months to reach near preinjury strength.[3] This demonstrates the importance of supporting wounds with buried sutures and adhesive wound-closure strips, including at the time of suture removal.

Types of Wounds

Two common types of skin wounds result from basic dermatologic surgery: a full-thickness wound that heals by primary intention and a partial-thickness wound that heals by secondary intention. However, even a full-thickness wound can be allowed to heal by secondary intention such as after a cancer removal on the scalp (Figure 25.1).

FULL-THICKNESS WOUNDS

The epidermis and full thickness of the dermis are lost. This is usually created by a full-thickness excision or injury. The wound heals slowly by granulation tissue formation, contracture, and reepithelialization from the wound edges. If the edges are approximated with sutures or adhesive tape (healing by primary intention), there will be less wound contracture and therefore less scarring.

PARTIAL-THICKNESS WOUNDS

The epidermis and part of the dermis are lost. This is usually created by shave excisions, curettage and electrodesiccation, CO_2 laser surgery, or chemical peels. If left to heal alone (healing by secondary intention), reepithelialization from the wound edges and adnexal structures in the base of the wound will quickly follow. The greater the depth of dermal injury, the more scarring.

Pressure Injury

Another type of wound commonly seen in the inpatient and outpatient setting is a pressure injury (ulcer). This is localized damage to skin and underlying soft tissue caused by pressure over a bony prominence or medical device. It can be painful and possibly affected by microclimates and patient comorbidities.[4] Risk factors for the development of a pressure injury include reduced mobility, sensory impairment, acute illness, level of consciousness, extremes of age, vascular disease, severe chronic or terminal illness, previous history of pressure damage, malnutrition, and dehydration.[5] Pressure injuries are divided into four main stages by the National Pressure Injury Advisory Panel (NPIAP; last updated in 2016, see https://npiap.com/page/PressureInjuryStages for more detailed descriptions and images) which help characterize the lesion and determine treatment.

- Stage 1: Intact skin with color or temperature change. The color can range from nonblanchable erythema to brown or black depending on the individual's normal skin color. It can be helpful to compare concerning areas to nonaffected skin in the individual patient if there are subtle changes (Figure 25.2).
- Stage 2: Partial-thickness loss of skin with exposed dermis. The epidermis is absent or elevated due to bullous

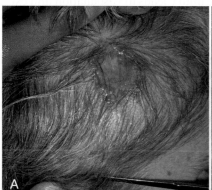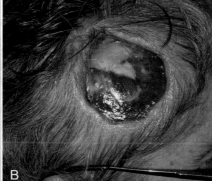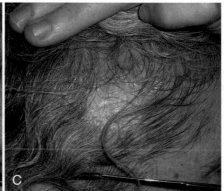

Figure 25.1 (A) Large nodular BCC on the scalp of a 37-year-old woman. **(B)** The BCC was resected in the operating room by ENT, and the patient preferred to allow the wound to heal by secondary intention rather than have a large flap done. This photo was taken 2 weeks after the surgery was completed when the patient removed the dressing for a postop check. **(C)** Six months later the wound was completely reepithelialized, and in the following year the scar retracted and shrunk in size so that it was no longer visible under her hair. (Copyright Richard P. Usatine, MD.)

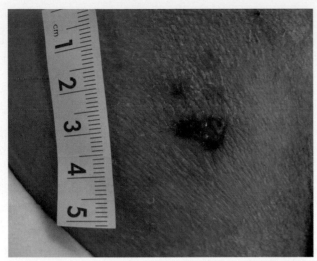

Figure 25.2 Stage 1 color changes and stage 2 sacral pressure injury. (Copyright Daniel Stulberg, MD.)

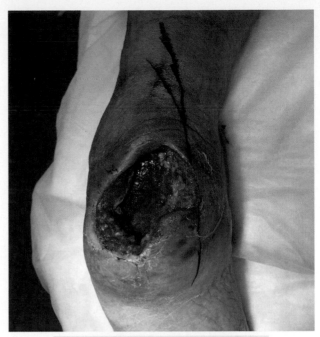

Figure 25.4 Stage 4 with exposed calcaneus.

change, but the dermis is still intact, so underlying subcutaneous fat and other structures are not visible. Risk is increased when sheer forces, pressure, and moisture combine especially in the sacral area. There are separate entities not due to pressure including age- and atrophy-associated skin tears, moisture-associated skin damage (MASD), tape injuries, or trauma (Figure 25.2).

- Stage 3: Full-thickness loss of skin revealing subcutaneous fat but no visible deep structures (fascia, muscle, tendon, or bone). Clinically it is useful to probe the area with a cotton-tipped applicator (CTA) to assess for the extent of the injury and tunneling under adjacent tissues (Figure 25.3).
- Stage 4: In addition to full-thickness skin and tissue loss, there is exposed fascia, muscle, tendon, ligament,

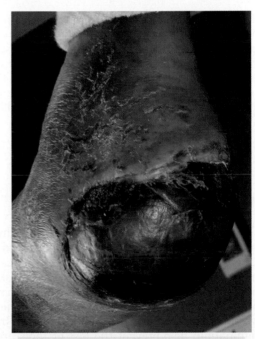

Figure 25.5 Stage 4 unstageable due to eschar.

cartilage, or bone in the injury field. Slough and/or eschar may be visible (Figure 25.4).

- Unstageable: Full-thickness skin and tissue loss, but the extent of tissue damage cannot be confirmed because of slough or eschar obscuring the depth. In contrast to previous practice, stable leathery eschar without signs of infection, drainage, or erythema should not be debrided unless there is a need to further assess underlying tissues (Figure 25.5).
- Deep tissue pressure injury (DTPI): Color, temperature, or texture change concerning for underlying tissue

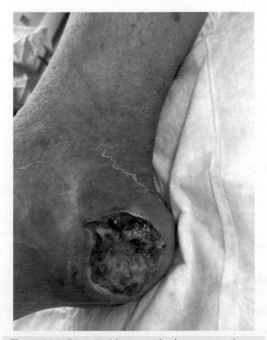

Figure 25.3 Stage 3 with exposed subcutaneous tissue.

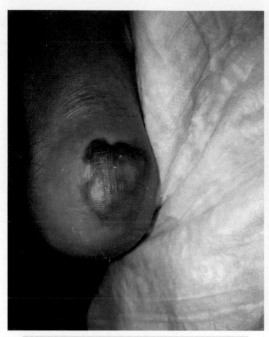

Figure 25.6 Deep pressure tissue injury of heel.

Table 25.1   Ideal Dressing Characteristics

Handling of excess exudate	Removal of toxic substances
Maintenance of moist environment	Barrier to microorganisms
Thermal insulation provided	Freedom from particulate contaminants
Removal without trauma to new tissue	Adheres well to a thin margin of surrounding skin
Does not adhere to wound	Nontoxic and nonreactive
Conforms well to body contours and motion	Promotes patient comfort and is not bulky
Readily available and inexpensive	Long shelf-life

From Freitag DS. Surgical wound dressings. In: Lask G, Moy R, eds. *Principles and Techniques of Cutaneous Surgery.* McGraw-Hill; 1996.

breakdown due to acute or subacute pressure injury before the skin and tissues have broken down or sloughed. Often the skin color is violaceous, but in dark-skinned individuals, careful inspection may show even darker tones and less redness (Figure 25.6). Over time the extent of the injury becomes apparent with tissue breakdown. This is a form of pressure injury and is different from traumatic or acute vascular injuries.

Prevention and treatment of pressure injuries will be discussed in further detail later.

Wound Care Dressings

The task of selecting an appropriate wound care dressing can be overwhelming due to the number of advanced dressings available on the market. To help ease this task it is important to reflect back on the functions of the skin, as the wound dressings are essentially serving as a skin substitute until the new epithelium is synthesized. The ideal dressing should provide a protective barrier against trauma or contamination, help prevent the loss of moisture, and facilitate healing by providing a controlled, moist healing environment. In addition, some advanced dressings will also include compressive properties. See Table 25.1 on Ideal Dressing Characteristics. There is evidence that occlusive dressings increase early epithelial migration on acute full-thickness biopsies in comparison to air-exposed wounds.[6,7] Furthermore, Madden and colleagues demonstrated that partial-thickness wounds treated under occlusion with hydrocolloid healed significantly faster and resulted in increased keratinocyte proliferation when compared to wounds covered with fine mesh gauze or silver sulfadiazine.[8] However, in clean sutured surgical incisions, an experimental animal trial showed no difference in infection or white cell infiltration when managed dressed or

undressed.[6] Hence, the following material mostly refers to complex open wound care.

Most dressings applied have three layers. The first layer, the contact layer, is the dressing applied directly onto the wound bed. It is important to take into consideration the ease of dressing removal when selecting the contact layer. Dressings with nonadherent properties such as petrolatum-impregnated gauze will help prevent unwanted trauma to the newly synthesized tissue during dressing removal. In addition, antimicrobial ointments or gels can be applied when the wound demonstrates clinical signs of infection. The absorbent layer above the contact layer assists in the management of wound exudate. Ideally, the absorbent layer will absorb and wick away wound exudate from the wound bed while controlling maceration of the surrounding intact skin. The combination of the contact and absorbent layers is known as the primary dressing. The role of the secondary or outer dressing is to cover, protect, and reinforce the primary dressings. Elastic bandages and multilayer wraps offer additional absorptive capabilities along with wound protection and compressive properties to aid in the management of edema when indicated.

The following is a list of the most common types of dressings available to providers. Depending on the wound characteristics and amount of drainage, some of these dressings can be used alone or can be combined to facilitate an optimal wound healing environment.

- Gauze dressings
- Transparent films
- Foams
- Hydrocolloids
- Alginate
- Composite dressings

Table 25.2, **Types of Dressings for Wound Characteristics and Quantity of Drainage**, lists some of the specific common dressings that are utilized based on the quantity of wound exudate or drainage for open wound management.

Wound Care

WOUND HEALING BY SECONDARY INTENTION

Partial-thickness wounds that are allowed to heal by secondary intention may be cleansed after procedures using a

Table 25.2   Types of Dressings for Wound Characteristics and Quantity of Drainage

	Necrotic Black/Brown/Dry/Hard	Mildly Exudative Pink/Red/Yellow/Tan	Moderately Exudative Pink/Red/Yellow/Tan	Highly Exudative Pink/Red/Yellow/Tan With Periwound Maceration
Bismuth Tribromoph/Petrolatum (Xeroform)		x	x	
Honey (Therahoney)		x	x	
Calcium Alginate (Aquacel)				x
Cadexomer Iodine (Iodosorb)			x	x
Povidone-Iodine (Betadine)	x			
Collagen (Puracol)			x	x

sterile CTA dipped in saline. The applicator is gently rolled over the wound to remove any loose debris and crusted exudate. Care should be taken not to rub or apply excessive friction to the wound bed. Although antiseptic use is recommended prior to procedures, a review by Punjataewakupt and Napavichayan warns against the potential toxicity of antiseptics such as hydrogen peroxide or chlorhexidine in open wounds because they are toxic to epithelial cells and delay wound healing.[9]

After cleaning the wound, it is dressed with an agent that facilitates a moist wound bed and environment as delineated above. Table 25.3, **Types of Antibacterial Agents**, lists common ointments that are used for open wounds. Patients with an allergy to antibiotic ointments should use only nonadherent dressings such as petroleum gauze. Because of the high potential for contact dermatitis, neomycin-containing ointments should be avoided[9] (Figure 25.7). Although there is literature that supports the use of antibiotic-containing ointments in contaminated wounds, data to support their superiority to petrolatum in clean wounds is insufficient.

Studies suggest that white petrolatum is as safe and effective as bacitracin with less risk for inducing allergy.[10,11] Furthermore, a review by Sheth and Weitzul recommended using petrolatum instead of antimicrobial ointment on clean wounds given that the rate of allergic contact dermatitis from antibacterial ointments (1.6% to 2.3%) is similar to the rate of postoperative infections (1% to 2%) in dermatologic surgery.[11]

If the wound is superficial and has a smaller surface area (<2 cm), patients are encouraged to use adhesive bandages to cover the wound. For superficial wounds with a larger surface area, they may be covered with a nonadherent dressing pad, such as a perforated foam absorbent (Telfa), and secured with a hypoallergenic tape. Superficial or partial-thickness wounds may be cleaned several times a week and dressed appropriately until the wound has epithelialized completely.

Full-thickness or deep wounds that are moderate to highly exudative such as leg ulcers can be managed with calcium alginate (e.g., Aquacel) or carboxymethylcellulose (e.g., Melgisorb). These dressings are then covered with a highly absorbent pad (ABD) and secured with rolled gauze (e.g., Kerlix). Next, a circumferential layer of cotton padding (e.g., Webril) may be applied and secured with a lightly compressive general elastic bandage (e.g., ACE). Note that highly exudative wounds may produce yellow or green foul-smelling strike-through on their dressings, which is not a sign of infection.

Due to the high quantity of exudate, these wounds typically require dressing changes every 2 to 3 days and can be changed less often as clinically indicated. As wounds become more superficial and less extensive, a transition to techniques utilized for superficial wounds may then take place.

WOUND HEALING BY PRIMARY INTENTION

To care for large wounds or incisions closed primarily with sutures, use a saline-soaked CTA gently rolling along the suture line to remove any crusted exudate. The sutured wound may then be covered with a nonadherent dressing and dry gauze. Topical antibiotic ointment may be applied for wounds that exhibit minimal exudative drainage prior to applying a nonadherent dressing. A Cochrane review published by Heal and Banks concluded that the number needed to treat to prevent wound infection with topical antibiotics versus no treatment applied to surgical wounds healing by primary intention was 50. However, the review included contaminated surgeries and notes that the case for the use of topical antibiotics in clean surgery is weaker.[12]

Smaller wounds and incisions may be primarily closed or approximated using semipermeable tape strips (e.g., Steri-Strips) and/or micropore tape across the incision site immediately after the procedure. These can also be placed on sutured wounds for reinforcement. This provides support and reduces tension along the per-iincisional area. These are then reapplied after sutures are removed. The 2-mm

Table 25.3   Types of Antibacterial Agents

Brand Name	Active Antimicrobial Ingredients
Bacitracin	Bacitracin zinc (covers staphylococci and streptococci)
Polysporin	Bacitracin zinc, Polymyxin B sulfate (covers gram-negative bacilli and Pseudomonas[8])
Neosporin	Neomycin sulfate (covers staphylococci and most gram-negative bacilli), Bacitracin zinc, Polymyxin B sulfate
Gentamicin	Gentamicin sulfate
Bactroban	Mupirocin (covers streptococci and staphylococci resistant to methicillin)

Note: All can cause contact dermatitis.

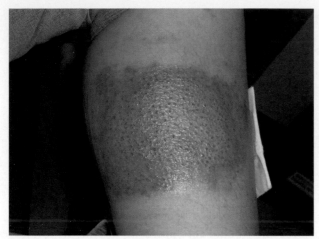

Figure 25.7 Contact dermatitis from neomycin applied broadly over a shave biopsy wound. The geometrical shape of the erythema is a clue to the etiology of a contact allergy. (Copyright Richard P. Usatine, MD.)

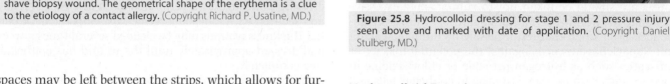

Figure 25.8 Hydrocolloid dressing for stage 1 and 2 pressure injury seen above and marked with date of application. (Copyright Daniel Stulberg, MD.)

spaces may be left between the strips, which allows for further exudate to drain and absorb into the overlying dressing. Tissue adhesives (e.g., Mastisol or Benzoin tincture) may be used to increase adherence of the strips.

Timing of suture removal depends on many factors but is generally 4 to 6 days for the head and neck, 7 to 10 days for upper limbs, 10 days for the trunk and abdomen, and 14 days for lower limbs. A nonadherent primary dressing may then be applied and secured in place with Medipore tape, cotton wadding, or rolled gauze. Light-to-medium pressure dressing can then be applied with cohesive or elastic bandage.

The use of pressure dressings is useful and important in reducing the risk of hematoma formation after the excision of large cysts or lipomas. A pressure dressing consists of generous amounts of absorbent gauze pads and is secured with rolled gauze, cotton cast padding, and elastic bandage. Patients may be instructed to remove the bulky outer pressure dressing 24 to 36 hours after the procedure. The underlying primary dressing is left undisturbed. It is not advisable to apply any pressure dressings to areas of suspected vascular compromise.

Hydrocolloid Dressing

Hydrocolloid (e.g., DuoDERM) may be used for occluding small and manageable wounds with minimal exudate (Figure 25.8). This product can be cut and sized to cover a wound 5 to 10 mm beyond the border in all directions. Hydrocolloid may also be used over small incisions where absorbable sutures were placed for primary wound closure. Absorbable sutures will eventually hydrolyze within the subcutaneous layers, whereas suture material above the surface will have embedded into the hydrocolloid. When the hydrocolloid is removed, the absorbable sutures detach with it.[11]

Hydrocolloid dressings are also useful for superficial wounds overlying anatomical prominences, the trunk, or digits, as wounds in these areas can be difficult to secure when compared to other wound care dressings that need to be secured with standard bandage tape (Figure 25.9A–C). Lastly, hydrocolloid is water resistant, which allows for light bathing.

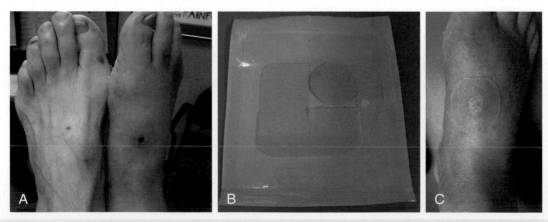

Figure 25.9 (A) Ulcer over a localized bony prominence. **(B)** Cutting hydrocolloid dressing for the size of the wound. **(C)** Applying hydrocolloid dressing with a 1-cm margin around the wound. (Copyright Daniel Stulberg, MD.)

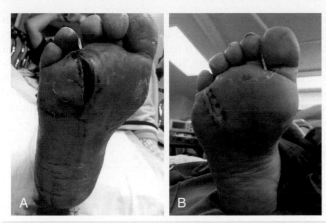

Figure 25.10 (A) Incision and drainage of abscess. **(B)** Subsequent delayed primary closure. (Copyright Eric Lew, DPM.)

WOUND HEALING BY TERTIARY INTENTION

Larger wounds and soft tissue deficits may require a longer period of healing before wound closure can be achieved. Usually these types of wounds are preceded by prior excisional debridement of all nonviable tissue to address tumors or infection. Advanced wound care modalities such as negative pressure therapy are often utilized to stimulate granulation tissue across a wound bed. This process and period of open wound management prepares the wound for eventual surgical intervention and wound closure with suturing, application of autologous skin grafting, or rotational free flap closure. This is referred to as tertiary intention or delayed primary closure (Figure 25.10A–B).

NEGATIVE PRESSURE WOUND THERAPY

Negative pressure wound therapy (NPWT), occasionally referred to as vacuum-assisted closure (VAC), uses differential suction to help close wounds and increase healing. After open surgical wounds or surgery complications involving wounds, a wound vacuum can be applied. This tool helps control exudates and increase wound contracture (Figure 25.11). Although commonly used in clinical practice based on expert opinion, there is no data to support NPWT for treating surgical wounds or pressure ulcers. NPWT has been shown to be of benefit in patients with wounds and diabetes mellitus.[13,14] A study included in a recent review illustrated that compared to saline there was an increased odds ratio for healing when using NPWT in diabetic wounds.[13]

WOUND CLEANING AND CARE FOR CHRONIC WOUNDS AND PRESSURE INJURIES

Wound cleaning may delay the development of biofilm and reduce bioburden. Debris remaining in the wound can lead to bacterial growth and delayed wound healing. Historically there have been various items used to clean wounds including water, saline, hydrogen peroxide, chlorhexidine, and povidone-iodine.[15] However, hydrogen peroxide, chlorhexidine, and povidone-iodine may be toxic to the local tissue and of limited efficacy. One study found Vulnopur spray (saline with aloe vera, silver chloride, and decyl glucoside) had benefit above standard saline for wound cleaning.[16] Otherwise tap water from a safe supply or standard saline is considered safe, effective, and nontoxic for wound care.

ALTERNATIVE THERAPIES

Honey has been shown to increase area of epithelization, wound contraction, skin-breaking strength, and tissue granulation. It appears to heal partial thickness burns and infected postoperative wounds more quickly than conventional treatment (which included polyurethane film, paraffin gauze, soframycin-impregnated gauze, sterile linen, and leaving the burns exposed). Beyond these comparisons, any evidence for differences in the effects of honey and comparators is of low or very low quality and does not form a robust basis for decision making.[17] Phenytoin, olive oil, and aloe vera are also less conventional therapies that have been used with wound healing. However, as with honey, studies with these items are limited, and the quality of evidence is low.[18,19]

Human Amniotic Membranes

Desiccated human amniotic membranes (HAMs) aid in the healing of chronic wounds by providing a suprastructure, supplying growth factors and cytokines. It can also decrease

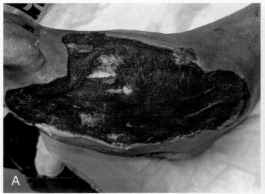
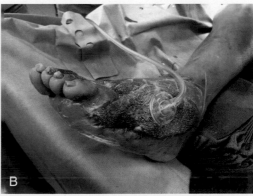

Figure 25.11 (A) Large postoperative debridement for osteomyelitis. **(B)** Wound vacuum for control of exudate and wound contraction. (Copyright Eric Lew, DPM.)

pain and fluid loss in burns. As a product, not a medication, it is not assessed by the FDA for the treatment of either burns or chronic wounds. It can be applied to clean wounds and covered with petrolatum or a nonadherent dressing (Adaptic), and it should be changed weekly.[20]

Prevention of Pressure Injuries

There are many tools or measures that are useful to prevent pressure injuries.[4]

- Nutritional supplements if impaired nutrition, otherwise they do not improve outcome
- Appropriate support surfaces – mattresses, overlays on operating tables, and specialized foam and sheepskin overlays
- Frequent repositioning – optimal schedule uncertain, usually recommended every 2 hours
- Moisturizers – specifically to the sacral area
- Prophylactic padding to bony prominences
- Silk-like fabric may reduce sheer forces vs cotton
- Float the heels – position heels to remove all contact between heels and surface by padding under the legs

There are also scales to predict the chance of a patient developing a pressure ulcer. The Braden scale was designed for neurointensive care patients and measures six categories to produce a score; a higher score correlates to a lower risk.[21] Prealbumin may also be used to estimate the clinical outcome of patients with a pressure ulcer; a level higher than 15 shows improvement, but that less than 5 indicates a poor prognosis.

Treatment of Pressure Injuries

General treatment for pressure injury is to remove the pressure from the affected area (Figure 25.12A–C). Antiseptics and alcohol should be avoided, and wet dressings should not be allowed to dry out since that leads to tissue desiccation. Routine cultures of wounds are not helpful as many microbial species can contaminate the wound without being the cause of a wound infection. Pentoxifylline and cilostazol should be considered for patients with arterial insufficiency, and hyperbaric oxygen can be considered in diabetics. Ultrasound, specific cleansers, and electromagnets have not been shown to be more helpful for treatment than standard measures. To monitor the healing of a pressure injury the Pressure Ulcer Scale for Healing (PUSH) can be utilized. To use the PUSH tool, the pressure ulcer is assessed and scored on the three elements in the tool: exudate amount, wound size, and tissue status.[4]

Special Circumstances

DIABETIC FOOT

Educating diabetic patients can help them understand that improving glycemic control may enhance wound healing. Hyperglycemia and reduced insulin results in diminished collagen synthesis, leading to stiffness and decreased tensile strength of tissues. They may have neuropathy, which can impact the ability to sense pain and make them prone to more injuries. Neuropathy can lead to altered bony structures, increasing the chance of developing wounds and ulcers in these locations (Figure 25.13A and B). It is important to offload pressure in a neuropathic foot when possible using diabetic shoes with inserts, total contact casts, custom walking boots, or other devices (Figure 25.14A–C).

VENOUS STASIS ULCERS

When treating venous stasis ulcers, compression is an important addition to dressings. Profore wrap, compression stockings, and the Unna Boot are examples of compressive devices (Figure 25.15). The Unna boot should not be used in patients with infected wounds, arterial insufficiency, or highly exudative wounds. A wound vacuum can be very helpful in highly exudative wounds (Figure 25.16A and B). Venous stasis ulcers should be compressed to 15 to 20 mmHg and elevated when possible; this should increase to 30 to 40 mmHg as the patient is able to tolerate.

There are technological advances associated with a multilayer compression system such as a combined Coban and foam layer (Coban-2). This system provides sustained, therapeutic compression and is simple to apply. The foam layer contours to the lower extremity and adheres to the outer cohesive compressive layer, making it less prone to slipping

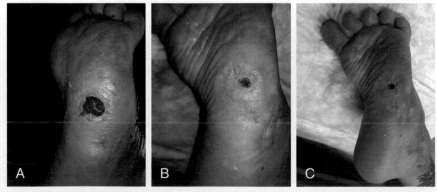

Figure 25.12 (A) Neuropathic ulcer at 5th metatarsal base. **(B)** After 2 weeks of offloading pressure. **(C)** Nearly healed after 4 weeks. (Copyright Eric Lew, DPM.)

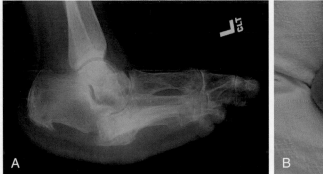
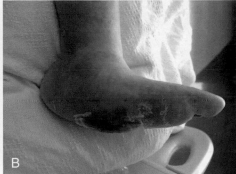

Figure 25.13 (A) X-ray of neuropathic AKA Charcot foot in diabetic patient. **(B)** Skin breakdown due to the bony changes of the Charcot foot. (Copyright Daniel Stulberg, MD.)

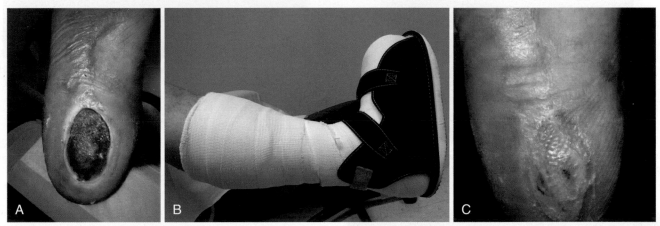

Figure 25.14 (A) Chronic neuropathic hindfoot ulceration on a 58-year-old female with diabetes. **(B)** The ulceration was offloaded in a total contact cast (TCC) for a period of 6 weeks. The TCC was changed weekly in conjunction with wound debridement and local wound care. **(C)** The ulceration fully epithelialized after offloading in the TCC. (Copyright Eric Lew, DPM.)

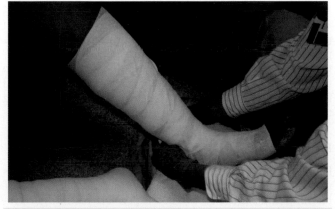

Figure 25.15 Application of an Unna boot. (Copyright Daniel Stulberg, MD.)

(Figure 25.17). This compression system also maintains a high working pressure when a patient is ambulatory. These multilayer compression systems are utilized for management of lymphedema in addition to venous leg ulcers. However, they should not be applied to patients with moderate or severe arterial insufficiency (ABI <0.8).

Moisture retentive dressing is beneficial in open or exudative wounds. Aspirin 300 mg/day and pentoxifylline 400 mg three times daily can both increase healing rates. Progressive resistance exercise has been shown to improve ulcer healing by 27%.[22] Lastly, adjunctive therapy with endovenous ablation added to compression therapy can be considered.[23]

NONHEALING WOUNDS

When wounds take longer to heal than anticipated, it is important to consider factors deterring optimal wound healing or other etiologies. These include but are not limited to osteomyelitis or infection, arterial insufficiency, noncompliance, continued pressure to the area, poor glycemic control, impaired nutrition, pyoderma gangrenosum (Figure 25.18), and malignancy. Consider biopsy for atypical and chronic leg ulcers that have been present for greater than approximately 3 months to rule out malignancy such as squamous or basal cell carcinoma or inflammatory conditions.[24]

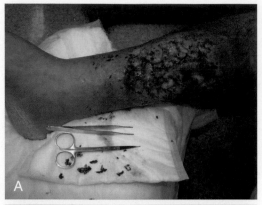

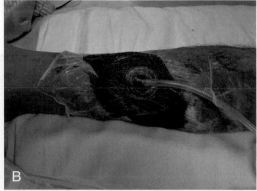

Figure 25.16 **(A)** A highly exudative leg wound. **(B)** Wound vacuum for control of exudate. (Copyright Daniel Stulberg, MD.)

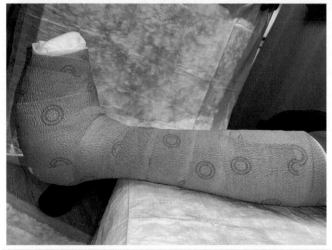

Figure 25.17 A combined foam layer with compressive cohesive bandage that is utilized for management of a patient with a chronic venous leg ulceration. (Copyright Regina Gallegos, MPT, CWS.)

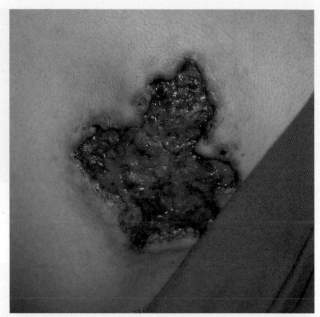

Figure 25.18 Pyoderma gangrenosum with metal gray color and ulceration with overriding borders. (Copyright Richard P. Usatine, MD.)

Postoperative Wound Care Patient Instructions

Postoperative patients are given instructions to keep their wound covered and dressings clean, dry, and intact. The primary dressing should neither get wet nor be removed until 24 to 48 hours postoperatively. For larger wounds and incisions that require splinting and immobilization, the dressing apparatus is usually kept protected for 5 to 7 days until reassessed in clinic during the first postoperative visit.

SHOWERING

Specific instruction on bathing and taking showers after a procedure is necessary to avoid a potential point of confusion for patients. Immersion of the wound in swimming pools or baths should be avoided. Many providers advise patients with sutured wounds to keep their dressings dry until suture removal. There is evidence, however, that there is no increased risk of infection in clean and clean-contaminated wounds when patients shower 48 hours after surgery.[25] After showering or bathing, patients should apply ointment and redress the wound appropriately. However, patients with peripheral neuropathy or comorbidities and immunocompromised status, which can lead to increased risk of operative site dehiscence or infection, should be advised to keep their dressings clean, dry, intact and to protect the wound from getting wet during bathing to avoid contaminating their surgical sites.

PAIN

For discomfort or pain following minor procedures, patients may take acetaminophen. Aspirin increases the risk of bleeding and should be avoided if possible with larger procedures. If the wound and patient are not at high risk of bleeding, an oral NSAID may be used. For patients who have a lower pain tolerance after procedures, a short course of opioid medication may be considered. However, if the patient has a problem with substance use, the provider should discuss alternative nonnarcotic methods for treating pain when possible. These recommendations should be adjusted based on an individual's allergies or underlying conditions.

BLEEDING

If bleeding occurs, the patient should apply firm pressure to the site for 5 to 20 minutes, without discontinuing the pressure to see if the bleeding has stopped. They may elevate an affected extremity if applicable. If the bleeding does not stop, then the patient should promptly return for care in the office or other setting as needed. Patients who have conditions requiring anticoagulants must undergo careful periprocedural management when undergoing more than simple skin procedures. Consulting with patients' other providers or consultants beforehand may be necessary, not only to discuss and estimate thromboembolic and bleeding risks but also for timing of interruption or bridging anticoagulation. Patients on warfarin require early discontinuation (usually 5 to 7 days) with normalization of the international normalized ratio (INR) before procedures. Typically, warfarin can be resumed 12 to 24 hours after procedures. Patients who are on direct oral anticoagulants may usually stop taking the medication 1 to 2 days before minor procedures and restart postprocedurally when hemostasis is achieved. Patients who are taking clopidogrel or aspirin typically can maintain their dosing for minor procedures, especially if they are at higher risk of coronary thrombosis.

INFECTION

Procedural and surgical site infections can occur but are less common in healthy individuals. Immunocompromised patients or those with medical comorbidities such as diabetes or tobacco use are at higher risk of developing surgical site infections and require attentive care periprocedurally. Utilizing sterile technique and optimizing patients prior to procedures can help reduce the risks of developing infection. Signs of infection include redness, swelling, warmth, purulent drainage, fever, or swollen lymph nodes. If a patient exhibits any of these signs and symptoms, they should be seen urgently or emergently. The most common bacteria infecting soft tissue are *staphylococcal* and *streptococcal.* Superficial wound swab cultures should be avoided as these can capture normal skin flora. Obtaining a deep tissue culture after thorough lavage is preferred. Most minor and superficial infections can be treated with culture-directed oral antibiotics. Hospital admission, parenteral antibiotic therapy, and operative procedures, such as an incision and drainage, or lavage and wound debridement may be necessary depending on the extent and severity of the infection.

WOUND HEALING

Patients should be educated on what to expect throughout the wound healing process at each stage of wound healing. Scar maturation and remodeling typically lasts 6 to 12 months or even longer in pediatric patients and adolescents. Patients may complain of pruritus and tightness. Scar hydration and massage with aloe vera or vitamin E may help alleviate these symptoms by preventing the wound from fissuring or peeling. Evidence showed improvement in dermal collagen organization but no reduction in scar hypertrophy with over-the-counter "scar gel" or topical ointment.[26] However, the products are massaged onto the scar, and scar massage has been shown to reduce hypertrophic scars,[27] so patients may utilize those products as desired. Scar hypertrophy, or keloids, may develop when scar tissue continues to develop after the skin heals. They are common in patients of African, Asian, or Hispanic descent. Patients may experience persistent itching or burning. If keloid formation is a concern, patients may tape the area continuously for 3 months with Micropore tape or another type of hypoallergenic nonsterile tape, because evidence suggests that this may reduce tension on the scar and reduce the tendency toward hypertrophy.[28] Multiple treatment modalities exist including intralesional or topical steroids, cryotherapy, radiotherapy, laser, or surgical excision. See Chapter 23, *Procedures to Treat Benign Conditions*, for additional details. Patients should also be educated that wound discoloration and redness can take 6 to 12 months to fade. They should avoid prolonged sun exposure as this may delay scar maturation and lead to hyperpigmentation. To prevent these changes, patients should keep the scar covered and/or apply sunscreen during scar maturation.

Special Locations

PERIORBITAL WOUNDS

Wounds that approach the cutaneous-conjunctival junction should not be cleaned with antiseptic solutions because they are potentially oculotoxic. If there is a chance that the ointment on the wound may get into the eye, a preparation specifically formulated for the eye (e.g., Polysporin ophthalmic ointment) should be used.

EAR

If cartilage is exposed, chondritis can occur from desiccation. To prevent this, petrolatum ointment should be applied liberally. Cotton should be placed in the external auditory meatus to prevent wound drainage that may lead to otitis externa.

DIGITS

When applying dressings to a finger or toe, two main types may be used: a tubular dressing or a bandage applied obliquely and attached at the wrists. Excessive pressure or circumferential tapes that do not allow for swelling and can constrict blood flow should be avoided.

Complications

Factors that negatively affect wound healing include the following:

- Excessive tension
- Hemostatic agents
- Antiseptic agents
- Infection
- Hypoxia
- Reactions to ointments
- Protein deficiency

- Deficiency of vitamins A and C, and zinc
- Immunocompromised state
- Nicotine use
- Steroids
- Vascular disease

The clinician should work to avoid or ameliorate these complicating factors.

CONTACT DERMATITIS

Erosions, bullae, contact dermatitis, and bruising may be associated with the use of adhesive tapes, particularly when used with tissue adhesives (Figure 25.19).

This commonly occurs on the facial skin of elderly patients and those patients on systemic steroid therapy. Wraps or elastic sleeves can be used to hold dressings in place instead of adhesives on the extremities of these high-risk individuals. Avoiding the use of topical antibiotics can minimize the risk of contact dermatitis.

OPTIMIZING OUTCOMES

- Avoid leakage of wound by using the proper dressing.
- Keep the wound moist with topical ointment and dressing.
- Remove necrotic tissue through debridement.
- Control pain.
- Ensure patient adherence to written and verbal instructions.

Conclusion

There are various methods and techniques to manage a wound and facilitate optimal wound healing. Providers may select their preferred method of wound dressing based

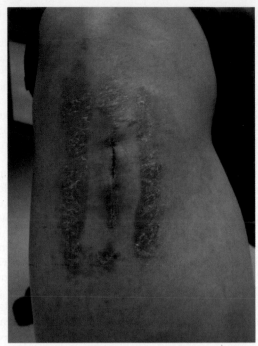

Figure 25.19 Contact dermatitis due to taped dressing following knee surgery. (Copyright Daniel L. Stulberg, MD.)

on the characteristics of the procedure and the resultant wound while taking into consideration patients' needs. Utilizing the principles discussed in this chapter will help produce optimal healing and reduce complications. For further information on potential complications of surgery and wound healing, see Chapter 26, *Complications: Postprocedural Adverse Effects and Their Prevention.*

| | **Patient Information Handout** |
| | **Care of Your Skin after Surgery** |

Supplies needed

- Clean petroleum jelly (a squeeze tube is cleaner than a tub) (Vaseline is one name brand) (Do not use Neosporin or Triple Antibviotic)
- Dressing or gauze that is made for wound care (Band-Aids are one name brand)
- Optimal-cotton-tipped applicators (Q-tips are one name brand)

Directions

- Keep the site clean and dry and do not remove the orignal dressing for 24 hours.
- After 24 hours you may shower daily. Gently wash the surgical site with soap and water in the shower or at least once daily.
- Apply petroleum jelly to the clean wound with a clean finger or cotton-tipped applicator one to two times per day.
- Use a dressing to cover the wound. While cleansing is only needed once or twice a day, additional petroleum jelly may be added as needed to keep the wound moist.
- Tylenol (acetaminophen) or ibuprofen can be taken for pain if needed. DO NOT start taking any medications with aspirin or aspirin products.

REPEAT THESE INSTRUCTIONS DAILY UNTIL THE WOUND IS HEALED. THIS MAY BE ANYWHERE FROM 5 TO 20 DAYS.

The wound will actually heal better and scar less if kept clean and covered with petroleum jelly.

Bleeding

If bleeding occurs, apply firm pressure to the site. Direct pressure should be applied to the wound. Five minutes should be adequate if the bleeding is minor and the wound is small. However, if the wound is larger and the bleeding is more severe, apply pressure for 10 minutes, timed by looking at a clock. If the bleeding continues, remove the pad and press directly with a clean gauze pad over the bleeding site. If bleeding soaks through the gauze or is not stopped by firm pressure, call and go to your doctor or an urgent care center.

Infection

If you notice pus or discharge coming from the wound this may be an infection. This is particularly worrisome if you develop a fever and the wound is red, painful, swollen, and warm. Other signs of infection could be red streaks from wound, increased pain, and painful or swollen, and warm. Other signs of infection could be red of having an infection, go to your doctor or an urgent care center.

Shower and washing

You may shower daily after the first 24 hours have passed. At first, you may leave the dressing on during the shower to protect the wound from the flow of water. Alternatively, if the wound needs cleaning, the shower is helpful to remove crusts and discharge. Dry the area gently and then apply the petroleum jelly and cover the healing wound as described above. We recommend not bathing in a tub or hot tub until the wound is completely healed over to avoid infection.

References

1. Demidova-Rice TN, Hamblin MR, Herman IM. Acute and impaired wound healing: pathophysiology and current methods for drug delivery, part 1: normal and chronic wounds: biology, causes, and approaches to care. *Adv Skin Wound Care*. 2012;25(7):304-314. doi:10.1097/01.ASW.0000416006.55218.d0.

2. Powers JG, Higham C, Broussard K, Phillips TJ. Wound healing and treating wounds. *J Am Acad Dermatol*. 2016;74(4):607-625. doi:10.1016/j.jaad.2015.08.070.

3. Byrne M, Aly A. The surgical suture. *Aesthet Surg J*. 2019;39 (suppl_2):S67-S72. doi:10.1093/asj/sjz036.

4. Edsberg LE, Black JM, Goldberg M, McNichol L, Moore L, Sieggreen M. Revised National Pressure Ulcer Advisory Panel Pressure Injury Staging System: revised pressure injury staging system. *J Wound Ostomy Continence Nurs*. 2016;43(6):585-597. doi:10.1097/WON.0000000000000281.

5. National Pressure Ulcer Advisory Panel, European Pressure Ulcer Advisory Panel and Pan Pacific Pressure Injury Alliance. In: Haesler E, ed. *Prevention and Treatment of Pressure Ulcers: Quick Reference Guide*. Osborne Park, Australia: Cambridge Media; 2014.

6. Davis SC, Li J, Gil J, et al. A closer examination of atraumatic dressings for optimal healing. *Int Wound J*. 2015;12(5):510-516. doi:10.1111/iwj.12144.

7. Agren MS, Karlsmark T, Hansen JB, Rygaard Jorgen. Occlusion versus air exposure on full-thickness biopsy wounds. *J Wound Care*. 2001;10(8):301-304.

8. Madden MR, Nolan E, Finkelstein JL, et al. Comparison of an occlusive and a semi-occlusive dressing and the effect of the wound exudate upon keratinocyte proliferation. *J Trauma*. 1989;29(7):924-930; discussion 930-931. doi:10.1097/00005373-198907000-00004.

9. Punjataewakupt A, Napavichayanun S, Aramwit P. The downside of antimicrobial agents for wound healing. *Eur J Clin Microbiol Infect Dis*. 2019;38(1):39-54. doi:10.1007/s10096-018-3393-5.

10. Inoue Y, Hasegawa M, Maekawa T, et al. The wound/burn guidelines – 1: wounds in general. *J Dermatol*. 2016;43(4):357-375. doi:10.1111/1346-8138.13276.

11. Sheth VM, Weitzul S. Postoperative topical antimicrobial use. *Dermatitis*. 2008;19(4):181-189.

12. Heal CF, Banks JL, Lepper PD, Kontopantelis E, van Driel ML. Topical antibiotics for preventing surgical site infection in wounds healing by primary intention. *Cochrane Database Syst Rev*. 2016;11(11):CD011426. doi:10.1002/14651858.CD011426.pub2.

13. Dumville JC, Owens GL, Crosbie EJ, Peinemann F, Liu Z. Negative pressure wound therapy for treating surgical wounds healing by secondary intention. *Cochrane Database of Syst Rev*. 2015;(6):CD011278.

14. Dumville JC, Webster J, Evans D, Land L. Negative pressure wound therapy for treating pressure ulcers. *Cochrane Database Syst Rev*. 2015;5(5):CD011334.

15. Wilkins RG, Unverdorben M. Wound cleaning and wound healing: a concise review. *Adv Skin Wound Care*. 2013;26(4):160-163. doi:10.1097/01.ASW.0000428861.26671.41.

16. Moore ZE, Cowman S. Wound cleansing for pressure ulcers. *Cochrane Database Syst Rev*. 2013;2013(3):CD004983. doi:10.1002/14651858.CD004983.pub3.

17. Jull AB, Cullum N, Dumville JC, Westby MJ, Deshpande S, Walker N. Honey as a topical treatment for wounds. *Cochrane Database Syst Rev*. 2015;(3):CD005083. doi:10.1002/14651858.CD005083.pub4.

18. Keppel Hesselink JM. Phenytoin repositioned in wound healing: clinical experience spanning 60 years. *Drug Discov Today*. 2018;23(2):402-408. doi:10.1016/j.drudis.2017.09.020.

19. Panahi Y, Izadi M, Sayyadi N, et al. Comparative trial of aloe vera/olive oil combination cream versus phenytoin cream in the treatment of chronic wounds. *J Wound Care*. 2015;24(10):459-465. doi:10.12968/jowc.2015.24.10.459.

20. Tenenhaus M. The use of dehydrated human amnion/chorion membranes in the treatment of burns and complex wounds: current and future applications. *Ann Plast Surg*. 2017;78(2 suppl 1):S11-S13. doi:10.1097/SAP.0000000000000983.

21. Wei M, Wu L, Chen Y, Fu Q, Chen W, Yang D. Predictive validity of the Braden Scale for Pressure Ulcer Risk in critical care: a meta-analysis. *Nurs Crit Care*. 2020;25(3):165-170. doi:10.1111/nicc.12500.

22. Jull A, Slark J, Parsons J. Prescribed exercise with compression vs compression alone in treating patients with venous leg ulcers: a systematic review and meta-analysis. *JAMA Dermatol*. 2018;154(11):1304-1311. doi:10.1001/jamadermatol.2018.3281.

23. Gohel MS, Heatley F, Liu X, et al. A randomized trial of early endovenous ablation in venous ulceration. *N Engl J Med*. 2018;378(22):2105-2114. doi:10.1056/NEJMoa1801214.

24. Senet P, Combemale P, Debure C, et al. Malignancy and chronic leg ulcers: the value of systemic wound biopsies: a prospective, multicenter, cross-sectional study. *Arch Dermatol*. 2012;148(6):704-708. doi:10.1001/archdermatol.2011.3362.

25. Hsieh PY, Chen KY, Chen HY, et al. Postoperative showering for clean and clean-contaminated wounds: a prospective, randomized controlled trial. *Ann Surg*. 2016;263(5):931-936. doi:10.1097/SLA.0000000000001359.

26. Saulis AS, Mogford JH, Mustoe TA. Effect of Mederma on hypertrophic scarring in the rabbit ear model. *Plast Reconstr Surg*. 2002;110(1):177-183; discussion 184-186. doi:10.1097/00006534-200207000-00029.

27. Khansa I, Harrison B, Janis JE. Evidence-based scar management: how to improve results with technique and technology. *Plast Reconstr Surg*. 2016;138(3 suppl):165S-178S. doi:10.1097/PRS.0000000000002647.

28. O'Reilly S, Crofton E, Brown J, Strong J, Ziviani J. Use of tape for the management of hypertrophic scar development: a comprehensive review. *Scars Burn Heal*. 2021;7:20595131211029206. doi:10.1177/20595131211029206.

26 Complications

RICHARD P. USATINE, MD, and DANIEL STULBERG, MD

POSTPROCEDURAL ADVERSE EFFECTS AND THEIR PREVENTION

SUMMARY

- Preparation, planning, and care can help mitigate complications and manage them when they occur.
- Communication before procedures and open lines of communication can help prepare patients' expectations and ability to report early signs of difficulties afterward.
- Prophylactic antibiotics are rarely indicated in routine skin surgery.
- The most common complication is bleeding, and infection rates are real but only 2%.
- The risk of infection is higher in complicated procedures, including large ellipses, flaps, and grafts.
- Immunocompromised patients and high-risk locations – lower leg, lip, or those involving cartilage – have higher rates of infection.
- Due to its benefits, appropriate anticoagulation should not be stopped for routine skin procedures, as bleeding can be managed by using lidocaine with epinephrine and intraoperative hemostasis.
- Postoperative infections are usually managed by removing sutures, expressing purulence, and usually empirically chosen systemic antibiotics if there is cellulitis or spreading infection.

Many adverse effects can occur during and after dermatologic procedures and skin surgeries. Some are predictable and inevitable, such as some pain and erythema, and others may fall into the category of complications such as nerve damage and infections. Whatever method we use to classify these adverse effects, one must be aware of the potential complications for each procedure in order to maximize prevention and early detection. Discussing possible complications with the patient is part of informed consent but is also part of the patient education that goes along with postoperative care. Patients need to know what they can do if a complication arises, and when they need to seek medical care. If postoperative patients have a concern about a possible complication, it is usually worthwhile to offer them an appointment that day. Whereas some complications can be handled over the phone, the offer of a face-to-face visit is useful and should be documented in the medical record.

Calling Patients to Check on Them After a Large Procedure

Calling a patient at home the evening after or day after a large skin surgery or procedure goes a long way toward preventing complications, building good relationships, and preventing malpractice claims. It is worthwhile to make sure you have a working phone number for patients before they leave your office, put the call on your "to do" list, and take that number home with you for the evening call. If the call is not made that evening, a call the following morning is equally appreciated. This also allows you to find out if the patient was able to sleep and whether he or she is having problems with pain or bleeding. Patients are delighted that you care enough to call. In addition, this is one way to diminish your anxiety about potential complications of the procedure.

Responding Quickly to Patients' Concerns After a Procedure

Being available to take your patients' calls is another positive way to build good relationships and deal with complications early before they become severe. If you do not have an answering service, consider giving out your cell phone number to select patients for whom your concerns are greatest. Remember, your call between 6 p.m. and 9 p.m. may eliminate their call between 9 p.m. and 6 a.m.!

The incidence of complications can be decreased with good procedural techniques and early recognition of problems before they become severe. Potential adverse effects and complications of skin procedures can be categorized by the time when they occur, as listed in Box 26.1.

An informed consent form covering the potential complications should be discussed with and signed by the patient. The informed consent form should cover the items in the list above that pertain to the surgical procedure for the specific site and patient. No absolute guarantees of cosmetic results should be made. See Chapter 1, *Preoperative Preparation*, and the sample consent form titled *Disclosure and Consent: Medical and Surgical Procedures* in Appendix A.

Box 26.1   Potential Adverse Effects and Complications of Skin Procedures

May Occur Within the First Few Weeks

- Pain
- Bleeding
- Hematoma
- Bruising and swelling
- Infection
- Dehiscence
- Suture spitting
- Flap necrosis

May Start Early and Become Permanent

- Distortion of normal anatomy around any facial feature
- Ectropion and entropion of eyelids
- Alopecia
- Nerve damage

Prolonged or Permanent

- Scarring
- Skin indentation
- Hypertrophic scars
- Keloid
- Hyperpigmentation
- Hypopigmentation
- Recurrence of the excised condition

Review of the Literature

In a prospective study of 3788 dermatologic surgery procedures, there were 236 complications (6%).[1] Most complications were minor, and bleeding was the most common (3%). Vasovagal syncope was the main anesthetic complication (51 of 54). Infectious complications occurred in 79 patients (2%). Complications requiring additional antibiotic treatment or repeat surgery accounted for only 22 cases (1%). No statistically significant correlation was found with the characteristics of the dermatologists, especially with respect to their training or amount of surgical experience. Multivariate analysis showed that anesthetic or hemorrhagic complications were independent factors that predicted infectious complications. Patients on anticoagulants or immunosuppressant medications, type of procedure performed, and duration exceeding 24 minutes were independent factors that predicted hemorrhagic complications.[1,2]

INFECTIONS

A study of 3491 dermatologic surgical procedures described postoperative infections in 67 patients (1.9%), with superficial suppuration accounting for 92.5% of surgical site infections.[3] The incidence was higher in the excision group with a reconstructive procedure (4.3%) than in excisions alone (1.6%). Infection control precautions varied according to the site of the procedure; multivariate analysis showed that hemorrhagic complications were an independent factor for infection in both types of surgical procedures. Male gender, immunosuppressive therapy, and not wearing sterile gloves were independent factors for infections occurring following excisions with reconstruction.[3]

Dixon et al. performed a prospective study of 5091 lesions (predominantly nonmelanoma skin cancer) treated on 2424 patients.[4] None of the patients was given prophylactic antibiotics, and warfarin or aspirin was not stopped. The overall infection rate was 1.47%. Individual procedures had the following infection incidence:

- Simple excision and closure: 0.5% (16/2974)
- Curettage: 0.7% (3/412)
- Skin flap repairs: 2.9% (47/1601)
- Wedge excision of lip and ear: 8.6% (3/35)
- Skin grafts: 8.7% (6/69).

Surgery below the knee had an infection incidence of 6.9% (31/448), and groin excisional surgery had an infection incidence of 10% (1/10). Patients with diabetes, those on warfarin and/or aspirin, and smokers showed no difference in infection incidence. In conclusion, all procedures below the knee, wedge excisions of the lip and ear, all skin grafts, and lesions in the groin had the highest rates of infection, and the authors suggest considering wound infection prophylaxis in these patients.[4]

In a prospective study of hospitalized patients undergoing diagnostic skin biopsies, infection, dehiscence, and/or hematoma occurred in 29% of the patients.[5] Complications occurred significantly more frequently when biopsies were performed below the waist, in the ward compared with the outpatient operating room, in smokers, and in those taking corticosteroids.[5] In addition, elliptical incisional biopsies developed complications more frequently when subcutaneous sutures were not used.[5] Current data does not support the belief that patients who smoke are at higher risk of infection.[3]

In one study of 1400 Mohs procedures, 25 infections were identified.[6] Statistically significant higher infection rates were found in patients with cartilage fenestration with second intent healing and patients with melanoma. There was no statistical difference in infection rates with all other measured variables including the use of clean, nonsterile gloves rather than sterile gloves during the tumor removal phase of surgery.[5] Sterile gloves were used by all surgeons during the repair phase.

Schlager et al. reviewed the literature regarding rates of postoperative wound infections based on body location. They found that the lower extremities and lips are at higher risk of wound infection and hands and ears may have a higher risk.[7] Additionally, a separate metanalysis also by Schlager found that immunosuppression and male gender were statistically significantly associated with an increase in postoperative infections for skin surgery, and diabetes had a tendency to increase this risk but did not reach statistical significance. They concluded that large controlled trials are needed to determine if the use of prophylactic antibiotics can reduce the rate of postoperative infections.[8] Although certain areas may be at higher risk for infection, a 2021 review by Strickler found no role for prophylactic antibiotics in routine dermatologic surgery or procedures.[2] As of March 2021, the American Heart Association, via their website (https://www.heart.org/en/health-topics/infective-endocarditis), recommends that antibiotic prophylaxis is indicated only for the highest-risk cardiac patients undergoing dental procedures. Patients undergoing other procedures including esophagogastroduodenoscopy, transesophageal echocardiography, cystoscopy, and colonoscopy only need antibiotic prophylaxis if there is active infection. In light of this, only patients with high-risk cardiac conditions, and a defined group of patients with prosthetic joints at high risk for hematogenous total joint infection, should be given prophylactic antibiotics and only when the surgical site is infected or when the procedure involves breach of the oral mucosa.[9]

Clinical Management and Evaluation of Possible Infection

Everyone is disappointed when the site of a skin procedure becomes infected. The highest risk for infection of skin procedures is for the larger elliptical excisions and flap procedures. The more cutting, undermining, and sewing that is done, the higher the risk of infection. Shave biopsies and intralesional injections are very low risk for infections, and these procedures can be performed as clean procedures without sterile gloves. All elliptical excisions and flaps should be performed with sterile technique. Unfortunately, there is little evidence-based information to guide how sterile these procedures should be. The spectrum ranges from sterile gloves and sterile equipment only, to the use of hair caps, face masks, sterile gowns, and full surgical scrubs before putting on the gloves. We all need to monitor infection rates in our practice and decide how much prevention and cost we want to assume.

Wound infections are most likely to manifest on postoperative days 2 to 4. If a patient has any complaints, it is best to examine the wound for evidence of infection. Wound infections may initially be subtle and appear like the erythema seen around a healing incision or biopsy (Figure 26.1). If you are uncertain about a possible infection, pressure applied with the gloved hand can be used to express pus hidden below the skin (Figure 26.2). If no pus is expressed but the suspicion for infection is great, consider removing a few stitches early and applying some pressure with a cotton-tipped applicator to detect pus. Unless the patient is immunosuppressed, no culture is usually performed as methicillin-resistant *Staphylococcus aureus* (MRSA) is so prevalent (Figure 26.2). The choice of antibiotics in purulent wound infections should cover for MRSA. If there is spreading

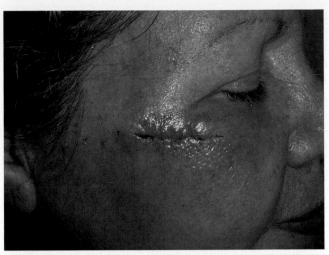

Figure 26.2 Erythema and swelling at the site of a wound infection caused by MRSA. (Copyright Richard P. Usatine, MD.)

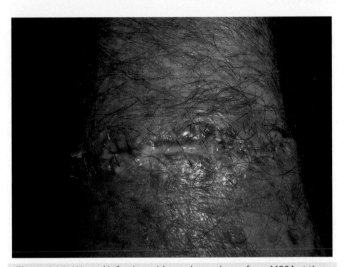

Figure 26.3 Wound infection with much purulence from MSSA at time of suture removal after SCC excision near wrist. (Copyright of Richard P. Usatine, MD.)

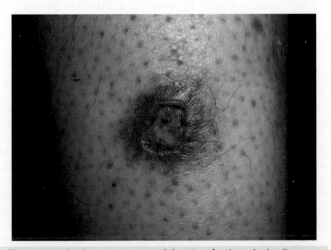

Figure 26.1 Erythema seen around the site of a shave bx healing normally on the leg. This is a variation of normal and not a wound infection. (Copyright of Richard P. Usatine, MD.)

erythema well beyond the expected mild erythema at the wound margins, then antibiotics covering *Streptococcus* should be used.

Sometimes symptoms become obvious around 5 to 7 days postoperatively or at the time of suture removal (Figure 26.3). If the wound is tender and fluctuant, removal of one or more sutures to allow drainage will speed up resolution of the infection.

Pain

Most skin procedures and surgeries will result in some pain when the anesthesia wears off. Explain to patients that they may safely use acetaminophen for pain relief unless they have severe liver disease, allergy to acetaminophen, or some other unusual contraindication. Ibuprofen or naprosyn should be safe unless the patient is anticoagulated or has another contraindication to the use of these or other nonsteroidal antiinflammatory drugs (NSAIDs). Aspirin should be avoided for pain control because it can increase the risk of bleeding and hematoma.

COMBINATIONS OF ACETAMINOPHEN AND NSAID FOR PAIN

Strickler's review of the literature found that combining NSAIDS and acetaminophen was the most effective regimen for pain control postoperatively and recommended minimizing the use of opioids for pain related to routine office-based skin surgery.[1] Acetaminophen and opioid combination products are generally not needed unless the procedure was large and particularly painful. When this is the case, it is helpful to write out that prescription before the patient leaves the office. A quick discussion about pain control can prevent unnecessary distress to the patient later and unnecessary phone calls to you at night. If a patient complains of increasing pain over time, a hematoma or infection should be considered, and it is best to see the patient in the office.

Bleeding

The most likely complication of dermatologic surgery is bleeding (accounting for half of a 6% complication rate).[1] Larger surgeries with more undermining are at highest risk of bleeding complications. Good intraoperative hemostasis, appropriate suturing techniques, and pressure dressings can help minimize bleeding complications. Aspirin can cause increased bleeding during surgery. Awtry reviewed the literature regarding the effects of aspirin on platelets. They found that aspirin has permanent effects on platelet cyclooxygenase reducing coagulation. The usual lifetime of platelets is 10 days; however, 10% of platelets are replaced every day, and after 2 days 20% of platelets present are unaffected, and the anticoagulation effects are mitigated.[10] Clinicians choosing to discontinue aspirin will often stop it 5 days before surgery. NSAIDs can also cause increased bleeding if not stopped 2 days before surgery. Warfarin (Coumadin) also increases the risk of bleeding intraoperatively and postoperatively (Figure 26.4). That said, most clinicians would not postpone skin surgery because the patient has recently taken aspirin or an NSAID. Often the risk of stopping warfarin or aspirin is greater to the patient (such as stroke) than dealing with the bleeding issues. In fact, in a study of 2424 patients undergoing dermatologic surgery, the warfarin or aspirin was not stopped in any of these patients.[4]

Isted's review of the literature regarding antiplatelet agents and anticoagulation found some increased bleeding risk with warfarin (Coumadin) and clopidogrel, but no increased difficulties with cosmetic outcomes, infection, or wound dehiscence. Isted noted that there was not enough information available yet regarding outcomes for patients taking Direct Acting Oral Anticoagulants (DOACs).[11] A metaanalysis by Columbo found that for noncardiac surgery patients there was no increased need for transfusion or additional interventions in people taking aspirin, clopidogrel, or both.[12] For further information on the risks of stopping anticoagulation before surgery see Chapter 1, *Preoperative Preparation*.

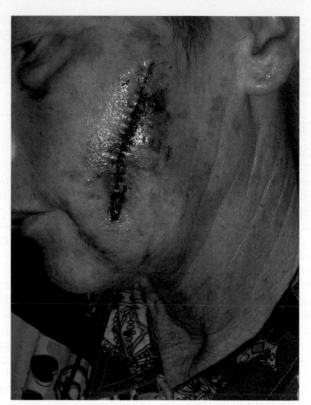

Figure 26.4 Bleeding and ecchymosis after the removal of a large squamous cell carcinoma on the face of a woman on Coumadin. Although this looked bad at this point in time, all healed well over time, and by continuing the Coumadin, she never had a stroke. (Copyright of Richard P. Usatine, MD.)

The risk of intraoperative bleeding can be decreased by waiting 10 minutes after injecting lidocaine and epinephrine to allow the epinephrine to have maximal vasoconstrictive effect before beginning the procedure. The risk of hematoma can be lessened with careful attention to hemostasis during surgery. However, excessive electrocoagulation can cause unnecessary tissue damage, leading to impaired wound healing. Although sutures that are placed tightly can cause suture marks, they can also stop bleeding. Tighter sutures might be used in a situation where the patient seems to be oozing or bleeding excessively. If the patient has intraoperative bleeding issues, undermining should be kept to the absolute minimum necessary.

Pressure dressings are helpful following most skin surgeries except most shave biopsies, which have little risk of bleeding. A good, firm pressure dressing will prevent many after-hour bleeding episodes. The pressure dressing may be constructed with gauze that is doubled up (or dental roll) and tape applied on top using firm pressure during the first 24 hours. Blood on the dressing is better than blood in the wound. Sending the patient home with gauze in hand along with instructions about what to do if bleeding occurs is also helpful. Although blood-soaked bandages can be one manifestation of excessive bleeding, internal bleeding can result in hematoma formation and/or ecchymosis (Figure 26.5A and B).

Postoperative bleeding usually occurs within the first 24 hours after surgery. It will occur more often in a patient who was taking aspirin but may also occur more often in a patient who has high blood pressure or who is physically

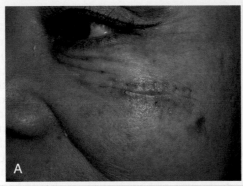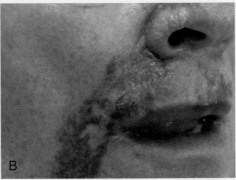

Figure 26.5 **(A)** Ecchymosis around the site of a BCC removal on the face. *(Copyright Richard P. Usatine, MD.)* **(B)** Ecchymosis around the site of an island pedicle flap. (Copyright of Ryan O'Quinn, MD.)

active. The usual scenario for postoperative bleeding is that the patient will contact the clinician with concerns of blood soaking through the bandage. The patient should be instructed to apply firm pressure for 20 minutes by the clock. This will usually stop the bleeding in a majority of situations. If not, the patient may need to come into the office or go to the emergency department.

HEMATOMA

Strickler's review of the literature found that the risk of hematoma formation is rare at less than 2.5%, but that there are multiple factors that increase the risk of hematomas.[2] These include:

- Hypertension
- Males
- Preoperative bleeding, or anemia
- Low body mass index
- Flap and graft reconstruction
- More than four current comorbidities

Hematomas can be prevented with good electrocoagulation of bleeding sites, the tying of large bleeders and large blood vessels, and the use of buried absorbable sutures to close dead space and a pressure bandage.

If the patient complains of increased pain and bulging around the surgical incision wound, the patient needs to be evaluated for a potential hematoma. If the hematoma is detected during the first 24 hours, the incision usually needs to be opened (Figure 26.6). All the sutures should be removed, and the bleeding should be stopped with electrocoagulation. The wound can then be sutured again, and the patient started on systemic antibiotics to prevent wound infection.

If the hematoma is detected more than 24 hours postoperatively and there does not seem to be active bleeding or an expanding hematoma, the wound may not need to be opened. Instead, a syringe with an 18-gauge needle may be used to extract the blood through the incision line. A pressure dressing is then applied, and the patient is started on antibiotics. Oral antibiotics are used because a hematoma is good bacterial growth media, and the risk of infection is higher. The use of a needle to decrease the size of the hematoma may not work after 1 week, when the blood from the hematoma has organized and formed a clot. If the hematoma has clotted, this must resolve with time.

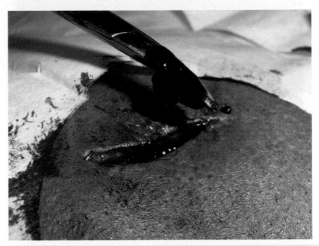

Figure 26.6 Evacuating a hematoma 1 day after lipoma resection. (Copyright of Richard P. Usatine, MD.)

Swelling and Bruising

Patients should be warned that surgery or procedures performed around the lids, nose, upper cheek, or forehead can cause swelling and bruising around the eyes (Figure 26.5A). It is even possible that the eyes may swell shut. The use of ice may help prevent some of this edema if it is used during the first few hours after surgery. The lips can also stay swollen for many weeks or months after surgery.

The best prevention for excessive bruising and swelling after facial surgery, especially around the eyes, is to have the patient sleep with the head elevated for the first 2 to 3 days. A reclining chair can be helpful, and propping the head and shoulders up with pillows on the bed is an alternative.

SUTURE REACTIONS

Suture reactions are frequently mistaken for infections and must be differentiated from them. These may arise in areas where buried sutures have been placed and can present as a small pustule or erosion in the suture line. The patient may complain of a "pimple" on the suture line or a piece of suture extruding from the incision line. This can occur when a buried suture is placed too close to the skin surface. Purulent material from these sites is sterile.

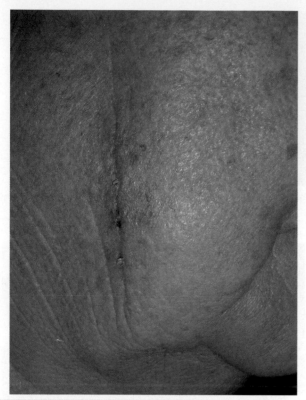

Figure 26.7 Spitting sutures along a facial repair. (Copyright of Richard P. Usatine, MD.)

Suture reactions can range from mild, with only a spicule of suture "spitting" (Figure 26.7), to more severe reactions in which the entire wound gets warm and boggy. These reactions are self-limited and can be calmed with intralesional injections of triamcinolone 2.5 mg/mL and warm compresses. Removal of reacting and spitting sutures can speed up resolution. Antibiotics are frequently given with severe reactions to cover the chance that there is also an element of infection. Suture reactions rarely affect the ultimate cosmetic outcome.

Scarring

Scarring can occur in any patient operated on by any clinician. In some situations, scarring is predictable and cannot be prevented. The deltoid area, the chest, and the back are prone to scarring because of either the skin tension in these areas, the thicker skin in these areas, or some unknown factor. Surgery on sebaceous skin, such as the type that appears on the nose, often leads to obvious incisional scars. The most important point is to warn the patient that in these areas excisional surgery will often result in scarring no matter who does the surgery. Therefore on the back, chest, and deltoid areas, a shave technique should be used when it is an acceptable alternative because it can offer a better cosmetic result than an excision with sutures. If a patient is overly concerned about a scar or expresses the unrealistic desire to have absolutely no scar, it is better to recommend a plastic surgeon before the procedure than after.

Excessive or increased skin tension leads to a widened scar. This is the reason why buried sutures that decrease tension can improve cosmetic results. The increased skin tension in younger patients probably contributes to the widened scars seen in young patients compared with the narrow fine scars seen in older patients. In Figure 26.8A, a widened scar is seen on a young woman's arm years after the wide excision of a melanoma.

Allowing sutures to remain in place for too long can also increase scarring. Complications such as infection, necrosis, or dehiscence can increase scarring (Figure 26.8B). Excessive skin tension often leads to dehiscence and scarring, and infection or necrosis can contribute to dehiscence. Dehiscence may be prevented by using good excision planning, undermining when necessary, and using deep absorbable sutures to decrease skin tension across a wound. Tying sutures too tightly can also cause scarring.

Depressed scars may result from a deep shave biopsy or scarring within the dermal layer of the skin. Depressed scars can be excised, or dermal fillers may be used.

The most important point when discussing potential scarring after surgery is to warn the patient about the risk of scarring or highly visible incision lines. The patient

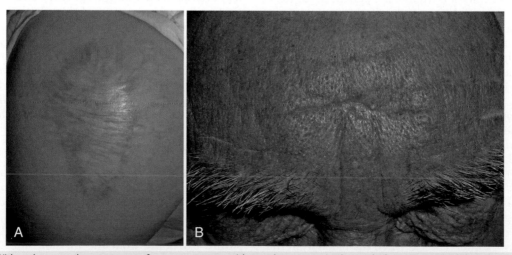

Figure 26.8 (A) Widened scar on the upper arm of a young woman with a melanoma excised years before. **(B)** Scarring that occurred after a wound infection. Note the milia seen at the wound edge, which can occur at sites of wound healing. (Copyright of Richard P. Usatine, MD.)

should understand that if scarring does occur, it can be treated with dermabrasion, intralesional steroids, laser resurfacing, or the yellow light laser used to treat persistent redness.

Wound Dehiscence

The rate of wound dehiscence for skin surgery cases is estimated at 8%. There is increased risk with advanced age, wounds in areas of increased tensions, smoking, infection, and after hematomas.[1] If a wound dehiscence occurs without evidence of infection, it might be advisable to resuture the wound with interrupted sutures and start the patient on antibiotics. The sutures may only have to be left in place for half the normal time because the fibroblasts have already initiated the wound site and the wound is partially healed. If the cause of the dehiscence was significant wound tension, a buried absorbable suture may decrease the wound tension and facilitate successful reclosure.

If infection or a hematoma is the cause of dehiscence, the wound should be opened and irrigated, and the patient should be started on antibiotics. The wound should be cleansed daily and left to heal by secondary intent. It will usually take at least 3 to 4 weeks before the wound healing is complete. The patient should be informed that a scar revision may be performed at a later time if desired.

Pigmentation Changes

Hypopigmentation is most likely to occur with the following procedures: cryosurgery, ED&C, and shave biopsies. Although it may be cosmetically more apparent in darker-skinned persons, it can occur in anyone. Patients must be warned of this complication, which can be permanent. Cryotherapy to treat nonmelanoma skin cancers is likely to cause hypopigmentation because of the long freeze times that are used (Figure 26.9A). Even a simple shave excision can lead to hypopigmentation (Figure 26.9B). Some patients, especially with darker skin types, will heal with hyperpigmentation. Postinflammatory hyperpigmentation often reduces over time. If it persists for a year or more, topical bleaching agents may help reduce the hyperpigmentation.

Flap Necrosis

A long, thin advancement flap in violation of the 3:1 ratio runs a high risk of distal flap tip necrosis (Figure 26.10). Patients who smoke excessively experience a much higher risk of flap tip necrosis and flap failure, and encouraging smoking cessation in the perioperative and postoperative course is helpful to achieve the best healing. The use of flaps must also be carefully weighed in those patients who may have underlying skin conditions that can lead to increased complications. Decreased flexibility and therefore impaired movement of skin can be seen in patients with extensive scarring from burns or other injuries, previous radiotherapy, or an underlying skin disease such as scleroderma. Decreased perfusion of skin leading to flap failure or infection can be seen in conditions such as diabetes mellitus, lung disease, or poor circulation secondary to atherosclerosis, especially in peripheral areas. Finally, the use of a flap may not be possible in patients with extremely thin skin that will not bear the stresses of flap movement such as elderly patients with extreme photodamage or long-term users of corticosteroids.

Nerve Damage

Numbness is a common complaint from patients after cutaneous surgery. It usually resolves in about 6 to 12 months after the nerves have regrown and arborized. The concern from cutaneous surgery is damaging a superficial motor nerve. The three motor nerves that are most vulnerable to damage are the temporal branch of the facial nerve, the spinal accessory nerve, and the marginal branch of the mandibular nerve.

The temporal branch of the facial nerve can be damaged by surgery to the temple area. The nerve lies just below the superficial musculoaponeurotic system (SMAS). It can be difficult to see, and there is enough anatomic variation that it can be unpredictable in its location. One way to locate the nerve is to draw an imaginary line from the tragus to the eyebrow and another imaginary line from the tragus to the upper forehead wrinkle area (Figure 26.11A–C). The area between these two lines within the temple area is where the temporal branch of the facial nerve is most superficial. If this nerve is cut, the patient will not be able to

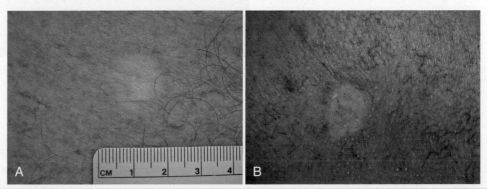

Figure 26.9 (A) Hypopigmentation that occurred after cryosurgery of a superficial BCC. **(B)** Hypopigmentation after the shave excision of a basal cell carcinoma on sun-damaged skin. (Copyright of Richard P. Usatine, MD.)

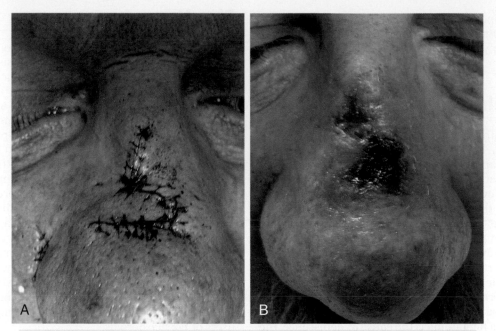

Figure 26.10 (A, B) Flap necrosis in a patient unable to quit smoking. (Copyright of Ryan O'Quinn, MD.)

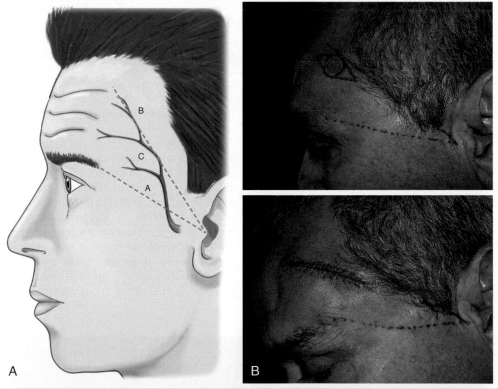

Figure 26.11 (A) Drawing of the temporal branch of the facial nerve. (From Usatine RP. *Skin Surgery: A Practical Guide.* Mosby; 1998.) **(B)** Planned BCC excision near the temporal branch of the facial nerve. **(C)** Repair following excision of BCC near the temporal branch of the facial nerve. (Copyright of Richard P. Usatine, MD.)

wrinkle the forehead because the innervation to the frontalis muscle is lost. The patient will also have a permanent inability to raise the upper eyelid (Figure 26.12A and B). If any surgery is performed in this area, it is important to discuss this risk with the patient in the informed consent process. Also explain that the anesthesia after surgery alone

can cause a temporary paralysis of this nerve (see Figure 11.2B in Chapter 11, *The Elliptical Excision*). When electrodesiccation and curettage is an option for a superficial skin cancer in this area, it may be a good choice. Mohs surgery is also an appropriate technique in this area because the tissue is removed layer by layer by an experienced surgeon.

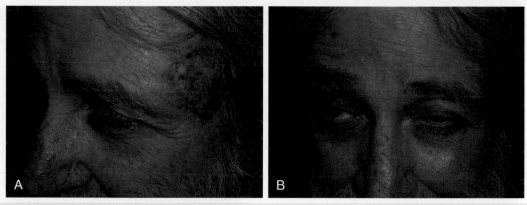

Figure 26.12 (A) Large BCC in the region of the temporal branch of the facial nerve. **(B)** Permanent inability to raise the eyebrow after the temporal branch of the facial nerve was cut during surgical excision of the BCC. (From Usatine RP. *Skin Surgery: A Practical Guide.* Mosby; 1998.)

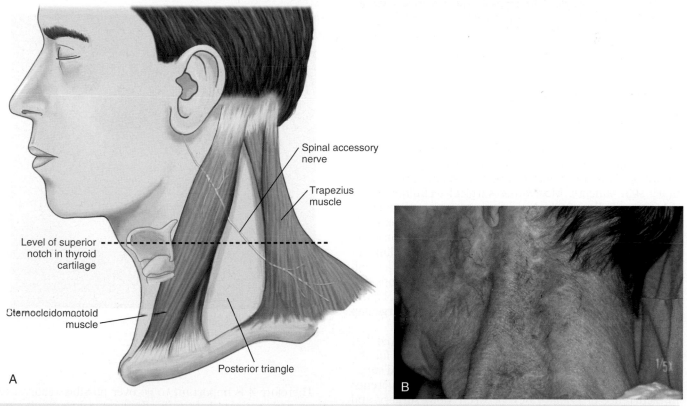

Figure 26.13 (A) Drawing of the spinal accessory nerve in the posterior triangle of the neck. **(B)** Recurrent BCC over the site of the spinal accessory nerve in the posterior triangle of the neck. Care must be taken to avoid cutting that nerve if possible. ([A] From Usatine RP. *Skin Surgery: A Practical Guide.* Mosby; 1998.)

The spinal accessory nerve lies within the posterior triangle posterior to the sternocleidomastoid muscle (Figure 26.13). The nerve can lie very superficially posterior to the sternocleidomastoid muscle at the level of the thyroid cartilage notch. If this nerve is cut, the patient will lose major innervation to the trapezius muscle, resulting in impaired mobility of the scapula and shoulder.

The marginal branch of the mandibular nerve (Figure 26.14) is the third nerve in the head and neck area that is vulnerable to injury during surgery. If it is cut, then motor innervation to the depressor anguli oris and depressor labii inferioris can be lost. This results in a cosmetic deformity and imbalance in the appearance of the mouth, especially when the mouth is opened or when the patient wants to frown. Fortunately, the nerve is not that superficial, but each clinician operating in the area of the lower mandible should be aware of this branch of the facial nerve.

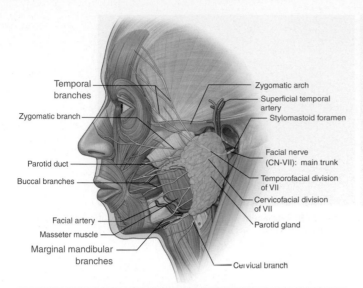

Figure 26.14 The branches of the facial nerve most prone to be cut during facial surgery include the temporal branches and the marginal mandibular branches. (From Vidimos A, Ammirati C, Poblete-Lopez C. *Dermatologic Surgery.* Saunders; 2008.)

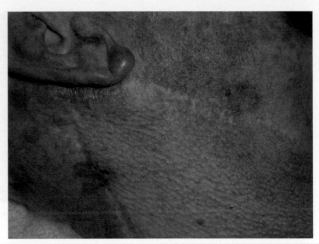

Figure 26.15 Recurrent BCC at two sites along the area of a large flap repair to an extensive BCC on the neck. (Copyright of Richard P. Usatine, MD.)

Recurrence of a Lesion or Skin Cancer

There is almost nothing in the practice of medicine that is a 100% guarantee. Mohs micrographic surgery for the removal of skin cancer has a cure rate of only 99% in primary skin cancers. Most other surgical techniques have cure rates of about 90%, depending on a number of factors. Lipomas, cysts, and nevi (especially if they are removed with a shave) can all recur. Although recurrent lesions may be considered a complication, the patient and clinician should both realize that recurrences will happen in a small percentage of cases. When a recurrent lesion develops, the lesion will usually need to be excised again. In Figure 26.15, a BCC recurred in the incision line after a large flap was placed on the neck.

With regard to recurrence of BCC, one study showed that Mohs surgery had significantly fewer recurrences for the treatment of facial *recurrent* BCC than after standard surgical excision.[13] However, there was no significant difference in recurrence of *primary* BCC between Mohs surgery and surgical excision in this study.[13]

In a systematic review of treatment modalities for primary BCC, the following recurrence rates were noted:

- Mohs micrographic surgery (three studies, $n = 2660$): recurrence rate 0.8 to 1.1.
- Surgical excision (three studies, $n = 1303$): recurrence rate was 2 to 8.1. The mean cumulative 5-year rate (all three studies) was 5.3.
- Cryosurgery (four studies, $n = 796$): recurrence rate 3.0 to 4.3. The cumulative 5-year rate (three studies) ranged from 0 to 16.5.
- Curettage and desiccation (six studies, $n = 4212$): recurrence rate ranged from 4.3 to 18.1. The cumulative 5-year rate ranged from 5.7 to 18.8.[14]

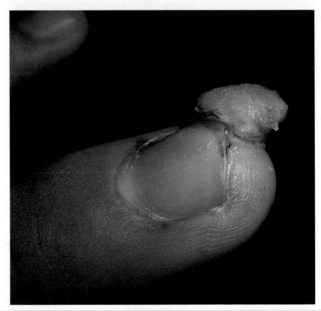

Figure 26.16 Recurrent pyogenic granuloma on the finger after previous excision. (Copyright of Richard P. Usatine, MD.)

Therefore it is important to go over possible recurrence rates with patients before the final procedure is chosen. Even benign lesions like pyogenic granulomas can recur if all of the abnormal tissue is not removed at the time of surgery (Figure 26.16).

Making Mistakes

As a clinician, it feels awful to make a mistake that leads to harming a patient. It may also feel bad when a patient gets a less-than-optimal cosmetic result after a surgical procedure. We all took the oath, "First, do no harm." In performing skin surgery, it is inevitable that you will have wounds that dehisce, scars that are larger than expected, flaps that necrose, and infections and hematomas that will occur in surgical sites. These are known complications of skin surgery and may not be caused by an error on your part. However, it is also possible for all of us to make mistakes. Postoperative infections and hematomas can occur even in the most carefully performed surgery. However, if a clinician is in a rush and uses less careful sterile technique or pays less attention to bleeding vessels, he or she may contribute to these complications. We have presented ways to minimize complications, but poor outcomes can and do happen. In all cases, the goal will be to provide the patient with the best possible outcome.

It is always important to express empathy to the patient and/or patient's family after an adverse surgical event. "I am sorry" is an appropriate expression of empathy that does not express fault. In the book *Sorry Works!* the authors make a strong case for using the phrase "I'm sorry" along with disclosure, apologies, and relationships to prevent medical malpractice claims.[15] They make the distinction that the phrase "I'm sorry" is an expression of empathy and "I apologize" is a communication that expresses responsibility along with empathy. They suggest to only apologize after due diligence has proven that a medical error occurred.

The authors make the case that it is better to disclose an error than to attempt to cover it up.[15] They state that "people can actually live with mistakes, but they do not accept or tolerate cover-ups." They suggest the use of honesty, candor, and a real commitment to fixing problems when something goes wrong. Showing empathy works by making a difficult situation a little better. To learn more about how to prevent lawsuits and improve relationships with patients during and after an adverse event, consult the book *Sorry Works!* and the website www.sorryworks.net.

Conclusion

Careful planning and execution of surgery can prevent most complications. Early recognition of complications and rapid treatment can minimize the potential adverse outcomes that can occur if complications are allowed to progress untreated.

References

1. Amici JM, Rogues AM, Lasheras A, et al. A prospective study of the incidence of complications associated with dermatological surgery. *Br J Dermatol.* 2005;153:967-971.
2. Strickler AG, Shah P, Bajaj S, et al. Preventing and managing complications in dermatologic surgery: procedural and postsurgical concerns. *J Am Acad Dermatol.* 2021;84(4):895-903. doi:10.1016/j.jaad.2021.01.037.
3. Rogues AM, Lasheras A, Amici JM, et al. Infection control practices and infectious complications in dermatological surgery. *J Hosp Infect.* 2007;65:258-263.
4. Dixon AJ, Dixon MP, Askew DA, Wilkinson D. Prospective study of wound infections in dermatologic surgery in the absence of prophylactic antibiotics. *Dermatol Surg.* 2006;32:819-826.
5. Wahie S, Lawrence CM. Wound complications following diagnostic skin biopsies in dermatology inpatients. *Arch Dermatol.* 2007;143:1267-1271.
6. Rhinehart MB, Murphy MM, Farley MF, Albertini JG. Sterile versus nonsterile gloves during Mohs micrographic surgery: infection rate is not affected. *Dermatol Surg.* 2006;32:170-176.
7. Schlager JG, Ruiz San Jose V, Patzer K, French LE, Kendziora B, Hartmann D. Are specific body sites prone for wound infection after skin surgery? A systematic review and meta-analysis. *Dermatol Surg.* 2022;48(4):406-410. doi:10.1097/DSS.0000000000003387.
8. Schlager JG, Hartmann D, Wallmichrath J, et al. Patient-dependent risk factors for wound infection after skin surgery: a systematic review and meta-analysis. *Int Wound J.* 2022;19(7):1748-1757. doi:10.1111/iwj.13780.
9. Wright TI, Baddour LM, Berbari EF, et al. Antibiotic prophylaxis in dermatologic surgery: advisory statement 2008. *J Am Acad Dermatol.* 2008;59:464-473.
10. Awtry EH, Loscalzo J. Aspirin. *Circulation.* 2000;101(10):1206-1218. doi:10.1161/01.cir.101.10.1206.
11. Isted A, Cooper L, Colville RJ. Bleeding on the cutting edge: a systematic review of anticoagulant and antiplatelet continuation in minor cutaneous surgery. *J Plast Reconstr Aesthet Surg.* 2018;71(4):455-467. doi:10.1016/j.bjps.2017.11.024.
12. Columbo JA, Lambour AJ, Sundling RA, et al. A meta-analysis of the impact of aspirin, clopidogrel, and dual antiplatelet therapy on bleeding complications in noncardiac surgery. *Ann Surg.* 2018;267(1):1-10. doi:10.1097/SLA.0000000000002279.
13. Mosterd K, Krekels GA, Nieman FH, et al. Surgical excision versus Mohs' micrographic surgery for primary and recurrent basal-cell carcinoma of the face: a prospective randomised controlled trial with 5-years' follow-up. *Lancet Oncol.* 2008;9:1149-1156.
14. Thissen MR, Neumann MH, Schouten LJ. A systematic review of treatment modalities for primary basal cell carcinomas. *Arch Dermatol.* 1999;135:1177-1183.
15. Wojcieszak D, Saxton W, Finklestein M. Sorry Works! Disclosure, *Apology, and Relationships Prevent Medical Malpractice Claims.* Bloomington: Author House, 2008.

27 When to Refer/Mohs Surgery

RYAN O'QUINN, MD, JOHN L. PFENNINGER, MD, and RICHARD P. USATINE, MD

SUMMARY

- Referrals and consults are primarily determined by the clinicians' level of expertise but are affected by medical-legal considerations and insurance coverages.
- Specific factors may also include the size of the lesion, patient and family requests for referral, and challenging patient relationships.
- Any clinician is more likely to refer a more aggressive cancer, a larger cancer, and a cancer in a high-risk area based on likelihood of recurrence and cosmetic challenges.
- These more difficult cancers are often referred for Mohs surgery or to surgical oncology.
- Mohs surgery is a technique where careful mapping of a malignant lesion (almost always a nonmelanoma skin cancer) is performed using mapping of the tumor with markers on the skin and dyed edges of the excised tissue.
- The advantage is that the entire tumor can be removed in a single setting with cure rates as high as 99%.
- Indications for Mohs surgery are reviewed, and a useful electronic app is highlighted.
- How to perform Mohs surgery is discussed so that the referring clinician can explain to the patient what to expect.

The primary care clinician handles a multitude of problems, and each person has their own level of comfort and expertise. There are no hard-and-fast guidelines to determine when a consultation/referral should be obtained. Some clinicians will feel very comfortable performing extensive flaps, while others are anxious about doing a fairly straightforward skin biopsy. In this chapter, some general guidelines will be provided to help gauge when, and if, the expertise of another clinician is needed.

In general, a *referral* means that the patient is being turned over to another physician for care. A *consult* asks for direction, but the patient remains under the care of the consulting physician. In practice, these two terms are often used interchangeably. The term *verbal consult* is often used to relay the fact that the case was discussed with someone else for input and direction as to proper care but not referred to formally. Although discouraged on a legal basis, it is commonly done, and for simple questions such as, "What should the margins of the excision be?", it functionally works well.

Medical-legal considerations are important. Hospitals may limit privileges and require that a referral be made for performing certain procedures in hospital-owned facilities. In such cases, it may not be a matter of expertise but rather of legal restriction as to what may be done.

HMOs and insurance companies may also limit the ability of a clinician to employ the full use of their skills. Some restrict payment to certain specialties only. It is not a matter of competence (despite the insurers' claims), but rather a matter of rules, regulations, and "protecting turf."

It is important that the clinician always have complete disclosure to the patient about their background and training. The patient must not be misled into thinking that the physician assistant, nurse practitioner, family physician, or internist is a dermatologist or plastic surgeon. The simplest procedure for professionals may appear very complex and a fearful ordeal to the patient. It is always appropriate to mention that a dermatologist, plastic surgeon, or referral to some other center is readily available, should the patient so desire. A statement such as, "This is a common procedure that has few complications. I perform it frequently, and I would be happy to do it for you. However, if you'd like to see someone else, I understand and can easily arrange a referral," goes a long way in putting the patient at ease. *Do not forget the family members* in the equation. Some may be extremely concerned about a scar, even though it involves an elderly parent. These issues need to be discussed and dealt with prior to performing any procedure. If the patient or the family appears to be hesitant, it is prudent to make a referral.

No clinician will ever feel totally comfortable in every situation that they encounter. Sometimes, too, a straightforward diagnosis and planned treatment becomes more complicated than expected. It is important to have *lines of communication open with other specialists* so that when these "complications" do arise, there is going to be support. Whether this consultant is a plastic surgeon, a dermatologist, a general surgeon, or another colleague who performs the same procedure, it is important to have the backup. Immediate complications will most likely involve bleeding or the inability to close a large, gaping wound; wound dehiscence; or nonhealing of a treated site. Rarely, a nerve may be transected, or the repair may leave the surrounding structures distorted. Long-term complications include hypertrophic or keloid scarring, missing a diagnosis, or recurrence.

Clinicians should not be hesitant to perform a skin biopsy. Multiple methods are available (see Chapters 8, 9, 10, and 11). Complications are so rare and the benefits are so great that all clinicians, especially those in primary care, should consider mastering this skill. If one wants to limit procedural acumen solely to skin biopsies, then referral would be necessary for most findings. However, the average primary care clinician should be able to evaluate and treat 95% of all dermatologic conditions that come into the office using the techniques described in this text. Cryotherapy, electrosurgery, injection techniques, laceration repair, and simple incisions/excisions will be adequate to treat the majority of conditions. When the excisions become larger and more complicated, it is then that many patients may need to be referred. Clinicians should learn to be comfortable performing biopsies even in challenging anatomic locations. Anxiety about performing eyelid biopsy, for example, should not delay the diagnosis of a malignant lesion. The biopsy should be performed, or the patient should be referred to a specialist who is comfortable doing an eyelid biopsy.

When diagnosing skin cancers, it is advisable to make use of digital photography to document the location of the biopsy. Patients very often forget where their biopsy was performed and can be unreliable historians in this regard. Especially with small lesions a biopsy site may completely heal over with minimal evidence for the referral surgeon to locate the lesion that needs to be treated. A simple digital photo can be taken and put in the patient's chart, which is an invaluable resource that can prevent wrong-site surgery. Since many healthcare systems do not share their EHRs with other systems, it is crucial to take photos of the biopsy site apart from what goes into the EHR. These photos can be taken with a smartphone or dedicated camera. The patients' smartphones can also be used to capture a photo that can be shared with the clinician that receives the referral. When referring to a Mohs surgeon, send these photos to them or their office staff.

With all the considerations noted above, *the clinician will individually define when a referral is indicated.* As expertise increases with training and experience, fewer consultations and referrals will be needed. General guidelines for when to consult and when to refer include the following:

1. *Lack of experience* with the method needed for diagnosis and/or treatment
2. Significant cosmetic concerns with the skills for removal beyond the practitioner's comfort level
3. *Large lesions,* whether benign or malignant, often need to be referred to a specialist. "Large" is relative and depends on the practitioner's expertise and the nature of the lesion (benign or malignant, location, new, or recurrent, etc.).
4. *Request by the patient or the family for a referral*
5. *A poor or questionable patient-doctor relationship*
6. *An uncooperative patient*
7. *Medical-legal or insurance requirements/regulations*
8. *Advanced and/or complicated disease.* In general, the major considerations for aggressiveness of a tumor are histological type, size, and location of the lesion. All factors should be considered in the decision for a referral. Skin cancers which cause the most concern for all of us can be categorized as follows:

Histologic type (from least to most aggressive):

Basal cell carcinoma (BCC)
- Superficial
- Nodular/ulcerative
- Micronodular
- Infiltrative
- Morpheaform (aggressive, sclerotic)

Squamous cell carcinoma (SCC)
- *In situ* (depending on size and location, generally does not need aggressive treatment)
- Invasive
- Perineural involvement
- Poorly differentiated

Melanoma
- *In situ*
- Superficial
- <1 mm invasion with no ulceration or neural involvement
- >1 mm invasion or with ulceration or neural involvement

More rare and potentially aggressive cancers include dermatofibrosarcoma protuberans, cutaneous T-cell lymphomas and Merkel cell carcinomas.) (see end of Chapter 24 for photographs and further information on these skin cancers).

The following are examples of when most primary care clinicians might consider referral: [1,2,3,6]

(a) *A melanoma with invasion 1 mm or deeper, or if there is neural involvement or ulceration.* Some would want to refer all melanomas. However, those less than 1 mm are generally treated with simple excision using 1-cm free margins. Once the melanoma has invaded 1 mm or more, then the work-up becomes much more extensive, often including a sentinel node biopsy. Surgical oncologists and melanoma clinics that deal with melanomas on a routine basis are more likely to provide the patient with more options for an improved outcome. Most dermatologists refer melanomas with Breslow depth over 1.0 mm as they do not do sentinel node biopsies.

(b) *Rare, unusual tumors, or metastatic disease* (e.g., dermatofibrosarcoma protuberans; Merkel cell carcinoma and any metastatic cancer to or from the skin) (Figure 27.1)

(c) *Recurrent skin cancers,* such as SCC which can metastasize. Even BCCs, which generally don't metastasize, can recur and require large margins for resection (Figure 27.2). Mohs micrographic surgery or radiation may be indicated in such cases.

(d) *Large nonmelanoma skin cancers* >1 cm in length or diameter, unless the clinician is capable of performing large excisions. Many basal cell carcinomas <1 cm in size can be treated with ablation/destruction techniques, such as electrodesiccation and curettage or cryotherapy. Small SCC <1 cm can be excised with 5-mm margins. Although some physicians refer all skin cancers for Mohs surgery, this is not a true cost-effective approach. A higher cure rate is sometimes cited to justify Mohs, but with lesions <1 cm

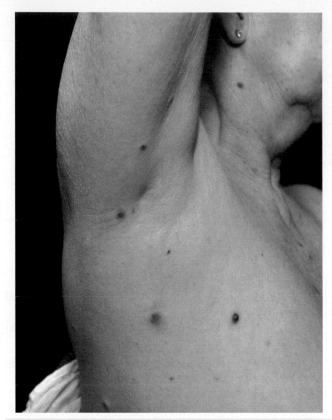

Figure 27.1 These scattered black nodules are caused by metastatic melanoma to the skin. The patient was referred directly to medical oncology. (Copyright Richard P. Usatine, MD.)

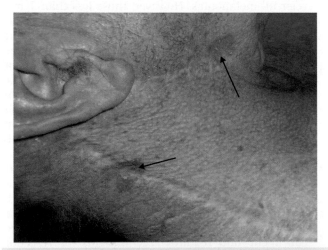

Figure 27.2 Two recurrent BCCs are seen along the scar from a previous large flap that was used after a large BCC was removed from the neck. The patient was referred for Mohs surgery. (Copyright Richard P. Usatine, MD.)

(BCCs and SCCs), the benefit is very small, and the scarring may be less with ablative techniques.

(e) *High-risk anatomic areas*: temporal (temporal branch of facial nerve); lateral neck (spinal accessory nerve); nasolabial groove with ablation (higher recurrence of skin cancers when size is over 0.6 cm); lacrimal duct area (scarring), excisions near eyelids (ectropion or entropion)

(f) *High-risk lesions*, such as SCC on the lips, temple, and ears, since there is a 10% rate of metastasis. SCC also requires more aggressive treatment if it is >2 cm, occurs in a scar, or there is evidence of perineural invasion.

(g) *High-risk patients*, such as those with chronic leukemia especially chronic lymphocytic leukemia (CLL), diabetes, immune suppression, obesity, peripheral vascular disease, stasis dermatitis/pedal edema with lower extremity lesions, alcoholics, HIV/AIDS, malnutrition

(h) *Areas where even normal scarring may be especially critical*, such as the eyelid margins; face, especially in the young/female patient; vermillion border

(i) Patients who are *hypertrophic- or keloid-scar formers*

(j) *Nonadherent patients or those with unrealistic expectations*

Mohs Surgery

Mohs surgery is a technique where careful mapping of a malignant lesion (almost always a nonmelanoma skin cancer) is performed using mapping of the tumor with markers on the skin and dyed edges of the excised tissue.[4,5] The lesion is excised and immediately processed histologically with frozen section pathology for quick results. The tissue is processed so that horizontally oriented frozen sections allow examination of the vast majority of the peripheral margin, unlike standard vertically oriented frozen sections. Once the histopathologic slides are completed, the Mohs surgeon can carefully evaluate the margins under light microscopy. If areas of residual tumor are identified under the microscope by the Mohs surgeon, further excision is completed in the specific areas needed. It is generally performed in an office under local anesthesia. The advantage is that the entire tumor can be removed in a single setting with cure rates as high as 99%. The disadvantages are the time and costs to perform the procedure.

Most reviews have found it to be cost-effective for high-risk cancers. Potential indications for Mohs are:

- High-risk anatomic locations (eyelids, nose, ears, lips, genitalia, fingers)
- Large tumors (2 cm or more in diameter) on the torso and extremities
- Recurrent tumors after previous excision or destruction
- Tumors with aggressive histologic patterns (sclerosing, infiltrative, or morphea-like growth in BCCs; perineural invasion, poorly differentiated histology or deep invasion in SCCs)
- Tumors in immunosuppressed patients
- Tumors occurring in previous sites of radiation therapy
- Tumors with involved borders or vague clinical margins, or incompletely excised tumors (positive histologic margins after resection).

Medicare will cover reimbursement for Mohs micrographic surgery for the diagnoses and indications listed in Box 27-1.

Box 27.1   Medicare Covers Reimbursement for Mohs Surgery for These Diagnoses*

1. Basal cell, squamous cell, or basalosquamous cell carcinomas in anatomic locations where they are prone to recur:
   - Central facial areas, periauricular, nose, and temple areas of the face (the so-called "mask area" of the face)
   - Lips, cutaneous and vermilion
   - Eyelids and periorbital areas
   - Auricular helix and canal
   - Chin and mandible
2. Other skin lesions:
   - Angiosarcoma of the skin
   - Keratoacanthoma, recurrent
   - Dermatofibrosarcoma protuberans
   - Malignant fibrous histiocytoma
   - Sebaceous gland carcinoma
   - Microcystic adnexal carcinoma
   - Extramammary Paget's disease
   - Bowenoid papulosis
   - Merkel cell carcinoma
   - Bowen's disease (squamous cell carcinoma *in situ*)
   - Adenoid type of squamous cell carcinoma
   - Rapid growth in a squamous cell carcinoma
   - Long-standing duration of a squamous cell carcinoma
   - Verrucous carcinoma
   - Atypical fibroxanthoma
   - Leiomyosarcoma or other spindle cell neoplasms of the skin

   - Adenocystic carcinoma of the skin
   - Erythroplasia of Queyrat
   - Oral and central facial, paranasal sinus neoplasm
   - Apocrine carcinoma of the skin
   - Malignant melanoma (facial, auricular, genital, and digital) when anatomic or technical difficulties do not allow conventional excision with appropriate margins
3. Basal cell carcinomas, squamous cell carcinomas, or basalo-squamous carcinomas that have one or more of the following features:
   - Recurrent
   - Aggressive pathology in the following areas: hands and feet, genitalia, and nail unit/periungual
   - Large size (2.0 cm or greater)
   - Positive margins on recent excision
   - Poorly defined borders
   - In the very young (<40 years old)
   - Radiation induced
   - In patients with proven difficulty with skin cancers or who are immunocompromised
   - Basal cell nevus syndrome
   - In an old scar (e.g., a Marjolin's ulcer)
   - Associated with xeroderma pigmentosum
   - Perineural invasion on biopsy
   - Deeply infiltrating lesion or difficulty estimating depth of lesion

*This is a simple guide to a complex coverage issue.

The physician performing Mohs surgery must serve both as surgeon and pathologist. Coverage is so complex that each Mohs surgery office should determine coverage for each case before surgery is begun. The best resource for the referring clinician is not this table but the app discussed in this chapter.

PATIENT SELECTION

Examples of patients that were referred for Mohs surgery including those with the following lesions:

- Pigmented BCC on the nose, newly diagnosed (Figure 27.3)
- BCC on the upper lip close to the vermilion border (Figure 27.4)
- Infiltrating BCC on the cheek (Figure 27.5)
- Recurrent SCC on the cheek (Figure 27.6)
- BCC on the ear, newly diagnosed (Figure 27.7)

PERFORMING MOHS SURGERY

See Videos 27.1 and 27.2.

1. Identification and marking of the malignant lesion or previous biopsy site
2. Local anesthetic with lidocaine and epinephrine is administered.
3. The tumor is debulked with a scalpel or curette and discarded.
4. Excise a saucer-shaped section, with a narrow margin, of the remaining tumor including lateral and deep margins (Figure 27.8). Small nicks on the margin edge retain specimen orientation.
5. Take this piece for processing, including inking of margins and divide into smaller specimens if the pieces are too large for a single slide.
6. Create map of the Mohs specimen indicating orientation, size and shape, and colors and ink location to maintain orientation.
7. The laboratory technician freezes and stains the segments with hematoxylin and eosin (Figure 27.9).
8. The Mohs surgeon reads the histology, looking at all margins.

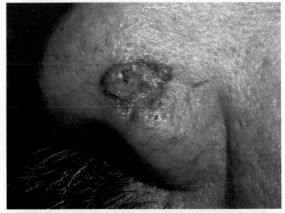

Figure 27.3 Resecting this pigmented BCC on the nose can easily result in a nasal deformity. The patient was referred for Mohs surgery to get the highest cure rates and the best cosmetic result. (Copyright Richard P. Usatine, MD.)

9. If there are any positive margins, a second stage is performed.
10. The process continues until there are completely clear margins.
11. The defect is repaired using Burow's triangles to create a simple ellipse or a more elaborate flap. A more complicated maneuver such as a full-thickness or split-thickness skin graft or a skin flap may be necessary. Some wounds may be allowed to heal by second intention (granulation) depending on location or other patient factors.

Standard pathology for an ellipse involves bread loaf examination of the tissue (Figure 27.10). Mohs surgery is

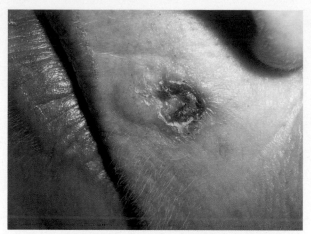

Figure 27.4 The BCC on the upper lip approaches the vermilion border. Unless you are experienced in facial flaps, this is a good patient to refer for Mohs surgery and a flap repair. (Copyright Richard P. Usatine, MD.)

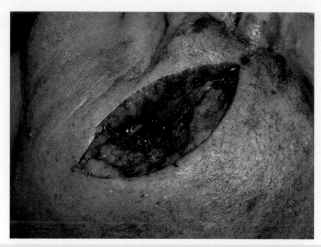

Figure 27.6 Squamous cell carcinoma was found to be recurrent along the excision scar on the face. When Mohs surgery was performed, the SCC was found to have infiltrated deeply and widely, resulting in the defect in this image. (Copyright Richard P. Usatine, MD.)

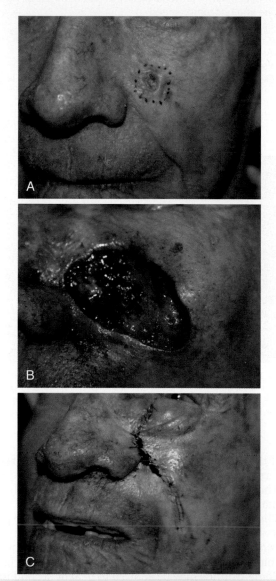

Figure 27.5 (A) This patient was referred for Mohs surgery to treat his sclerosing BCC. **(B)** The BCC had extensively infiltrated his cheek and required three stages to get clear margins. **(C)** A repair was able to close the defect to heal by primary intention. (Courtesy of Ryan O'Quinn, MD.)

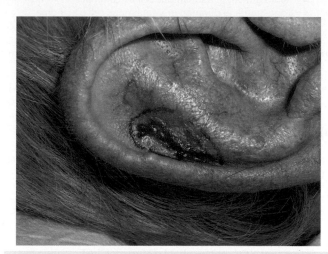

Figure 27.7 A new BCC was diagnosed on the pinna, and the patient was referred for Mohs surgery. See next figures. (Copyright Richard P. Usatine, MD.)

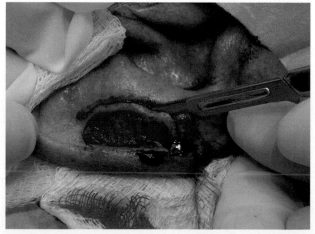

Figure 27.8 After debulking the tumor, the Mohs surgeon carefully removes a segment of the skin with margins laterally and deep. (Copyright Richard P. Usatine, MD.)

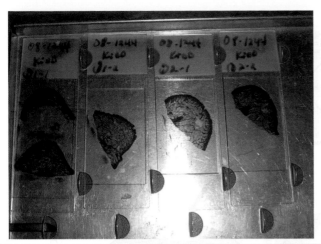

Figure 27.9 Mohs slides in the tray ready to be viewed under the microscope. (Copyright Richard P. Usatine, MD.)

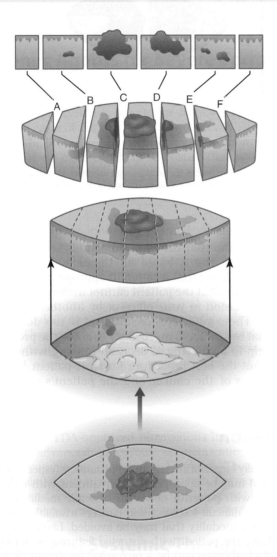

Figure 27.10 A standard elliptical excision of tumor followed by vertical sectioning "bread loafing." Here, all margins appear to be clear based on the sections evaluated at the top of the figure. However, the positive margin between sections B and C was not evaluated, hence the higher risk of recurrence with an ellipse rather than Mohs surgery. (From Vidimos A, Ammirati C, Poblete-Lopez C. *Dermatologic Surgery.* Saunders; 2008.)

done with a more complete examination of the margin (Figure 27.11).

WHO TO REFER FOR MOHS

One way to consider who to refer is to look at Figure 27.12 for the levels of recurrence risk. The H-zone resembles the letter "H" and is the highest-risk area.

In general, Mohs surgery is accepted in all cases of patients who are immunosuppressed due to a medical regimen or those with underlying conditions that cause immunosuppression such as HIV infection or CLL. Other factors include tumors arising in areas of skin that have been previously irradiated or in traumatic/burn scars or areas of osteomyelitis or chronic inflammation. Likewise, Mohs is appropriate in patients with genetic syndromes that predispose patients to BCC and SCC formation such as basal cell nevus (Gorlin) syndrome or xeroderma pigmentosum. However, with the availability of hedgehog pathway inhibitors such as vismodegib and sonidegib, patients with Gorlin syndrome can be treated with these oral agents to avoid numerous surgical procedures.

Appropriate Use Criteria Guideline and a Free App

Beyond these factors, Appropriate Use Criteria (AUC) Guidelines have been developed for determining when to refer nonmelanoma skin cancers for Mohs micrographic surgery. The guidelines take into consideration anatomic location, diagnosis, tumor histology, tumor size, and whether a tumor is recurrent following previous treatment.

The Mohs AUC app is an invaluable free tool for the smartphone or tablet to determine whether a particular patient is appropriate for referral to Mohs surgery (Figure 27.13).

- https://apps.apple.com/us/app/mohs-surgery-appropriate-use-criteria/id692790649
  AUC Guidelines (have three main anatomic subsets:
- Area H – higher risk
- Area M – moderate risk
- Area L – lower risk

Area H is composed of anatomic sites that are deemed to be critical for cosmesis, tissue sparing, or because they are areas associated with higher rates of recurrent carcinomas following treatment. Area H includes the areas of the face that most need tissue sparing such as the eyelids, nose, lips, and ears. It also extends onto the temples and down the central face to the chin. These areas are also highly correlated with increased rates of recurrence following standing excision or destructive modalities such as curettage. Other anatomic locations contained in Area H include the hands, feet, and genital/perineum and perianal skin. Mohs surgery is indicated for nearly all BCCs and SCCs of Area H regardless of size of the tumor or health of the patient.

Area M includes areas that are still cosmetically sensitive and where tissue sparing is a consideration. The scalp, forehead, neck, jawline, cheeks, and pretibial skin (anteriorly, not the posterior calves) are all included in Area M. Mohs is often indicated for treatment of BCCs and SCCs in Area M except for very small primary tumors that can be adequately

28 Coding Common Skin Procedures

JONATHAN B. KARNES, MD

SUMMARY

- Coding procedures precisely will help you avoid risk, receive fair compensation, and provide financial support for performing surgical offerings valuable to your patients.
- Coding for biopsies is divided into these categories: tangential, punch, incisional, and special codes based on special areas.
- The destruction of lesions is coded based upon whether the lesion is benign, premalignant, a skin tag, or malignant. Destruction of benign lesions in special body sites and with special methods are separated out into different codes.
- Excision coding is based upon the benign or malignant nature of the lesion, the size of the lesion measured at the longest diameter, the margins excised to achieve adequate removal, and the location of the excision.
- There is additional coding based on whether a surgical repair is simple, intermediate, or complex.
- Global periods and modifiers are covered.
- Soft tissue tumors and cosmetic removals are reviewed.
- Measure and record what you do, review what gets denied by insurers, and learn to adjust accordingly.

A few unfortunate souls may have entered medicine for money. No one enters medical practice drawn by the nuanced intricacies of coding. Thankfully, coding common outpatient procedures accurately can be straightforward. Additionally, coding procedures precisely will help you avoid risk, receive fair compensation, and provide financial slack to continue performing surgical offerings valuable to your patients. This chapter should help develop the skill and confidence needed to select the correct codes and move on to the next patient who needs real help. Use this chapter as a tool. It should decrease the work and time it takes to perform this necessary task and shed a little light on a dim subject. It is, after all, much easier to perform procedures when the lights stay on.

Medicine and coding work best in teams. Whether in a small private practice or a giant academic center, get to know everyone who reviews, enters, or audits your codes. They are making claims on your behalf. Communicating well with patients is crucial, and communicating well with your coding team, if you have one, is essential to translate the work that you do into the cold languages of Current Procedural Terminology (CPT), dollars, and cents. Coding schemes are updated frequently, and there are more procedures that you may perform than are discussed in this chapter. If you do an unusual procedure and aren't sure about the code, ask a coding expert or a colleague who performs that procedure more often than you for help.

Appropriate coding for the most common skin procedures including skin biopsy, excision, repair, and destruction of benign and malignant lesions is reviewed below with tables that can be used as a quick reference.

Comparing Medical Work

Work relative value units (wRVUs), facility relative values (FAC RVUs), and nonfacility relative value units (nFAC RVUs) attempt to fairly compare the value and cost of medical work and have become a common way to judge the financial productivity of healthcare providers across varied fields. The wRVUs account for direct physician effort, skill, and time while the other components account for material costs and overhead. These values are updated regularly by the Centers for Medicare & Medicaid Services, and the most current fee schedules can be accessed at www.cms.gov/Medicare/Medicare-Fee-for-Service-Payment/PhysicianFeeSched/PFS-Relative-Value-Files.[1]

One useful takeaway of comparing wRVUs of various procedures is that they may guide how much time to regularly allot to a particular procedure. While evaluation and management codes aren't discussed in depth in this chapter, it is worth noting the wRVUs for common Evaluation and Management codes (Table 28.1) for comparison to current wRVUs for procedures. One conclusion from reviewing these codes and comparing them with biopsy codes is that setting aside an hour for a visit in which a single biopsy will be performed will earn fewer wRVUs and dollars than the same amount of time devoted to follow-up visits. While scheduling this way may be clinically appropriate in some situations and settings, learning how to integrate a biopsy into an acute visit or a shorter amount of time will prove more sustainable. Excisions and repairs, however, may be sustainably scheduled for longer amounts of time.

Table 28.1 Work RVUs for Common E/M Codes

E/M Code	Description	wRVUs
99202	Outpatient visit new straightforward 15–29 minutes	0.93
99203	Outpatient visit new low complexity 30–44 minutes	1.6
99204	Outpatient visit new moderate complexity 45–59 minutes	2.6
99212	Outpatient visit established straight-forward 10–19 minutes	0.7
99213	Outpatient visit established low complex-ity 20–29 minutes	1.3
99214	Outpatient visit established moderate complexity 30–39 minutes	1.92

Table 28.2 Site-Specific Biopsy Codes

CPT	Location	wRVUs
11755	Nail unit	1.25
30100	Intranasal	0.94
41100	Tongue, anterior two-thirds	1.42
41105	Tongue, posterior third	1.47
54100	Penis, cutaneous	1.90
56605	Vulva or perineum, single lesion	1.10
56606	Vulva or perineum, each additional lesion	0.55
57100	Vagina, simple	1.2
57105	Vagina, extensive	1.74
67810	Eyelid margin	1.18
68100	Conjunctiva	1.35
69100	Pinna	0.81
69105	Ear canal	0.85

Biopsies

When the purpose of the procedure is to sample a lesion in whole or in part for pathologic examination, the correct procedure code is a biopsy – whether shave biopsy, punch biopsy, or incisional biopsy. If the intent is to completely remove the lesion, even if it may be sent for pathologic examination, a different code may be more appropriate, such as the excision series or the less frequently used shave removal codes.[2] Biopsy codes do not differentiate the nature of the lesion – whether benign or malignant. This is after all the purpose of the biopsy.

SHAVE BIOPSY (SEE CHAPTER 9)

The first lesion is coded separately with each additional shave biopsy coded additionally. A patient undergoing five shave biopsies will have five separate codes, 11102 (once) and 11103 (four times).

- 11102 (0.66 wRVUs): tangential biopsy of the skin, single lesion
- 11103 (0.38 wRVUs): tangential biopsy of the skin, each additional lesion

PUNCH BIOPSIES (SEE CHAPTER 10)

Like coding shave biopsies, the first lesion is coded differently from subsequent punch biopsies.

- 11104 (0.83 wRVUs): punch biopsy of the skin, single lesion
- 11105 (0.38 wRVUs): punch biopsy of the skin, each additional lesion

Biopsies by different methods are coded separately. A patient undergoing a single shave biopsy and a single punch biopsy would be coded 11102 and 11104.

INCISIONAL BIOPSY (SEE CHAPTER 11, *ELLIPTICAL EXCISION*)

- 11106 (1.01 wRVUs): incisional biopsy of the skin, single lesion
- 11107 (0.54 wRVUs): incisional biopsy of the skin, each additional lesion

SPECIAL BIOPSY SITES

- Special sites have specific biopsy codes listed in Table 28.2.
- As these are based on the location only, the type of biopsy is not an issue in the coding.

Destructions of Lesions (See Chapters 13, 14)

The destruction of lesions is coded based upon whether the lesion is benign, as in a seborrheic keratosis, premalignant, as in an actinic keratosis, or malignant, as in the electrodesiccation and curettage of a superficial basal cell carcinoma. Destruction of benign lesions in special body sites and with special methods are separated out into different codes.

DESTRUCTION OF BENIGN LESIONS OTHER THAN SKIN TAGS

These typically include warts, condyloma, molluscum, seborrheic keratoses, angiomas, and sebaceous hyperplasia. Choose only one code based on the number treated. If fewer than 15 lesions are treated, choose 17110. If 15 or more lesions are treated, choose 17111. Never code both on the same patient at the same visit.

- 17110 (0.7) Destruction of 1-14 benign lesions by any method
- 17111 (0.97) Destruction of 15 or more benign lesions by any method

DESTRUCTION OF SKIN TAGS

The first 15 lesions are coded, then for any component of an additional 10 lesions, the 11201 code is added. For example, treating 26 lesions would be coded 11200 + 11201 + 11201.

- 11200 Removal of up to 15 lesions
- 11201 Removal of up to 10 additional lesions

DESTRUCTION OF PREMALIGNANT LESIONS (ACTINIC KERATOSIS)

The first lesion treated is coded 17000. Each additional lesion treated is coded separately up to 14 lesions total (17000 + 17003 +17003 +17003 would code 4 lesions treated). If more than 14 lesions are treated, only code 17004.

- 17000 (0.61) Destruction of a premalignant lesion
- 17003 (0.04) Destruction of each additional premalignant lesion up to 14
- 17004 (1.37) Destruction of 15 or more premalignant lesions

Destructions of benign lesions in special sites and by special methods have special codes (Table 28.3). There are not hard-and-fast rules for when a destruction is extensive versus simple. In the case of benign lesions on the rest of the skin, this differentiation is made at 15 lesions, so this can be a rough guide. Some equivalence of volume, number, or effort should be documented to justify why the extensive code is chosen. The small differences in wRVUs in the table below may not reflect the significant difference in facility codes between methods of destruction. This has to do with some accounting of the overhead costs of a given method. A cryosurgery spray canister and a storage Dewar may cost several hundred to a couple thousand dollars, but some LASERs are well over $100,000 to purchase and maintain.

DESTRUCTION OF MALIGNANT LESIONS[1]

Destruction of malignant lesions is often carried out with electrodesiccation and curettage or cryotherapy. The location and size of the lesion itself, without a margin, is what determines the code (Table 28.4).

- Measure and record sizes at the time of surgery. Sometimes the true size of a lesion is not obvious until after curettage.

Table 28.3 Destruction of Benign Lesions in Special Sites[1]

CPT	Description	wRVUs
46916	Simple cryotherapy, anus	1.91
46924	Extensive cryotherapy, anus	2.81
54050	Penis, chemical	1.29
54055	Penis, electrosurgery	1.25
54056	Penis, cryosurgery	1.29
54057	Penis, LASER	1.29
54060	Penis, excision	1.98
54065	Penis, extensive	2.47
56501	Vulva, simple	1.58
56515	Vulva, extensive	3.08
57061	Vagina, simple	1.3
57065	Vagina, extensive	2.66
67850	Eyelid lesion	1.74
68135	Conjunctival lesion	1.89

Table 28.4 Destruction of Malignant Lesions[1]

Location	CPT	Size	wRVUs
Trunk, arms, legs	17260	Less than 0.5 cm	0.96
	17261	0.6–1.0 cm	1.22
	17262	1.1–2.0 cm	1.63
	17263	2.1–3.0 cm	1.84
	17264	3.1–4.0 cm	1.99
	17266	More than 4.0 cm	2.39
Scalp, neck, hands, feet	17270	Less than 0.5 cm	1.37
	17271	0.6–1.0 cm	1.54
	17272	1.1–2.0 cm	1.82
	17273	2.1–3.0 cm	2.10
	17274	3.1–4.0 cm	2.64
	17276	More than 4.0 cm	3.25
Face, ears, nose, lips	17280	Less than 0.5 cm	1.22
	17281	0.6–1.0 cm	1.77
	17282	1.1–2.0 cm	2.09
	17283	2.1–3.0 cm	2.69
	17284	3.1–4.0 cm	3.2
	17286	More than 4.0 cm	4.48

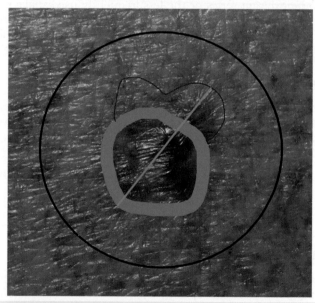

Figure 28.1 A BCC treated with destruction by electrodesiccation and curettage. The thick blue circle represents the initial clinical size of the lesion. After curettage, it is apparent that the true size of the lesion includes the area outlined in thin red. The black line represents the farthest extent curettage and desiccation are carried out. The appropriate size of the lesion to be measured and coded is designated by the thin green diagonal line, which is the longest diameter of the tumor. It does not include the margin treated. This differs from the coding of excisions in which the margins are added to the longest diameter of the tumor.

- The longest diameter of the true size of the malignant lesion is what determines the code. Note that a margin is not included in the size determination (Figure 28.1).
- Sizing and selecting destruction codes differ from sizing and selecting excision codes for malignant lesions.
- A biopsy and a destruction cannot be coded on the same lesion even if both are performed.

Shave Removal

The sharp removal of skin lesions without going all the way through the dermis by transverse or horizontal slicing can be coded distinctly. These are somewhat unusual in practice because virtually all benign tumors treated this way are sent for pathology and therefore could qualify as a tangential shave biopsy. There are risks of not sending the specimen for pathology and risks of insurance not paying for these codes if they determine that the procedure was only for cosmetic reasons. That said, these codes are useful when the primary purpose isn't diagnostic (as in biopsy codes) and the level of removal is above the subcutis. These codes (Table 28.5) are reimbursed at a somewhat higher rate than tangential shave biopsies if the lesion is larger than 0.5 cm or outside the trunk and extremities. However, it is worth repeating that if the purpose of the procedure is diagnostic, the biopsy codes are correct.

Excisions (See Chapter 11, *Elliptical Excision*, and Chapter 12, *Cysts and Lipomas*)

Excisions are defined as cutting through the dermis into the subcutaneous tissue with the intent to completely remove a lesion. There are several factors to consider when selecting the appropriate code for an excision including the size of the lesion measured at the longest diameter, the margins excised to achieve adequate removal, the location of the excision, and the benign or malignant nature of the lesion.

Excisions of malignant lesions are reimbursed at a higher rate than benign lesions, and if the nature of the lesions isn't known, it is common to hold the submission of the bill for a few days until the pathology report can confirm the correct code to use. If a lesion is known to be malignant by biopsy, the correct excision code is for an excision of a malignant lesion even if the histology on the final pathology

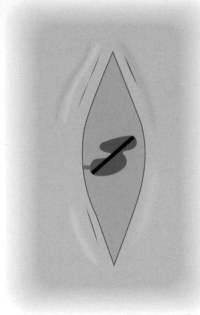

Figure 28.2 A tumor in pink has the outline as shown. The longest diameter in blue is added to twice the smallest margin shown in green to establish the correct size for coding purposes. Additionally, if the tumor is malignant, a pathology report must be available to justify using the malignant excision coding.

report does not show any remaining malignant cells. SCC in situ and melanoma in situ are malignant and should be coded that way.

The steps of measuring correctly include the following:

1. Before operating measure the longest diameter of the lesion being excised. This may be perpendicular or diagonal to the narrowest margin in an elliptical excision (Figure 28.2).
2. Measure the narrowest margin to be taken and double it.
3. Add together the two measurements and select the code corresponding to the nature of the lesion, body site, and this size, which includes the lesion and margins (Tables 28.6 and 28.7).

Skin Repairs (See Chapter 7, *Laceration Repair*, and Chapter 11, *Elliptical Excision*)

Skin repairs are coded by location, length, and complexity.

SIMPLE REPAIR (AS IN LACERATION) (TABLE 28.8)

- Involves a single layer of sutures approximating or closing a defect
- A simple repair may be coded when a laceration is repaired with a single layer of sutures.
- An excision INCLUDES a simple closure, so in the case of an excision closed with a single layer of sutures only the appropriate excision code is submitted.

Table 28.5 Shave Removal Codes[1]

CPT	Location	Size	wRVUs
11300	Trunk, arms, or legs	0.5 cm or less	0.60
11301	Trunk, arms, or legs	0.6 to 1 cm	0.90
11302	Trunk, arms, or legs	1.1 to 2 cm	1.05
11303	Trunk, arms, or legs	Over 2 cm	1.25
11305	Scalp, neck, hands, feet, genitals	0.5 cm or less	0.80
11306	Scalp, neck, hands, feet, genitals	0.6 to 1 cm	0.96
11307	Scalp, neck, hands, feet, genitals	1.1 to 2 cm	1.20
11308	Scalp, neck, hands, feet, genitals	Over 2 cm	1.46
11310	Face, ears, eyelids, nose, lips, mucous membranes	0.5 cm or less	0.80
11311	Face, ears, eyelids, nose, lips, mucous membranes	0.6 to 1 cm	1.10
11312	Face, ears, eyelids, nose, lips, mucous membranes	1.1 to 2 cm	1.30
11313	Face, ears, eyelids, nose, lips, mucous membranes	Over 2 cm	1.68

Table 28.6   Excisions of Benign Lesions[1]

Location	CPT	Size	wRVUs
Trunk and extremities	11400	Less than or equal to 0.5 cm	0.9
	11401	0.6 to 1 cm	1.28
	11402	1.1 to 2 cm	1.45
	11403	2.1 to 3 cm	1.84
	11404	3.1 to 4 cm	2.11
	11406	Over 4 cm	3.52
Hands, feet, neck, or scalp	11420	Less than or equal to 0.5 cm	1.03
	11421	0.6 to 1 cm	1.47
	11422	1.1 to 2 cm	1.68
	11423	2.1 to 3 cm	2.06
	11424	3.1 to 4 cm	2.48
	11426	Over 4 cm	4.09
Face, eyelids, ears, nose, lips	11440	Less than or equal to 0.5 cm	1.05
	11441	0.6 to 1 cm	1.53
	11442	1.1 to 2 cm	1.77
	11443	2.1 to 3 cm	2.34
	11444	3.1 to 4 cm	3.19
	11446	Over 4 cm	4.80

Table 28.7   Excisions of Malignant Lesions[1]

Location	CPT	Size	wRVUs
Trunk and extremities	11600	Less than or equal to 0.5 cm	1.63
	11601	0.6 to 1 cm	2.07
	11602	1.1 to 2 cm	2.27
	11603	2.1 to 3 cm	2.82
	11604	3.1 to 4 cm	3.17
	11606	Over 4 cm	5.02
Hands, feet, neck, or scalp	11620	Less than or equal to 0.5 cm	1.64
	11621	0.6 to 1 cm	2.08
	11622	1.1 to 2 cm	2.41
	11623	2.1 to 3 cm	3.11
	11624	3.1 to 4 cm	3.62
	11626	Over 4 cm	4.61
Face, eyelids, ears, nose, lips	11640	Less than or equal to 0.5 cm	1.67
	11641	0.6 to 1 cm	2.17
	11642	1.1 to 2 cm	2.62
	11643	2.1 to 3 cm	3.42
	11644	3.1 to 4 cm	4.34
	11646	Over 4 cm	6.26

Table 28.8   Simple Wound Repair Codes[1]

CPT	Location	Length	wRVUs
12001	Scalp, neck, axilla, genitals, trunk	Less than or equal to 2.5 cm	0.84
12002	Scalp, neck, axilla, genitals, trunk	2.5 to 7.5 cm	1.14
12004	Scalp, neck, axilla, genitals, trunk	7.6 to 12.5 cm	1.44
12005	Scalp, neck, axilla, genitals, trunk	12.6 to 20 cm	1.97
12006	Scalp, neck, axilla, genitals, trunk	20.1 to 30 cm	2.39
12007	Scalp, neck, axilla, genitals, trunk	More than 30 cm	2.90
12011	Face, ears, eyelids, nose, lips, or mucous membranes	Less than or equal to 2.5 cm	1.07
12013	Face, ears, eyelids, nose, lips, or mucous membranes	2.6 to 5 cm	1.22
12014	Face, ears, eyelids, nose, lips, or mucous membranes	5.1 to 7.5 cm	1.57
12015	Face, ears, eyelids, nose, lips, or mucous membranes	7.6 to 12.5 cm	1.98
12016	Face, ears, eyelids, nose, lips, or mucous membranes	12.6 to 20 cm	2.68
12017	Face, ears, eyelids, nose, lips, or mucous membranes	20.1 to 30 cm	3.18
12018	Face, ears, eyelids, nose, lips, or mucous membranes	More than 30 cm	3.61

INTERMEDIATE REPAIR (AS IN TWO-LAYER CLOSURE OF AN ELLIPSE) (TABLE 28.9)

- Helpful to reduce wound tension created by an excision or local skin characteristics
- Involves a two-layered closure or closure of a heavily contaminated wound requiring extensive irrigation/cleaning
- May involve limited undermining defined as less than the diameter of the initial defect
- When used to close an excision rather than a laceration, can be coded in addition to the excision code
- Often reimbursed at a rate comparable to the excision itself and can take about as much time or more when done carefully

- Failing to code for this portion of an excision and repair when performed is a costly oversight.

COMPLEX REPAIR (TABLE 28.10)

Complex repairs of wounds require meeting the characteristics of an intermediate closure and one of the following features[2]:

- Exposure of bone, cartilage, or named nerve or vessel
- Debridement of wound edges unsuitable for closure due to trauma or avulsion
- Undermining equal to or greater than the width of the wound perpendicular to the final closure
- Involvement of special anatomic/cosmetic sites, including the helical rim, vermillion border, and nasal rim

Table 28.9 Intermediate Wound Repair Codes

CPT	Location	Length	wRVUs
12031	Scalp, axilla, trunk	Less than or equal to 2.5 cm	2.00
12032	Scalp, axilla, trunk	2.6 to 7.5 cm	2.52
12034	Scalp, axilla, trunk	7.6 cm to 12.5 cm	2.97
12035	Scalp, axilla, trunk	12.6 cm to 20 cm	3.50
12036	Scalp, axilla, trunk	20.1 cm to 30 cm	4.23
12037	Scalp, axilla, trunk	More than 30 cm	5.00
12041	Neck, hands, feet, genitals	Less than or equal to 2.5 cm	2.10
12042	Neck, hands, feet, genitals	2.6 to 7.5 cm	2.79
12044	Neck, hands, feet, genitals	7.6 cm to 12.5 cm	3.19
12045	Neck, hands, feet, genitals	12.6 cm to 20 cm	3.75
12046	Neck, hands, feet, genitals	20.1 cm to 30 cm	4.30
12047	Neck, hands, feet, genitals	More than 30 cm	4.95
12051	Face, ears, eyelids, nose, lips, or mucous membranes	Less than or equal to 2.5 cm	2.33
12052	Face, ears, eyelids, nose, lips, or mucous membranes	2.6 to 5 cm	2.87
12053	Face, ears, eyelids, nose, lips, or mucous membranes	5.1 to 7.5 cm	3.17
12054	Face, ears, eyelids, nose, lips, or mucous membranes	7.6 to 12.5 cm	3.50
12055	Face, ears, eyelids, nose, lips, or mucous membranes	12.6 to 20 cm	4.50
12056	Face, ears, eyelids, nose, lips, or mucous membranes	20.1 to 30 cm	5.30
12057	Face, ears, eyelids, nose, lips, or mucous membranes	More than 30 cm	6.00

Table 28.10 Complex Wound Repair Codes

CPT	Location	Length	wRVUs
13100	Trunk	1.1 to 2.5 cm	3.00
13101	Trunk	2.6 to 7.5 cm	3.50
13102	Trunk	Each additional 5 cm or less	1.24
13120	Scalp, arms, and/or legs	1.1 to 2.5 cm	3.23
13121	Scalp, arms, and/or legs	2.6 to 7.5 cm	4.00
13122	Scalp, arms, and/or legs	Each additional 5 cm or less	1.44
13131	Forehead, cheeks, chin, mouth, neck, axillae, genitals, hands, and/or feet	1.1 to 2.5 cm	3.73
13132	Forehead, cheeks, chin, mouth, neck, axillae, genitals, hands, and/or feet	2.6 to 7.5 cm	4.78
13133	Forehead, cheeks, chin, mouth, neck, axillae, genitals, hands, and/or feet	Each additional 5 cm beyond 7.5 cm	2.19
13151	Eyelids, nose, ears, and/or lips	1.1 to 2.5 cm	4.34
13152	Eyelids, nose, ears, and/or lips	2.6 to 7.5 cm	5.34
13153	Eyelids, nose, ears, and/or lips	Each additional 5 cm or less	2.38

- Use of retention sutures
- Like intermediate closures, these are coded in addition to an excision if one has been performed.

MULTIPLE REPAIRS

- When multiple repairs are performed of the same complexity (simple, intermediate, or complex) and in the same body site, their lengths are added together into a single repair code.
- When multiple repairs are performed in different body sites or with different complexities, they are coded separately.

- When multiple procedures are coded, a modifier -59 is added to the less significant procedures.

Incision and Drainage (See Chapter 16) (Table 28.11)

INTRALESIONAL INJECTIONS (SEE CHAPTER 15)

Intralesional injection of steroids for the treatment of alopecia areata, psoriasis, cystic acne, and hidradenitis is an effective and valuable tool. Intralesional candida antigen

Table 28.11   Selection of Incision and Drainage Codes[1]

CPT	Location/Description	wRVUs
10040	Acne surgery (milia, comedones, small cysts)	0.91
10060	Simple I&D	1.22
10061	Complex or multiple I&D	1.45
10080	Pilonidal cyst, single	1.22
10081	Pilonidal cyst, multiple or complex	2.5
10140	Drainage of hematoma (other than nail)	1.58
10160	Puncture aspiration of a hematoma, bulla, or cyst	1.25
10180	I&D Postoperative wound infection	2.30
11740	Subungual hematoma	0.37
26010	Finger, simple I&D	1.59
26011	Finger, complex I&D	2.24
40800	Vestibule of mouth, simple	1.23
40801	Vestibule of mouth, complicated	2.63
41000	Lingual	1.35
41005	Sublingual, superficial	1.31
41006	Sublingual, deep, supramylohyoid	3.34
41800	Gums	1.27
46040	I&D Ischiorectal or perirectal (deep procedure)	5.37
46050	I&D Superficial anus	1.24
55100	I&D Scrotum	2.45
56405	I&D Vulva or perineum	1.49
56420	Bartholin's gland	2.89
67700	Eyelid	1.4
69000	I&D External ear, simple	1.5
69005	I&D External ear, complex	2.16
69020	I&D External ear canal	1.53

Table 28.12   Foreign Body Removal[1,2]

CPT	Location/Description	wRVUs
10120	Subcutaneous, simple	1.22
10121	Subcutaneous, complicated	2.74
20520	Muscle/tendon sheath, simple	1.9
23330	Shoulder, subcutaneous	1.9
24200	Upper arm/elbow, subcutaneous	1.81
27086	Pelvis/hip, subcutaneous	1.92
28190	Foot, subcutaneous	2.01
28192	Foot, deep	4.78
30300	Intranasal	1.09
40804	Vestibule of the mouth	1.3
65205	External eyelid, conjunctiva, superficial	0.49
69200	External ear canal without general anesthesia	0.77

GLOBAL PERIODS

The code for a procedure may include all following related care bundled into the procedure code for a period of time. This means that if a patient returns for a wound check, repacking an I&D, or complication of a procedure before the global period is over, this care receives no further provider compensation. This global period may be either 0 days, 10 days, or 90 days.[3]

- Biopsies have a 0-day global period.
- Destruction of lesions (benign, premalignant, or malignant), excisions, intermediate repairs, and incision and drainage have 10-day global periods.
- Complex repairs (and flaps and grafts not discussed in this chapter) have a 90-day global period.

MODIFIERS (TABLE 28.13)

Modifiers are appended to procedural CPTs or E/M codes to express "exceptional" situations. Below are several common modifiers encountered in coding outpatient procedures. Modifier 25 is the most commonly used code in dermatology.

SOFT TISSUE TUMORS (TABLE 28.14)

The soft tissue tumor code series is an optional coding method for the removal of lipomas and other subcutaneous tumors that don't originate in the dermis or epidermis. These codes are based upon the size of the subcutaneous tumor and the location of the tumor. These codes include closure, and so unlike the skin excision codes in which an intermediate closure could be added to an excision code, these codes stand alone and assume appropriate closure. The reimbursement is comparable to or higher than a skin excision of the same size with an intermediate closure though an intermediate closure isn't required. Due to the high wRVUs, it is more likely that these codes may be rejected or questioned.

for the treatment of warts, condyloma, or molluscum is additional use of this code series.

- 11900 (0.52 wRVUs) up to 7 lesions
- 19001 (0.8 wRVUs) more than 7 lesions
- Many medications have a specific J-code that can also be added in a non-hospital-based clinic.
- These codes do not apply to local anesthesia.

Sometimes, injection of chemotherapy into a malignant tumor is an excellent nonsurgical option. An example would include intralesional methotrexate or 5-fluorouracil injected into a squamous cell carcinoma.

- 96405 (0.52 wRVUs) up to 7 lesions
- 96406 (0.8 wRVUs) more than 7 lesions

Foreign Body Removal (Table 28.12)

Foreign body removals are coded by location and complexity.

Cosmetic Removals

Patients often request removal of skin lesions known to be benign. This is rarely covered unless the lesion is causing

Table 28.13 Common Modifiers[2]

Modifier	Description	Example
-22	Increased procedural service.	A patient with severe lymphedema undergoing an excision in the lower leg requiring preoperative compression of the surgical field and significant additional tissue handling for adequate closure
-24	Unrelated F/M service by the same physician/provider during a postoperative period	A day after a skin excision, a patient comes in for evaluation and treatment of a strep throat.
-25	Significant separately identifiable service by the same physician/provider on the same day of the procedure	A patient presenting with a new rash requiring a history and physical exam for evaluation and then undergoes a biopsy for this rash.
-50	Bilateral procedure	Two excisions on the right and left upper arms are performed on the same day.
-51	Additional procedure during the same session, on a different site, or performed multiple separate times	A patient undergoes an excision of 2 benign nevi on the back. One excision is 8 mm and one excision is 1.5 cm. A 51 modifier is added to indicate that multiple distinct procedures were performed by the same physician at the same visit. The modifier is added to the lowest RVU procedure.
-59	Distinct procedural service. Under the -59 umbrella, there are X modifiers, XE, XP, XS, and XU, that help describe in what way the service is distinct. Modifiers more specific -XE: a separate service is performed during a separate encounter -XP: a separate service is performed by a different provider -XS: a service is distinct because it was performed on a separate structure or organ -XU: unusual nonoverlapping service[4]	You biopsy a suspicious lesion and also perform cryosurgery on actinic keratoses.
-79	Separate procedure performed during a postoperative period. Mirrors -24 but for procedures instead of E/M services.	A patient undergoes an excision. During the suture removal visit prior to 10 days, they undergo an incision and drainage of a paronychia.

Table 28.14 Soft Tissue Tumor Removal Codes[1,2]

CPT	Size/Location	wRVUs
21011	Face or scalp, subcutaneous; <2cm	2.99
21012	Face or scalp, subcutaneous; ≥2 cm	4.45
21555	Neck or anterior thorax, subcutaneous; <3 cm	3.96
21552	Neck or anterior thorax, subcutaneous; ≥3 cm	6.49
21930	Back or flank, subcutaneous; <3 cm	4.94
21931	Back or flank, subcutaneous; ≥3 cm	6.88
22902	Abdominal wall, subcutaneous; <3 cm	4.42
22903	Abdominal wall, subcutaneous; ≥3 cm	6.39
23075	Shoulder, subcutaneous; <3 cm	4.21
23071	Shoulder, subcutaneous; ≥3 cm	5.91
24075	Upper arm or elbow, subcutaneous; <3 cm	4.24
24071	Upper arm or elbow, subcutaneous; ≥3 cm	5.70
25075	Forearm and/or wrist, subcutaneous; <3 cm	3.96
25071	Forearm and/or wrist, subcutaneous; ≥3 cm	5.91
26115	Hand or finger, subcutaneous; <1.5 cm	3.96
26111	Hand or finger, subcutaneous; ≥1.5 cm	5.42
27047	Pelvis or hip, subcutaneous; <3 cm	4.94
27043	Pelvis or hip, subcutaneous; ≥3 cm	6.88
27327	Thigh or knee, subcutaneous; <3 cm	3.96
27337	Thigh or knee, subcutaneous; ≥3 cm	5.91
27618	Leg or ankle, subcutaneous; <3 cm	3.96
27632	Leg or ankle, subcutaneous; ≥3 cm	5.91
28043	Foot or toe, subcutaneous; <1.5 cm	3.96
28039	Foot or toe, subcutaneous; ≥1.5 cm	5.42

pain, severe itching, or bleeding. Cryotherapy for seborrheic keratoses and skin tags are common examples. If you treat lesions for cosmetic purposes, develop a logical and fair fee schedule that you can present to a patient quickly and clearly. Sometimes in a big system, this is a tough challenge. In my experience, being kind and blunt with this information is best.

For more complicated surgical removals and possible repairs, work with someone in your office who can give patients the most accurate cost based on expected procedure codes and free you up to move on to other tasks/patients. If needed, have the patient sign an advance beneficiary notice that the service they are requesting is unlikely to be covered by insurance and the fee they will be required to pay. Patients will "forget" that this was discussed between the exam room and the cash register and treat staff very differently from the doctor.

Another option to consider is to not charge for a minor cosmetic procedure as a favor to build rapport with a patient that has limited means. For example, after freezing a number of covered AKs, freeze an additional 1 to 2 skin tags on the neck to make the patient happy. This also saves you and your staff time haggling over dollars with the patient.

Measure, Review, and Learn

Measure and record what you do, review what gets denied by insurers, and learn to adjust accordingly. Work as a team when you can, and ask for help when you are doing something new or encounter something difficult or unexpected. Just as in the rest of medicine, prevention is the key to minimizing financial harm.

References

1. CMS. *2022 National Physician Fee Schedule Relative Value File January Release*. Microsoft Excel spreadsheet. Washington, D.C.: Department of Health and Human Services; 2022. Available at: https://www.cms.gov/medicaremedicare-fee-service-paymentphysicianfeeschedpfs-relative-value-files/rvu22a. Accessed February 10, 2022.
2. *Physicians Current Procedural Terminology 2022*. Chicago, IL: American Medical Association; 2021.
3. Medicare Learning Network. *Global Surgery Booklet*. Accessed February 10, 2022. Available at: https://www.cms.gov/outreach-and-education/medicare-learning-network-mln/mlnproducts/downloads/globallsurgery-icn907166.pdf.
4. Medicare Learning Network. *MLN Factsheet: Proper Use of Modifiers 59 & -X{EPSU}*. Available at: https://www.cms.gov/files/document/proper-use-modifiers-59-xepsu.pdf. Accessed February 10, 2022.

Disclosure and Consent

Medical and Surgical Procedures

TO THE PATIENT: You have the right, as a patient, to be informed about your condition and the recommended surgical, medical or diagnostic procedure to be used so that you may make the decision whether or not to undergo the procedure after knowing the risks and hazards involved. This disclosure is not meant to scare or alarm you; it is simply an effort to make you better informed so you may give or withhold your informed consent to the procedure.

I (we) voluntarily request Dr. _____

As my physician, and such associates, technical assistants and other health care providers as they may deem necessary to treat my condition which has been explained to me as _____
_____

I (we) understand that the following surgical, medical and/or diagnostic procedures are planned for me and **I (we)** voluntarily consent and authorize these procedures:

☐ shave ☐ punch biopsy ☐ excision ☐ cryotherapy ☐ electrosurgery ☐ electrosurgery and curettage
☐ intralesional injections ☐ incision ☐ acne surgery ☐ other _____

I (we) understand that my physician may discover other or different conditions which require additional or different procedures than those planned. **I (we)** authorize my physician, and such associates, technical assistants and other health care providers to perform such other procedures which are advisable in their professional judgment.

Just as there may be risks and hazards in continuing my present condition without treatment, there are also risks and hazards related to the performance of the surgical, medical and/or diagnostic procedures planned for me. **I (we)** realize that common to surgical, medical and/or diagnostic procedures is the potential for infection, blood clots in veins and lungs, hemorrhage, allergic reactions, and even death. **I (we)** also realize that the following risks and hazards may occur in connection with this particular procedure: **ACUTE PAIN AND CHRONIC PERSISTENT PAIN, BLEEDING, INFECTION, SCARRING, CHANGE IN PIGMENTATION, RE-GROWTH, SLOW HEALING, CHANGE IN ANATOMICAL APPEARANCE, SKIN INDENTATION, SKIN PROTRUSION AND LOCAL NERVE DAMAGE (numbness or loss of muscle function)**

I (we) understand that anesthesia involves additional risks and hazards but **I (we)** request the use of anesthetics for the relief and protection from pain during the planned and additional procedures. **I (we)** realize the anesthesia may have to be changed possibly without explanation to me (us). **I (we)** understand that certain complications may result from the use of any anesthetic including respiratory problems, drug reactions, paralysis, brain damage, or even death. Other risks and hazards which may result from the use of general anesthetics range from minor discomfort to injury to vocal chords, teeth, or eyes. **I (we)** understand that other risks and hazards resulting from spinal or epidural anesthetics include headache and chronic pain.

I (we) have been given an opportunity to ask questions of my physicians about my condition, alternative forms of anesthesia and treatment, risks of non-treatment, the procedures to use, and the risks and hazards involved, and **I (we)** believe that **I (we)** have sufficient information to give this informed consent.

I (we) certify this form has been fully explained to me, that **I (we)** have read it or have had it read to me, that the blank spaces have been filled in, and that **I (we)** understand its contents.

PATIENT Signature: _____

Or other Legally Responsible Person's Signature: _____ / **Relationship:** _____

Date: _____ **Time:** _____ ( )AM ( )PM

Witness: _____ **Date:** _____ **Time:** _____ ( )AM ( )PM

I have explained to the patient or legal representative the disclosure and consent required for the medical, surgical, and/or diagnostic procedures planned as well as the patient's right to withhold consent.

Physician's Signature: _____ **Date:** _____

Divulgación y Consentimiento

Procedimientos Médicos y Quirúrgios

PARA EL PACIENTE: Usted, como paciente, tiene derecho a ser informado sobre su condición y sobre los recomendados procedimientos quirúrgicos, médicos, o diagnósticos que serán utilizados para que así usted tome la decisión de aceptar realizarse el procedimiento o no, una vez que sepa los riesgos y peligros involucrados. Esta declaración no tiene la intención de asustario o alarmarlo, es simplemente un esfuerzo para que usted esté mejor informado para poder dar o negar su consen- timiento para el procedimiento.

Yo (nosotros) solicito (amos) de manera voluntaria que el Dr. _____
como mi médico, junto con sus socios, ayudantes técnicos y otros proveedores médicos que consideren necesarios, me proporcionen el tratamiento para mi condición, el cual se me ha explicado como.

_____

Yo (nosotros) entiendo (entendemos) que se ha planeado se me realicen los siguientes procedimientos quirúrgicos, médicos y / o diagnósticos, y yo (nosotros) voluntariamente acepto y autorizo se me realicen los siguientes procedimientos:
□ afeitado   □ crioterapia   □ electrocirugía   □ electrocirugía y legrado   □ abstracción   □ biopsia por punción
□ inyección intralesional   □ incisión   □ cirugía por acné   □ otros_____

Yo (nosotros) entiendo (entendemos) que mi médico podria descubrir condición adicionales o distintos, que requieran procedimientos adicionales o distintos a los previstos. Yo (nosotros) autorizo (autorizamos) a mi médico, junto con sus socios, ayudantes técnicos y otros proveedores médicos realicen dichos procedimientos adicionales que a su juicio profesional sean prudentes.

Así com pueden existir riesgos y peligros en seguir con mi condición actual sin tratamiento, también existen riesgos y peligros relaciona- dos con la realización de los procedimientos quirúrgicos, médicos y / o diagnósticos planeados para mí. Yo (nosotros) entiendo (entendemos) que con los procedimientos quirúrgicos, médicos y / o diagnósticos existe la posibilidad de infección, formación de coágu- los de sangre en venas y pulmones, hemorragias, reacciones alérgicas e incluso al muerte. Yo (nosotros) también entiendo (entendemos) que pueden presentarse los siguientes riesgos y peligros en conexión con este procedimiento en particular:

DOLOR AGUDO Y DOLOR CRÓNICO Y PERSISTENTE, SANGRANDO, INFECCIÓN, CICATRICES, CAMBIO DE PIGMENTACIÓN, NUEVO CRECIMIENTO, CURACIÓN LENTA, CAMBIO EN LA APARIENCIA ANATÓMICA, HENDIDURA EN

LA PIEL, PROTRUSIÓN DE LA PIEL Y DAÑO A LOS NERVIOS LOCALES (sensación de entumecimiento o pérdida de la función muscular)

Yo (nosotros) entiendo (entendemos) que la anestesia involucra reisgos y peligros adicionales, pero yo (nosotros) solicito (solicitamos) el uso de anestésicos para el alivio y la protección conra el dolor durante los procedimientos previstos y los adicionales. Yo (nosotros) comprendo (comprendemos) que la anestesia puede tener que ser cambiada, posiblemente sin que se dé una explicación a mí (nosotros). Yo (nosotros) entiendo (entendemos) que con el uso de cualquier anestésico pueden surgir ciertas complicaciones, incluy- endo problemas respiratorios, reacción adversa a medicamentos, parálisis, daño cerebral o incluso la muerte.

Se me (nos) ha ofrecido la oportunidad de hacer preguntas sobre mi padecimiento., las formas alternativas de anestesia y tratamiento, los riesgos por no recibir tratamiento, los procedimientos que se utilizarán y los riesgos y peligros involucrados, y creo (creemos) que tengo (tenemos) la información suficiente para dar este consentimiento informado.

Yo (nosotros) certifico (certificamos) que este formulario se me (nos) ha sido plenamente explicado., que **yo (nosotros)** lo he leído o se me ha leído, que los espacios en blanco han sido llenados y que **yo (nosotros)** entiendo (entendemos) su contenido.

FIRMA DEL PACIENTE: _____

O de otra persona legalmente responsable: _____   **Parentesco:** _____

Fecha: _____   **Hora:** _____   ( )AM   ( )PM

Testigo: _____   **Fecha:** _____   **Hora:** _____   ( )AM   ( )PM

Le he explicado al paciente o su representate legal la divulgación y consentimiento necesarios para la realización de los proced- imientos médicos, quirúrgicos y / o diagnósticos programados, así como el derecho del paciente a rehusar su consentimiento.

Firma del Médico: _____   **Fecha:** _____

Patient Information Handout

Care of Your Skin after a Shave Biopsy

Supplies needed

- Clean petroleum jelly (a squeeze tube is cleaner than a tub) (Vaseline is one name brand) (Do not use Neosporin or Triple Antibiotic)
- Dressing or gauze that is made for wound care (Band-Aids are one name brand)
- Optional – cotton-tipped applicators (Q-tips are one name brand)

Directions

- Keep the site clean and dry and do not remove the original dressing for 24 hours.
- After 24 hours you may shower daily. Gently wash the surgical site with soap and water in the shower or at least once daily.
- Apply petroleum jelly to the clean wound with a clean finger or cotton-tipped applicator one to two times per day.
- Use a dressing to cover the wound. While cleansing is only needed once or twice a day, additional petroleum jelly may be added as needed to keep the wound moist.
- Tylenol (acetaminophen) or ibuprofen can be taken for pain if needed. DO NOT start taking any medications with aspirin or aspirin products.

REPEAT THESE INSTRUCTIONS DAILY UNTIL THE WOUND IS HEALED. THIS MAY BE ANYWHERE FROM 5 TO 20 DAYS.

The wound will actually heal better and scar less if kept clean and covered with petroleum jelly.

Bleeding

If bleeding occurs, apply firm pressure to the site. Direct pressure should be applied to the wound. Five minutes should be adequate if the bleeding is minor and the wound is small. However, if the wound is larger and the bleeding is more severe, apply pressure for <u>10 minutes</u>, timed by looking at a clock. It is best not to discontinue pressure to see if the bleeding has stopped until 10 minutes have passed. If the bleeding continues, remove the pad and press directly with a clean gauze pad over the bleeding site. If bleeding soaks through the gauze or is not stopped by firm pressure, call and go to your doctor or an urgent care center.

Infection

If you notice pus or discharge coming from the wound this may be an infection. This is particularly worrisome if you develop a fever and the wound is red, painful, swollen, and warm. Other signs of infection could be red streaks from wound, increased pain, and painful or swollen lymph nodes (glands). If you have any suspicion of having an infection, go to your doctor or an urgent care center.

Shower and washing

You may shower daily after the first 24 hours have passed. At first, you may leave the dressing on during the shower to protect the wound from the flow of water. Alternatively, if the wound needs cleaning, the shower is helpful to remove crusts and discharge. Dry the area gently and then apply the petroleum jelly and cover the healing wound as described above. We recommend not bathing in a tub or hot tub until the wound is completely healed over to avoid infection.

Wound healing

After the wound looks healed over you can stop daily dressing changes. The wound may remain red and will slowly fade over the next few weeks or months. Sometimes it can take 6 months to 1 year for the redness to fade completely.

You may experience a sensation of tightness as your wound heals. This is normal and will gradually go away. After the wound has healed, frequent, gentle massaging of the area will help to loosen the scar. Sometimes the surgery involves small nerves and may take up to a year before feeling returns to normal. Only rarely will the area remain numb permanently.

Your healed wound may be sensitive to temperature changes (such as cold air). This sensitivity improves with time, but if you are experiencing a lot of discomfort, try to avoid temperature extremes. You may experience itching after your wound appears to have healed. This is due to the healing that continues underneath the skin. Petroleum jelly may help to relieve this itching. Try not to scratch the wound since this may cause it to reopen.

IF YOU HAVE ANY CONCERNS NOT ANSWERED BY THIS INFORMATION, PLEASE CALL: _____ OR GO TO ANOTHER MEDICAL FACILITY IF WE ARE CLOSED.

Patient Information Handout

Care of Your Skin after a Punch Biopsy

Supplies needed

- Clean petroleum jelly (a squeeze tube is cleaner than a tub) (Vaseline is one name brand) (Do not use Neosporin or Triple Antibiotic)
- Dressing or gauze that is made for wound care (Band-Aids are one name brand)
- Optional – cotton-tipped applicators (Q-tips are one name brand)

Directions

- Keep the site clean and dry and do not remove the original dressing for 24 hours.
- After 24 hours you may shower daily. Gently wash the surgical site with soap and water in the shower or at least once daily.
- Apply petroleum jelly to the clean wound with a clean finger or cotton-tipped applicator one to two times per day.
- Use a dressing to cover the wound especially if the wound was not sutured. While cleansing is only needed once or twice a day, additional petroleum jelly may be added as needed to keep the wound moist. Sutured (stitched) wounds may be left uncovered without petroleum jelly after two days.
- Tylenol (acetaminophen) or ibuprofen can be taken for pain if needed. DO NOT start taking any medications with aspirin or aspirin products.

For wounds that were not sutured (stitched), these will actually heal better and scar less if kept clean and covered with petroleum jelly.

Bleeding

If bleeding occurs, apply firm pressure to the site. Direct pressure should be applied to the wound. Five minutes should be adequate if the bleeding is minor and the wound is small. However, if the wound is larger and the bleeding is more severe, apply pressure for 10 minutes, timed by looking at a clock. It is best not to discontinue pressure to see if the bleeding has stopped until 10 minutes have passed. If the bleeding continues, remove the pad and press directly with a clean gauze pad over the bleeding site. If bleeding soaks through the gauze or is not stopped by firm pressure, call and go to your doctor or an urgent care center.

Infection

If you notice pus or discharge coming from the wound this may be an infection. This is particularly worrisome if you develop a fever and the wound is red, painful, swollen, and warm. Other signs of infection could be red streaks from wound, increased pain, and painful or swollen lymph nodes (glands). If you have any suspicion of having an infection, call and go to your doctor or an urgent care center.

Shower and washing

You may shower daily after the first 24 hours have passed. At first, you may leave the band-aid on during the shower to protect the wound from the forceful flow of water. Alternatively, if the wound needs cleaning, the shower is helpful to remove crusts and discharge. Dry the area gently and then apply petroleum jelly if the wound was not sutured. We recommend not bathing in a tub or hot tub until the wound is completely healed over to avoid infection.

Wound healing

After the wound looks healed over you can stop daily dressing changes. The wound may remain red and will slowly fade over the next few weeks or months. Sometimes it can take 6 months to 1 year for the redness to fade completely.

You may experience a sensation of tightness as your wound heals. This is normal and will gradually fade. After the wound has healed, frequent, gentle massaging of the area will help to loosen the scar. Sometimes the surgery involves small nerves and may take up to a year before feeling returns to normal. Only rarely will the area remain numb permanently.

Your healed wound may be sensitive to temperature changes (such as cold air). This sensitivity improves with time, but if you are experiencing a lot of discomfort avoid temperature extremes. You may experience itching after your wound appears to have healed. This is due to the healing that continues underneath the skin. Petroleum jelly may help to relieve this itching. Try not to scratch the wound since this may cause it to reopen.

SPECIAL INSTRUCTIONS FOR WOUNDS WITH SUTURES
- After surgery, go home and take it easy (avoid exertion, lifting, bending, or straining).
- Be very careful not to accidentally cut the sutures, especially while shaving.

SPECIAL INSTRUCTIONS FOR WOUNDS ON THE FACE WITH SUTURES

It is perfectly normal to have bruising or discoloration around the surgery site, especially if the wound is around the eye area. Do not be alarmed by this; it will eventually fade and return to normal color.

IF YOU HAVE ANY CONCERNS NOT ANSWERED BY THIS INFORMATION, PLEASE CALL: _____ OR GO TO ANOTHER MEDICAL FACILITY IF WE ARE CLOSED.

Patient Information Handout

Care of Your Skin after Surgery

Supplies needed

- Clean petroleum jelly (a squeeze tube is cleaner than a tub) (Vaseline is one name brand) (Do not use Neosporin or Triple Antibiotic)
- Dressing or gauze that is made for wound care (Band-Aids are one name brand)
- Optional – cotton-tipped applicators (Q-tips are one name brand)

Directions

- Keep the site clean and dry and do not remove the original dressing for 24 hours.
- After 24 hours you may shower daily. Gently wash the surgical site with soap and water in the shower or at least once daily.
- Apply petroleum jelly to the clean wound with a clean finger or cotton-tipped applicator one to two times per day.
- Use a dressing to cover the wound. While cleansing is only needed once or twice a day, additional petroleum jelly may be added as needed to keep the wound moist.
- Tylenol (acetaminophen) or ibuprofen can be taken for pain if needed. DO NOT start taking any medications with aspirin or aspirin products.

REPEAT THESE INSTRUCTIONS DAILY UNTIL THE WOUND IS HEALED. THIS MAY BE ANYWHERE FROM 5 TO 20 DAYS.

The wound will actually heal better and scar less if kept clean and covered with petroleum jelly.

Bleeding

If bleeding occurs, apply firm pressure to the site. Direct pressure should be applied to the wound. Five minutes should be adequate if the bleeding is minor and the wound is small. However, if the wound is larger and the bleeding is more severe, apply pressure for 10 minutes, timed by looking at a clock. It is best not to discontinue pressure to see if the bleeding has stopped until 10 minutes have passed. If the bleeding continues, remove the pad and press directly with a clean gauze pad over the bleeding site. If bleeding soaks through the gauze or is not stopped by firm pressure, call and go to your doctor or an urgent care center.

Infection

If you notice pus or discharge coming from the wound this may be an infection. This is particularly worrisome if you develop a fever and the wound is red, painful, swollen, and warm. Other signs of infection could be red streaks from wound, increased pain, and painful or swollen lymph nodes (glands). If you have any suspicion of having an infection, go to your doctor or an urgent care center.

Shower and washing

You may shower daily after the first 24 hours have passed. At first, you may leave the dressing on during the shower to protect the wound from the flow of water. Alternatively, if the wound needs cleaning, the shower is helpful to remove crusts and discharge. Dry the area gently and then apply the petroleum jelly and cover the healing wound as described above. We recommend not bathing in a tub or hot tub until the wound is completely healed over to avoid infection.

Wound healing

After the wound looks healed over you can stop daily dressing changes. The wound may remain red and will slowly fade over the next few weeks or months. Sometimes it can take 6 months to 1 year for the redness to fade completely.

You may experience a sensation of tightness as your wound heals. This is normal and will gradually fade. After the wound has healed, frequent, gentle massaging of the area will help to loosen the scar. Sometimes the surgery involves small nerves and may take up to a year before feeling returns to normal. Only rarely will the area remain numb permanently.

Your healed wound may be sensitive to temperature changes (such as cold air). This sensitivity improves with time, but if you are experiencing a lot of discomfort, try to avoid temperature extremes. You may experience itching after your wound appears to have healed. This is due to the healing that continues underneath the skin. Petroleum jelly may help to relieve this itching. Try not to scratch the wound since this may cause it to reopen.

Avoid sunlight to the scar by keeping it covered and/or using sunscreen. Prolonged sun exposure may turn the pink scar to a darker red or purple color and delay healing.

Continued

Patient Information Handout

Care of Your Skin after Surgery (continued)

SPECIAL INSTRUCTIONS FOR ALL WOUNDS WITH STITCHES (SUTURES)

- After surgery, go home and take it easy (avoid exertion, lifting, bending, or straining).
- Be very careful not to accidentally cut the sutures, especially while shaving.
- For one month, avoid heavy lifting or vigorous exercise that could cause your wound to pull apart.
- Contact the clinic if the incision pulls apart.

SPECIAL INSTRUCTIONS FOR WOUNDS ON THE FACE WITH STITCHES

- Keep your head elevated for the first 2 nights even while sleeping.
- Avoid sleeping on the same side of the body as the wound.
- Do not bend over with your head lower than your heart level. Bend at the knees to stoop down. Be careful not to lift anything heavy or do anything that might cause strain on the sutures.
- It is perfectly normal to have bruising or discoloration around the surgery site, especially if the wound is around the eye area. There can be a lot of swelling and dark bruising around the eyes at first but it will eventually fade and return to normal color.

IF YOU HAVE ANY CONCERNS NOT ANSWERED BY THIS INFORMATION, PLEASE CALL: _____ OR GO TO ANOTHER MEDICAL FACILITY IF WE ARE CLOSED.

B Procedures to Consider for Benign, Premalignant, and Malignant Conditions

Table 1 Procedures to Consider for Benign Conditions

Benign	Cryo	Curettement	Electrodestruction[a]	Electrosection	Shave/Snip	Surgery[b]	Topical Meds[c]	Intralesional[d]
Acne	O	N	N	N	N	O (AS)	P	O
Acrochordons (skin tags)	P	N	O	O	P	N	N	N
Angiokeratoma	P	O	P	P	P	O	N	N
Angiomas (cherry)	O	O	P	P	O	N	N	N
Angiomas (small spider on face)	N	N	P	N	N	N	N	N
Chondrodermatitis nodularis helicis	O	O	O	O	O	P	N	O
Condyloma acuminata	P	O	O	P	O	O	P	O
Cutaneous horn	N	N	N	O	P	P	N	N
Dermatofibroma	O	N	N	N	O	P	N	N
Dermatosis papulosa nigra	P	O	O	O	O	O	N	N
Digital mucous cyst	P	N	N	N	P	P	N	O
Granuloma annulare	O	N	N	N	N	N	N	P
Hemangiomas	O	O	N	N	O	O	N	N
Hypertrophic scar	P	N	N	N	O	O	O	P
Keloids	P	N	N	N	O	O	O	P
Lentigines	P	N	N	N	O	N	O	N
Lichen planus	O	N	N	N	N	N	P	O
Milia	O	N	N	N	N	P (AS)	O	N
Molluscum contagiosum	P	P	N	N	O	O	P	N
Mucocele	O	N	O	O	P	P	N	O
Neurofibromas	N	N	O	O	P	P	N	N
Nevi	N	N	N	O	P	P	N	N
Pearly penile papules	P	N	N	O	O	N	N	N
Pilomatricoma	N	N	N	N	N	P	N	N
Prurigo nodularis	P	N	N	N	O	O	P	P
Pyogenic granuloma	O	P	P	P	P	P	N	N
Sebaceous hyperplasia	O	O	P	O	P	O	O	N
Seborrheic keratosis	P	O	O	O	O	O	N	N
Skin tags (acrochordons)	P	N	O	O	P	O	N	N
Stucco keratoses	P	O	O	O	O	O	N	N
Syringomas	O	N	P	P	O	O	N	N
Telangiectasias	N	N	P	N	N	N	N	N
Trichoepithelioma	N	O	N	N	P	P	N	N

Continued

Table 1   Procedures to Consider for Benign Conditions—cont'd

Benign	Cryo	Curettement	Electrodestruction[a]	Electrosection	Shave/Snip	Surgery[b]	Topical Meds[c]	Intralesional[d]
Vascular malformations (port-wine stain)	O	N	N	N	N	N	N	N
Venous lake	P	N	O	O	N	O	N	N
Verruca, common	P	O	O	O	O	O	P	O
Verruca, flat	P	O	O	O	O	N	P	N
Verruca, plantar	P	O	O	O	O	O	P	O
Xanthelasma	O	O	O	O	O	O	N	N

Code: N = not recommended, O = optional, P = preferred.
AS = acne surgery, ED&C = electrodessication and curettage.
Disclaimer: Note that this table was created by the two editors using available evidence, but much evidence is incomplete and missing. Therefore it is important to not take this table as a set of rigid recommendations to follow, but to use the information along with your clinical judgment and patient preferences to make real time clinical decisions.
[a]Electrodestruction includes ED&C and use of small electrodes for destruction of small vascular lesions.
[b]Surgery includes all types of excisions and acne surgery.
[c]Topical meds include 5-FU, imiquimod, hydroquinone, and acne meds.
[d]Intralesional includes steroids, candida antigen, HPV vaccine.

Table 2   Procedures to Consider for Premalignant and Malignant Conditions

Premalignant	Cryo	Curettement	Electrodestruction (including ED&C)[a]	Shave/Snip	Surgery[b]	Topical Meds[c]	Mohs Surgery
Actinic cheilitis	P	N	O	O	O	P	N
Actinic keratosis	P	O	O	O	O	P	N
BCC (superficial or small nodular)	O	O	O	O	O	O	O
BCC (sclerosing, infiltrating)	N	N	N	N	P	N	P
Keratoacanthoma	O	O	P	P	P	N	O
SCC in situ (Bowen's disease)	O	O	P	O	O	O	O
SCC (small and early)	O	O	P	P	P	O	O
SCC (large, aggressive)	N	N	N	N	P	N	P
Recurrent BCC or SCC	N	N	N	N	P	N	P
Melanoma	N	N	N	N	P	N	O
Merkel cell carcinoma	N	N	N	N	P	N	P

Code: N = not recommended, O = optional, P = preferred.
ED&C = electrodessication and curettage.
Disclaimer: Note that this table was created by the two editors using available evidence, but much evidence is incomplete and missing. Therefore it is important to not take this table as a set of rigid recommendations to follow, but to use the information along with your clinical judgment and patient preferences to make real time clinical decisions.
[a]Electrodestruction includes ED&C
[b]Surgery includes all types of excisions and acne surgery.
[c]Topical meds include 5-FU, imiquimod, hydroquinone, and acne meds.

Index

Note: Page numbers followed by *f* refer to figures; page numbers followed by *t* refer to tables; page numbers followed by *b* refer to boxes.

A

Abscess. *See also* Incision and drainage
  breast, 220f
  with cellulitis, 219, 220f
  complications, 226
  formation, 219, 220f
  incision of, 222f
  packing with strip gauze, 223f
Absorbable gelatin foam sponge, 38
Absorbable staples, 45
Absorbable sutures, 36f, 45, 46t
Accentuated heart shape, buried vertical
    mattress sutures with, 55, 55f
Acetaminophen, 390
Acne
  keloidalis nuchae, 207–208, 209f
  nodules and cysts, 207
  scarring, 211
  surgery, 330, 331f
Acral lentiginous melanoma, 238, 239f,
    366–367, 366f
Acral melanomas, 281t
Acrochordons (skin tags), 330–332
  cryo tweezers and, 331
  diagnosis of, 330, 331f
  electrosurgery and, 198, 332
  snip with iris scissors, 331
  special considerations/pathology/billing, 332
  treatment of, 330–332
Actinic keratoses, 92, 180–181, 181f, 181t,
    355–359
  cryosurgery and, 356–357
  curettage, 357
  diclofenac gel, 357
  fluorouracil, 357
  imiquimod, 357
  management of, 356–357t
  photodynamic therapy, 357
  topical medications, 357
  treatment of, 356–357
Adhesives, 45–46
Adson forceps, 14
Advancement flaps, 309–312
  bilateral advancement flap (H-plasty),
    311, 311f
  blood supply and, 310, 310f
  conceptual, 309–310
  L-plasty, 311, 312f
  redirection of tissue movement, 309, 309f
  reorientation of tissue redundancy, 309, 310f
  single-pedicle advancement flap (U-plasty),
    310, 310f
  step-by-step instructions and, 311–312, 312f
  T-plasty (O-T flap), 311, 311f
Adverse effects. *See* Procedural complications
Alopecia, 97–98, 114, 115f
Alopecia areata, intralesional injections and,
    208–209, 209f
Aluminum chloride, 18, 18f, 34–35, 34f, 35f,
    101, 104
Amelanotic melanomas, 93, 94f, 367, 367f
Anesthesia, 190. *See also* Local anesthesia;
    Topical anesthetics
  elliptical excision and, 137

Anesthesia *(Continued)*
  field or ring blocks, 28, 31f
  laceration repair and, 72–73
  local anesthesia by injection, 23–24, 23t
  most useful anesthetics, 31
  needles and, 31
  nerve blocks, 27–28, 27b, 29f
  office setup and, 18
  pregnancy and lactation and, 28–29
  syringes and, 31
  topical anesthetics, 21–22, 22f, 22t
  topical refrigerants/cryoanesthesia, 22–25
Angiofibromas
  diagnosis of, 332, 333f
  electrodesiccation for small lesions and, 332
  lasers and, 333
  treatment of, 332–333
Angiokeratomas
  diagnosis of, 332
  electrodesiccation for small lesions and, 332
  lasers and, 333
  treatment of, 332–333, 332f
Angiomas. *See also* Cherry angiomas; Spider
    angiomas
  diagnosis of, 332
  electrodesiccation for small lesions and, 332
  lasers and, 333
  treatment of, 332–333, 332f
Antianxiety medications, 6–7
Antibiotic prophylaxis, 5–6, 5t
Antibiotics, skin infections and, 71
Anticoagulation/antiplatelet therapy, 3–4
Antiseptics, preoperative preparation and, 7
Aspirin therapy, 4
Asteatotic eczema, 285
Atypical dots, 271, 272f
Atypical moles, 341
Atypical pigment network, 270–271, 271f
Atypical vessels, 273, 273f
Autoimmune bullous diseases, 88–89
Axial pattern flaps, 307

B

Bacitracin, 235
Bartholin's duct cyst, 154f
Basal cell carcinoma, 24f, 93, 93f, 167, 190
  biopsy choice and, 89
  cryosurgery, 364
  dermoscopic features, 262–263t
  diagnosis of, 261–264, 361–362, 361f
  electrodesiccation and curettage, 364
  elliptical excision, 363
  Mohs micrographic surgery, 364, 364f
  photodynamic therapy, 365
  punch biopsy and, 116f
  radiation therapy, 364
  recurrent, 396f
  shave biopsy and, 101–103, 102f, 112, 112f
  special consideration, 365
  systemic agents for severe forms, 405
  topical immunotherapy, 364
  treatment of, 362–365, 362t
Benign conditions, 421–422t

Benign lesions, electrosurgery and, 193–196
Benign nevi, 92
  patterns, 267–269t
Benign *vs.* malignant subcutaneous
    masses, 328
Bilateral advancement flap (H-plasty), 311, 311f
Bilateral O-Z rotation flap, 314, 314f
Biopsy. *See also* Cancer determination
  anterior shin and, 97
  basal cell carcinoma and, 89
  biopsy site, 87–91
  bullous lesions and, 97, 97f
  chest and buttocks and, 97
  curcttement biopsy and, 87, 87f
  direct immunofluorescence biopsies, 88f, 89t
  ears, eyelids, nose, and lips, 98
  erythroderma and, 95–97, 96f
  five biopsy methods, 84f
  general principles and, 83–87
  hands and feet and, 97
  incisional and excisional biopsy and, 85–86
  infiltrative disorders and, 95, 95f
  inflammatory disorders and, 94–95, 94f
  margin assessment, 99, 99b
  melanoma and, 90–91
  partial, 85
  punch biopsy and, 85
  rash or inflammatory process and, 87
  scalp and, 97–98
  scattered lesions and, 87–88
  shave biopsy and, 83
  site, documentation of, 91
  specific anatomic areas and, 97–98
  squamous cell carcinoma and, 89
  suspected infectious rash and, 97
  type, size, and requested laboratory tests, 90t
  vesicular-bullous reaction and, 87
Bipolar forceps, 36, 36f, 187f
Blades, scalpel, 12, 13, 13f
Bleeding, intraoperative, 390–391
Bleeding, postoperative, 390–391, 390f
Bloody field work, 36–37
Blue-white veil, raised, 272, 272f
Bovie Bantam PRO electrosurgical unit, 189f
Bovie DERM 942 electrosurgical unit, 189f
Bowen's disease, treatment of, 358–359
Branchial cleft cyst, 154f
Bruising, postoperative, 391–392, 391f
Bulla, 117
Bullous impetigo, 97
Bullous lesions, 97, 97f, 115f
Bullous lichen planus, 117f
Bullous pemphigoid, 97, 97f, 115f
Buried, hemostasis, 37
Buried vertical mattress sutures, 54, 54f
  with accentuated heart shape, 55, 55f
Burns, 192
Burton Nova Exam® LED exam light, 11–12, 12f
Buttocks, biopsy choice and, 97

C

Cancer determination, 91–97. *See also* Biopsy
  actinic keratoses and, 92

Cancer determination *(Continued)*
   amelanotic melanomas and, 93, 94f
   basal cell carcinoma and, 93, 93f
   benign nevi and, 92
   keratoacanthomas and, 92–93, 93f
   lentigo maligna and, 92, 92f
   nonpigmented lesions and, 92–93
   pigmented lesions and, 91–92
   seborrheic keratoses and, 92, 92f
   squamous cell carcinomas and, 93, 93f
Candida antigen injections, 215–217, 216f,
      217b, 217f
   periungual warts, 217f
Capillaritis, 289–290, 289f, 290f
Capillary angiomas. *See* Cherry angiomas
Catgut (absorbable) sutures, 45
Cellulitis, 326
Cellulose, 39
Chalazion clamp, 39, 40f
Chemical hemostatic agents, 33–35
   aluminum chloride, 34–35, 34f, 35f
   general principles and, 33–35
   Monsel's solution, 35
   silver nitrate, 35
Chemical matrixectomy, 236b
Chemicals, 18, 18f
Cherry angiomas, 193–194, 332
Chest, biopsy choice and, 97
Chlorhexidine, 7, 138, 231
Chondrodermatitis nodularis helicis, 333–334
   cryosurgery and, 334
   diagnosis of, 333, 333f
   electrodesiccation and curettage and, 334
   elliptical excision and, 334
   injection and, 334
   lasers and, 334
   treatment of, 333–334
Clamps, 39, 40f
Clean cotton-tipped applicators, 16–17
Cleansing, wound, 73
Closed probes, 176–177
Coding common skin procedures, 406–414
   cosmetic removals, 412–413
   destructions of lesions, 407–408
   excisions, 409
   foreign body removal, 412, 412t
   global periods, 412
   incisional biopsy, 407
   incision and drainage, 411–412, 412t
   measure, review, and learn, 413
   medicine, 406
   modifiers, 412, 413t
   punch biopsy, 407
   shave biopsy, 407
   shave removal, 409, 409t
   skin repairs, 409–411
   soft tissue tumors, 412, 413t
   special biopsy site, 407
   work relative value units, 406, 407t
Color Doppler, 318
Common warts, 290, 290f
Complications. *See* Procedural complications
Compound nevi, 341
Compressive sutures, 63, 65f
Condyloma, 177–178
Condyloma acuminata, 116f, 177–178,
      177f, 178f, 194–195, 195f. *See also*
      Genital warts
Connective tissue diseases, 89
Consent forms, 415t
Contamination, laceration repair and, 72
Conventional cutting needles, 43
Corner (tip) stitch, 59–60, 59f
Cosmetic results, of shave biopsy, 84
Cotton-tipped applicators (CTAs), 34, 171, 221
Crescent excision, 147, 147f

Cryoanesthesia, 22–25
Cryocones, 172–173
Cryogun, 171
CryoPen, 176–177
Cryoplate, 172, 172f
Cryoprobe, 175f
Cryosurgery, 167, 187
   actinic keratoses, 180–181
   advantages, 167
   aftercare, 183
   basal cell carcinoma and, 364
   benign lesions, 168t
   chondrodermatitis nodularis helicis
      and, 334
   closed probes, 176–177
   coding and billing pearls, 183–184
   complications, 177
   contraindications, 167, 169t
   Cryo Tweezers, 170, 170f, 175–176
   with curettage for superficial basal cell
      carcinoma (BCC), 183
   dermatosis papulosis nigra, 178
   disadvantages, 169
   equipment for liquid nitrogen, 169–170
   factors affecting freezing of tissue, 171t
   forms of cryogens and temperatures, 171t
   freezing times, 173
   halo diameters, 173
   hypertrophic scars, 178
   indications, 167
   keloids and, 178, 336–337
   key events during freezing, 168t
   learning the techniques and, 183
   liquid nitrogen and, 170–177
   liquid nitrogen probes and, 175
   liquid nitrogen spray and, 173–175, 174f
   malignant lesions, 181–183
   methods, 170–177
   molluscum contagiosum, 178–179, 179f
   mucocele and, 340
   palliation, 183
   pitfalls in, 177b
   premalignant and malignant conditions, 169t
   premalignant lesions, 180–183
   principles, 170
   pyogenic granuloma and, 180, 180f, 344
   seborrheic keratosis, 179, 180f
   skin tags and, 176f, 331, 331f
   solar lentigines, 179
   specific lesions, 177–183
   spray tips for, 170f
   syringomas and, 348
   thaw times, 173
   vascular conditions and, 169t
   vascular lesions and, 180
   venereal warts, 351
   venous lakes, 180, 181f
   warts, 179
   warts, common, 349–350
Cryotherapy, 167
   digital mucous cysts and, 161, 161f
   equipment for, 18, 18f, 19f
   sebaceous hyperplasia and, 346
Cryo Tweezers, 170, 170f, 175–176, 175f,
      176f, 331
Curettage, recommended hemostasis methods
      for, 41t
Curettement biopsy, 87, 87f
Curettes, 14, 14f
Cutaneous horn, 92, 93f, 334
   diagnosis of, 334
   treatment of, 334
Cutaneous lupus, 209
Cutaneous sarcoidosis, 115f
Cutaneous T-cell lymphomas, 95, 95f,
      368–369, 368f

Cutting instruments, 12–14
Cyst removal. *See* Minimal excision technique
      for cysts
Cysts. *See specific cyst type*

D
Dead space, wound closure, 73
Debridement, 73
Deep horizontal mattress suture, 55, 55f
Deep nodular melanoma, 87f
Deep or buried sutures, 54
Deep shave biopsy
   melanoma and, 84f, 91
   superficial *versus*, 83–85, 84f
Deep shave saucerization technique, 106–108,
      107–108f, 108f
Deep suture removal, 55
Deep (buried) sutures, 42
Deep suture with inverted knot or buried
      stitch, 74–75, 75f
Delayed primary closure, 77
Dermal curettes, 14, 14f
Dermatitis, 284–285, 286f
Dermatofibroma, 257–258, 257f, 334–336
   diagnosis of, 334
   special considerations/pathology/billing, 336
   treatment of, 334–335, 335f
Dermatofibrosarcoma protuberans, 369–370
   diagnosis of, 369–370, 370f
   treatment and prognosis, 370
Dermatomyositis, 116f
Dermatosis papulosa nigra, 198, 198f,
      346–348
   cryosurgery of, 347
   diagnosis of, 346–347
   electrodesiccation without local
      anesthesia, 347
   special considerations/billing, 347–348
   treatment of, 347
Dermatosis papulosis nigra, 178
Dermoid cysts, 155f, 159
Dermoscopy, 239
   advantages, 101
   comedo-like openings, 258, 258f
   of darker nevus with dark center, 270f
   dermatofibroma, 257–258, 257f
   equipment, 253
   evidence for, 253
   fissures and ridges, 258–261, 258f
   hemangiomas, 258–261, 259f
   infectious skin diseases, 290–293
   inflammatory diseases, 284–290
   intradermal nevi, 259–261, 259f,
      260f, 261f
   learn and perform algorithms, 253–254
   of melanoma, 282f
   original two-step algorithm, 254
   parameters, 284
   sebaceous hyperplasia, 259, 259f
   seborrheic keratoses, 258, 258f
   for skin cancer criteria, 261–279, 262f
   TADA, 254–258
   top-down two-step approach, 254
   triage amalgamated dermoscopic algorithm,
      253–254
Digital block, 27–28, 27b, 29f, 230, 232f
Digital mucous (myxoid) cysts, 155f, 160, 325
   causing nail deformity, 160f
   coding and billing pearls, 165
   indications for treating, 160
   needling and cryotherapy, 161, 161f
Direct immunofluorescence (DIF) biopsies, 88,
      88f, 89t, 97
   ear, 80, 80f
Discoid lupus erythematosus, 289, 289f

Disseminated sporotrichosis, 118f
Drapes, 7–8
Dressings
    hydrocolloid dressing, 378, 378f
    wound care, 376
Dysplastic nevi (atypical mole), 341, 342–343

E
Ear, 299–300
    biopsy choice and, 98
    lacerations of, 80, 80f
Ear lacerations, 80, 80f
Ecchymosis, 391f
Eczema. See Dermatitis
Electric shock, electrosurgery, 192
Electrocoagulation, 35–36, 35f, 36f, 101, 105,
    111, 185, 186f
Electrodesiccation, 185, 186f
    sebaceous hyperplasia and, 346
    small lesions and, 332
    syringomas and, 348
    venereal warts, 351
Electrodesiccation and curettage, 148, 190,
    201–202, 202f, 203f
    basal cell carcinoma and, 364
    chondrodermatitis nodularis helicis and, 334
Electrosection, 185, 187f
Electrosurgery, 185, 187
    accessories, 189–190
    advantages, 185
    anesthesia, 190
    angiomas (cherry) and, 193–194
    angiomas (spider) and, 194, 194f
    benign lesions, 193–196
    coding and billing pearls, 204
    condyloma acuminata and, 194–195, 195f
    disadvantages, 186
    electric shock, 192
    electrodesiccation and curettage, 201–202,
        202f, 203f
    electrosurgical units, 188–189
    equipment and, 18–19, 19f, 36, 188–189
    fire and burns, 192
    high-frequency units, 188–189
    Hyfrecator, 189
    implanted electrical devices, 193
    indications, for use of, 190
    infection transmission through, 192
    learning the techniques, 202–204
    malignant lesions, 201
    nevi (moles) benign and, 195–196, 196f
    pacemaker problems, 193
    potential hazards, 191–192
    power settings and, 190, 191b, 191t
    practicing radiosurgery, 203–204
    practicing with Hyfrecator, 202–203
    precautions, 190
    pyogenic granuloma, 196, 197f
    radiosurgery practical pearls, 190–191
    safety measures with, 191–193
    scalpel vs., 188
    sebaceous hyperplasia, 196–198, 197f
    seborrheic keratosis, 197–198, 198f
    shave, 106, 106f
    skin tags and, 198, 199f, 332, 332f
    smoke evacuators, 189–190, 190f
    smoke plume, 192–193
    spattering blood, 192–193
    standard electrosurgical units, 188
    telangiectasias, 199–200
    thermal pencil/battery cautery, 188
    treating specific lesions, 193–201
    unipolar and bipolar current and, 185
    units, 185, 188–189
    warts (verruca vulgaris) and, 200–201

Ellipse geometry, elliptical excision
    and, 134–136, 136f
Ellipse or large excision sets, 16–17, 17f
Elliptical biopsy method, 86
Elliptical excision, 342
    aftercare and, 146
    alternatives to, 147–148, 158, 159f
    anesthesia and, 137
    avoiding vital structures and, 131–132
    chondrodermatitis nodularis helicis and, 334
    cleaning and dressing wound and, 146
    coding and billing pearls, 150–151
    contraindications for, 130
    crescent excision and, 147, 147f
    danger zones and, 132
    ellipse geometry and, 134–136, 136f
    equipment and, 130–131, 131f
    hemostasis and, 141–142, 142f
    incision and, 138–141, 139–140f,
        140f, 141f
    incision line placement and, 132, 134f
    indications for, 130
    infection and, 146–147
    lateral forehead and, 132, 132f
    lateral midface and, 132, 133f
    lateral neck and, 132, 133f
    lipomas and, 165
    M-plasty and, 147, 148f
    mucocele and, 340
    partial closure and, 147, 148f
    planning and designing and, 131–137
    pyogenic granuloma and, 344
    recommended hemostasis methods for, 41t
    relaxed skin tension lines and, 132, 135f
    room, patient, and equipment preparation
        and, 138, 138f
    side-to-side closure and, 136
    S-plasty and, 147, 148f
    standing cones (dog-ear) repair, 145–146,
        146f
    steps and principles, 131–146
    suggestions for learning, 148–150
    surgical margin and, 132–134, 135t
    suturing and, 145, 145f
    tagging specimen and, 141, 141f
    tissue distortion and, 136–137
    undermining and, 142–143, 142f,
        143f, 144f
    variations and, 147, 149–150f
    wound closure and, 143–146, 144f, 145f
Elliptical excisional biopsy, 86, 87f
EMLA cream, 21
Endarterectomy scissors, 13
Endocarditis prophylaxis, 6, 6t
Epidermal inclusion cysts, 152, 158f,
    323, 323f
    central punctum, 153f
    coding and billing pearls, 165
    cyst removal contraindications, 153
    cyst removal indications, 152–153
    differential diagnosis and, 154b
    minimal excision technique and, 156,
        158–160
Epinephrine, 23, 33, 299f
    adverse reactions to, 26
    elliptical excision and, 137, 137f, 138f
    pregnancy and lactation and, 29
Erythema nodosum, 94–95, 95f
Erythematous lesions, 118f
Erythroderma, 88f, 95–97, 96f, 127, 127f
Ethyl chloride spray, 22
Evaporative liquids, 176
Exam rooms. See Office setup
Excisional biopsy, 85–86, 87f, 91
Excisional elliptical biopsies, 86
External sutures, 42

Extremities suture recommendations, 47, 47t
Eyelid lacerations, 79
Eyelids, biopsy choice and, 98

F
Face, 278, 278f
    suture recommendations and, 46, 47t
Feet, biopsy choice and, 97
Felon, 226, 226f
Field block, 28, 31f
Figure-of-eight sutures, 35–36, 36f, 60, 60f
Fingernails. See Nail procedures
Fire, 192
Flaps
    advancement, 309–312
    coding and billing pearls, 316–317, 317b
    contraindications and, 308–309
    island pedicle, 312–314
    learning the techniques, 316
    necrosis and, 393, 394f
    planning of, 309
    rhombic transposition flap, 315–316
    rotation flaps, 314–315
    terminology and, 307–308
    transposition flap, 315, 316
    Zitelli bilobed transposition flap, 316
Flat warts, 290–291, 291f
Floor lamps, 11–12, 12f
5-Fluorouracil (5-FU), 212
Forceps, 14, 50, 51f
Forearms, suture recommendations, 48
Fragile skin, suturing techniques for, 59–63, 59f
Fulguration, 185, 186f
Full nail plate removal, 237
Full-thickness nail matrix biopsy, 244
Full-thickness wounds, 374
Fusiform, 130

G
Ganglion cysts, 325
Gelatin sponges, 38–39
Genitalia, 302
Genital warts, 291, 291f
Glandular rosacea, 289
Globules, 271, 272f
Glues, 64
Gradle scissors, 13
Granuloma annulare, 95, 95f
    intralesional injections and, 210, 210f
Granulomatous rosacea, 289

H
Hailey-Hailey disease, 118f
Hair preparation, preoperative, 7, 7f
Hand instruments, 12–15
    curettes, 14, 14f
    cutting and, 12–14
    forceps, 14
    hemostats, 15
    needle holders, 15–16, 16f
    punches, 14, 14f
    razor blades, 13
    scalpels, 12–13, 13f
    scissors, 13, 13f
    skin hooks, 14–15, 15f
    small instrument sets, 16–17
    staplers, 16
    surgical skin markers, 17
    suture-cutting scissors, 16
    tissue holding and, 14–15
    undermining and, 15
    wound closure and, 15–16
Hands, biopsy choice and, 97

Hemangiomas, 258–261, 259f
Hematoma, 391
Hemorrhagic blisters, 177f
Hemostasis
    chemical hemostatic agents, 33–35
    electrocoagulation and, 35–36, 35f, 36f
    elliptical excision and, 141–142, 142f
    and eye, 37
    mechanical hemostasis, 37
    physical agents and, 38–39, 38f, 39f
    punch biopsy and, 120–124, 123f
    recommended methods and, 41t
    shave biopsy and, 109
    types of, 33
Hemostats, 15
Hidradenitis suppurativa, 226
    intralesional injections and, 210
    unroofing/deroofing, 226–227, 227–228f
Hidrocystomas, 155f, 159, 160f
High-frequency units, 188–189
Horizontal mattress sutures, 38, 38f, 56–57,
    58f, 75, 76f
H-plasty, 311, 311f
Human amniotic membranes, 379–380
Human papilloma virus, 187
Hyfrecator, 36–37, 37f, 189, 189f
Hypertrophic scars
    cryosurgery, 178, 179t
    intralesional injections, 210–212, 211f
Hypopigmentation, shave biopsy and, 110, 111f
H-zone, 403, 404f

I

Imiquimod, 351
Immunotherapy, 350
Implantable cardioverter-defibrillator, 193
Implanted electrical devices, 193
Incisional biopsy, 85–86, 407
Incision and drainage (I&D), 72, 158, 219
    advantages, 220
    aftercare and packing of, 222–223
    coding and billing pearls, 228
    contraindications and cautions, 219–220
    disadvantages, 221
    equipment, 221
    felon, 226
    indications for procedure, 219
    of inflamed and infected cysts, 158–159
    loop drainage technique, 223, 225f
    paronychia, 223–226
    procedure, 221–222
    recommended hemostasis methods for, 41t
    special populations, 227
    specific lesions, 227
    unroofing/deroofing hidradenitis
        suppurativa (HS), 226–227, 227–228f
Infectious skin diseases
    common warts, 290, 290f
    flat warts, 290–291, 291f
    genital warts, 291, 291f
    molluscum contagiosum, 291, 291f, 292f
    scabies, 291–292, 292f, 293f
    tinea corporis, 292–293, 293f
Infiltrative disorders, biopsy choice and, 95, 95f
Infiltrative skin conditions, 114
Inflammatory diseases
    capillaritis, 289–290, 289f, 290f
    dermatitis, 284–285, 286f
    discoid lupus erythematosus, 289, 289f
    lichen planus, 286, 287f
    pityriasis rosea, 286–287, 287f, 288f
    porokeratosis, 287, 288f
    prurigo nodularis, 287–288, 288f
    psoriasis, 284, 285f
    rosacea, 288–289, 289f

Inflammatory phase, of wound healing, 373
Inflammatory process, biopsy choice and, 87
Inflammatory skin disease, 114
Information handouts. See Patient education
    handouts
Informed consent, 3, 387
    intralesional injections, 206
Infraorbital blocks, 28, 28b, 30f, 31f
Ingrown toenail. See Nail procedures
Injections, intralesional. See Intralesional
    injections
Injection technique, 25
Injury method, laceration repair and, 72
Instrument sterilization, 8
Instrument tie, 50–51, 52f
Intense pulsed light, 194
Intradermal nevi, 259–261, 259f, 260f,
    261f, 341
Intralesional candida antigen, 351
Intralesional injections, 206, 208t
    acne keloidalis nuchae, 207–208, 209f
    acne nodules and cysts, 207
    aftercare, 217
    alopecia areata, 208–209, 209f
    Candida antigen injections, 215–217, 216f
    coding and billing pearls, 217
    complications of steroid injections, 214–215
    contraindications, 206
    cutaneous lupus, 209
    equipment, 206
    granuloma annulare, 210, 210f
    hidradenitis suppurativa, 210
    hypertrophic scars and keloids, 210–212
    indications, 206
    informed consent, 206
    intralesional treatments, 215
    keloids and, 206, 207t
    lichen planus, 213
    localized dermatitis, 212
    psoriasis, 212–213
    psoriatic nail disease, 213
    sarcoidosis, 214
    steroid strength, 206–207
    tattoo reactions, 214
    treating specific lesions, 207–214
Inverted figure-of-eight suture, 60
Iris scissors, 13
Irrigation, wound, 73
Island pedicle flaps, 312–314
    conceptual, 312–313
    step-by-step instructions and, 313–314, 313f

J

Junctional nevi, 341

K

Keloidal or hypertrophic scarring, 97
Keloids, 336–338
    cryosurgery, 178, 179t
    cryosurgery and, 336
    diagnosis of, 336
    excision of, 336–337
    injection and, 336
    intralesional injections, 206, 207t,
        210–212, 211f
    lasers and, 337
    special considerations/pathology/billing,
        337–338
    treatment of, 336–337
Keratoacanthoma, 92–93, 93f, 102f,
    360–361
    diagnosis of, 360–361, 361f
Key suture, flap, 307–308
Knobology, 318–320

L

Laceration repair
    closure technique, 73–77
    coding and billing and, 80
    coexisting conditions and, 71–72
    complications and, 77
    contamination and, 72
    contraindications for, 70
    ear, 80, 80f
    eyelids and, 79
    indications for, 70
    initial assessment and, 71, 71t
    lips and, 79, 79f
    local and regional anesthesia an, 72–73
    location and, 72
    method of injury and, 72
    nail bed and, 80, 81f
    nose and, 79–80
    postprocedure patient education and, 77–79
    preprocedure patient preparation and, 71–73
    supplies and equipment and, 70–71
    suture choice and, 74
    sutured repairs, 74
    suturing pearls for, 81b
    wound preparation and, 73
Lactation, local anesthetics and, 28–29
Lasers
    angiofibromas and, 333
    angiokeratomas and, 333
    angiomas and, 333
    chondrodermatitis nodularis helicis and, 334
    keloids and, 337
    sebaceous hyperplasia and, 346
    syringomas and, 348
    venereal warts, 351
Lateral forehead, elliptical excision
    and, 132, 132f
Lateral longitudinal excision, 244–245, 245f
Lateral midface, elliptical excision
    and, 132, 133f
Lateral neck, elliptical excision and, 132, 133f
Lentigines (solar), 338
    diagnosis of, 338
    special considerations/pathology, 338
    treatment of, 338
Lentigo maligna melanoma, 92, 92f, 103,
    103f, 179, 366, 366f
    face with circle in circle pattern, 279f
    face with rhomboidal structures, 279f
Lentigo maligna, progression model for, 279f
Lesions. See also Malignant lesions; Pigmented
    lesions
    benign lesions, 193–196
    bullous lesions, 97, 97f
    electrodesiccation for small lesions, 332
    erythematous lesions, 118f
    malignant lesions, 181–183
    nail procedures, 245–248
    nonpigmented lesions, 92–93
    premalignant lesions, 180–183
    recurrence of, 396
    scattered lesions, 87–88
    vascular lesions, 180
Less common benign adnexal tumors, 352
Leukocytoclastic vasculitis, 115f
Leukoplakia, 116f
Lichen planus, 94, 94f, 116f, 286, 287f
    intralesional injections and, 213, 214f
Lichen sclerosis, 95, 96f
Lidocaine, 178, 231, 299f
    adverse reactions to, 26
    allergies and, 27
    with epinephrine, 23, 33
    maximal doses and, 23, 24t
    pregnancy and lactation and, 29
    topical, 21

Lighting, office, 11–12
Lipomas, 162–164, 324
  coding and billing pearls, 165
  diagnosis, 162
  elliptical excision of, 165
  examination and pathology and, 164
  general considerations, 162
  incision and pressure method and, 163–164, 163f
  preoperative measures and, 163
  punch (enucleation) technique and, 164–165, 165f
  removal complications and, 165
  removal indications, 162
Liposarcomas, 324
Lips, 300–301
  biopsy choice and, 98
  lacerations of, 79, 79f
Liquid nitrogen, 22, 23
  equipment, 169–170, 170f
Liquid nitrogen alternatives, 176–177
  closed probes, 176–177
  evaporative liquids, 176
LMX4, 21
LMX5, 21
Local anesthesia, 23–24, 23t. *See also* Anesthesia
  adverse reactions and, 26
  basal cell carcinoma and, 24f
  decreasing the pain of, 23–24
  epinephrine, 23
  injection technique, 25
  laceration repair and, 72–73
  one percent lidocaine with epinephrine, 23
Localized dermatitis, intralesional injections, 212
Location, laceration repair and, 72
Longitudinal melanonychia, 230
Loop drainage technique, 223, 225f
L-plasty, 311, 312f
Lupus, 116f
  punch biopsy and, 128, 128f

M
Magnification devices, 17, 17f
Malignant conditions, 421–422t
Malignant lesions. *See also* Lesions
  cryosurgery, 181–183
  electrosurgery, 201
  flap use following treatment of, 308
Mandibular nerve, 395, 396f
Mayo stands, 12
McKesson anesthetic spray, 22
Mechanical hemostasis, 37
  tourniquets, clamps, and instruments and, 39–40, 39f, 40f
Melanocytes, 167
Melanoma, 102f, 115f, 365
  ABCDE guidelines for diagnosing, 238, 238b
  acral lentiginous melanoma, 238, 239f
  biopsy choice and, 90–91
  deep shave biopsy and, 84
  dermoscopic features, 275–277t
  differential diagnosis and, 91–92
  dysplastic nevus and, 341
  features, 270
  specific structures, 270–271
  streaks in, 271f
Mental nerve blocks, 28, 28b, 30f
Merkel cell carcinoma, 370, 370f
Metzenbaum scissors, 13, 15
Microfibrillar collagen, 39
Milia
  diagnosis of, 338, 339f
  special considerations/pathology/billing, 339
  treatment of, 338–339, 339f

Minimal excision technique for cysts, 156
  advantages, 156
  alternatives to, 158–160
  dermoid cysts, 159
  disadvantages, 156
  equipment, 156
  hidrocystomas, 159, 160f
  pathology and, 157
  performing procedure, 157
  preoperative measures, 156–157
Mistakes, clinician, 396–397
Mohs micrographic surgery, 364, 364f, 400–403
  appropriate use criteria, 354–355
  basal cell carcinoma and, 402f
  freezing and staining segments, 403f
  H-zone and, 403, 404f
  Medicare reimbursement for, 401b
  patient selection and, 401
  performing surgery, 401–403, 403f
  squamous cell carcinoma and, 402f
  standard pathology and, 401–403, 403f, 404f
Moles. *See* Nevi
Molluscum contagiosum, 291, 291f, 292f
  cryosurgery, 178–179, 179f
  diagnosis of, 339
  special considerations/pathology/billing, 340
  treatment of, 339–340, 339f
Monocryl™ sutures, 45
Monsel's solution, 35
Morphea, 95, 96f, 127, 128f
M-plasty, 147, 148f
Mucinous cystadenoma, 155f
Mucocele
  cryosurgery and, 340
  diagnosis of, 340, 340f
  elliptical excision and, 340
  shave excision and, 340
  treatment, 340
Mucosa suture recommendations, 47t
Mupirocin, 219
Mycobacterium abscessus infection, 119f

N
Nail avulsion, 237, 237f
Nail bed lacerations, 80, 81f
Nail matrix biopsy, 29f
Nail matrix destruction, 235–237
  chemical matrixectomy, 236b
  phenol application and, 235
  physical matrixectomy, 235–237, 236f
  wound dressings, 237
Nail procedures, 230–232
  algorithm, 249, 249f
  anatomy of nail unit, 230, 231f
  biopsies to diagnose pigment nail changes, 237–245
  coding and billing pearls, 251
  common steps and, 230–231
  complications of nail surgery, 248
  destruction of nail matrix, 235–237
  digital block, 230, 232f
  equipment, 230
  full nail plate removal, 237
  full-thickness nail matrix biopsy, 244
  glove use for tourniquet and sterile field, 231–232, 233f
  lateral longitudinal excision, 244–245, 245f
  lesions, 245–248
  nail plate dermatopathology, 251
  partial nail plate excision, 232–235, 234f
  postop directions for patients, 251
  punch biopsy of nail matrix, 240–242, 241f
  shave biopsy of nail matrix, 242
  trichloroacetic acid, 235f
  wing block, 230

National Institute for Occupational Safety and Health (NIOSH), 192
Neck, suture recommendations and, 47t, 48
Needles, 43, 43f
  body of, 43
  length of, 43, 44f
  needle holders, 15–16, 16f, 50, 51f
  types of points/tips, 43
Negative network, 271, 271f
Neosporin, 235
Nerve blocks, 27–28, 27b, 29f
Nerve damage, 393–395, 394f, 395f, 396f
Neurofibromas
  diagnosis of, 343
  treatment of, 343
Nevi
  acquired nevi, 341
  with age, 92
  compound nevi, 341
  congenital nevi, 343
  electrosurgery and, 195–196, 196f
  with hair, 92
  intradermal nevi, 341
  junctional nevi, 341
Nevi (moles) benign, 195–196
Nodular melanoma, 366, 366f
Nonabsorbable staples, 45
Nonabsorbable sutures, 45, 46t
Nonaggressive nonmelanoma skin cancers, 167
Nonhealing wounds, 381
Nonmelanoma skin cancers, 109, 190, 354
Nonpigmented lesions, cancer suspicions and, 92–93
Nonstop bleeding in surgery, 40
Nose, 298–299
  biopsy choice and, 98
  lacerations of, 79–80
NSAIDS, 390
Nylon, 45, 46t

O
Off-centered blotch, 271, 272f
Office setup
  cryotherapy equipment, 18, 18f, 19f
  for each exam room, 19–20
  electrosurgery equipment, 18–19, 19f
  hand instruments, 12–15
  injectable medications and chemicals, 18
  lighting, 11–12
  magnification devices, 17, 17f
  Mayo stands, 12
  personal protective equipment, 17
  stools, 12
  surgical tables, 12
Onychogryphosis, 245
Onychomatricoma, 245–247, 247f
Onychopapilloma, 247, 247f
Oozing on edges, hemostasis, 38–39, 38f
OptiVisor, 17, 17f
Oral, 301–302
Oral biopsies, 301–302
Osteomas, 327–328
O-T flap, 311, 311f

P
Pacemaker problems, electrosurgery, 193
Pain, postprocedural, 389–390
Palliation, cryosurgery, 183
Palmoplantar psoriasis, punch biopsy and, 127, 127f
Palms, 278–279
Papulopustular rosacea, 289
Parallel ridge pattern (PRP), 279–282
Paronychia, 223–226, 225f

Partial biopsy, 85
Partial closure, elliptical excision and, 147, 148f
Partial nail plate excision, 232–235, 234f
Partial-thickness wounds, 374
Patient calls, 387
Patient education handouts, 415t
PDS™ sutures, 45
Pemphigus, 117, 118f
Pemphigus foliaceous, 118f
Penis, 302–304, 303f
Peppering, 273, 273f
Periodic acid Schiff (PAS) stains, 97
Peripheral tan structureless areas, 272, 272f
Periungual fibroma, 247, 248f
Personal protective equipment, 17
Personna DermaBlade, 104
Personna Plus Microcoat blades, 13
Petrolatum, 235, 235f
Phenol EZ SWABS, 235
Physical agents, hemostasis, 38–39, 38f
Physical matrixectomy (electrodestruction),
    235–237, 236f
Pigmentation changes, 393
Pigmented basal cell carcinomas, 93, 93f
Pigmented lesions, 91–92, 105f, 109
Pigmented purpuric dermatoses. See
    Capillaritis
Pilar cysts, 152, 153f, 159f
Pilomatricoma, 344
Pilomatrixomas, 324–325
Pilonidal cyst, 155f
Pincer nails, 245, 245f
Pityriasis rosea, 286–287, 287f, 288f
Podofilox, 351
Point-of-care ultrasound (POCUS), 318
Polybuster, 46t
Polyester, 46t
Polypropylenes, 44, 46t
Porokeratosis, 287, 288f
Povidone-iodine, 7
Power Doppler, 318
Power settings, electrosurgery, 190, 191b, 191t
Pregnancy, local anesthetics and, 28–29
Premalignant conditions, 421–422t
Premalignant lesions, cryosurgery, 180–183
Preoperative medical evaluation, 2–3
    informed consent and, 3
    medical contraindications, 3
    medical history, 2–3
Preoperative preparation
    complex surgery scheduling and, 2
    drapes and, 7–8
    hair and, 7
    medications and, 3–7
    preoperative medical evaluation and, 2–3
    skin and, 7
    standby medications and equipment, 7
    sterile technique, 8
    surgical planning and, 2
    universal precautions, 3
Pressure dressings, 390
    hemostasis, 38
Pressure injuries
    prevention of, 380
    treatment of, 380
Prilocaine, 178
Primary defect, 307–308
Primary motion, flap, 307–308
Procedural complications
    bleeding, 390–391, 390f
    clinical management and evaluation of
        possible infection, 389, 389f
    flap necrosis, 393
    hematoma, 391
    informed consent forms and, 387

Procedural complications (Continued)
    lesion or skin cancer recurrence, 396
    literature review and, 388–389
    making mistakes, 396–397
    nerve damage, 393–395
    pain, 389–390
    patient calls and, 387
    patients, responding quickly to, 387
    pigmentation changes, 393
    potential adverse effect and complications,
        388b
    scarring, 392–393
    suture reactions, 391–392
    swelling and bruising, 391–392
    wound dehiscence, 393
Proliferative phase of wound healing,
    373–374
Prurigo nodularis, 287–288, 288f
    intralesional injections and, 212, 213f
Pseudopods, 271, 271f
Psoriasis, 284, 285f
    intralesional injections, 212–213, 213f
    shave biopsy and, 112–113, 112f
Psoriatic nail disease, intralesional injections
    and, 213, 214f
Punch biopsy, 299f, 305f, 407
    advantages of, 117
    basal cell carcinoma and, 116f
    biopsy choice and, 85
    of blue nevus, 124–126, 124f
    choosing punch size, 119
    coding and billing pearls and, 128–129, 128t
    complications and, 127, 128
    contraindications and cautions for, 116
    cutting the biopsy, 120, 121f, 122f
    disadvantages of, 117–118
    dressing and aftercare, 125–126, 126b
    equipment and, 119–120, 119f
    erythroderma and, 127, 127f
    gelatin foam and, 125
    hemostasis and repair, 120–124, 123f
    indications for, 114–115
    inflammatory disorders and, 94
    lupus and, 128, 128f
    making diagnosis and, 117–118
    morphea and, 127, 128f
    nail matrix, 240–242, 241f
    palmoplantar psoriasis and, 127, 127f
    preoperative measures and, 120
    recommended hemostasis methods for, 41t
    steps and principles, 120–124
    stretching the skin and, 120, 122–123f
    suggestions for learning, 127
    suturing and, 119–120, 124f
    tamponade on, 125, 125f
Punches, 14, 14f
Punch excision, 341–342
Punch or small excision sets, 16, 16f
Punch (enucleation) technique, lipoma
    removal and, 164–165, 165f
Purse string suture, 63, 64f, 65f
Pustular psoriasis, punch biopsy and, 127, 127f
Pyoderma gangrenosum, 117f
Pyogenic granuloma, 36–37, 37f, 102f,
    344–345
    cryosurgery and, 180, 180f, 181f, 344
    diagnosis of, 344, 345f
    electrosurgery and, 196, 197f
    elliptical excision and, 344
    recurrent, 396f
    shave biopsy and, 101, 102f, 112, 112f
    shave, curettage, and electrodesiccation, 344
    silver nitrate, 344
    special considerations/billing, 345
    treatment, 344

Q
Quickloop, 223, 225f

R
Radial streaming, 271
Radiation referrals, 404
Radiation therapy, basal cell carcinoma
    and, 364
Radiofrequency, 188
Randomized controlled study, 196
Random pattern flaps, 307–308, 308f
Rash, 87, 97, 114, 128
    diagnosis of, 94–97
Razor blades, 13, 105, 105f
Recurrent nevus, 103f, 110
Referrals, 398–405
    appropriate use criteria guideline, 403–404,
        405f
    clinical examples and, 399–400
    complete disclosure and, 398
    general guidelines and, 399
    insurance considerations and, 398
    medical-legal considerations and, 398
    radiation and, 404
    skin cancers and, 399
    systemic therapies for advanced
        melanoma, 405
Regional anesthesia, laceration repair and,
    72–73
Regional nerve blocks, 27–28, 27b, 29f
Relaxed skin tension lines, 132, 135f
Remaining tissue, shave biopsy and, 109, 109f
Remodeling, wound healing and, 374
Reverse cutting needles, 43, 44f
Rhombic transposition flap, 315–316, 316f
Ring blocks, 28, 31f
Rosacea, 288–289, 289f
Rotation flaps, 314–315
    bilateral O-Z rotation flap, 314, 314f
    conceptual, 314
    single rotation flaps, 314, 314f
    step-by-step instructions, 314–315, 315f
Running horizontal mattress sutures,
    58–59, 58f
Running locked sutures, 38, 38f
Running simple sutures, 55–56, 56f
Running subcuticular sutures, 60–62, 61–62f

S
Sarcoidosis, 95, 95f
    intralesional injections and, 214
Saucerization, 341
    biopsy, 83–100, 83, 84f, 91f, 106–108, 107f
Scabies, 291–292, 292f, 293f
Scalp
    challenges to overcome, 296
    elliptical excision, 297, 297f
    instrument tamponade, 297
    punch biopsies and excisions, 296, 297
    suture recommendations and, 47, 47t
    choice and, 97–98
Scalpel, 12–13, 13f, 188
    blade use, 105, 106f
Scarring, 392–393, 392f
Scattered lesions, biopsy choice and, 87–88
Scheduling, complex surgeries and, 2
Scissors, 13, 13f
Sclerosing basal cell carcinomas, 93
"Scoop" biopsy, 83
Scoop shave, 106–108, 107–108f
Sebaceous hyperplasia, 259, 259f, 345–346
    cryotherapy and, 346
    diagnosis of, 345, 346f

Sebaceous hyperplasia *(Continued)*
   electrodesiccation and, 346
   electrosurgery and, 196–198, 197f
   lasers and, 346
   shave excision and, 346
   special considerations/billing, 346
   treatment of, 346
Seborrheic dermatitis, 285
Seborrheic keratosis, 92, 92f, 102f, 179, 188, 258, 258f, 346–348
   cryosurgery, 179, 180f, 347
   diagnosis of, 346–347
   electrodesiccation with local anesthesia, 347
   electrosurgery, 197–198, 198f
   special considerations/billing, 347–348
   treatment of, 347
Secondary defect, 307–308
Secondary motion, flap, 307–308
Senile angiomas. *See* Cherry angiomas
Sentinel lymph node biopsy (SLNB), 84
Shank, needle, 43
Shave biopsy, 242, 299f, 407
   advantages of, 101–103
   aftercare and, 109, 109f
   biopsy choice and, 83
   coding and billing pearls and, 113, 113t
   contraindications for, 101
   cosmetic results and, 111
   critical steps in, 104
   differential diagnosis and, 111–112
   disadvantages of, 103
   electrosurgical shave and, 106, 106f
   equipment and, 103–104, 104f
   hemostasis and, 109
   hypopigmentation and, 110, 111f
   indications for, 101
   learning suggestions and, 109, 111f
   less than optimal outcomes and, 110, 111f
   pathology and follow-up and, 109
   preoperative measures and, 104, 105f
   psoriasis and, 112–113, 112f
   pyogenic granuloma and, 112, 112f
   razor blade use and, 105, 105f
   recommended hemostasis methods for, 41t
   remaining tissue after, 109, 109f
   saucerization, 106–108, 107f
   scalpel blade use and, 105
   scoop shave and, 106–108, 107–108f
   snip excision with scissors, 105–106, 106f
   stabilization techniques and, 108–109, 108f, 109f
Shave excision, 341
   nevi and, 333
   sebaceous hyperplasia and, 346
Shin, biopsy choice and, 97
Shiny white lines, 271
Side-to-side closure, elliptical excision and, 136
Silk, 46t
Silver nitrate, 35, 344
Simple interrupted suture, 51–54, 52f, 53f, 54f, 74, 75f
Simple running stitch, 74, 75f
Single-pedicle advancement flap (U-plasty), 310, 310f
Single rotation flaps, 314, 314f
Skin cancer, 354
Skin cancer recurrence, 396, 396f
Skin hooks, 14–15, 15f
Skin markers, surgical, 17
Skin preparation, preoperative, 7
Skin repairs
   complex repair, 410–411, 411t
   intermediate repair, 410, 411t
   multiple repairs, 411, 411t
   simple repair, 409, 410t

SkinStitch adhesives, 77, 78f
Skin stretching, punch biopsy and, 120, 122–123f
Skin tags, 198, 199f, 332, 332f
Skin tape, 46
Skin tension lines, 134f
Smaller sutures, 42
Small instrument sets, 16–17
Smoke evacuators, 189–190, 190f
Smoke plume, 192–193
Snip excision of pedunculated acrochordo, 331
Snip excision with scissors, 105–106, 106f
Sodium hydroxide (NaOH), 235
Soft tissue tumors, 412, 413t
Solar lentigines, 179
Sole of foot, 304, 304f, 305f
Soles, 278–279
Solid cystic hidradenoma, 154f
Spattering blood, 192–193
Specimen submissions, 98–99
Spider angiomas, 194, 194f, 348
Spinal accessory nerve, 395, 395f
S-plasty, 147, 148f
Sporotrichosis, 118f
Spray tips, cryosurgical, 169, 170f
Squamous cell carcinoma, 87f, 93, 93f, 102f, 157, 167, 190
   biopsy choice and, 89
   dermoscopic features, 264–266t
   diagnoses of, 359–360, 359f
   diagnostic criteria, 264, 264f
   nonsurgical therapy, 360t
   special considerations, 360
   systemic agents for severe forms, 405
   treatment of, 360, 360t
Stabilization techniques, shave biopsy and, 108–109, 108f, 109f
Standard electrosurgical units, 188
Standby medications and equipment, 7
Standing cones (dog-ear) repair, 145–146, 146f
Standing cutaneous cones, 307–308
Staplers, 16
Staples, 45, 77
Stasis dermatitis, 285
Steatocystoma multiplex, 156f
Sterile technique, 8
Steri-strips, 76
Steroid strength, intralesional injections, 206–207
Stools, 12
Streaks, 271, 271f
   in melanoma, 271f
Subcutaneous fat necrosis, 327
Subcuticular running suture, 76, 76f
Subcuticular sutures, 42
Subungual hematoma evacuation, 247–248, 248f
Superficial basal cell carcinoma, 183
Superficial, hemostasis, 37
Superficial spreading melanoma, 366, 366f
Superficial *versus* deep shave biopsy, 83–85, 84f
Supraorbital/supratrochlear nerve blocks, 27b, 28, 30f
Surgery
   ears, 299–300
   genitalia, 302
   lips, 300–301
   nose, 298–299
   oral, 301–302
   periocular, 298
   scalp, 296–297
   sole of the foot, 304
Surgical adhesive strips, 76

Surgical lamps, 11
Surgical margins, lesion types and, 132–134, 135t
Surgical planning, 2
Surgical-site infection, antibiotic prophylaxis and, 5–6, 5t
Surgical skin markers, 17
Surgical strips, 46
Surgical tables, 12
Surgical time-outs, 8–9
Suture materials, 44–45
   characteristics and properties, 44–45
   types by their degradation, 45
Sutures, 42. *See also* Suturing techniques
   absorbable, 36f
   anatomy of, 43, 43f
   capillarity, 44
   choice of, 74, 74t
   coating, 44
   coefficient of friction, 44
   configuration, 44
   deep or buried, 54
   ease of handling and, 44
   elasticity, 44
   elliptical excision and, 145, 145f
   figure-of-eight suture, 35–36, 36f
   horizontal mattress sutures, 38, 38f
   knot security, 45
   by location, 48, 49t
   materials, 44–45
   memory, 44
   needles. *See* Needles
   nonabsorbable, 45, 46t
   origin of, 44
   plasticity, 44
   pliability, 44
   punch biopsy and, 119–120, 124f
   reactions to, 391–392, 392f
   removal of, 63
   running locked suture, 38, 38f
   selection of, 46–48, 47t, 48t
   size of, 44, 74t
   spacing between, 54
   spitting potential, 45
   suture-cutting scissors, 16
   tensile strength, 44
   time of removal and, 74t
   tissue reactivity, 45
   visibility, 44
   wound healing and, 42–48
Suturing techniques
   accentuated heart shape, buried vertical mattress sutures with, 55, 55f
   advantages and disadvantages of, 66t
   basic skills, 50–51
   buried vertical mattress sutures, 54, 54f
   compressive sutures, 63, 65f
   corner (tip) stitch, 59–60, 59f
   deep horizontal mattress suture, 55, 55f
   deep suture with inverted knot or buried stitch, 74–75, 75f
   delayed primary closure, 77
   figure-of-eight sutures, 60, 60f
   glues, 64
   horizontal mattress sutures, 58–59, 58f, 75, 76f
   inverted figure-of-eight suture, 60
   loading the needle holder, 50, 51f
   performing an instrument tie, 50–51, 52f
   practice tips and, 64, 66f
   purse string suture, 63, 64f, 65f
   removing a deep suture, 55
   running horizontal mattress sutures, 58–59, 58f
   running simple sutures, 55–56, 56f, 74, 75f

Suturing techniques (*Continued*)
running subcuticular sutures, 60–62, 61–62f, 76, 76f
simple interrupted suture, 51–54, 52f, 53f, 54f, 74, 75f
staples, 77
surgical adhesive strips, 76
three-point or half-buried mattress suture, 76
tips for working with fragile skin, 59–63, 59f
tissue adhesives, 76–77, 78f
two-layer closure, 62–63, 62f
using forceps in the nondominant hand, 50, 51f
vertical mattress sutures, 56, 57f, 75, 75f
wound closure tapes, 63, 65f
Swage, needle, 43
Swelling, postoperative, 391–392, 391f
Syringomas, 348, 348f
Systemic lupus erythematosus (SLE), 94, 94f

T
TADA, 254–258
Tapes, wound closure, 63, 65f
Tattoo reactions, intralesional injections and, 214, 214f
Telangiectasias, 102f, 199–200, 348
Tenotomy scissors, 13
Thermal pencil/battery cautery, 188
Three-point or half-buried mattress suture, 76
Thyroglossal duct cysts, 155f, 325–326
Time-outs, surgical, 8–9
Tinea corporis, 292–293, 293f
Tissue adhesives, 45–46, 76–77, 78f
Tissue destruction, electrosurgery and, 35
Tissue distortion, elliptical excision and, 136–137
Tissue freezing. *See* Cryosurgery
Tissue holding, 14–15
Toenails. *See* Nail procedures
Topical anesthetics, 21–22, 22f, 22t. *See also* Anesthesia
Topical lidocaine, 21
Topical refrigerants, 22–25
Tourniquets, 39, 39f
T-plasty (O-T flap), 311, 311f
Transposition flap, 315, 316
conceptual, 315
rhombic transposition flap, 315–316, 316f
step-by-step instructions and, 316, 317f
Zitelli bilobed transposition flap, 316, 316f
Transthecal anesthesia, 230–231, 233f
Triage Amalgamated Dermoscopic Algorithm, 253–254, 255f

Triamcinolone, 212
Triamcinolone acetonide suspension, 206, 207f
Triamcinolone dilutions, 208t
Trichloroacetic acid, 234
Trichoepithelioma, 348–349
Tridocaine gel, 21
Trunk suture recommendations, 47, 47t
Two-layer closure, 62–63, 62f

U
Ulcer, 117, 117f
Ultrasound
acoustic enhancement, 318, 319f
applications, 323–328, 323f, 323t, 324f
color Doppler, 318
hyperechoic structures, 318
hypoechoic structures, 318
isoechoic structures, 318
mirror artifact, 318
normal anatomy, 320–321, 321f, 322f
Power Doppler, 318
Undermining, 15, 73, 142–143, 142f, 143f, 144f
Universal precautions, 3
U-plasty, 310, 310f

V
Vascular lesions, cryosurgery, 180
Vasculitis, 89
Venous lakes, cryosurgery, 180, 181f
Venous stasis ulcers, 380–381
Vertical mattress sutures, 56, 57f, 75, 75f
Vesicular-bullous reaction, biopsy choice and, 87
Vicryl™ sutures, 45
Vulva, 303–304, 304f
Vulvar intraepithelial neoplasia, 116f

W
Warfarin, 3, 4
Warts, 179
Candida antigen injections, 217b
common, 349–350
electrosurgery, 200–201
filiform, 350
intralesional treatments, 215
plantar, 350–351
venereal, 351
Wickham's striae, 116f, 286
Wing blocks, 28, 29f, 230

Wood's lamp, 12
Work relative value units, 406, 407t
Wound care, 73
alternative therapies, 379
bleeding, 383
cleaning and care, 379
cleansing and, 73
complications, 383–384
contact dermatitis, 384
debridement and, 73
determining intervention needs and, 73
digits, 383
dressings, 376
ear, 383
elliptical excision and, 143–146, 144f, 145f
full-thickness wounds, 374
hand instruments and, 15–16
healing phases and, 70
hydrocolloid dressing, 378
infection, 383
inflammatory phase and, 373
irrigation and, 73
negative pressure wound therapy, 379
optimizing outcomes, 384
pain, 382
partial-thickness wounds, 374
periorbital wounds, 383
postoperative patient instructions, 382–383
pressure injury, 374–376
by primary intention, 377–378
proliferative phase and, 373–374
remodeling phase and, 374
by secondary intention, 376–377
showering, 382
tapes and, 63, 65f
by tertiary intention, 379
undermining and, 73
wound assessment and, 71, 71t
Wound closure materials, 45–46
skin tape or surgical strips, 46
staples, 45
tissue adhesives, 45–46
Wound healing, and sutures, 42–48

X
Xanthelasma, 351

Z
Zerowet Klenzalac system, 71f
Zitelli bilobed transposition flap, 316, 316f